Probiotics: Application in Food and Pharmacology

Probiotics: Application in Food and Pharmacology

Editor: Rocio Perkins

AMERICAN
MEDICAL PUBLISHERS
www.americanmedicalpublishers.com

AMERICAN
MEDICAL PUBLISHERS
www.americanmedicalpublishers.com

Cataloging-in-Publication Data

Probiotics : application in food and pharmacology / edited by Rocio Perkins.
p. cm.
Includes bibliographical references and index.
ISBN 979-8-88740-393-9
1. Probiotics. 2. Probiotics--Health aspects. 3. Probiotics--Physiological effect.
4. Probiotics--Nutritional aspects. 5. Pharmacology. 6. Dietary supplements.
7. Diet therapy. 8. Probiotics--Therapeutic use. I. Perkins, Rocio.
RM666.P835 P764 2023
615.329--dc23

American Medical Publishers,
41 Flatbush Avenue,
1st Floor, New York,
NY 11217, USA

ISBN 979-8-88740-393-9 (Hardback)

Contents

Preface

Over the recent decade, advancements and applications have progressed exponentially. This has led to the increased interest in this field and projects are being conducted to enhance knowledge. The main objective of this book is to present some of the critical challenges and provide insights into possible solutions. This book will answer the varied questions that arise in the field and also provide an increased scope for furthering studies.

Probiotics refer to the living microorganisms, whose consumption is regarded to have health benefits, generally by restoring and improving gut flora. They are safe to consume but they may result in side effects and bacteria-host interactions in some situations. Probiotic-fortified foods, fermented dairy products and other fermented foods contain live probiotic cultures. Lactic acid bacteria (LABs), that are food fermenting bacteria, prevent food from spoilage and can increase the nutritional content of the foods they live in. There are several fermented products, which contains LAB, such as pao cai, kimchi, sauerkraut, pickled vegetables, etc. They are assumed to be beneficial in decreasing gastrointestinal discomfort, relieving constipation and evading the common cold. This book contains some path-breaking studies on probiotics. It strives to provide a fair idea about their applications in food and pharmacology. This book aims to serve as a resource guide for students and experts alike and contribute to the growth of research in this area of study.

I hope that this book, with its visionary approach, will be a valuable addition and will promote interest among readers. Each of the authors has provided their extraordinary competence in their specific fields by providing different perspectives as they come from diverse nations and regions. I thank them for their contributions.

Editor

1

Lactobacillus fermentum Postbiotic-Induced Autophagy as Potential Approach for Treatment of Acetaminophen Hepatotoxicity

Miroslav Dinić[1], Jovanka Lukić[1]*, Jelena Djokić[1], Marina Milenković[2], Ivana Strahinić[1], Nataša Golić[1] and Jelena Begović[1]

[1] Laboratory for Molecular Microbiology, Institute of Molecular Genetics and Genetic Engineering, University of Belgrade, Belgrade, Serbia, [2] Department of Microbiology and Immunology, Faculty of Pharmacy, University of Belgrade, Belgrade, Serbia

***Correspondence:**
Jovanka Lukić
lukicjovanka@imgge.bg.ac.rs

The aim of this study was to investigate the potential of postbiotics originated from *Lactobacillus fermentum* BGHV110 strain (HV110) to counteract acetaminophen (APAP)-induced hepatotoxicity in HepG2 cells. This strain was selected according to its autophagy inducing potential, based on previous studies reporting protective role of autophagy in APAP caused cellular damage. Cell viability was assessed using MTT and LDH assays, while autophagy was monitored by qPCR analysis of *BECN1*, *Atg5*, *p62/SQSTM1,* and *PINK1* mRNA expression and by Western blot analysis of p62/SQSTM1 and lipidated LC3 accumulation. Our results showed that detrimental effect of APAP on cell viability was suppressed in the presence of HV110 which was linked with increased conversion of LC3 protein and p62/SQSTM1 protein degradation. Additionally, higher *p62/SQSTM1* and *PINK1* mRNA transcription were noticed in cells co-treated with APAP/HV110, simultaneously. In conclusion, this study suggests that HV110 enhances activation of PINK1-dependent autophagy in HepG2 cells and its eventual co-supplementation with APAP could be potentially used for alleviation of hepatotoxic side effects caused by APAP overdose.

Keywords: autophagy, *Lactobacillus fermentum*, postbiotics, acetaminophen, hepatotoxicity

INTRODUCTION

Acetaminophen [paracetamol, *N*-acetyl-*p*-aminophenol (APAP)] is widely used analgesic and antipyretic drug which is safe and effective at a therapeutic dose (Lee, 2004). However, acute or cumulative overdose can cause hepatic necrosis and liver failure (Larson et al., 2005). The mechanisms of APAP-induced liver injury described to this moment include generation of reactive metabolite, *N*-acetyl-*p*-benzoquinone imine (NAPQI) and *p*-aminophenol (PAP) (Miyakawa et al., 2015). Given an important role of autophagy in elimination of damaged organelles, including mitochondria, it has been shown that activation of autophagy could serve as a cellular adaptive mechanism to counteract APAP-induced hepatotoxicity (Igusa et al., 2012; Ni et al., 2012).

Autophagy is tightly regulated and highly inducible catabolic cellular process involved in degradation of organelles and long-living proteins. During this process double-membrane vesicles (autophagosomes) are formed and fused with lysosomes while enclosed material is degraded. Literature data suggest that deregulation of autophagy is highly associated with various liver diseases. For example, in liver ischemia reperfusion injury autophagy exhibits prosurvival activity, while in hepatocellular carcinoma autophagy level is decreased (Rautou et al., 2010). Therefore, therapeutics capable to induce autophagy could be beneficial for liver associated pathological conditions.

In addition to well-known autophagy promoting stimuli (e.g., starvation, rapamycin, hormones), upregulation of autophagy can occur in bacterial, viral, and parasitic infections (Lum et al., 2005; Mizushima et al., 2010). Irving et al. (2014) demonstrated that peptidoglycan derived from *Helicobacter pylori* and *Pseudomonas aeruginosa* promotes autophagy in epithelial cells via NOD1 receptor activation. Moreover, several studies reported potential of some *Bifidobacteria* and *Lactobacillus* species to stimulate or suppress autophagy (Wu et al., 2013; Lin et al., 2014; Motevaseli et al., 2016).

Lactobacilli are beneficial bacteria, commonly used as probiotics. It has been shown that certain *Lactobacillus* strains were associated with suppression of liver injury caused by oxidative stress, pathogens, hepatic encephalopathy, and alcoholic liver disease (Segawa et al., 2008; Forsyth et al., 2009; Rishi et al., 2009). However, novel trends in probiotic supplementation are oriented toward replacement of live bacteria with non-viable bacterial extracts and metabolic by-products, termed postbiotics (Konstantinov et al., 2013; Patel and Denning, 2013). This new approach reduces health risks associated with consumption of live bacteria, especially concerning their high immune stimulating potential (Tsilingiri et al., 2012). Recent data showed that postbiotics can modulate different cellular pathways. Sharma et al. (2011) reported the cyto-protective activity of supernatants obtained from probiotics *Enterococcus lactis* IITRHR1 and *Lactobacillus acidophilus* MTCC447 against APAP induced hepatotoxicity. Particularly, the authors showed that the postbiotics have potential to restore glutathione level, reduce generation of major oxidative stress markers and to enhance production of anti-apoptotic (Bcl-2) protein.

Considering the fact that mitochondrial damage is a critical event in APAP-induced oxidative stress and cellular necrosis, activation of PINK1-Parkin signaling pathway is crucial for upregulation of mitochondrial autophagy. PINK1 is required for Parkin recruitment to damaged mitochondria when mitochondrial membrane potential is impaired, causing recruitment of p62/SQSTM1, an autophagy adaptor molecule, which is essential for final mitochondrial clearance (Williams and Ding, 2015).

In the light of above presented facts, we assessed the potential of autophagy inducing postbiotics originated from *Lactobacillus fermentum* BGHV110 strain to improve the viability of human hepatoma HepG2 cells exposed to APAP. Hence, according to our knowledge the results of this study for the first time suggest on the cyto-protective effect of postbiotics in APAP mediated hepatotoxicity.

MATERIALS AND METHODS

Bacterial Strain and Preparation of the Bioactive Lysate (Postbiotic)

Lactobacillus fermentum BGHV110, a human isolate from Laboratory collection, was used in the study. Determination of the species identity was performed by 16S rDNA sequencing using UNI16SF and UNI16SR primers complementary to 16S rDNA (Jovcic et al., 2009). PCR amplification was performed using KAPA *Taq* DNA polymerase kit (Kapa Biosystems, Wilmington, MA, USA). Reaction mixture contained: 20 mM Tris-HCl (pH 8.4), 50 mM KCl, 3 mM MgCl2, 50 mM each of the dNTPs, 1 U of *Taq* polymerase, 5 pM of each primer (for multiplex PCR 0.25 μM of each primer), and 0.1 μg of template DNA in a final volume of 50 μl. The PCR product was purified with QIAquick PCR Purification KIT (Qiagen, Hilden, Germany) and sequenced by Macrogen (Seoul, South Korea). The BLAST algorithm[1] was used to determine the most related DNA sequences in the NCBI GenBank database.

Bacteria were cultured in MRS broth (Merck, Darmstadt, Germany) at 37°C under anaerobic conditions using Anaerocult A (Merck). In order to obtain bioactive lysate overnight culture was pelleted (5000 rpm, 10 min) and washed twice with phosphate-buffered saline (PBS). Bacterial pellet was 10 times concentrated in PBS followed by homogenization in a French press (three passages). Homogenized bacterial suspension was lyophilized (Alpha 1–4 LSC Plus Freeze dryer, Martin Christ, Germany) and stored at +4°C until further use.

Cell Culture and Treatments

Human hepatoma cell line HepG2 was cultured in low glucose DMEM supplemented with 10% fetal bovine serum (FBS), 100 U/ml penicillin and 100 μg/ml streptomycin and 2 mM l-glutamine (Gibco, Life Technologies). The cells were maintained in 75 cm^2 flasks at 37°C in a humidified atmosphere containing 5% CO_2 and split at 80% confluence every 5 days. Cells were seeded in 24-well plate (2×10^5 cells) and incubated at 37°C overnight followed by cells pretreatment with complete DMEM containing high glucose concentration in order to downregulate autophagy (Kobayashi et al., 2012). After 6 h, cells were treated with different concentrations of postbiotics obtained from *Lactobacillus fermentum* BGHV110 strain (HV110) in order to select appropriate dose for further experiments. Postbiotic was dissolved in complete DMEM medium and added to the cells in specific final concentration. In all other experiments seeded cells were treated with 50 mM APAP (Sigma-Aldrich, Germany) alone or co-treated with 50 mM APAP and selected dose of lyophilized HV110. To analyze autophagic flux, simultaneously with treatments, cells were exposed to lysosomotropic agent chloroquine (Sigma-Aldrich) at a concentration of 25 μM, to inhibit autophagosome–lysosome fusion. After 16 h of incubation, cells were subjected to following analysis.

Metabolic Activity of HepG2 Cells

Metabolic activity of HepG2 cells was examined by MTT [3-(4,5-dimethylthiazol-2-yl)-2,5-diphenyl tetrazolium bromide] assay (Serva, Electrophoresis GmbH, Heidelberg, Germany) as described by Mosmann (1983). After the treatment, the cells were washed with PBS and MTT dissolved in complete media was added at the final concentration of 0.5 mg/ml. After 4 h of incubation, at 37°C with 5% CO_2, the media was aspirated and 10% SDS-0.01 N HCl was added to dissolve formazan.

[1] http://www.ncbi.nlm.nih.gov/BLAST

The absorbance was measured with a microplate reader (Tecan Austria GmbH, Grödig, Austria) at a wavelength of 570 nm. Results are presented as percentage of metabolic activity of treated cells compared to control.

Cytotoxicity Assay

The level of cytotoxicity in the cell cultures was measured by lactate dehydrogenase (LDH) Cytotoxicity Assay Kit (Thermo Scientific) which detects LDH released from dead cells. After treatments, supernatants were collected and LDH activity was determined by following the manufacturer's instructions. The absorbance was measured at 450 nm on a microplate reader (Tecan). Since there is an interference between APAP and LDH assay (Xu et al., 2003) only the treatments where APAP is used in the same dose are compared and results are presented as absorbance at 450 nm.

Western Blotting

Following the different treatments, cells were lysed with RIPA buffer (50 mM Tris-HCl pH = 7.4; 150 mM NaCl; 1% NP-40; 0.25% sodium deoxycholate) containing Protease Inhibitor Cocktail Tablets (Roche, Basel, Switzerland) and 1 mM phenylmethyl sulfonyl fluoride (Sigma-Aldrich), for 30 min on ice. Cell lysate was centrifuged at 12000 rpm for 15 min at 4°C and the protein concentration was measured using Bradford reagent (Bio-Rad Laboratories). Total cell proteins (20 μg) were separated on 12% SDS-PAGE and transferred to 0.2 μm nitrocellulose membrane (GE Healthcare) using a Bio-Rad Mini *trans*-blot system (Bio-Rad, Hercules, CA, USA). In case of p62 detection, proteins were transferred to 0.45 μm PVDF membrane (Millipore Corporation, Billerica, MA, USA). Immunoblots were blocked in a 10% non-fat dry milk in TBS-Tween (50 mM Tris-HCl, pH 7.4; 150 mM NaCl, and 0.05% Tween-20) overnight at 4°C followed by 2 h incubation at room temperature with the primary antibodies; anti-LC3 (1:2000; Thermo Fischer Scientific), anti-p62 (1:1000; Progen Biotechnik GmbH, Heidelberg, Germany) and anti-β-actin (1:1000; Thermo Fischer Scientific). The membranes were subsequently washed and incubated with appropriate HPR-conjugated secondary antibodies (goat anti-rabbit; 1:10000; Thermo Fischer Scientific and goat anti-guinea pig; 1:10000; Novex Life Technologies) for 1 h at room temperature. Proteins were detected by enhanced chemiluminescence (Immobilon Western, Merck Milipore). The intensity of the bands was quantified using ImageJ software. p62 was normalized to β-actin loading control. Autophagy induction was measured by calculation of LC3-II/LC3-I ratio.

Quantitative Real-time PCR

Total RNA was extracted from HepG2 cells as previously described by Lukic et al. (2013) with slight modifications. Cells were washed with PBS and lysed in denaturing solution (4 M guanidine thiocyanate, 25 mM sodium citrate, 0.1 M β-mercaptoethanol, 0.5% [wt/vol] *N*-lauroylsarcosinate sodium salt) followed by acid phenol (pH 4) extractions and isopropanol precipitation. cDNA was generated from 0.5 μg total RNA according to the reverse transcriptase manufacturer's protocol (Thermo Scientific). Quantitative PCR was carried out on 7500 real-time PCR system (Applied Biosystems, Waltham, MA, USA) using KAPA SYBR Fast qPCR Kit (Kapa Biosystems, Wilmington, MA, USA) under the following conditions: 3 min at 95°C activation, 40 cycles of 15 s at 95°C and 60 s at 60°C. All used primers (**Table 1**) were purchased from Thermo Fisher Scientific.

Statistical Analysis

All data are presented as mean values ± standard error of the mean (SEM). One-way ANOVA with the Tukey's *post hoc* test were used to compare multiple groups. The differences between control and experimental groups were compared using Student's t-test. Values at $p < 0.05$ or less were considered to be statistically significant. All experiments were repeated at least three times. Statistical analysis was carried out using SPSS 20.0 for Windows. Graphs were drawn in the GraphPad Prism software (trial version).

RESULTS

HV110 Exhibits Dose-dependent Effect on Cell Viability

We initially investigated in which way HV110 affects metabolic activity of HepG2 cells. The results of MTT assay showed dose-dependent effect of HV110 on HepG2 metabolic activity. Doses of 5 and 7 mg/ml of HV110 significantly ($p < 0.05$) decreased cell metabolic activity to 88.11 ± 0.43% and 83.06 ± 0.35%, respectively (**Figure 1A**). As detected decrease in metabolic activity could point on cell death, the level of LDH released in the cell culture was examined in order to determine the HV110 cytotoxicity. Only when applied in dose of 7 mg/ml, significantly higher ($p < 0.05$) LDH level in supernatants of the treated cells was detected in comparison to control (**Figure 1B**). Since the dose of 3 mg/ml didn't change cell metabolic activity or cause cell damage, this dose was used in further experiments.

HV110 Protects Cells against APAP-Induced Hepatotoxicity

In order to explore the potential cyto-protective role of selected dose of HV110 in APAP-induced hepatotoxicity, cell viability

TABLE 1 | The list of primers used in this study.

Primer name	Primer sequence 5′–3′	Reference
β-Actin forward	TTGCTGACAGGATGCAGAAGGAGA	Li et al., 2015
β-Actin reverse	TCAGTAACAGTCCGCCTAGAAGCA	
BECN1 forward	CTGGGACAACAAGTTTGACCAT	Liu et al., 2014
BECN1 reverse	GCTCCTCAGAGTTAAACTGGGTT	
ATG5 forward	CACAAGCAACTCTGGATGGGATTG	He et al., 2013
ATG5 reverse	GCAGCCAC GGACGAAACAG	
p62/SQSTM forward	GCCAGAGGAACAGATGGAGT	Sahani et al., 2014
p62/SQSTM reverse	TCCGATTCTG GCATCTGTAG	
PINK1 forward	GGGGAGTATGGAGCAGTCAC	Kim et al., 2013
PINK1 reverse	CATCAGGGTAGTCGACCAGG	

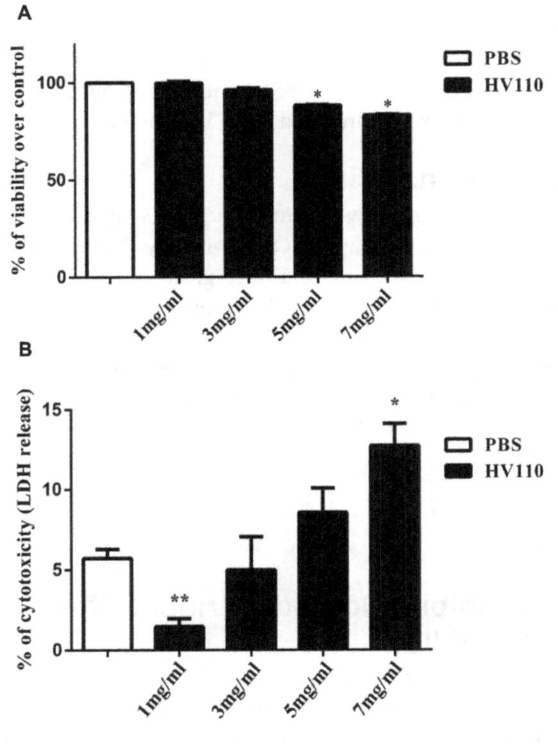

FIGURE 1 | Dose-dependent effect of HV110 on HepG2 cells viability after 16 h of treatment assessed by MTT assay (**A**; $n = 3$) and LDH assay (**B**; $n = 3$). All values are presented as mean ± SEM. Student's *t*-test was used to compare treated groups relative to control (*$p < 0.05$, **$p < 0.01$).

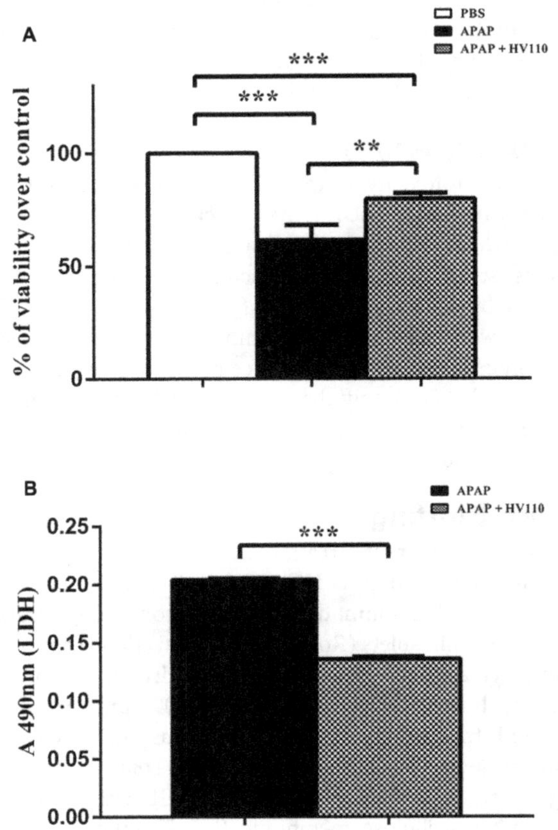

FIGURE 2 | HV110 protects cells against APAP-induced hepatotoxicity. Viability of HepG2 cells treated with 50 mM APAP and 3 mg/ml of HV110 for 16 h was examined by MTT (**A**, $n = 4$) and LDH assay (**B**, $n = 3$). LDH results are presented only as absorbance values indicating that higher absorbance correlates with the elevated cytotoxicity. All values are mean ± SEM. One-way ANOVA with the Tukey's *post hoc* test was used to compare multiple groups (**$p < 0.01$, ***$p < 0.001$).

in the presence of APAP was assessed using MTT and LDH assays. As expected, MTT assay shows that APAP in a dose of 50 mM significantly ($p < 0.001$) reduced cell viability to 61.5 ± 6.65%. Interestingly, the significant ($p < 0.01$) increase in cell viability to 79.7 ± 2.47% was observed in the APAP/HV110 co-treated cells, compared to APAP treated cells (**Figure 2A**). In parallel, LDH release in the media was measured and the results showed significantly lower ($p < 0.001$) toxic effect of APAP in the presence of HV110. Due to interference between APAP and LDH assay, the results of LDH assay are presented only as absorbance values, indicating that higher absorbance correlate with the increased cytotoxicity (**Figure 2B**).

The Influence of HV110 on Autophagy in HepG2 Cells

One of the key cellular adaptive mechanisms involved in attenuation of APAP-induced liver injury is autophagy. To investigate whether autophagy is correlated with protective effect of HV110 on HepG2 cells several factors involved in autophagy process were monitored. At first, conversion of the soluble LC3-I to lipid-bound LC3-II form of LC3 protein, a commonly used marker of autophagosomes formation associated with number of autophagosomes, was assessed by Western blot analysis. The potential of HV110 alone to trigger protective autophagy in HepG2 cells was investigated. Results revealed the significant increase ($p < 0.05$) of LC3-II/LC3-I conversion compared to the control cells (**Figures 3A,B**). In addition, the expression of *BECN1* a gene involved in nucleation step, and *Atg5* gene, involved in elongation step of autophagy process, were determined. The results showed that the expression of *BECN1* was significantly increased ($p < 0.05$) in cells treated with HV110, while the expression of *Atg5* remained unchanged, in comparison to control untreated cells (**Figure 3C**).

Further, the LC3-II/LC3-I ratio in APAP/HV110 co-treatment of HepG2 cells was followed. The results showed significant increase of LC3-II/LC3-I conversion in APAP/HV110 treated cells compared to cells treated with APAP alone ($p < 0.01$) and untreated control cells ($p < 0.001$), respectively (**Figures 4A,B**). Interestingly, although the treatment with APAP alone induced conversion of LC3 protein, it should be noted that this induction was not statistically significant in comparison to untreated cells.

Next, we investigated p62/SQSTM1 protein degradation by autophagy machinery. As a cargo receptor, p62/SQSTM1 binds to LC3 protein and contributes to clearance of ubiquitinated proteins. Consistent with the above mentioned results, APAP treatment as well as APAP/HV110 co-treatment caused

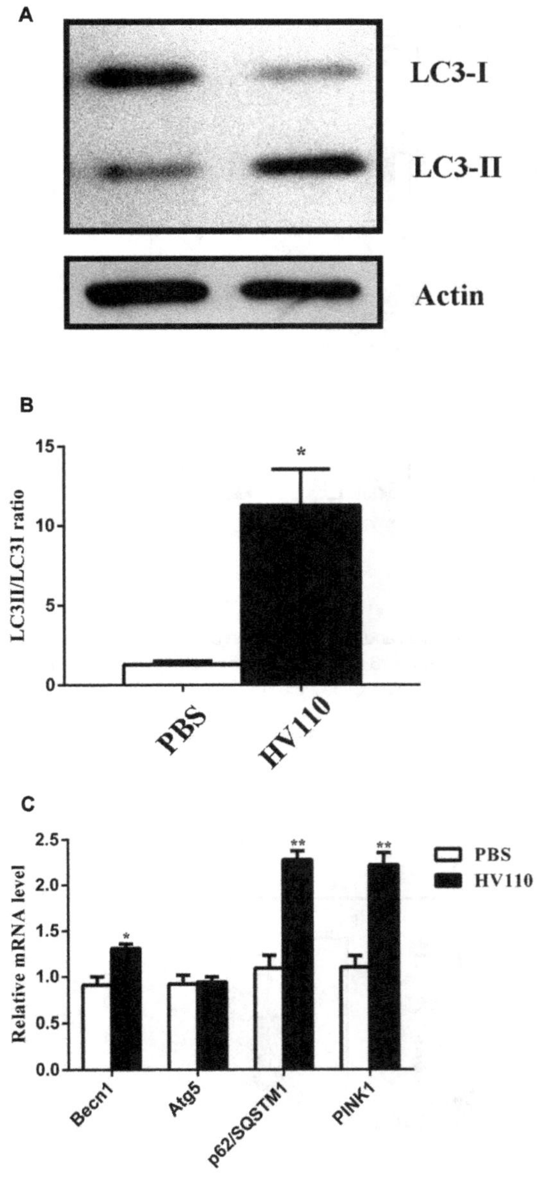

FIGURE 3 | The influence of HV110 on autophagy in HepG2 cells. Representative western blot **(A)** and densitometric analysis (**B**, $n = 4$) of LC3 conversion in HepG2 cells. Quantification of *BECN1*, *Atg5*, *p62/SQSTM1* and *PINK1* mRNA levels (**C**, $n = 3$). HepG2 cells were treated with 3 mg/ml of HV110 for 16 h. Student's *t*-test was used to compare experimental group relative to control (*$p < 0.05$, **$p < 0.01$).

significant degradation of p62/SQSTM1 protein compared to control, respectively ($p < 0.01$, $p < 0.001$). However, difference in p62/SQSTM1 degradation between APAP treatment and APAP/HV110 co-treatment is visible on western blot, but didn't reach statistically significance (**Figures 4C,D**).

Autophagosomes' accumulation could be a consequence either of autophagy activation or inhibition of downstream autophagy steps. Therefore, assessment of autophagy flux, which reflects the dynamics of the process, is essential. Results of autophagy flux monitoring showed significant increase conversion of LC3 marker and accumulation of LC3-II in the APAP/HV110 co-treated cells compared to chloroquine treated control ($p < 0.01$; **Figures 5A,B**), supporting the above mentioned evidence of autophagy activation.

However, levels of mRNA of *BECN1* and *Atg5* genes were decreased after 6 h and reached statistical significant decrease after 16 h of treatment ($p < 0.05$, $p < 0.01$) with no differences between APAP and APAP/HV110 co-treated groups (**Figures 4E,F**).

Autophagy Inhibition Decreases the Protective Effect of HV110

With the aim of the final confirmation of involvement of HV110-induced autophagy in protective effect on HepG2 cells against APAP, the autophagy was inhibited by chloroquine. The results of MTT assay showed that chloroquine added to the APAP/HV110 co-treated HepG2 cells decreased cell survival compared to the same treatment without chloroquine. More precisely, the difference between bars representing the percentage of viable cells after APAP/HV110 co-treatment and the percentage of viable cells after APAP treatment, without added chloroquine, was significantly higher (27.42 ± 1.86%) than in the presence of chloroquine (15.07 ± 1.21%) ($p < 0.01$; **Figure 5C**). This result supports our assumption of autophagy involvement in survival of cells treated with HV110. Additionally, LDH levels in supernatants of the cells treated with APAP, HV110 and chloroquine were much higher compared to treatment with no chloroquine added, but statistical significance wasn't achieved (**Figure 5D**). Considering the fact, that APAP/HV110 co-treated cells in the presence of chloroquine, still exhibit significantly higher viability rate compared to only APAP treated cells (MTT; $p < 0.05$ and LDH; $p < 0.001$) in the presence of chloroquine, the additional mechanism(s) involved in protective effect of HV110 on APAP-induced hepatotoxicity could be assumed.

Gene Expression Profile Revealed the Activation of PINK1 Autophagy Pathway

To analyze whether the PINK1-Parkin signaling pathway could be responsible for autophagy activation, we followed the expression of *PINK1* and *p62/SQSTM1* genes by qPCR. Results revealed that *PINK1* and *p62/SQSTM1* mRNAs were significantly induced in cells treated only with HV110 ($p < 0.01$) (**Figure 3C**).

Next, the expression profile of *PINK1* and *p62/SQSTM1* in APAP-induced hepatotoxicity was studied. The expression of the analyzed genes was not changed after the APAP treatment, regardless of the exposure time. Interestingly, the levels of *PINK1* and *p62/SQSTM1* mRNAs were increased in cells co-treated with both APAP and HV110 for 6 h, compared to control and APAP treated cells ($p < 0.01$; **Figure 4E**). After 16 h of APAP/HV110 treatment, the genes' expression returned to the control level (**Figure 4F**).

DISCUSSION

The literature data regarding the involvement of probiotics in autophagy activation are still limited. Most of the research in this

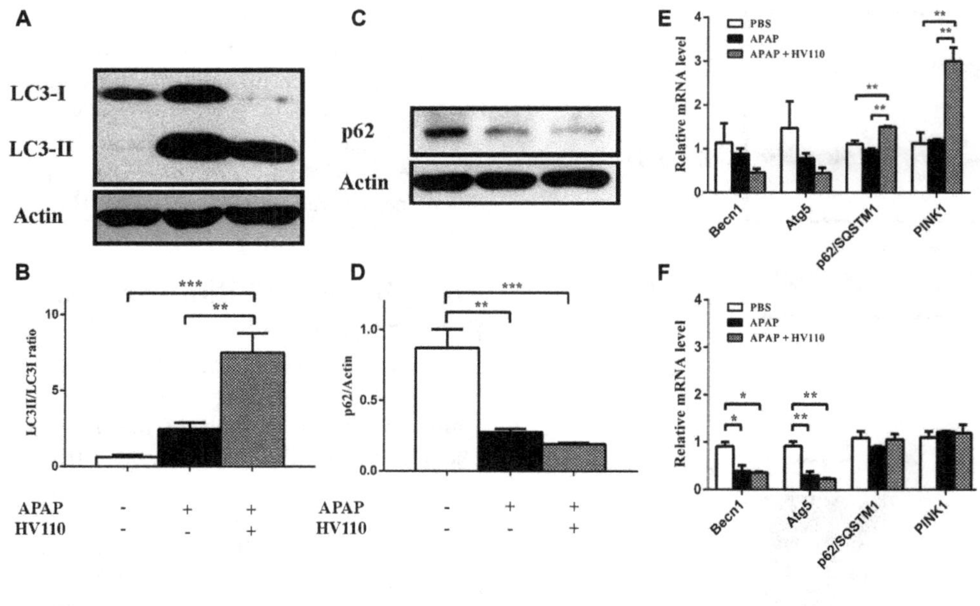

FIGURE 4 | Correlation between autophagy and HV110 protective effects. Evaluation of LC3 conversion and p62 degradation by immunoblot **(A,C)** and densitometric analysis (**B**, $n = 5$; **D**, $n = 4$) in HepG2 cells treated with 50 mM APAP and 3 mg/ml of HV110 for 16 h. The mRNA expression levels of *BECN1*, *Atg5*, *p62/SQSTM1* and *PINK1* after 6 h (**E**, $n = 3$) and 16 h (**F**, $n = 3$) of treatments with APAP and HV110. Values are expressed as mean ± SEM. One-way ANOVA with the Tukey's *post hoc* test were used to compare multiple groups (*$p < 0.05$, **$p < 0.01$, ***$p < 0.001$).

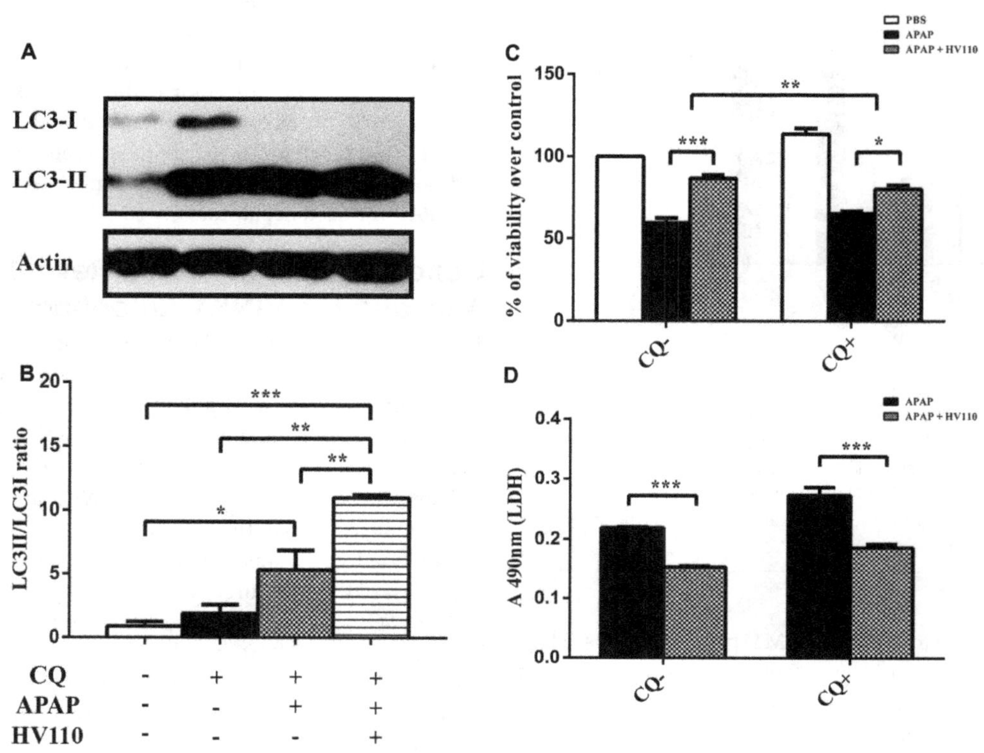

FIGURE 5 | Autophagy flux assessment. Representative western blot **(A)** and densitometric analysis (**B**, $n = 3$) of LC3 conversion in HepG2 cells treated for 16 h with 50 mM APAP and 3 mg/ml of HV110 in the absence or presence of chloroquine (CQ, 25 μM). In parallel, cell viability of HepG2 cells were evaluated using MTT assay (**C**, $n = 3$) and LDH assay (**D**, $n = 3$). All values are presented as mean ± SEM. For comparison of multiple groups, one-way ANOVA with the Tukey's *post hoc* test were used (*$p < 0.05$, **$p < 0.01$, ***$p < 0.001$).

field has been focused on the influence of pathogenic bacteria on autophagy machinery, while little space was given to the research on potential of beneficial bacteria to stimulate autophagy (Escoll et al., 2016; Zhang et al., 2016). This is the first report indicating that postbiotic HV110, originated from *Lactobacillus fermentum* BGHV110 strain, is potent inducer of autophagy in HepG2 cells, as demonstrated by increased LC3 lipidation and mRNA expression of *BECN1*, *PINK1*, and *p62/SQSTM1*. Bacterial lysates are rich in different pathogen associated molecular patterns (PAMPs) which can trigger autophagy through Toll-like receptor (TLR) signaling (Delgado et al., 2008). TLRs play an important role in liver physiology and pathophysiology due to the liver's exposure to gut-derived bacterial products and they are expressed in all cells present in the liver (Seki and Brenner, 2008; Mencin et al., 2009). Also, research over the last few years identified another class of pattern recognition receptors (PRRs), NOD-like receptors, involved in autophagy (Oh and Lee, 2014). On the other side, it has been described that overstimulation of PRRs can lead to induction of apoptosis. For example, TLR2 and TLR4 ligands present in the mycobacterial cell wall were identified as active ingredients of BCG treatment of superficial bladder tumors (Salaun et al., 2007; Subramaniam et al., 2016). This could be a reason for dose dependent decreased of cell viability caused by HV110 which was obtained in this study. However, involvement of PRRs in HV110 induced autophagy and impact on cell viability should be tested in further experiments.

Our finding that HV110 exhibits potential to induce protective autophagy served as the starting point to examine its cyto-protective effects against APAP-induced hepatotoxicity, which was shown that could be alleviated by autophagy induction (Ni et al., 2012). APAP exerts its toxic effects by two mechanisms: by CYP450-dependent NAPQI generation and by formation of PAP, as the result of APAP deacetylation (Miyakawa et al., 2015). CYP450-dependent pathway is activated immediately after APAP exposure and it lasts for the first several hours of exposure. However, after prolonged exposure to APAP, PAP-mediated pathway is activated with higher impact on cell viability compared to CYP450-dependent pathway. We thus assume that, in spite of lower expression of CYP450 enzymes in HepG2 cells (Westerink and Schoonen, 2007), our experimental setup provided enough and sustainable damage in HepG2 cells.

Though numerous studies investigated the effects of cytoprotective agents applied to hepatocytes before or after the addition of cytotoxic agents, our study was concerned with simultaneous HV110/APAP application. According to the results presented by Sharma et al. (2011) post-treatment with cytoprotective probiotics could not effectively reduce hepatocyte damage after APAP exposure, though pre and co-treatment were shown to be effective in the same study. This indicates that cell damage inflicted by high APAP doses is irreversible, as also evident from case studies reporting liver failure after intake of high APAP doses. Eventually, incorporation of postbiotics in formulations containing hepatotoxic drugs could significantly reduce the side effects and the degree of intoxication.

HV110 succeeded to alleviate APAP induced cell damage, as evidenced from MTT and LDH assays. Although APAP exposure *per se* induced protective autophagy in HepG2 cell line, induction of autophagy was threefold higher in APAP/HV110 co-treated cells, according to the degree of LC3 protein conversion and 1.5-fold higher based on the p62/SQSTM1 protein degradation. Chloroquine also favored the formation of autophagic vesicles containing cellular components in cells stimulated with HV110. Moreover, presence of chloroquine resulted in decreased survival of the cells exposed to APAP/HV110, suggesting the role of HV110-induced autophagy in the cells' protection. However, after chloroquine treatment, percentage of viable cells exposed to APAP/HV110 has not decreased to the viability level of those treated only with APAP, suggesting involvement of other protective mechanisms.

According to the results of mRNA expression, APAP/HV110 treated cells elevated mRNA levels of *p62/SQSTM1* and *PINK1* after 6 h. The main role of PINK1 in cells is to promote Parkin-mediated mitophagy by recruiting Parkin to damaged mitochondria (Williams and Ding, 2015). Along with its protective function and the potential to activate mitophagy, it was shown that PINK1 may also have an important role in activation of basal and starvation-induced autophagy by interacting with Beclin-1 protein (Michiorri et al., 2010). On the other hand, p62/SQSTM1 is a molecular adapter between degradation substrates and molecules involved in autophagosome formation and antioxidant defense (Lamark et al., 2009; Rautou et al., 2010; Ichimura et al., 2013). Elevated *p62/SQSTM1* mRNA synthesis in cells co-treated with APAP/HV110 implies activation of NF-E2-related factor 2 (Nrf-2), an important transcription factor that regulates the expression of antioxidant specific genes. Recent data showed that p62/SQSTM1 also plays important role in regulation of Nrf2 activity. The p62 binds to Kelch-like ECH-associating protein 1 (Keap1) causing release of Nrf2 and consequent transcription of genes, including those involved in xenobiotic and ROS (reactive oxygen species) detoxification (Ichimura et al., 2013). Jones et al. (2015) provided evidence that lactobacilli can elicit their beneficial influences in the gut through direct contact with NADPH oxidases on a cell surface, resulting in ROS generation and consequential activation of Nrf2 signaling. However, according to our knowledge this is the first study that reports link between postbiotics and p62/SQSTM1 as possible new mechanism of postbiotics activation of Nrf2 pathway in hepatocytes. *PINK1* gene upregulation suggests that HV110 treatment triggers a low sub-lethal level of oxidative stress that could be reflected at the level of transcription of *PINK1* which is highly sensitive to subtle changes in intracellular environment.

Although APAP/HV110 co-application induced changes in *PINK1* and *p62/SQSTM1* mRNA expression after 6 h treatment, the values returned to basal levels after prolonged treatment (16 h). It was shown that antioxidants produced by cells as response to oxidative damage, in this case caused by APAP, inhibit Nrf2 dependent gene transcription, via negative feedback (Murata et al., 2015). Considering the fact that *PINK1* regulation, as well as regulation of *p62/SQSTM1* transcription is dependent on Nrf2 protein, this could explain downregualtion of *PINK1* and *p62/SQSTM* mRNA expression after 16 h treatment, which was obtained in this study (Jain et al., 2010; Murata et al., 2015). Interestingly, we did not detect any changes in *PINK1* and *p62/SQSTM1* expression, in cells treated only with APAP, neither after 6 h nor after 16 h of treatment. This suggests that mechanisms which lead to acute cellular response were more intensively activated in the presence of HV110. It could be assumed that rapid activation of these mechanisms might have elevated cellular defensive system, including autophagy response which aided cellular survival, as demonstrated in MTT and LDH assays. All above mentioned results are consistent with the concept of "hormesis," a response to xenobiotic and environmental stimuli, where low stress levels are protective against more destructive stimuli. This concept has generally been given as an explanation for beneficial effects of microbes upon the host (Jones et al., 2015).

In spite of their well-known role in autophagy induction, we surprisingly noticed a decrease of *BECN1* and *Atg5* transcription in APAP treated cells, for which increased LC3 lipidation was obtained. This was irrespective of HV110 presence. Beclin-1, in complex with class III phosphatidylinositol 3-kinase (PI3K) is crucial for the nucleation phase of autophagosome formation, while Atg5 conjugates to Atg12 and facilitates the lipidation of LC3 protein (Rautou et al., 2010; Otomo et al., 2013). Aside from being indispensable for autophagy, Beclin-1 has additional roles not related to autophagosomes formation. Beclin-1 is known as haplo-insufficient tumor-suppressor and accumulating evidence of data suggests its down-regulation in cancers (Li et al., 2013; Huang et al., 2014). Findings of Li et al. (2013) show that down-regulation of Beclin-1 triggered autophagy, decreased apoptosis and stimulated proliferation of cells exposed to gemcitabine in Miapaca2 tumor cells. Therefore, lower levels of *BECN1* mRNA in APAP-treated cells could be explained as a cellular attempt to overcome toxicity caused by very high APAP dose. In the case of *Atg5* gene downregulation, the results could be explained by the role of Atg5 protein to regulate its own transcription through a feedback inhibition loop, as demonstrated by Hu et al. (2011).

CONCLUSION

Our study demonstrated protective effect of autophagy activated by postbiotic HV110 originated from *Lactobacillus fermentum* BGHV110 strain in APAP induced cytotoxicity in HepG2 cells. To the best of our knowledge, this is the first study to correlate autophagy inductive potential of lactobacilli to their protective effects against drug-induced toxicity. Taken together, this could be of special relevance for designing of new analgetic drug formulations with added postbiotic for prevention of possible hepatotoxic side effects, although the safety and health promoting efficacy of such drugs should be further tested.

AUTHOR CONTRIBUTIONS

MD: performed main work, analyzed, interpreted the data and draft the work; JL: conception and design of experiments, performed part of the experiments, analyzed, interpreted the data and critically revised the manuscript; JD: performed part of the experiments, analyzed and interpreted the data; MM: supervised the work, analyzed the data and critically revised the manuscript; IS: analyzed, interpreted and critically revised the manuscript; NG: supervised the work, analyzed and interpreted the data, draft the work; JB: conception and design of the work, supervised the work, analyzed and interpreted the data and critically revised the manuscript. All authors finally approved the version to be published and agreed to be accountable for all aspects of the work in ensuring that questions related to the accuracy or integrity of any part of the work are appropriately investigated and resolved.

FUNDING

This work was supported by Ministry of Education, Science and Technological Development of the Republic of Serbia (grant no. 173019).

ACKNOWLEDGMENT

MD is grateful to Nemanja Mirkovic from the Faculty of Agriculture, University of Belgrade, Belgrade, Serbia, for liophilization of HV110 postbiotic.

REFERENCES

Delgado, M. A., Elmaoued, R. A., Davis, A. S., Kyei, G., and Deretic, V. (2008). Toll-like receptors control autophagy. *EMBO J.* 27, 1110–1121. doi: 10.1038/emboj.2008.31

Escoll, P., Rolando, M., and Buchrieser, C. (2016). Modulation of host autophagy during bacterial infection: sabotaging host munitions for pathogen nutrition. *Front. Immunol.* 7:81. doi: 10.3389/fimmu.2016.00081

Forsyth, C. B., Farhadi, A., Jakate, S. M., Tang, Y., Shaikh, M., and Keshavarziana, A. (2009). *Lactobacillus* GG treatment ameliorates alcohol-induced intestinal oxidative stress, gut leakiness, and liver injury in a rat model of alcoholic steatohepatitis. *Alcohol* 43, 163–172. doi: 10.1016/j.alcohol.2008.12.009

He, Z., Liu, H., Agostini, M., Yousefi, S., Perren, A., Tschan, M. P., et al. (2013). p73 regulates autophagy and hepatocellular lipid metabolism through a transcriptional activation of the ATG5 gene. *Cell Death Differ.* 20, 1415–1424. doi: 10.1038/cdd.2013.104

Hu, Z., Zhang, J., and Zhang, Q. (2011). Expression pattern and functions of autophagy-related gene atg5 in zebrafish organogenesis. *Autophagy* 7, 1514–1527. doi: 10.4161/auto.7.12.18040

Huang, X., Qi, Q., Hua, X., Li, X., Zhang, W., Sun, H., et al. (2014). Beclin 1, an autophagy-related gene, augments apoptosis in U87 glioblastoma cells. *Oncol. Rep.* 31, 1761–1767. doi: 10.3892/or.2014.3015

Ichimura, Y., Waguri, S., Sou, Y. S., Kageyama, S., Hasegawa, J., Ishimura, R., et al. (2013). Phosphorylation of p62 activates the Keap1-Nrf2 pathway during selective autophagy. *Mol. Cell.* 51, 618–631. doi: 10.1016/j.molcel.2013.08.003

Igusa, Y., Yamashina, S., Izumi, K., Inami, Y., Fukada, H., and Komatsu, M. (2012). Loss of autophagy promotes murine acetaminophen hepatotoxicity. *J. Gastroenterol.* 47, 433–443. doi: 10.1007/s00535-011-0500-0

Irving, A. T., Mimuro, H., Kufer, T. A., Lo, C., Wheeler, R., Turner, L. J., et al. (2014). The immune receptor NOD1 and kinase RIP2 interact with bacterial peptidoglycan on early endosomes to promote autophagy and inflammatory signalling. *Cell Host Microbe* 15, 623–635. doi: 10.1016/j.chom.2014.04.001

Jain, A., Lamark, T., Sjottem, E., Larsen, K. B., Awuh, J. A., Overvatn, A., et al. (2010). p62/SQSTM1 is a target gene for transcription factor NRF2 and creates a positive feedback loop by inducing antioxidant response element-driven gene transcription. *J. Biol. Chem.* 285, 22576–22591. doi: 10.1074/jbc.M110.118976

Jones, R. M., Desai, C., Darby, T. M., Luo, L., Wolfarth, A. A., Scharer, C. D., et al. (2015). Lactobacilli modulate epithelial cytoprotection through the Nrf2 pathway. *Cell Rep.* 12, 1217–1225. doi: 10.1016/j.celrep.2015.07.042

Jovcic, B., Begovic, J., Lozo, J., Topisirovic, L., and Kojic, M. (2009). Dynamic of sodium dodecyl sulfate utilization and antibiotic susceptibility of strain *Pseudomonas* sp. ATCC19151. *Arch. Biol. Sci.* 61, 159–165. doi: 10.2298/ABS0902159J

Kim, S. J., Khan, M., Quan, J., Till, A., Subramani, S., and Siddiqui, A. (2013). Hepatitis B virus disrupts mitochondrial dynamics: induces fission and mitophagy to attenuate apoptosis. *PLoS Pathog.* 9:e1003722. doi: 10.1371/journal.ppat.1003722

Kobayashi, S., Xu, X., Chen, K., and Liang, Q. (2012). Suppression of autophagy is protective in high glucose-induced cardiomyocyte injury. *Autophagy* 8, 577–592. doi: 10.4161/auto.18980

Konstantinov, S. R., Kuipers, E. J., and Peppelenbosch, M. P. (2013). Functional genomic analyses of the gut microbiota for CRC screening. *Nat. Rev. Gastroenterol. Hepatol.* 10, 741–745. doi: 10.1038/nrgastro.2013.178

Lamark, T., Kirkin, V., Dikic, I., and Johansen, T. (2009). NBR1 and p62 as cargo receptors for selective autophagy of ubiquitinated targets. *Cell Cycle* 8, 1986–1990. doi: 10.4161/cc.8.13.8892

Larson, A. M., Polson, J., Fontana, R. J., Davern, T. J., Lalani, E., and Hynan, L. S. (2005). Acetaminophen-induced acute liver failure: results of a United States multicenter, prospective study. *Hepatology* 42, 1364–1372. doi: 10.1002/hep.20948

Lee, W. M. (2004). Acetaminophen and the US acute liver failure study group: lowering the risks of hepatic failure. *Hepatology* 40, 6–9. doi: 10.1002/hep.20293

Li, X., Xu, M., Liu, M., Ji, Y., and Li, Z. (2015). TNF-alpha and IL-6 inhibit apolipoprotein A-IV production induced by linoleic acid in human intestinal Caco2 cells. *J. Inflamm.* 12:22. doi: 10.1186/s12950-015-0069-0

Li, X., Yan, J., Wang, L., Xiao, F., Yang, Y., Guo, X., et al. (2013). Beclin1 inhibition promotes autophagy and decreases gemcitabine-induced apoptosis in Miapaca2 pancreatic cancer cells. *Cancer Cell Int.* 13, 26. doi: 10.1186/1475-2867-13-26

Lin, R., Jiang, Y., Zhao, X. Y., Guan, Y., Qian, W., Fu, X. C., et al. (2014). Four types of *Bifidobacteria* trigger autophagy response in intestinal epithelial cells. *J. Dig. Dis.* 15, 597–605. doi: 10.1111/1751-2980.12179

Liu, K., Shi, Y., Guo, X., Wang, S., Ouyang, Y., Hao, M., et al. (2014). CHOP mediates ASPP2-induced autophagic apoptosis in hepatoma cells by releasing Beclin-1 from Bcl-2 and inducing nuclear translocation of Bcl-2. *Cell Death Dis.* 5:e1323. doi: 10.1038/cddis.2014.276

Lukic, J., Strahinic, I., Milenkovic, M., Golic, N., Kojic, M., Topisirovic, L., et al. (2013). Interaction of *Lactobacillus fermentum* BGHI14 with rat colonic mucosa: implications for colitis induction. *Appl. Environ. Microbiol.* 79, 5735–5744. doi: 10.1128/AEM.01807-13

Lum, J. J., Bauer, D. E., Kong, M., Harris, M. H., Li, C., Lindsten, T. C., et al. (2005). Growth factor regulation of autophagy and cell survival in the absence of apoptosis. *Cell* 120, 237–248. doi: 10.1016/j.cell.2004.11.046

Mencin, A., Kluwe, J., and Schwabe, R. F. (2009). Toll-like receptors as targets in chronic liver diseases. *Gut* 58, 704–720. doi: 10.1136/gut.2008.156307

Michiorri, S., Gelmetti, V., Giarda, E., Lombardi, F., Romano, F., Marongiu, R., et al. (2010). The Parkinson-associated protein PINK1 interacts with Beclin1 and promotes autophagy. *Cell Death Differ.* 17, 962–974. doi: 10.1038/cdd.2009.200

Miyakawa, K., Albee, R., Letzig, L. G., Lehner, A. F., Scott, M. A., Buchweitz, J. P., et al. (2015). A cytochrome P450-independent mechanism of acetaminophen-induced injury in cultured mouse hepatocytes. *J. Pharmacol. Exp. Ther.* 354, 230–237. doi: 10.1124/jpet.115.223537

Mizushima, N., Yoshimorim, T., and Levine, B. (2010). Methods in mammalian autophagy research. *Cell* 140, 313–326. doi: 10.1016/j.cell.2010.01.028

Mosmann, T. (1983). Rapid colorimetric assay for cellular growth and survival: application to proliferation and cytotoxicity assays. *J. Immunol. Methods* 65, 55–63. doi: 10.1016/0022-1759(83)90303-4

Motevaseli, E., Azam, R., Akrami, S. M., Mazlomy, M., Saffari, M., Modarressi, M. H., et al. (2016). The effect of *Lactobacillus crispatus* and *Lactobacillus rhamnosus* culture supernatants on expression of autophagy genes and HPV E6 and E7 oncogenes in the HeLa cell line. *Cell J.* 17, 601–607.

Murata, H., Takamatsu, H., Liu, S., Kataoka, K., Huh, N. H., and Sakaguchi, M. (2015). NRF2 regulates PINK1 expression under oxidative stress conditions. *PLoS ONE* 10:e0142438. doi: 10.1371/journal.pone.0142438

Ni, H. M., Bockus, A., Boggess, N., Jaeschke, H., and Ding, W. X. (2012). Activation of autophagy protects against acetaminophen-induced hepatotoxicity. *Hepatology* 55, 222–232. doi: 10.1002/hep.24690

Oh, J. E., and Lee, H. K. (2014). Pattern recognition receptors and autophagy. *Front. Immunol.* 5:300. doi: 10.3389/fimmu.2014.00300

Otomo, C., Metlagel, Z., Takaesu, G., and Otomo, T. (2013). Structure of the human ATG12~ATG5 conjugate required for LC3 lipidation in autophagy. *Nat. Struct. Mol. Biol.* 20, 59–66. doi: 10.1038/nsmb.2431

Patel, M. R., and Denning, W. P. (2013). Therapeutic use of prebiotics, probiotics, and postbiotics to prevent necrotizing enterocolitis: What is the current evidence? *Clin. Perinatol.* 40, 11–25. doi: 10.1016/j.clp.2012.12.002

Rautou, P.-E., Mansouri, A., Lebrec, D., Durand, F., Valla, D., and Moreau, R. (2010). Autophagy in liver diseases. *J. Hepatol.* 53, 1123–1134. doi: 10.1016/j.jhep.2010.07.006

Rishi, P., Mavi, S. K., Bharrhan, S., Shukla, G., and Tewari, R. (2009). Protective efficacy of probiotic alone or in conjunction with a prebiotic in *Salmonella*-induced liver damage. *FEMS Microbiol. Ecol.* 69, 222–230. doi: 10.1111/j.1574-6941.2009.00703.x

Sahani, M. H., Itakura, E., and Mizushima, N. (2014). Expression of the autophagy substrate SQSTM1/p62 is restored during prolonged starvation depending on transcriptional upregulation and autophagy-derived amino acids. *Autophagy* 10, 431–441. doi: 10.4161/auto.27344

Salaun, B., Romero, P., and Lebecque, S. (2007). Toll-like receptors' two-edged sword: when immunity meets apoptosis. *Eur. J. Immunol.* 37, 3311–3318. doi: 10.1002/eji.200737744

Segawa, S., Wakita, Y., Hirata, H., and Watari, J. (2008). Oral administration of heat-killed *Lactobacillus brevis* SBC8803 ameliorates alcoholic liver disease in ethanol-containing diet-fed C57BL/6N mice. *Int. J. Food Microbiol.* 128, 371–377. doi: 10.1016/j.ijfoodmicro.2008.09.023

Seki, E., and Brenner, D. A. (2008). Toll-like receptors and adaptor molecules in liver disease: update. *Hepatology* 48, 322–335. doi: 10.1002/hep.22306

Sharma, S., Singh, R. L., and Kakkar, P. (2011). Modulation of Bax/Bcl-2 and caspases by probiotics during acetaminophen induced apoptosis in primary hepatocytes. *Food Chem. Toxicol.* 49, 770–779. doi: 10.1016/j.fct.2010.11.041

Subramaniam, M., In, L. L., Kumar, A., Ahmed, N., and Nagoor, N. H. (2016). Cytotoxic and apoptotic effects of heat killed *Mycobacterium indicus pranii* (MIP) on various human cancer cell lines. *Sci. Rep.* 28, 19833. doi: 10.1038/srep19833

Tsilingiri, K., Barbosa, T., Penna, G., Caprioli, F., Sonzogni, A., Viale, G., et al. (2012). Probiotic and postbiotic activity in health and disease: comparison on a novel polarised ex-vivo organ culture model. *Gut* 61, 1007–1015. doi: 10.1136/gutjnl-2011-300971

Westerink, W. M., and Schoonen, W. G. (2007). Cytochrome P450 enzyme levels in HepG2 cells and cryopreserved primary human hepatocytes and their induction in HepG2 cells. *Toxicol. In Vitro* 21, 1581–1591. doi: 10.1016/j.tiv.2007.05.014

Williams, J. A., and Ding, W. X. (2015). Targeting Pink1-Parkin-mediated mitophagy for treating liver injury. *Pharmacol. Res.* 102, 264–269. doi: 10.1016/j.phrs.2015.09.020

Wu, S., Yuan, L., Zhang, Y., Liu, F., Li, G., Wen, K., et al. (2013). Probiotic *Lactobacillus rhamnosus* GG mono-association suppresses human rotavirus-induced autophagy in the gnotobiotic piglet intestine. *Gut Pathog.* 5:22. doi: 10.1186/1757-4749-5-22

Xu, J., Ma, M., and Purcell, W. M. (2003). Characterisation of some cytotoxic endpoints using rat liver and HepG2 spheroids as in vitro models and their application in hepatotoxicity studies. I. Glucose metabolism and enzyme release as cytotoxic markers. *Toxicol. Appl. Pharmacol.* 189, 100–111. doi: 10.1016/S0041-008X(03)00089-9

Zhang, Y., Li, Y., Yuan, W., Xia, Y., and Shen, Y. (2016). Autophagy is associated with pathogenesis of haemophilus parasuis. *Front. Microbiol.* 7:1423. doi: 10.3389/fmicb.2016.01423

2

Health-Associated Niche Inhabitants as Oral Probiotics: The Case of *Streptococcus dentisani*

*Arantxa López-López†, Anny Camelo-Castillo†, María D. Ferrer, Áurea Simon-Soro and Alex Mira**

Department of Health and Genomics, Center for Advanced Research in Public Health, FISABIO Foundation, Valencia, Spain

Correspondence:
Alex Mira
mira_ale@gva.es

†These authors have contributed equally to this work.

Oral diseases, including dental caries and periodontitis, are among the most prevalent diseases worldwide and develop as a consequence of a microbial dysbiosis. Several bacterial strains are being tested as potential oral health-promoting organisms, but usually they are species isolated from niches other than the site where they must exert its probiotic action, typically from fecal samples. We hypothesize that oral inhabitants associated to health conditions will be more effective than traditional, gut-associated probiotic species in key aspects such as colonization of the oral site where disease takes place or the possession of oral health promoting functions, as well as more practical issues like safety and toxicity, and establishing proper doses for administration. As an example of these *active colonizers*, we describe the case of *Streptococcus dentisani*, a new streptococcal species isolated from dental plaque of caries-free individuals. We have detected it in 98% of dental plaque samples from healthy individuals and, as expected, it does not produce any toxic secondary metabolite and does not survive a simulated stomach digestion, preventing potential secondary effects. Besides, this species has a double probiotic action, as it inhibits the growth of major oral pathogens through the production of bacteriocins, and also buffers acidic pH (the primary cause of dental caries) through an arginolytic pathway. We propose the use of *S. dentisani* as a promising probiotic against tooth decay.

Keywords: probiotics, dental caries, pH buffering, arginolytic pathway, bacteriocins, *Streptococcus dentisani*

INTRODUCTION

Oral diseases such as dental caries (tooth decay) and periodontitis (gum disease) are caused by microorganisms. However, they are currently not considered infectious diseases in classical terms because their etiology is clearly polymicrobial (Fejerskov, 2004; Simón-Soro and Mira, 2015), and because the pathogenic bacteria involved are also found at lower proportions in healthy individuals (Hajishengallis and Lamont, 2012; Camelo-Castillo et al., 2015). Thus, it has been pointed out that antimicrobial strategies may not be effective against oral diseases, and new preventive or therapeutic approaches based on restoring the microbial ecological balance in the oral cavity have been proposed (Marsh, 2015; Marsh et al., 2015). Those new preventive measures could include the use of prebiotic compounds to promote the growth of health-associated bacteria (Santarpia et al., 2014), or the application of probiotic bacteria with beneficial features (Saha et al., 2012). In the case of dental caries, health-associated microbial communities have been identified using omics approaches (Zaura et al., 2009; Belda-Ferre et al., 2011; Alcaraz et al., 2012), and therefore culturing those microorganisms could provide potential beneficial bacteria to prevent oral diseases.

However, due to the greater development of probiotics in gut pathologies, and the strong safety evidence accumulated for gut bacteria, many microorganisms isolated from human or animal fecal samples with beneficial properties are being developed as potential probiotics to promote oral health. These often include strains of lactobacilli and bifidobacteria, which had previously been shown to have inmunomodulatory, anti-inflammatory and anti-bacterial properties in different *in vitro* studies and also in clinical trials (see **Table 1**; Reid et al., 2011; Cagetti et al., 2013). However, the use of many of these strains in oral diseases like dental caries can be problematic because both *Lactobacillus* and *Bifidobacterium* species have been shown to be acidogenic and to be involved in tooth decay (Badet and Thebaud, 2008; Mantzourani et al., 2009a). Even if weak acidogenic strains are selected, the capacity of gut bacteria to colonize the oral niche and to produce anti-caries effects has still to be demonstrated, and the use of gut probiotics in the oral cavity has been criticized. For instance, when the strain *Lactobacillus salivarius* W24 was tested in an *in vitro* oral biofilm model, it was shown that this strain further lowered the pH and affected the compositional stability of oral communities (Pham et al., 2009). Thus, the identification of novel strains isolated from the oral cavity itself could be instrumental for the development of efficient probiotics applied to oral health.

In the current manuscript, we describe the potential probiotic features of the new species *Streptococcus dentisani* that we recently isolated from the dental plaque of caries-free individuals (Camelo-Castillo et al., 2014). There are currently six isolates for which the genome sequence is available and that robust phylogenomic analysis include within the *dentisani* cluster (Jensen et al., 2016). This cluster forms part of the *S. oralis* clade and differs from the *S. oralis* and *S. tigurinus* clusters mainly in their ability to hydrolyze arginine (Jensen et al., 2016). In this manuscript, we study strains 7746 and 7747^T, which were isolated from two different individuals and that were shown to be different by comparison of their genomes (Camelo-Castillo et al., 2014). We describe their ability to inhibit the growth of caries-producing bacteria, as *Streptococcus mutans* and *Streptococcus sobrinus*, and to buffer extracellular acidic pH, which is the underlying cause of tooth decay. In addition, we show that, being a commensal species in the oral cavity of healthy individuals, their safety features are robust and the appropriate dose for probiotic treatment can be easily determined experimentally.

MATERIALS AND METHODS

Inhibition Assays with *S. dentisani* Supernatants

Inhibition experiments against cariogenic bacteria were carried out with concentrated supernatants of well grown cultures of *S. dentisani* 7746 and 7747 (stationary phase). In order to obtain 5 ml of the concentrated supernatants, single colonies of each *S. dentisani* strain were inoculated into 50 ml of brain hearth infusion broth (BHI, Biolife) and incubated aerobically at 37°C without agitation during 48 h, or until they reached an optical density of around 1.5 at 610 nm (O.D. $_{610}$). After the incubation period, the cultures were centrifuged at 4000 rpm 10 min and the pellets discarded. The obtained supernatants were filtered throughout 0.2 μm pore-size filters (Millipore) and ten-fold concentrated by rotary evaporation on a RV 10 digital device (VWR) with the following settings: heating bath at 40°C, 70 rpm of rotation, 100 mbar of pressure, and 30 min of operating time. The resulting 5 ml of concentrated supernatants were filtered throughout 0.2 μm pore-size filters (Millipore) and stored at −20°C until use.

The inhibitory activity of the supernatants was determined by monitoring the growth of *S. mutans* ATCC 25175 and *S. sobrinus* CECT 4034 in the presence/absence of the potential inhibitor by means of optical density measurements. Pre-inocula of *S. mutans* and *S. sobrinus* were obtained by inoculating a single colony of each strain in 10 ml of BHI liquid medium and incubated aerobically overnight at 37°C without agitation. The O.D. $_{610}$ of the pre-inocula was measured in a spectrophotometer (BioPhotometer, Eppendorf) and diluted with BHI liquid medium to obtain an optical density of 0.1. To assess the inhibitory effect of *S. dentisani* on the growth of *S. mutans* and *S. sobrinus*, 160 μl of the bacterial suspensions were mixed with 40 μl of the concentrated supernatants and loaded by triplicate into a Nunc Microwell 96-well microplate by triplicate. As controls, 160 μl of the bacterial suspensions were mixed with 40 μl of 10-fold concentrated BHI and loaded by triplicate into the 96-well microplate. The microplate was loaded into a microplate reader (Infinite 200 PRO, Tecan) and incubated at 37°C during 24 h. The O.D. $_{610}$ of each inoculated well was measured every 30 min during the incubation time.

To determine the active size fraction, the concentrated supernatant was size-fractionated by sequential filtering throughout 10 KDa and 3 KDa filters (Amicon), following the manufacturer's recommendations. By this way, we obtained three size fractions (>10 KDa, 3–10 KDa, and <3KDa) that were tested by triplicate against *S. mutans* cultures by the same methodology explained above. To confirm the peptidic nature of the inhibitory compounds and discard that the inhibition was produced by hydrogen peroxide we proceed as described in Zhu and Kreth (2012). Briefly, *S. dentisani* was grown on a BHI plate for 24 h and peroxidase (40 μg), peptidase (64 μg), or phosphate-buffered saline were applied beside each colony for 10 min before the other species were inoculated at the same spot. *S. mutans* and *S. sanguinis* were used as controls of proteinaceus inhibitory substance and H_2O_2, respectively.

Besides, we used scanning electron microscopy (SEM) to directly observe the effect of the *S. dentisani* supernatants on the three type strains *S. mutans* ATCC 25175, *Prevotella intermedia* NCTC 13070, and *Fusobacterium nucleatum* DSMZ 20482 cells. Briefly, 160 μl of the bacterial cultures in exponential phase (O.D. $_{610}$ = 0.6) were mixed with 40 μl of the concentrated supernatant and incubated for 30, 60, and 90 min at 37°C. After the incubation period, the suspensions were centrifuged at 4000 rpm 10 min and the supernatant discarded. The pellets were fixed in 2.5% paraformaldehyde and 0.5% glutaraldehyde,

TABLE 1 | Bacteria tested in clinical trials as oral care probiotics.

Strain	Origin	Brand	Disease	Reference[1]
Lactobacillus rhamnosus GG	Human intestinal tract		Caries	Aminabadi et al., 2011
Lactobacillus rhamnosus LB21	Human intestinal tract		Caries	Stecksén-Blicks et al., 2009
Lactobacillus reuteri 55730 + PTA 5289	Woman breast milk	Prodentis™	Ginvival health, plaque reduction and caries	Krasse et al., 2006; Caglar et al., 2008a
Lactobacillus brevis CD2	Dairy products	Inersan®	Periodontal disease and caries	Riccia et al., 2007; Campus et al., 2014
Lactobacillus paracasei SD1	Human oral cavity		Caries	Ritthagol et al., 2014
Bifidobacterium animalis DN-173 010	Dairy products	ACTIVIA®	Caries	Caglar et al., 2005
Bifidobacterium animalis subsp. lactis BB-12®	Dairy cultures	BB-12®	Caries	Caglar et al., 2008b
Streptococcus salivarius M18	Saliva of a healthy child	BLIS M18®	Plaque reduction	Burton et al., 2013
Lactobacillus salivarius WB21	Mammalian digestive tract		Gingival health, periodontal disease, halitosis and caries	Shimauchi et al., 2008; Mayanagi et al., 2009; Iwamoto et al., 2010; Suzuki et al., 2014
Streptococcus oralis KJ3®, *Streptococcus uberis* KJ2® and *Streptococcus rattus* JH145®	Healthy mouths	ProBiora(3)®	Caries, periodontal disease and halitosis	Zahradnik et al., 2009
Weissella cibaria CMU, CMS-1, CMS-2 and CMS-3	Children's saliva		Halitosis and plaque reduction	Kang et al., 2006a,b
Lactobacillus reuteri DSM 17938 + PTA 5289	Human saliva	BioGaia ProDentis	Halitosis	Keller et al., 2012
Lactobacillus plantarum 7481 and *Lactobacillus brevis* 7480	Children's saliva	AB:Dentis®	Halitosis and gingivitis	WO 2012022773 A1*
Streptococcus salivarius K12	Children's saliva	BLIS K12®	Halitosis	Burton et al., 2006
Lactobacillus acidophilus NK1 + 100ash + K3III24	Human intestinal tract	Acilact (solely Russia)	Periodontal disease	Pozharitskaia et al., 1994
Bifidobacterium bifidum N1 and *Lactobacillus acidophilus* NK1	Human intestinal tract	Bifidumbacterin + Acilact (solely Russia)	Periodontal disease	Grudianov et al., 2002
Lactobacillus casei 37	Human intestinal tract		Periodontal disease	Volozhin et al., 2004
Lactobacillus paracasei GMNL-33 (ADP-1)	Human oral cavity	Dental-Lac™	Periodontal disease	Chuang et al., 2011
Lactobacillus salivarius TI 2711 (LS 1)	Human saliva		Periodontal disease	Matsuoka et al., 2006
Lactobacillus rhamnosus GG (53103) + LC705	Human intestinal tract		Oral candidasis	Hatakka et al., 2007

[1]*Reference = Publication with results of clinical trial; *Patent number.*

washed three times with PBS buffer and exposed to 1% osmium tetroxide in PBS buffer for 1 h. The samples were rinsed with PBS buffer three more times and then moved through a gradual process of dehydration, starting with 30% ethanol and ending with absolute ethanol (multiple rinse steps at each 30, 50, 70, 80, 90, and 100% ethanol). Finally, the samples were mounted on scanning electron micrograph stubs, sputter coated with gold, and viewed on a JEOL JSM 840 scanning electron microscope.

pH Range of Growth and Resistance of *S. dentisani* to the Digestive Process

To know the optimal and pH growth range of *S. dentisani* strains 7746 and 7747 we prepared BHI broth at different pHs (4.7, 5.5, 6, 6.5, 7, and 7.5) by adding NaOH 10 N or HCl 10 N to the commercial medium (Biolife). Pre-inocula were obtained as explained above. Two-hundred microliters of the BHI broths at different pHs were inoculated by triplicate with 20 μl of the inocula into a Nunc Microwell 96-well microplate. The O.D. $_{610}$ of each inoculated well was measured every 2 h and plotted versus the time of incubation to obtain the growth curves.

To evaluate the resistance of *S. dentisani* to the digestive process, the viability of the strains 7746 and 7747 was checked after a treatment with the salivary enzyme alpha amylase, followed by digestion with gastric enzymes under progressive acidic conditions to simulate digestion, following the protocol described in Khalf et al. (2010) and Martínez et al. (2011). The assays were performed in an *in vitro* model stomach (or dynamic digester) by the external services of the Food Industry Research Association AINIA (Valencia, Spain). Each strain was tested by duplicate whereas the control was assayed once. Colony forming units (CFU) counts were obtained in BHI agar before any treatment (reference cultures), after the chewing step, and during the gastric digestion at three different times (30, 60, and 120 min). The plates were incubated at 37°C during 24–48 h. As the medium used for CFU counts was not selective for *S. dentisani*, the same assay was made without inoculation and used as blank to discount any contamination, obtaining 0 CFUs in this control.

Growth of *S. dentisani* in an Arginine Enriched Medium

Streptococcus dentisani 7746 was grown in 300 ml of BHI medium amended with 5 g/l of L-arginine monohydrochloride 98% (Alfa-Aesar). The pre-inoculum was obtained by inoculating a single colony of the strain in 10 ml of BHI broth and incubating overnight at 37°C without agitation. Inoculation was made with the volume required to obtain an initial O.D. $_{610}$ of 0.02. For comparison, the same volume was used to inoculate 300 ml of BHI without arginine. In both conditions the initial pH was set at 7.3. The cultures were incubated at 37°C during 24 h and aliquots of 1 ml were taken every hour for measuring the pH and the O.D. $_{610}$. Both conditions were assayed by triplicate.

Prevalence of *S. dentisani* and Other Oral Probiotics in the Dental Plaque of Healthy Individuals

To assess the prevalence of *S. dentisani* in the dental plaque of healthy individuals we compared the genomic sequences of the *S. dentisani* strains 7746 and 7747 (1.98 and 1.74 Mb, respectively) against 118 metagenomes of the dental plaque of healthy individuals available at The Human Microbiome Project Consortium (HMP, Turnbaugh et al., 2007). The metagenomic reads were mapped against the sequenced reference genomes using the NUCmer and PROmer v3.06 alignment algorithms (Kurtz et al., 2004) with the default parameters, following the methodology of Belda-Ferre et al. (2011). We considered that *S. dentisani* was present in a sample if at least 20 sequences >100 bp of the metagenome showed a similarity equal to or higher than 99% with the sequenced genomes. For comparison, the same approach was used to analyze the prevalence of *S. salivarius* in dental plaque.

The presence of the genus *Lactobacillus* in different parts of the oral cavity was performed by the analysis of the oral 16S rDNA sequences deposited in the Human Microbiome Project database in year 2014[1]. The niches analyzed were the keratinized gingiva, buccal mucosa, hard palate, palatine tonsils, saliva, supra- and subgingival plaque, and tongue dorsum. The analyses were carried out with a total of 4.3×10^8 sequences. The taxonomic affiliation was performed using the Megablast tool implemented in the NCBI against the SILVA ribosomal database[2], with the following parameters: *e* value $<1e{-}^{10}$, percent identity >97%, alignment length >350 bp.

Quantification of *S. dentisani* in the Dental Plaque of Healthy Individuals

Two healthy volunteers, named MG01 and MG02, were selected for sampling. They were males aged 20–30 years, non-smokers, with 28 teeth excluding third molars, with good dental and periodontal health: in both, absence of caries (non-cavitated level), DMF = 0, OHI = 0, GI = 1, and CPI = 1 (following nomenclature by World Health Organization [WHO], 1997). They had not been treated with antibiotics in the 6 months prior to the study nor presented antecedents of routine use of oral antiseptics. The two donors signed a written informed consent and the sampling procedure was approved by the Ethics Committee from the DGSP-CSISP (Valencian Health Authority), with reference 10/11/2009. Supragingival and subgingival dental plaque samples were taken from vestibular (buccal) and lingual (palatine) surfaces of 28 teeth in each volunteer. *Streptococcus dentisani* was quantified in individual free surfaces of each tooth type (incisor, canine, premolar, and molar) from one quadrant and the absolute numbers calculated by multiplying the obtained value by the number of each tooth type in the mouth. The same procedure was followed for the total bacterial content quantification.

Dental plaque samples were resuspended in 100 μl of PBS buffer and DNA was extracted with the MagnaPure LC JE379 instrument and the MagnaPure LC DNA Isolation Kit (Roche). The quantification of the DNA was done with the Quant-iT PicoGreen dsDNA Assay Kit (Invitrogen), and real-time PCR was performed in a LightCycler 480 System with the LightCycler 480 SYBR Green I Master Mix (Roche). In every step, we followed the manufacturer's recommendations.

The specific primers used for the quantification of *S. dentisani* were designed for this study and targeted the genes for the carbamate kinase (*arcC*): CkSdF 5′-GTAAC CAACCGCCCAGAAGG-3′ and CkSdR 5′-CCGCTTTCGGA CTCGATCA-3′; and the ORF540: Orf540F (5′-ATGTTCA TCGGCTTGACAGGCTT-3′) and Orf540R (5′- TAAGCAA GCATAGAACCGCGCC-3′). Primers specificity was predicted *in silico* by the primerBLAST tool implemented in the NCBI[3] and confirmed by absence of amplification by qPCR with 5 ng/μl DNA from *S. mutans, S. sobrinus, S. sanguinis, S. salivarius, S. mitis, S. pneumoniae, S. infantis, and S. oralis.* The specificity of the primers was also checked by scrutinizing the melting profiles after every assay. Primers for the Ck gene did not amplify any of the tested streptococcal species. Primers for the ORF540 amplified only the DNA of *S. pneumoniae*, which is a rare inhabitant of dental plaque. Amplification was performed in a 20 μl final volume containing 1 μl of template DNA (at concentrations 5–22 ng/μl), 10 μl of the LightCycler 480 SYBR Green I Master Mix, 0.4 μl of each primer, and 7.2 μl of nuclease-free water. The thermocycling protocol used was as follows: an initial step of 95°C for 5 min, and 40 cycles of 10 s at 95°C, 20 s at 65°C, and 25 s at 72°C. All the quantifications were made by duplicate.

The concentration of *S. dentisani* in each sample was calculated by comparison with the Cq values obtained from a standard curve. This was generated using serial 10-fold dilutions of DNA extracted from 2×10^7 CFUs/ml (counted by serial dilutions in agar plates). Finally, the Cq values obtained with the plaque samples were replaced in the standard equation and expressed in absolute numbers per tooth type analyzed.

[1] http://hmpdacc.org

[2] http://www.arb-silva.de

[3] www.ncbi.nlm.nih.gov/tools/primer-blast

RESULTS

Inhibitory Activity of the *S. dentisani* Supernatants

As shown in **Figure 1A**, the addition of the *S. dentisani* 7746 concentrated supernatant produced a marked inhibitory effect on the growth of both *S. mutans* and *S. sobrinus*, as compared to the curves obtained when only concentrated BHI was added. Similarly, the concentrated supernatant completely inhibited the growth of other *S. mutans* strains (strains OMZ175 and ATCC 700610, data not shown). Regarding the curves obtained with the different size fractions, the <3 KDa fraction retained the inhibitory activity when tested against *S. mutans* ATCC 25175, while the 3–10 KDa and >10 KDa fractions did not (**Figure 1B**). The last two even enhanced the growth of *S. mutans*, probably due to a higher availability of nutrients coming from the concentrated culture medium and/or the *S. dentisani* metabolism. The same results were obtained with strain 7747 (data not shown).

Microscopy visualizations revealed that after 30 min of incubation with concentrated supernatants of *S. dentisani*, the cells of *S. mutans*, *F. nucleatum*, and *P. intermedia* were clearly affected, showing pores in the surface of the cells (*S. mutans*), changes in the cell walls' structure (*P. intermedia*) and cell lysis (*F. nucleatum*) (**Figures 2A–C**).

Proteinase treatment of the supernatant provoked the absence of growth inhibition when tested against *S. mutans*, while the peroxidase treatment did not affect the inhibitory activity (**Figure 3**). Taken together, the results indicated that the inhibition is not due to the production of hydrogen peroxide, and supports the idea that *S. dentisani* inhibit oral pathogenic bacteria by the production of inhibitors of peptidic nature, such as bacteriocin-like peptides.

pH Tolerance and Resistance of *S. dentisani* to the Digestive Process

Streptococcus dentisani was tested for its ability to grow at different pHs. The growth curves obtained showed that both strains displayed a very similar behavior, with an optimal growth pH close to 7 (**Supplementary Figures S1A,B**). It is noteworthy that they were able to grow at pH values between 6 and 7.5 but not between 4.7 and 5.5, indicating that *S. dentisani* can endure moderately acidic conditions but is not an acidophilic organism. Surprisingly, the growth of both strains at pH 6 was better than at 6.5, suggesting the activation of a buffering metabolic pathway at pH values around 6 (see Section "pH Buffering Capacity of *S. dentisani*" below).

Regarding the simulated digestive process, and as expected from the pH curves obtained before, *S. dentisani* was not able to maintain the initial viability during digestion simulations. As starting values of viability we obtained 6.5×10^8 and 3.9×10^8 CFUs/ml for the strains 7746 and 7747, respectively. After the chewing simulation with salivary enzymes these values decreased in only two to three orders of magnitude, showing that both strains could remain in the mouth at high levels after chewing, whereas the gastric digestion strongly inhibited their growth, even after the first step of the simulation (30 min, see **Table 2**). As neither strain of *S. dentisani* survived the gastric process, the simulation of an intestinal digestion was not performed.

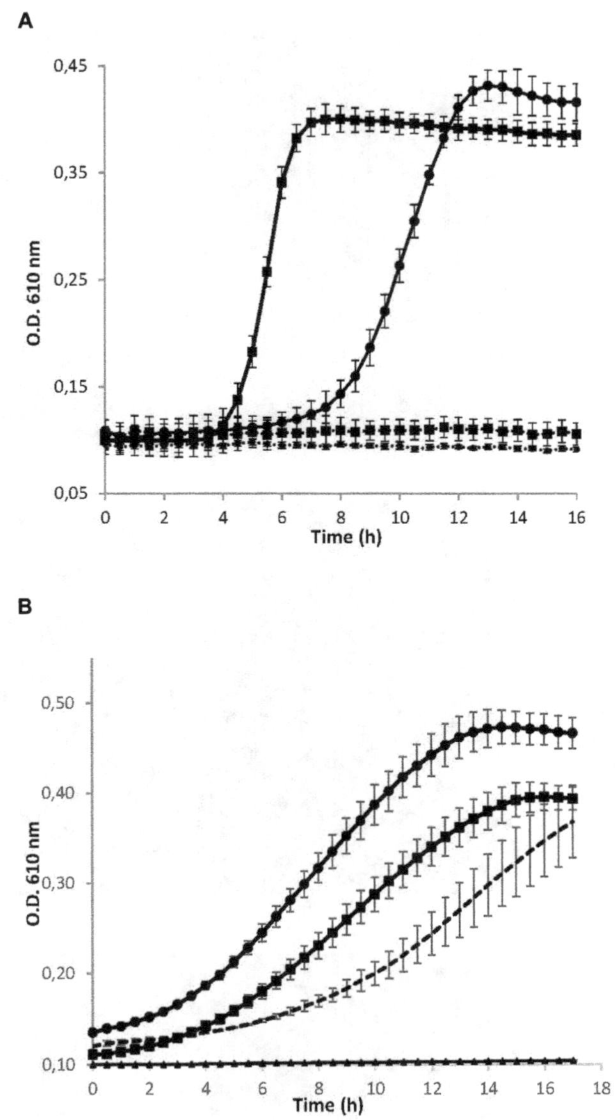

FIGURE 1 | (A) Growth curves of the cariogenic bacteria *Streptococcus mutans* ATCC 25175 (squares) and *S. sobrinus* CECT 4034 (circles) in the presence (dotted lines) and absence (solid lines) of concentrated supernatant of *S. dentisani* strain 7746. **(B)** Growth curves of *S. mutans* ATCC 25175 in the presence of different size fractions of the 10× concentrated supernatant of *S. dentisani* 7746. Circles correspond to the fraction >10 KDa, squares to the 3–10 KDa fraction, and triangles to the fraction <3 KDa. For comparisons, *S. mutans* was grown in the presence of 10x concentrated BHI medium (dotted line). Means ± SD from three independent replicates are plotted.

pH Buffering Capacity of *S. dentisani*

Figure 4 depict the growth curves obtained by triplicate when *S. dentisani* 7746 was grown in presence/absence of arginine. During the initial 6 h of incubation, the growth seemed to be fueled by the sugars present in the BHI medium, as the growth

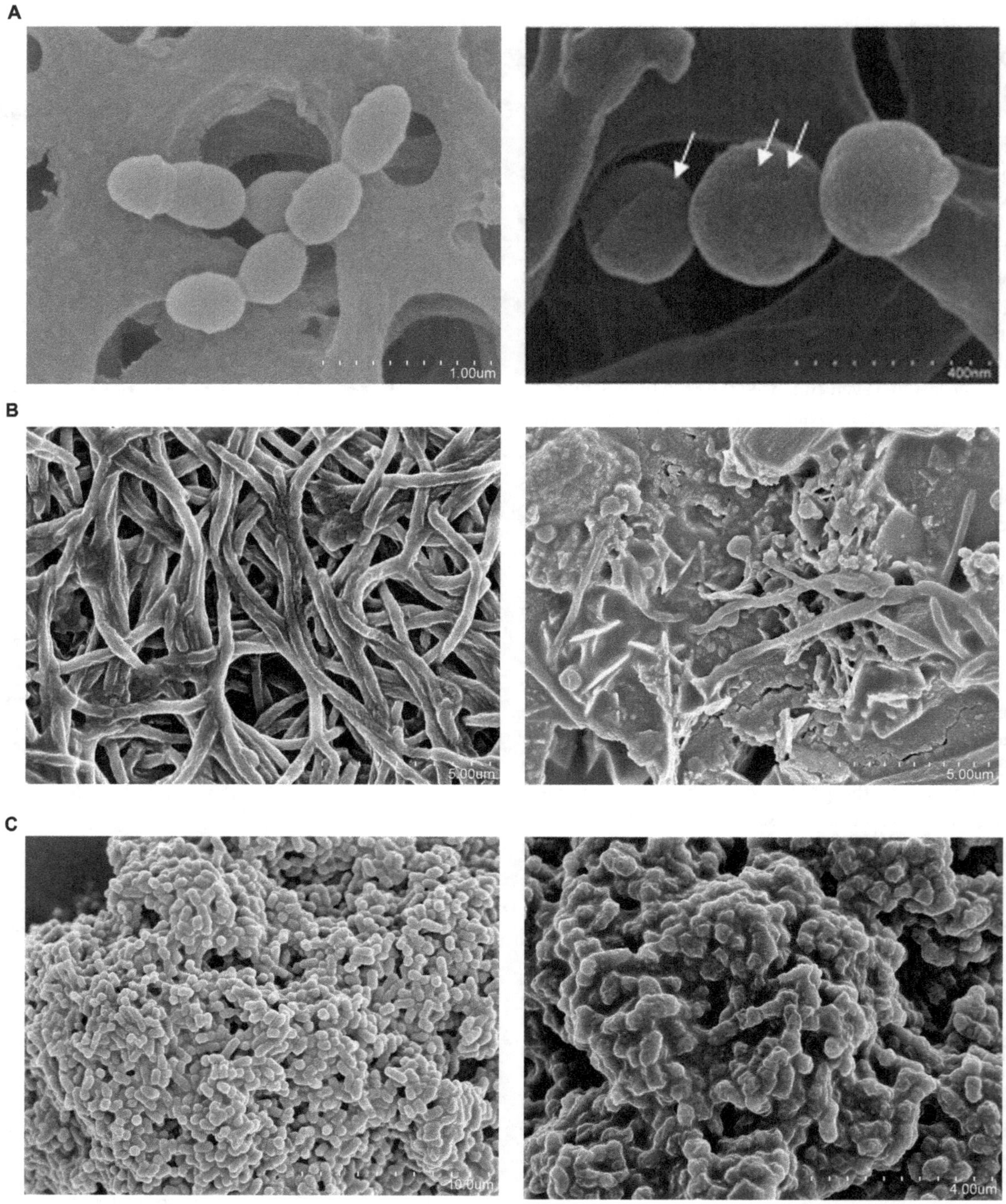

FIGURE 2 | Scanning electron microscopy (SEM) of three oral pathogens before (left) and after (right) a 30-min treatment with 10-fold concentrated supernatant of *S. dentisani* strain 7746. (A) *Streptococcus mutans* (pores are pointed with arrows). **(B)** *Fusobacterium nucleatum*. **(C)** *Prevotella intermedia*.

curves were identical in both conditions (with and without arginine), and the culture pH dropped from 7.3 to about 6.2. Soon after completion of this first phase, in the cultures containing arginine the pH starts to rise, reaching almost the initial pH value 12 h after inoculation. Contrarily, in the medium without arginine the pH continuously decreased to reach a value of about 6.2. In both conditions the O.D. $_{610}$ measurements were similar, with a maximum value of around 1.3 after 12 h of incubation.

The analysis of the genome of *S. dentisani* showed that strains 7746 and 7747^{T} contain the key genes of the arginine deiminase system: *arcA* (arginine deiminase, locus tag HK29_RS02275), *arcC* (carbamate kinase, locus tag HK29_RS02285), and *arcB* (ornithine carbamoyltransferase, locus tag HK29_RS02280),

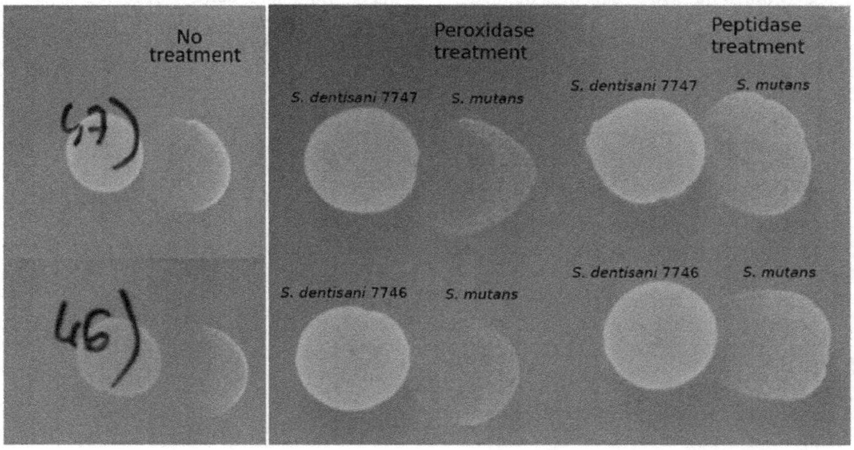

FIGURE 3 | Inhibition of *S. mutans* by *S. dentisani* in the presence of peroxidase and proteinase. The tests were performed with *S. dentisani* strains 7746 and 7747, treating with the enzymes the spots where *S. mutans* would later be grown. The controls on the left panel show the inhibition without treatment.

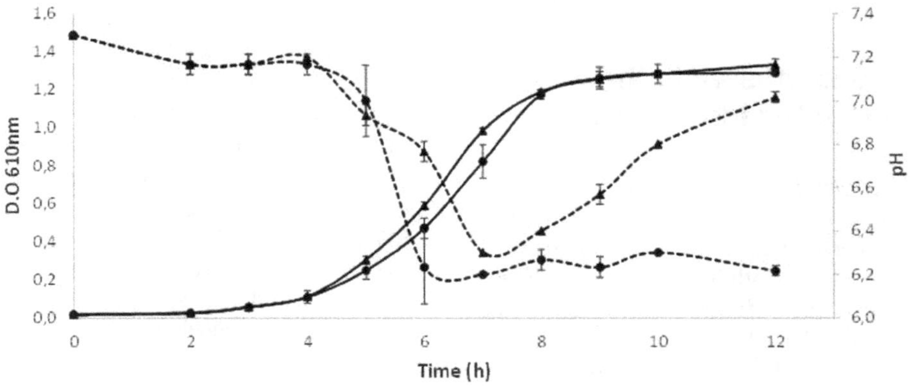

FIGURE 4 | Growth curves of *S. dentisani* strain 7746 in a medium with (triangles) and without (circles) the addition of 5 g/l of arginine. The mean ± SD of O.D. $_{610}$ (solid lines) and pH of the culture (dotted lines) from three replicates are depicted.

involved in the ammonia generation through arginine metabolism, a mechanism that releases ammonnia extracellularly producing the alkalinization of the environment (Liu et al., 2008, 2012).

Prevalence of *S. dentisani* in the Dental Plaque of Healthy Individuals

The recruitment analyses showed that sequences of *S. dentisani* were present in most of the analyzed metagenomes (direct, whole-sequenced DNA coming from dental plaques of healthy individuals at the Human Microbiome Project). At least 20 metagenomic sequences > 100 bp were found to have a similarity ≥99% compared with the 7746 genome in 116 out of 118 individuals, and in the strain 7747 this threshold was fulfilled in all 118 individuals. Contrarily, the species *S. salivarius* that has been proposed as a probiotic agent against caries was only detected in three of these metagenomes, in agreement with this species inhabiting mucosal surfaces and not the hard tissues. In addition, we have analyzed the *Lactobacillus* 16S rRNA gene sequences from oral samples contained in the HMP database, as this genus contains species commonly used as oral probiotics (namely *L. acidophilus*, *L. reuteri*, and *L. rhamnosus*). The results showed that *Lactobacillus* spp. is present in very low numbers in the oral cavity, accounting for less than 0.05% of the bacterial genera in the buccal mucosa, hard palate, palatine tonsils, saliva, tongue, and supragingival plaque. The highest numbers of *Lactobacillus* 16S rDNA sequences were obtained in the subgingival plaque, but even here this genus accounted for only 0.94% of the total bacterial population. We analyzed in the same oral niches the prevalence of the genus *Streptococcus*, which was found to be present at very high numbers in the keratinized gingiva, buccal mucosa, hard palatine, palatine tonsil, tongue dorsum, and saliva (59.5, 58.8, 54, 27.1, 26.8, and 19.7 per cent of the total bacterial members, respectively). Furthermore, the percentage of the genus *Streptococcus* in the subgingival and supragingival plaques was high (18.8 and 20.2%, respectively). Overall, the results showed that the genus *Streptococcus* is much more abundant than *Lactobacillus* in every analyzed oral niche, and particularly in those directly affected by the cariogenic processes, being *Streptococcus* between 20 and 600 times more

TABLE 2 | Viability, expressed in CFU/ml, of the two strains of *S. dentisani* after the chewing and gastric digestion processes (G.D.) at three different times.

Strain	Starting culture	Chewing pH 6.9	G.D. 30 min pH 3	G.D. 60 min pH 2.1	G.D. 120 min pH 1.7
S. dentisani 7746	$6.5 \times 10^8 \pm 3.05 \times 10^8$	$5.3 \times 10^6 \pm 2.8 \times 10^8$	<10	<10	<10
S. dentisani 7747	$3.9 \times 10^8 \pm 4 \times 10^7$	$1 \times 10^6 \pm 9.8 \times 10^5$	<10	<10	<10

The values shown are the mean of two independent replicates and the standard deviation is specified.

TABLE 3 | Total cell counts of *S. dentisani* on supragingival dental plaque in the vestibular (V) and lingual (L) parts of different tooth types in two caries-free individuals (MG01 and MG02).

	Incisor	Canine	Premolar	Molar
MG01 (V)	$2.1 \times 10^5/2.8 \times 10^4$	$4.7 \times 10^5/7.9 \times 10^4$	$2.9 \times 10^5/3.46 \times 10^4$	$3.1 \times 10^5/3.1 \times 10^4$
(L)	$2.8 \times 10^5/2.7 \times 10^4$	$1.4 \times 10^5/4.1 \times 10^5$	$4.6 \times 10^5/9.8 \times 10^6$	$4.3 \times 10^5/6.9 \times 10^4$
MG02 (V)	$5.5 \times 10^2/7.5 \times 10^3$	$2.7 \times 10^3/4.4 \times 10^3$	$1.2 \times 10^3/1.3 \times 10^4$	$2.5 \times 10^4/4.5 \times 10^4$
(L)	$3.4 \times 10^4/5.1 \times 10^4$	$2.8 \times 10^4/5.9 \times 10^3$	$7.1 \times 10^4/5.0 \times 10^5$	$4.7 \times 10^4/1.7 \times 10^7$

Data show the estimates of bacterial numbers obtained by qPCR with two different sets of S. dentisani-specific primers (orf540/CK).

abundant than *Lactobacillus* in the subgingival and supragingival plaque, respectively.

Quantification of *S. dentisani* in the Dental Plaque of Healthy Individuals by q-PCR

The absolute numbers of *S. dentisani* cells were obtained for the teeth's free surfaces of two healthy volunteers by the use of two set of *S. dentisani*-specific primers, which provided similar estimates (**Table 3**). The results showed that both individuals contain very similar values of abundance of *S. dentisani* (1.04×10^7 and 3.14×10^7 cells for MG01 and MG02, respectively, as estimated by the ORF540 primers; 4.46×10^7 and 6.94×10^7 cells for MG01 and MG02, as estimated by the carbamate kinase primers). However, although the calculated *S. dentisani* numbers in the mouth of both individuals was highly similar, its distribution was very different. As shown in **Table 3**, MG01 did not show important differences in the amounts of *S. dentisani* between tooth types nor between the lingual and vestibular surfaces. Patient MG02 however, had a more heterogeneous distribution, with higher proportions of *S. dentisani* in premolars and molars, and on the lingual surfaces of every tooth type.

DISCUSSION

Dental caries is considered the most prevalent disease worldwide, with up to 80% of the human population being affected at some point during their lives (Petersen and Lennon, 2004). There are however no efficient means to prevent it, as the polymicrobial nature of the infection and its complex etiology make passive and active immunization strategies (e.g., a caries vaccine) ineffective (Fejerskov, 2004; Simón-Soro and Mira, 2015). Thus, new strategies directed towards the re-establishment of the natural balance in the oral microbiome like the use of pre- and probiotics have been proposed (Marsh et al., 2015). However, as shown in **Table 1**, most of the probiotics proposed to promote oral health are bacteria isolated from environments other than the oral cavity, usually the human gut (Cagetti et al., 2013). In addition, the most commonly used probiotic bacteria to treat dental caries are lactobacilli, due to their well-proven safety characteristics. However, the use of non-oral bacteria may prevent efficient colonization of the oral niche, which is a vital and desirable feature of probiotics. This is supported by the low frequencies of lactobacilli detected in tooth tissues by molecular methods, as reported in the current manuscript. In addition, lactobacilli are important acid-producers and long known to be associated to dental caries lesions (Badet and Thebaud, 2008; Plonka et al., 2012), as well as bifidobacteria (Mantzourani et al., 2009b; Beighton et al., 2010), which are also common oral probiotics. This can be the reason why *in vitro* experiments with these bacteria, even if low-acid producing strains are selected, may result in pH acidification (Pham et al., 2009). These results underline the need to use potential probiotics from the oral cavity, and therefore the isolation of a bacteriocin-producing probiotic *Streptococcus salivarius* which inhibited the cariogenic agent *S. mutans* was promising (Wu et al., 2015). However, the comparison of the *S. salivarius* genome against a high number of metagenomes from supragingival plaque presented in the current manuscript reveals its absence in the tooth, in agreement with its soft-tissues-associated nature. *Streptococcus salivarius* is a typical inhabitant of the buccal epithelium, tongue, and dorsal epithelium (Bowden et al., 1979; Power et al., 2008) and comprises an important part of the total cultivable flora on the soft tissues of the mouth (Wilson, 2005). Probably for this reason, it has been proposed as a probiotic for the pharyngeal mucosa (Guglielmetti et al., 2010) but its inability to colonize the tooth surface may hamper its potential as an anti-caries probiotic. The high heterogeneity of environments in the mouth and the resulting adaptation of microorganisms to those specific microniches (Simon-Soro et al., 2013) underscores the importance of selecting oral bacteria adapted to live in hard tissues as probiotics against dental caries to guarantee a proper colonization. In agreement with this view, our data show that *Streptococcus dentisani*, which was isolated from supragingival dental plaque of caries-free

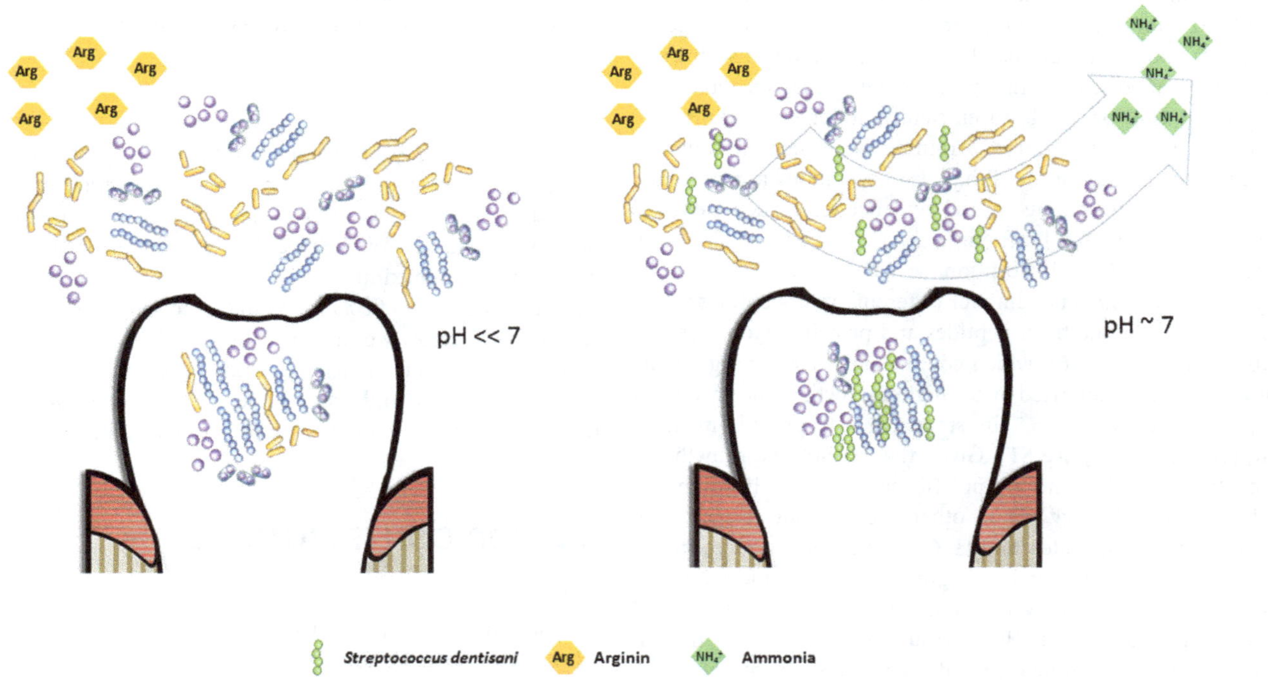

FIGURE 5 | Potential buffering effect in the oral cavity due to the enrichment of the dental plaque bacterial community with *Streptococcus dentisani*. When arginine is available (either as an added prebiotic or as a product of peptide degradation) and *S. dentisani* is established on the tooth surfaces, the pH drop caused by the accumulation of organic acids can be buffered by the production of NH_4^+ through the arginolytic pathway, maintaining the pH close to neutrality (right panel). In the absence of *S. dentisani*, or if present at low proportions, the buffering effect would be diminished, with the consequent acidification and enamel damage. This would be the perfect scenario for the proliferation of acidogenic/cariogenic microorganisms (left panel).

individuals (Belda-Ferre et al., 2011; Camelo-Castillo et al., 2014), was widespread among dental plaque samples from healthy subjects.

Apart from dental colonization, we show that an important probiotic feature of *S. dentisani* is its anti-microbial properties, inhibiting the growth of important oral pathogens like *S. mutans*, *S. sobrinus*, or *Prevotella intermedia*. In addition, the killing of *Fusobacterium nucleatum* is unusual among oral probiotics and may provide an important beneficial effect, as this organism is responsible for a large number of co-aggregation patterns with many oral species and is considered the main "bridge" bacteria between early and late colonizers of dental plaque (Kolenbrander et al., 2002). Thus, its inhibition could contribute to impede the adhesion of pathogenic organisms that co-aggregate with this bacterium and by doing so hamper dental plaque development, whose maturity has been shown to considerably increase the drop in pH after a meal (Firestone et al., 1987). In addition, *F. nucleatum* itself has been associated with halitosis due to the production of volatile sulfur compounds (Krespi et al., 2006), and therefore its growth inhibition should be investigated in the future as a way to diminish the severity of this condition.

The different experiments performed in the current work suggest a peptidic nature of the inhibitory molecules, as the inhibitory effect was significantly reduced by proteinase treatment but was unaffected by peroxidase, indicating that the inhibition was not due to the production of hydrogen peroxide as it is common in other streptococci (Zhu and Kreth, 2012). This, together with the small size of the molecules responsible for the inhibition (<3 KDa) and the appearance of pores in the membrane of sensitive bacteria as identified by SEM, strongly suggest that the inhibition is caused by bacteriocins, and future work should be directed towards identifying and characterizing such antimicrobial peptides.

Dental caries, as well as other oral diseases like periodontitis or halitosis are not considered typical infectious diseases in classical terms, as there is more than one species responsible for their etiology, the microbial consortia causing the disease varies considerably between individuals and even between lesions of the same patient, and pathogenic organisms normally can be isolated also from healthy individuals (Hajishengallis and Lamont, 2012; Simon-Soro et al., 2014; Camelo-Castillo et al., 2015; Marsh et al., 2015; Simón-Soro and Mira, 2015). For these reasons, antimicrobial properties of probiotics may not be sufficient for effectively preventing dental caries (ten Cate and Zaura, 2012) and the ability to restore the microbial ecological balance after pH acidification, for instance by alkali production, is a promising probiotic feature (Huang et al., 2015). Production of ammonia from urea or arginine by several oral bacteria has been shown to efficiently buffer salivary pH and has been associated to a reduction in caries risk (Reyes et al., 2014; Moncada et al., 2015). The analysis of the genome of *Streptococcus dentisani* revealed all genes from the arginolytic pathway, including the arginine deiminase and the carbamate kinase, a feature which appears to be common to all members of the cluster (Jensen et al., 2016). In addition, the agmatine deiminase gene, involved in the production of ammonia (Liu et al., 2012) was also present in both analyzed strains. In agreement with this, our data show that *S. dentisani* was able to efficiently buffer extracellular pH in the presence of arginine. Arginine is present in saliva in variable concentrations and it has also been added as a prebiotic to toothpaste, with strong clinical evidence for reducing enamel demineralization and buffering acidic pH (Yin et al., 2013; Santarpia et al., 2014). In addition, we have found in the genome of *S. dentisani* genes encoding for different aminopeptidases that can liberate arginine from peptides and proteins (Gonzales and Robert-Baudouy, 1996), which could then enter the arginolytic pathway. This is supported by the higher growth of the bacterium at pH 6 than at pH 6.5 in standard BHI growth medium (**Supplementary Figure S1**). Given that its optimal growth pH is neutral, and that the arginolytic pathway has been shown to be activated by low pH in other species (Liu et al., 2008), the higher growth rates at pH 6 are probably the result of protein degradation liberating arginine, which would allow the production of NH_4, as well as the production of ATP derived from this metabolic route. These results also suggest that the full activation of the arginine degradation genes occurs at pH < 6.5, and the regulation of this pathway should be studied in the future. In **Figure 5**, we have illustrated the buffering effect that could take place in the oral cavity due to the enrichment of the dental plaque bacterial community with *S. dentisani*. When acidification occurs as a consequence of the consumption of dietary carbohydrates, and the pH drops to values around 6, *S. dentisani* would be able to activate the ADS system producing ammonia and, consequently, buffering the pH of its close environment.

The double beneficial action of *S. dentisani* (i.e., anti-microbial and anti-acid) makes it a promising probiotic bacterium. These benefits, together with its dental colonization capacity, derive to a big extent from its oral inhabitance. In addition, the choice of a dental plaque species as probiotic allows the quantification of the species in caries-free individuals, in order to use those levels as the appropriate administration dose, instead of using the dosages normally delivered for gut probiotics. In the current manuscript, we have quantified *S. dentisani* amounts in dental plaque for just two individuals and similar estimates for larger sample sizes could serve to accurately determine the dosage for an appropriate treatment.

For all these reasons, we propose the use of probiotics which are *active colonizers*, that is microorganisms which inhabit the site where the disease takes place, and that are isolated from healthy individuals. We believe that the administration of these organisms will maximize the chance of colonization and the potential beneficial effects for human and animal health. In the case of dental caries, we encourage the search of probiotic bacteria that are normal inhabitants of the human supragingival plaque in healthy individuals and propose the use of *S. dentisani* in clinical trials to test its potential in promoting oral health.

AUTHOR CONTRIBUTIONS

AM conceived the work, was implied in the analyses and interpretation of data and wrote the manuscript together with AL-L. AL-L, AC-C, and MF worked in the designing and performance of the experiments, data acquisition, analyses, and interpretation of the results. AS-S collected the plaque samples and made the bioinformatic analyses.

ACKNOWLEDGMENT

The research leading to these results has received funding from the Spanish Government under grant agreements BIO2012-40007 and CSD2009-0006.

SUPPLEMENTARY MATERIAL

FIGURE S1 | Growth curves of *Streptococcus dentisani* strains 7746 (A) and 7747 **(B)** in BHI medium at different starting pHs: 4.7 (red), 5.5 (orange), 6 (yellow), 6.5 (light blue), 7 (dark blue), and 7.5 (purple).

REFERENCES

Alcaraz, L. D., Belda-Ferre, P., Cabrera-Rubio, R., Romero, H., Simón-Soro, A., Pignatelli, M., et al. (2012). Identifying a healthy oral microbiome through metagenomics. *Clin. Microbiol. Infect.* 18, 54–57. doi: 10.1111/j.1469-0691.2012.03857.x

Aminabadi, N. A., Erfanparast, L., Ebrahimi, A., and Oskouei, S. G. (2011). Effect of chlorhexidine pretreatment on the stability of salivary lactobacilli probiotic in six- to twelve-year-old children: a randomized controlled trial. *Caries Res.* 45, 148–154. doi: 10.1159/000325741

Badet, C., and Thebaud, N. B. (2008). Ecology of Lactobacilli in the oral cavity: a review of literature. *Open Microbiol. J.* 2, 38–48. doi: 10.2174/1874285800802010038

Beighton, D., Al-Haboubi, M., Mantzourani, M., Gilbert, S. C., Clark, D., Zoitopoulos, L., et al. (2010). Oral Bifidobacteria: caries-associated bacteria in older adults. *J. Dent. Res.* 89, 970–974. doi: 10.1177/0022034510369319

Belda-Ferre, P., Alcaraz, L. D., Cabrera, R., Simon-Soro, A., Romero, H., Pignatelli, M., et al. (2011). The oral metagenome in health and disease. *ISME J.* 6, 46–56. doi: 10.1038/ismej.2011.85

Bowden, G. H. W., Ellwood, D. C., and Hamilton, I. R. (1979). "Microbial ecology of the oral cavity," in *Advances in Microbial Ecology*, ed. M. Alexander (New York, NY: Plenum Press), 135–217. doi: 10.1007/978-1-4615-8279-3_4

Burton, J. P., Chilcott, C. N., Moore, C. J., Speiser, G., and Tagg, J. R. (2006). A preliminary study of the effect of probiotic *Streptococcus salivarius* K12 on oral malodour parameters. *J. Appl. Microbiol.* 100, 754–764. doi: 10.1111/j.1365-2672.2006.02837.x

Burton, J. P., Drummond, B. K., Chilcott, C. N., Tagg, J. R., Thomson, W. M., Hale, J. D., et al. (2013). Influence of the probiotic *Streptococcus salivarius* strain M18 on indices of dental health in children: a randomized double-blind, placebo-controlled trial. *J. Med. Microbiol.* 62, 875–884. doi: 10.1099/jmm.0.056663-0

Cagetti, M. G., Marstroberardino, S., Milia, E., Cocco, F., Lingström, P., and Campus, G. (2013). The use of probiotic strains in caries prevention:

a systematic review. *Nutrients* 5, 2530–2550. doi: 10.3390/nu5072530

Caglar, E., Kuscu, O. O., Cildir, S. K., Kuvvetli, S. S., and Sandalli, N. (2008a). A probiotic lozenge administered medical device and its effect on salivary mutans streptococci and lactobacilli. *Int. J. Paedr. Dent.* 18, 35–39.

Caglar, E., Kuscu, O. O., Selvi Kuvvetli, S., Kavaloglu Cildir, S., Sandalli, N., and Twetman, S. (2008b). Short-term effect of ice-cream containing *Bifidobacterium lactis* Bb-12 on the number of salivary mutans streptococci and lactobacilli. *Acta Odontol. Scand.* 66, 154–158. doi: 10.1080/00016350802089467

Caglar, E., Sandalli, N., Twetman, S., Kavaloglu, S., Ergeneli, S., and Selvi, S. (2005). Effect of yogurt with *Bifidobacterium* DN-173 010 on salivary mutans streptococci and lactobacilli in young adults. *Acta Odontol. Scand.* 63, 317–320. doi: 10.1080/00016350510020070

Camelo-Castillo, A., Benítez-Páez, A., Belda-Ferré, P., Cabrera-Rubio, R., and Mira, A. (2014). *Streptococcus dentisani* sp. nov., a novel member of the Mitis group. *Int. J. Syst. Appl. Microbiol.* 64, 60–65. doi: 10.1099/ijs.0.054098-0

Camelo-Castillo, A., Mira, A., Pico, A., Nibali, L., Henderson, B., and Tomás, I. (2015). Subgingival microbiota in health compared to periodontitis and the influence of smoking. *Front. Microbiol.* 6:119. doi: 10.3389/fmicb.2015.00119

Campus, G., Cocco, F., Carta, G., Cagetti, M. G., Simark-Mattson, C., Strohmenger, L., et al. (2014). Effect of a daily dose of *Lactobacillus brevis* CD2 lozenges in high caries risk schoolchildren. *Clin. Oral Investig.* 18, 555–561. doi: 10.1007/s00784-013-0980-9

Chuang, L. C., Huang, C. S., Ou-Yang, L. W., and Lin, S. Y. (2011). Probiotic *Lactobacillus paracasei* effect on cariogenic bacterial flora. *Clin. Oral Investig.* 15, 471–476. doi: 10.1007/s00784-010-0423-9

Fejerskov, O. (2004). Changing paradigms in concepts on dental caries: consequences for oral health care. *Caries Res.* 38, 182–191. doi: 10.1159/000077753

Firestone, A. R., Imfeld, T., Schiffer, S., and Lutz, F. (1987). Measurement of interdental plaque pH in humans with an indwelling glass pH electrode following a sucrose rinse: a long-term retrospective study. *Caries Res.* 21, 555–558. doi: 10.1159/000261066

Gonzales, T., and Robert-Baudouy, J. (1996). Bacterial aminopeptidases: properties and functions. *FEMS Microbiol. Rev.* 18, 319–344. doi: 10.1111/j.1574-6976.1996.tb00247.x

Grudianov, A. I., Dmitrieva, N. A., and Fomenko, E. V. (2002). Use of probiotics *Bifidumbacterin* and Acilact in tablets in therapy of periodontal inflammations [Article in Russian]. *Stomatologiia (Mosk)* 81, 39–43.

Guglielmetti, S., Taverniti, V., Minuzzo, M., Arioli, S., Stuknyte, M., Karp, M., et al. (2010). Oral bacteria as potential probiotics for the pharyngeal mucosa. *Appl. Environ. Microbiol.* 76, 3948–3958. doi: 10.1128/AEM.00109-10

Hajishengallis, G., and Lamont, R. J. (2012). Beyond the red complex and into more complexity: the polymicrobial synergy and dysbiosis (PSD) model of periodontal disease etiology. *Mol. Oral Microbiol.* 6, 409–419. doi: 10.1111/j.2041-1014.2012.00663.x

Hatakka, K., Ahola, A. J., Yli-Knuuttila, H., Richardson, M., Poussa, T., Meurman, J. H., et al. (2007). Probiotics reduce the prevalence of oral candida in the elderly–A randomized controlled trial. *J. Dent. Res.* 86, 125–130. doi: 10.1177/154405910708600204

Huang, X., Schulte, R. M., Burne, R. A., and Nascimento, M. M. (2015). Characterization of the arginolytic microflora provides insights into pH homeostasis in human oral biofilms. *Caries Res.* 49, 165–176. doi: 10.1159/000365296

Iwamoto, T., Suzuki, N., Tanabe, T., Takeshita, T., and Hirofuji, T. (2010). Effects of probiotic *Lactobacillus salivarius* WB21 on halitosis and oral health: an open-labeled pilot trial. *Oral Surg. Oral Med. Oral Pathol. Oral Radiol. Endod.* 110, 201–208. doi: 10.1016/j.tripleo.2010.03.032

Jensen, A., Scholz, C. F. P., and Kilian, M. (2016). Re-evaluation of the taxonomy of the Mitis group of the genus *Streptococcus* based on whole genome phylogenetic analyses, and proposed reclassification of *Streptococcus dentisani* as *Streptococcus oralis* subsp. dentisani comb. nov., *Streptococcus tigurinus* as *Streptococcus oralis* subsp. tigurinus comb. nov., and *Streptococcus oligofermentans* as a later synonym of *Streptococcus cristatus*. *Int. J. Syst. Evol. Microbiol.* 66, 4803–4820. doi: 10.1099/ijsem.0.001433

Kang, M. S., Chung, J., Kim, S. M., Yang, K. H., and Oh, J. S. (2006a). Effect of *Weissella cibaria* isolates on the formation of *Streptococcus mutans* biofilm. *Caries Res.* 40, 418–425.

Kang, M. S., Kim, B. G., Chung, J., Lee, H. C., and Oh, J. S. (2006b). Inhibitory effect of *Weissella cibaria* isolates on the production of volatile sulphur compounds. *J. Clin. Periodontol.* 33, 226–232.

Keller, M. K., Bardow, A., Jensdottir, T., Lykkeaa, J., and Twetman, S. (2012). Effect of chewing gums containing the probiotic bacterium *Lactobacillus reuteri* on oral malodour. *Acta Odontol. Scand.* 70, 246–250. doi: 10.3109/00016357.2011.640281

Khalf, M., Dabour, N., Kheadr, E., and Fliss, I. (2010). Viability of probiotic bacteria in maple sap products under storage and gastrointestinal conditions. *Bioresour. Technol.* 101, 7966–7972. doi: 10.1016/j.biortech.2010.05.053

Kolenbrander, P. E., Andersen, R. N., Blehert, D. S., Egland, P. G., Foster, J. S., and Palmer, R. J. Jr. (2002). Communication among oral bacteria. *Microbiol. Mol. Biol.* 66, 3486–3505. doi: 10.1128/MMBR.66.3.486-505.2002

Krasse, P., Carlsson, B., Dahl, C., Paulsson, A., Nilsson, A., and Sinkiewicz, G. (2006). Decreased gum bleeding and reduced gingivitis by the probiotic *Lactobacillus reuteri*. *Swed. Dent. J.* 30, 55–60.

Krespi, Y. P., Shrime, M. G., and Kacker, A. (2006). The relationship between oral malodor and volatile sulfur compound-producing bacteria. *Otolaryngol. Head Neck Surg.* 135, 671–676. doi: 10.1016/j.otohns.2005.09.036

Kurtz, S., Phillippy, A., Delcher, A. L., Smoot, M., Shumway, M., Antonescu, C., et al. (2004). Versatile and open software for comparing large genomes. *Genome Biol.* 5:R12. doi: 10.1186/gb-2004-5-2-r12

Liu, Y., Dong, Y., Chen, Y. Y., and Burne, R. A. (2008). Arginine deiminase gene regulation in *Streptococcus gordonii*. *J. Dent. Res.* 87, 714–721.

Liu, Y. L., Nascimento, M., and Burne, R. A. (2012). Progress toward understanding the contribution of alkali generation in dental biofilms to inhibition of dental caries. *Int. J. Oral Sci.* 4, 135–140. doi: 10.1038/ijos.2012.54

Mantzourani, M., Fenlon, M., and Beighton, D. (2009a). Association between Bifidobacteriaceae and the clinical severity of root caries lesions. *Mol. Oral Microbiol.* 24, 32–37. doi: 10.1111/j.1399-302X.2008.00470.x

Mantzourani, M., Gilbert, S. C., Sulong, H. N., Sheehy, E. C., Tank, S., Fenlon, M., et al. (2009b). The isolation of bifidobacteria from occlusal carious lesions in children and adults. *Caries Res.* 43, 308–313. doi: 10.1159/000222659

Marsh, P. D. (2015). The commensal microbiota and the development of human disease–an introduction. *J. Oral Microbiol.* 7:29128. doi: 10.3402/jom.v7.29128

Marsh, P. D., Head, D. A., and Devine, D. A. (2015). Ecological approaches to oral biofilms: control without killing. *Caries Res.* 49, 46–54. doi: 10.1159/000377732

Martínez, R. C. R., Aynaou, A., Albrecht, S., Schols, H. A., De Martinis, E. C. P., Zoetendal, E. G., et al. (2011). In vitro evaluation of gastrointestinal survival of Lactobacillus amylovorus DSM 16698 alone and combined with galactooligosaccharides, milk and/or *Bifidobacterium animalis* subsp. lactis Bb-12. *Int. J. Food Microbiol.* 149, 152–158. doi: 10.1016/j.ijfoodmicro.2011.06.010

Matsuoka, T., Sugano, N., Takigawa, S., Takane, M., Yoshimura, N., Ito, K., et al. (2006). Effect of oral *Lactobacillus salivarius* TI 2711 (LS1) administration on periodontopathic bacteria in subgingival plaque. *J. Jpn. Soc. Periodontol.* 48, 315–324. doi: 10.2329/perio.48.315

Mayanagi, G., Kimura, M., Nakaya, S., Hirata, H., Sakamoto, M., Benno, Y., et al. (2009). Probiotic effects of orally administered *Lactobacillus salivarius* WB21-containing tablets on periodontopathic bacteria. *J. Clin. Periodontol.* 36, 506–513. doi: 10.1111/j.1600-051X.2009.01392.x

Moncada, G., Maureira, J., Neira, M., Reyes, E., Oliveira Junior, O. B., Faleiros, S., et al. (2015). Salivary urease and ADS enzymatic activity as endogenous protection against dental caries in children. *J. Clin. Pediatr. Dent.* 39, 358–363. doi: 10.17796/1053-4628-39.4.358

Petersen, P. E., and Lennon, M. A. (2004). Effective use of fluorides for the prevention of dental caries in the 21st century: the WHO approach. *Community Dent. Oral Epidemiol.* 32, 319–321. doi: 10.1111/j.1600-0528.2004.00175.x

Pham, L. C., van Spanning, R. J. M., Roling, W. F. M., Prosperi, A. C., Terefework, Z., ten Cate, J. M., et al. (2009). Effects of probiotic *Lactobacillus salivarius* W24 on the compositional stability of oral microbial communities. *Arch. Oral Microbiol.* 54, 132–137. doi: 10.1016/j.archoralbio.2008.09.007

Plonka, K. A., Pukallus, M. L., Barnett, A. G., Walsh, L. J., Holcombe, T. F., and Seow, W. K. (2012). A longitudinal study comparing mutans streptococci and lactobacilli colonisation in dentate children aged 6 to 24 months. *Caries Res.* 46, 385–393. doi: 10.1159/000339089

Power, D. A., Burton, J. P., Chilcott, C. N., Dawes, P. J., and Tagg, J. R. (2008). Preliminary investigations of the colonisation of upper respiratory tract tissues of infants using a paediatric formulation of the oral probiotic *Streptococcus salivarius* K12. *Eur. J. Clin. Microbiol. Infect. Dis.* 27, 1261–1263. doi: 10.1007/s10096-008-0569-4

Pozharitskaia, M. M., Morozova, L. V., Mel'nichuk, G. M., and Mel'nichuk, S. S. (1994). The use of the new bacterial biopreparation Acilact in the combined treatment of periodontitis [Article in Russian]. *Stomatologiia (Mosk)* 73, 17–20.

Reid, G., Younes, J. A., Van der Mei, H. C., Gloor, G. B., Knight, R., and Busscher, H. J. (2011). Microbiota restoration: natural and supplemented recovery of human microbial communities. *Nat. Rev. Microbiol.* 9, 27–38. doi: 10.1038/nrmicro2473

Reyes, E., Martin, J., Moncada, G., Neira, M., Palma, P., Gordan, V., et al. (2014). Caries-free subjects have high levels of urease and arginine deiminase activity. *J. Appl. Oral Sci.* 22, 235–240. doi: 10.1590/1678-775720130591

Riccia, D. D., Bizzini, F., Perilli, M., Polimeni, A., Trinchieri, V., Amicosante, G., et al. (2007). Anti-inflammatory effects of *Lactobacillus brevis* (CD2) on periodontal disease. *Oral Dis.* 13, 376–385. doi: 10.1111/j.1601-0825.2006.01291.x

Ritthagol, W., Saetang, C., and Teanpaisan, R. (2014). Effect of probiotics containing *Lactobacillus paracasei* SD1 on salivary mutans Streptococci and Lactobacilli in orthodontic cleft patients: a double-blinded, randomized, placebo-controlled study. *Cleft Palate Craniofac. J.* 51, 257–263. doi: 10.1597/12-243

Saha, S., Tomaro-Duchesneau, C., Tabrizian, M., and Prakash, S. (2012). Probiotics as oral health biotherapeutics. *Exp. Opin. Biol. Ther.* 12, 1207–1220. doi: 10.1517/14712598.2012.693474

Santarpia, P., Lavender, S., Gittins, E., Vandeven, M., Cummins, D., and Sullivan, R. (2014). A 12-week clinical study assessing the clinical effects on plaque metabolism of a dentifrice containing 1.5% arginine, an insoluble calcium compound and 1,450 ppm fluoride. *Am. J. Dent.* 27, 100–105.

Shimauchi, H., Mayanagi, G., Nakaya, S., Minamibuchi, M., Ito, Y., Yamaki, K., et al. (2008). Improvement of periodontal condition by probiotics with *Lactobacillus salivarius* WB21: a randomized, double-blind, placebo-controlled study. *J. Clin. Periodontol.* 35, 897–905. doi: 10.1111/j.1600-051X.2008.01306.x

Simon-Soro, A., Guillen-Navarro, M., and Mira, A. (2014). Metatranscriptomics reveals overall active bacterial composition in caries lesions. *J. Oral Microbiol.* 6:25443. doi: 10.3402/jom.v6.25443

Simón-Soro, A., and Mira, A. (2015). Solving the etiology of dental caries. *Trends Microbiol.* 23, 76–82. doi: 10.1016/j.tim.2014.10.010

Simon-Soro, A., Tomás, I., Cabrera-Rubio, R., Catalan, M. D., Nyvad, B., and Mira, A. (2013). Microbial geography of the oral cavity. *J. Dent. Res.* 92, 616–621. doi: 10.1177/0022034513488119

Stecksén-Blicks, C., Sjöström, I., and Twetman, S. (2009). Effect of long-term consumption of milk supplemented with probiotic lactobacilli and fluoride on dental caries and general health in preschool children: a cluster-randomized study. *Caries Res.* 43, 374–381. doi: 10.1159/000235581

Suzuki, N., Yoneda, M., Tanabe, K., Fujimoto, A., Iha, K., Seno, K., et al. (2014). *Lactobcaillus salivarius* WB21-containing tablets for the treatment of oral malodor: a double blind, randomized, placebo-controlled crossover trial. *Oral Surg. Oral Med. Oral Pathol. Oral Radiol.* 117, 462–470. doi: 10.1016/j.oooo.2013.12.400

ten Cate, J. M., and Zaura, E. (2012). The numerous microbial species in oral biofilms: how could antibacterial therapy be effective? *Adv. Dental Res.* 24, 108–111. doi: 10.1177/0022034512450028

Turnbaugh, P. J., Ley, R. E., Hamady, M., Fraser-Liggett, C., Knight, R., and Gordon, J. I. (2007). The human microbiome project: exploring the microbial part of ourselves in a changing world. *Nature* 18, 804–810. doi: 10.1038/nature06244

Volozhin, A. I, Il'in, V. K., Maksimovskiĭ, IuM, Sidorenko, A. B., Istranov, L. P., Tsarev, V. N., et al. (2004). Development and use of periodontal dressing of collagen and *Lactobacillus casei* 37 cell suspension in combined treatment of periodontal disease of inflammatory origin (a microbiological study). *Stomatologiia (Mosk)* 83, 6–8.

World Health Organization [WHO] (1997). *Oral Health Surveys: Basic Methods.* Geneva: World Health Organization.

Wilson, M. (2005). *Microbial Inhabitants of Humans: Their Ecology and Role in Health and Disease.* Cambridge: Cambridge University Press.

Wu, C. C., Lin, C. T., Wu, C. Y., Peng, W. S., Lee, M. J., and Tsai, Y. C. (2015). Inhibitory effect of *Lactobacillus salivarius* on *Streptococcus mutans* biofilm formation. *Mol. Oral Microbiol.* 30, 16–26. doi: 10.1111/omi.12063

Yin, W., Hu, D. Y., Li, X., Fan, X., Zhang, Y. P., Pretty, I. A., et al. (2013). The anti-caries efficacy of a dentifrice containing 1.5% arginine and 1450 ppm fluoride as sodium monofluorophosphate assessed using Quantitative Light-induced Fluorescence (QLF). *J. Dent.* 41(Suppl. 2), S22–S28. doi: 10.1016/j.jdent.2010.04.004

Zahradnik, R. T., Magnusson, I., Walker, C., McDonell, E., Hillman, C. H., and Hillman, J. D. (2009). Preliminary assessment of safety and effectiveness in humans of ProBiora3, a probiotic mouthwash. *J. Appl. Microbiol.* 107, 682–690. doi: 10.1111/j.1365-2672.2009.04243.x

Zaura, E., Keijser, B. J. F., Huse, S., and Crielaard, W. (2009). Defining the healthy "core microbiome" of oral microbial communities. *BMC Microbiol.* 9:259. doi: 10.1186/1471-2180-9-259

Zhu, L., and Kreth, J. (2012). The role of hydrogen peroxide in environmental adaptation of oral microbial communities. *Oxid. Med. Cell. Longev.* 2012:717843. doi: 10.1155/2012/717843

3

Respiratory Commensal Bacteria *Corynebacterium pseudodiphtheriticum* Improves Resistance of Infant Mice to Respiratory Syncytial Virus and *Streptococcus pneumoniae* Superinfection

Paulraj Kanmani[1,2†], Patricia Clua[3,4†], Maria G. Vizoso-Pinto[5], Cecilia Rodriguez[6], Susana Alvarez[3,4], Vyacheslav Melnikov[7,8], Hideki Takahashi[9,10], Haruki Kitazawa[1,2] and Julio Villena[1,3,4*]*

[1] Food and Feed Immunology Group, Laboratory of Animal Products Chemistry, Graduate School of Agricultural Science, Tohoku University, Sendai, Japan, [2] Livestock Immunology Unit, International Education and Research Center for Food and Agricultural Immunology, Graduate School of Agricultural Science, Tohoku University, Sendai, Japan, [3] Immunobiotics Research Group, Tucuman, Argentina, [4] Laboratory of Immunobiotechnology, Reference Centre for Lactobacilli (CERELA-CONICET), Tucuman, Argentina, [5] Faculty of Medicine, INSIBIO (UNT-CONICET), National University of Tucuman, Tucuman, Argentina, [6] Laboratory of Genetics, Reference Centre for Lactobacilli (CERELA-CONICET), Tucuman, Argentina, [7] Gabrichevsky Institute of Epidemiology and Microbiology, Moscow, Russia, [8] Central Research Institute of Epidemiology, Moscow, Russia, [9] Laboratory of Plant Pathology, Graduate School of Agricultural Science, Tohoku University, Sendai, Japan, [10] Plant Immunology Unit, International Education and Research Center for Food and Agricultural Immunology, Graduate School of Agricultural Science, Tohoku University, Sendai, Japan

***Correspondence:**
Haruki Kitazawa
haruki.kitazawa.c7@tohoku.ac.jp
Julio Villena
jcvillena@cerela.org.ar

† These authors have contributed equally to this work.

Corynebacterium pseudodiphtheriticum is a Gram-positive bacterium found as a member of the normal microbiota of the upper respiratory tract. It was suggested that *C. pseudodiphtheriticum* may be potentially used as a next-generation probiotic for nasal application, although no deep studies were performed in this regard. We hypothesized that human isolate *C. pseudodiphtheriticum* strain 090104 is able to modulate the respiratory innate immune response and beneficially influence the resistance to viral and bacterial infections. Therefore, in the present study we investigated how the exposure of infant mice to nasal priming with viable or non-viable *C. pseudodiphtheriticum* 090104 influences the respiratory innate immune response triggered by Toll-like receptor (TLR)-3 activation, the susceptibility to primary Respiratory Synsytial Virus (RSV) infection, and the resistance to secondary *Streptococcus pneumoniae* pneumonia. We demonstrated that the nasal priming with viable *C. pseudodiphtheriticum* 090104 differentially modulated TLR3-mediated innate antiviral immune response in the respiratory tract of infant mice, improving their resistance to primary RSV infection, and secondary pneumococcal pneumonia. In association with the protection against RSV-pneumococcal superinfection, we found that viable *C. pseudodiphtheriticum* improved lung $CD3^+CD4^+IFN\text{-}\gamma^+$, and $CD3^+CD4^+IL\text{-}10^+$ T cells as well as $CD11c^+SiglecF^+IFN\text{-}\beta^+$ alveolar macrophages. Of interest, non-viable bacteria did not have the same protective effect, suggesting that *C. pseudodiphtheriticum* colonization is needed for achieving its protective effect. In conclusion, we present evidence that nasal application of viable *C. pseudodiphtheriticum* could be thought as an alternative to boost defenses against RSV and secondary pneumococcal pneumonia, which should be further studied and validated in clinical trials. Due to the absence of a long-lasting immunity, re-infection with RSV throughout life is common. Thus, a possible perspective use could be a seasonal application of a nasal probiotic spray to boost respiratory innate immunity in immunocompetent subjects.

Keywords: *Corynebacterium pseudodiphtheriticum*, TLR3, Respiratory Synsytial Virus, *Streptococcus pneumoniae*, respiratory immunity, nasal probiotic

INTRODUCTION

Corynebacterium pseudodiphtheriticum is a non-lipophilic, non-fermentative, urease- and nitrate-positive Gram-positive bacterium with variable shape (rods and cocci), which is found as a member of the normal microbiota of the human skin and upper respiratory tract (Ahmed et al., 1995; Burke et al., 1997; Bittar et al., 2010; Olender and Niemcewicz, 2010). Although there are clinical case reports pointing out at this bacterium as an opportunistic pathogen, it was suggested that *C. pseudodiphtheriticum,* being a natural member of the normal microbiota of nares and throat, may be potentially used as a probiotic for nasal application. In this regard, it has been demonstrated that *C. pseudodiphtheriticum* 090104 "Sokolov" is able to reduce *Staphylococcus aureus* colonization in humans (Uehara et al., 2000). There is also an inverse association between *S. aureus* and corynebacteria suggesting microbial competition during colonization (Liu C. M. et al., 2015). Controversially, some probiotic properties such as adherence to epithelial cells, biofilm formation, certain degree of immune stimulation, competition for nutrients, and adhesion sites are also shared by pathogens. For instance, some of the most known and used species of probiotic bacteria such as *Lactobacillus rhamnosus, L. plantarum, Enterococcus faecium, E. faecalis,* and even *E. coli* strain Nissle were also reported, though exceptionally, in clinical case reports. In any case, it has been established that security aspects such as antibiotic resistance or the presence of virulence factors are strain specific. Therefore, in order to propose *C. pseudodiphtheriticum* 090104 as a probiotic strain detailed studies evaluating both its functional properties and security aspects are necessary.

Respiratory syncytial virus (RSV) is a main respiratory pathogen responsible of bronchiolitis and pneumonia causing high morbidity and mortality in children under 3 years old. Currently, there are no available vaccines to prevent RSV infections or specific therapeutic treatments. Both viral and host factors are involved in disease severity. RSV cytopathogenicity is limited, but it elicits a strong immune response, which may result in tissue injury, loss of function and even death (Rutigliano and Graham, 2004; Bem et al., 2011). When exacerbated, immune response turns pathological, and in the case of RSV infection is characterized by high levels of pro-inflammatory chemokines and cytokines such as interleukin (IL)-6, IL-8, macrophage inflammatory protein (MIP)-1, tumor necrosis factor (TNF)-α, monocyte chemotactic protein (MCP)-1, and RANTES. At the very early stages of RSV infection, these pro-inflammatory factors participate in virus clearance, but their continuous production leads to increased injury (Rutigliano and Graham, 2004; Bem et al., 2011). In addition, secondary bacterial pneumonia is an important complication responsible for high morbidity and mortality of respiratory infections in infants and children (Liu et al., 2012; Bosch et al., 2013; Liu L. et al., 2015). The prevalence of bacteremia in children with RSV infection reported in the literature is low, ranging between 0.6 and 1.1% when conventional cultures were performed (Levine et al., 2004; Hishiki et al., 2011). However, a recent study showed that one out of every 10 previously healthy children hospitalized due to RSV had bacteremia, and these patients experienced a more severe disease (Cebey-Lopez et al., 2016). The rates of concurrent bacteremia was 10 times higher (10.6%) when molecular methods were applied. These findings are of importance because studies in clinical trials (Weinberger et al., 2013; Cebey-Lopez et al., 2016) and animal models of RSV-*Streptococcus pneumoniae* superinfection (Hament et al., 2005; Smith et al., 2014) showed that enhanced lung injuries and elevated levels of bacteremia are critical factors that determine the severity of infection and the rate of mortality.

Finding alternative strategies for the prevention of primary viral respiratory infections and secondary pneumococcal pneumonia in populations at risk is mandatory. In this regard, we have evaluated the possibility of administering probiotics to enhance the natural respiratory host defenses. In previous work, we showed that oral or nasal application of the probiotic strain *L. rhamnosus* CRL1505 protects adult and infant mice from RSV lethal challenge (Chiba et al., 2013; Tomosada et al., 2013). The main mechanism responsible for protection induced by the CRL1505 strain was enhancement of the mucosal antiviral innate immunity and the reduction of immunopathology. We hypothesized that a commensal bacterium from the respiratory tract such as *C. pseudodiphtheriticum* 090104 would modulate the respiratory antiviral innate immune response and beneficially influence the resistance to secondary bacterial infections. Therefore, in the present study we investigated how the exposure of infant mice to nasal priming with viable or non-viable human isolate *C. pseudodiphtheriticum* 090104 influences the respiratory innate immune response triggered by Toll-like receptor (TLR)-3 activation, the susceptibility to primary RSV infection, and the resistance to secondary *S. pneumoniae* pneumonia.

MATERIALS AND METHODS

Microorganisms

Corynebacterium pseudodiphtheriticum 090104 was cultured in trypticase soy broth and harvested by centrifugation at 3,000 × g for 10 min, washed three times with sterile 0.01 M phosphate buffer saline (PBS, pH 7.2), and resuspended in sterile PBS. Non-viable *C. pseudodiphtheriticum* 090104 was obtained as described previously (Tomosada et al., 2013). Briefly, bacteria were killed by tyndallization in a water bath at 80°C for 30 min and the lack of bacterial growth was confirmed by plating on to soy broth agar plates.

Safety Studies

In order to evaluate the susceptibility to antimicrobials of *C. pseudodiphtheriticum* 090104, the broth microdilution method was followed as recommended by the CLSI for infrequently isolated or fastidious bacteria (M45-A, CLSI-2006). The antimicrobial agents were penicillin (PEN), cefotaxime (CTX), ceftriaxone (CRO), meropenem (MER), vancomycin (VAN), gentamicin (GEN), ciprofloxacin (CIP), erythromicin (ERY), tetracycline (TET). MIC results were interpreted following CLSI guidelines (M45-A, CLSI-2006). Evaluation of bacterial translocation in infant mice was monitored by determining the presence of *C. pseudodiphtheriticum* lung, blood and spleen samples.

Animals and Feeding Procedures

Female 3-week-old BALB/c mice were obtained from the closed colony kept at CERELA (San Miguel de Tucumán, Argentina) or Tohoku University (Sendai, Japan). They were housed in plastic cages at room temperature. Mice were housed individually during the experiments. Viable and non-viable *C. pseudodiphtheriticum* 090104 were nasally administered to mice for 5 consecutive days at a dose of 10^8 cells/mouse/day in 50 μl of PBS. All groups were fed a conventional balanced diet *ad libitum*. This study was carried out in strict accordance with the recommendations in the Guide for the Care and Use of Laboratory Animals of the Guidelines for Animal Experimentation of CERELA and all efforts were made to minimize suffering. The Institutional Animal Welfare Committee of CERELA reviewed and approved the protocols used in this study.

Intranasal Administration of Poly(I:C)

Administration of the viral pathogen molecular pattern poly(I:C) was performed on day 6, after a 5 days treatment with viable or non-viable *C. pseudodiphtheriticum* 090104. Mice were lightly anesthetized and 100 μl of PBS, containing 250 μg poly(I:C) (equivalent to 10 mg/kg body weight), was administered dropwise, via the nares (Tomosada et al., 2013). Control animals received 100 μl of PBS. Mice received three doses of poly(I:C) or PBS with 24 h rest period between each administration.

Respiratory Syncytial Virus Primary Infection

Human RSV strain A2 was grown in Vero cells as described by Murawski et al. (2009). Briefly, Vero cells were infected with RSV at a multiplicity of infection (MOI) of 1 in 5 ml of Dulbecco's modified Eagle's medium (DMEM). Cells were infected for 2.5 h at 37°C and 5% CO_2. After infection, 7 ml of DMEM with 10% FBS (Sigma, Tokyo, Japan), 0.1% penicillin–streptomycin (Pen/Strep) (Sigma, Tokyo, Japan), and 0.001% ciprofloxacin (Bayer) were added to the flask and further incubated. When extensive syncytia formed, cells were scraped from the flask and sonicated three times, 5 s per pulse, at 25 W on ice. Cell lysates were centrifuge at 700 × *g* for 10 min at 4°C. Cell-free virus stocks were stored in 30% sucrose at −80°C. Uninfected cells were treated identically to generate a virus- and cell-free supernatant control. Mice were slightly anesthetized and intranasally challenged with 2.4 × 10^6 PFU RSV strain A2 or an equivalent volume of Vero cell lysate on day 6 after viable or non-viable *C. pseudodiphtheriticum* 090104 treatment.

Intact lung tissue was removed and stored in 30% sucrose for plaque assays. RSV immune-plaque assay was done as previously explained (Chiba et al., 2013). Briefly, lungs were homogenized using a pellet pestle and centrifuged at 2,600 × *g* for 10 min at 4°C. Twenty-four-well tissue culture plates were seeded with 1.5 × 10^5 Vero cells/well in DMEM (10% FBS, 0.1% Pen/Strep, and 0.001% ciprofloxacin) and virus plaques assays were performed in triplicate. Plates were incubated at 37°C and 5% CO_2 for 2.5 h. After incubation, supernatant was removed, and 1 ml of fresh DMEM medium supplemented with 10% FBS, 0.1% Pen/Strep, and 0.001% ciprofloxacin was overlaid on monolayers. When extensive syncytia developed, the overlay was removed and monolayers were fixed with ice-cold acetone:methanol (60:40). Primary RSV anti-F (clones131-2A; Chemicon) and anti-G (Mouse monoclonal [8C5 (9B6)] to RSV glycoprotein, Abcam) antibodies were added to wells for 2 h, followed by secondary horseradish peroxidase anti-mouse immunoglobulin antibody (Anti-mouse IgG, HRP-linked Antibody #7076, Cell signaling Technology) for 1 h. Plates washed twice with PBS containing 0.5% Tween 20 (Sigma) after each antibody incubation step. Individual plaques were developed using a DAB substrate kit (ab64238, Abcam) following manufacture's instructions. Results for immune-plaque assay were expressed as $\log_{10}$ PFU/g of lung.

Streptococcus pneumoniae Secondary Infection

Streptococcus pneumoniae serotype 6B (ANLIS, Argentina) was obtained from the respiratory tract of a patient from Hospital del Niño Jesús, Tucumán, Argentina. Pneumococci were grown on blood agar for 18 h. Colonies were suspended in Todd Hewitt broth (Oxoid), incubated overnight at 37°C, harvested and washed with sterile PBS. Cell density was adjusted to 4 × 10^7 CFU/ml. Challenge with pneumococci was performed 5 days after the last administration of poly(I:C) or RSV challenge. Viable or non-viable *C. pseudodiphtheriticum*-treated as well as control infant mice were challenged intranasally with the pathogen by dripping 25 μl of inoculums containing 10^3 CFU (log phase) in PBS into each nostril.

Treated and control mice were sacrificed 2 days after *S. pneumoniae* infection. Lungs were excised, weighed and homogenized in sterile peptone water. Homogenates were diluted appropriately, plated in duplicate on blood agar and incubated for 18 h at 37°C. *Streptococcus pneumoniae* was identified by standard techniques and the results were expressed as log of CFU/g of lung. Bacteremia was monitored in blood samples obtained by cardiac puncture which were plated on blood agar. Results were reported as negative or positive hemocultures.

Cytokine Concentrations in Broncho-Alveolar lavages (BAL)

BAL samples were obtained as described previously (Villena et al., 2005) by performing lavages of lungs with sterile PBS. After centrifugation, cell-free supernatants were kept at −70°C. Tumor necrosis factor (TNF)-α, interferon (IFN)-γ, IFN-β, IFN-α, interleukin (IL)-6, and IL-10 concentrations in serum and BAL were measured by enzyme-linked immunosorbent assay (ELISA) following the manufacturer's recommendations (R&D Systems, MN, USA) (Salva et al., 2011).

Lung Cell Suspensions

Single lung cells were prepared using the previously described method (Villena et al., 2012). Briefly, mice were anesthetized and lungs were removed, finely minced and incubated for 90 min with 300 U of collagenase (Yakult Honsha Co., Tokyo, Japan) in 15 ml of RPMI 1640 medium (Sigma, Tokyo, Japan). After removal of debris, erythrocytes were depleted by hypotonic lysis. The cells were washed with RPMI medium supplemented with 0.1% Pen/Strep and suspended in a medium supplemented with 10% heat-inactivated fetal calf serum (FCS). Cells were counted using Trypan Blue and adjusted to 5×10^6 cells/ml.

Flow Cytometry Studies

Single lung cells from mice were prepared as previously described (Villena et al., 2012; Zelaya et al., 2014, 2015). Lungs were removed, finely minced and incubated for 90 min with 300 U of collagenase (Yakult Honsha Co., Tokyo, Japan) in 15 ml of RPMI 1640 medium (Sigma, Tokyo, Japan). To dissociate the tissue into single cells, collagenase-treated minced lungs were gently tapped into a plastic dish. After removal of debris, erythrocytes were depleted by hypotonic lysis. The cells were washed with RPMI medium supplemented with 100 U/ml of penicillin and 100 mg/ml of streptomycin and then resuspended in a medium supplemented with 10% heat-inactivated fetal calf serum (FCS). Cells were counted using Trypan Blue exclusion and then resuspended at 5×10^6 cells/ml.

Lung cell suspensions were pre-incubated with anti-mouse CD32/CD16 monoclonal antibody (Fc block) for 15 min at 4°C. Cells were incubated in the antibody mixes for 30 min at 4°C and washed with FACS buffer. Then, cells were stained with fluorochrome-conjugated antibodies against CD3, CD4, CD8, CD11c, CD11b, CD103, MHC-II, IFN-γ, IL-10, sialic acid-binding immunoglobulin-like lectin F (SiglecF) (BD Bioscience), IFN-β, and CD45 (eBioscience). Cells were then acquired on a BD FACSCalibur™ flow cytometer (BD Biosciences) and data were analyzed with FlowJo software (TreeStar). The total number of cells in each population was determined by multiplying the percentages of subsets within a series of marker negative or positive gates by the total cell number determined for each tissue (Villena et al., 2012; Zelaya et al., 2014, 2015).

Lung Tissue Injury Studies

To measure increased permeability of the bronchoalveolar–capillarity barrier, we quantified albumin and protein content in cell-free BAL. Furthermore, lactate dehydrogenase (LDH) activity was quantified as an indicator of general cytotoxicity (Villena et al., 2012; Zelaya et al., 2014, 2015). Lung wet:dry weight ratio was determined as described before. Briefly, mice were euthanized and exsanguinated; lungs were removed, weighed (wet weight), dried at 55°C for 7 days, and weighed again (dry weight). The wet:dry weight ratio is a measure of intrapulmonary fluid accumulation. Histopathological examination was also performed in order to evaluate tissue damage during respiratory superinfection. Lungs were aseptically removed, fixed in 4% formalin and embedded in histowax (Leica Microsystems). Histopathological assessment was performed on five-micron tissue sections stained with hematoxylin-eosin.

Statistical Analysis

Experiments were performed in triplicate and results were expressed as mean ± standard deviation (SD). Five to six animals were used in each replicate per experimental group. Normal distributed data were tested by 2-way ANOVA was used. Tukey's test (for pairwise comparisons of the means) or the Fisher's least significant difference (LSD) test (for multi-comparison) were used to evaluate the differences between the groups. Differences were considered significant at $p < 0.05$.

RESULTS

Influence of Viable and Non-viable *C. pseudodiphtheriticum* on Respiratory Immune Response

In order to determine whether viable or non-viable *C. pseudodiphtheriticum* could modulate mucosal immune responses in the respiratory tract, we quantified key cytokines in broncho-alveolar lavages (BAL) and serum samples as well as immune cell populations in lungs. Both treatments elicited an increase in the levels of the proinflammatory cytokines TNF-α and IL-6 in serum and BAL (**Figure 1**). Furthermore, *C. pseudodiphtheriticum* induced a significant increase in the production of IFN-γ and a slight but still significant enhancement of IFN-β, while no effect was observed in IFN-α levels. The immunoregulatory cytokine IL-10 was also detected at higher concentrations in viable or non-viable *C. pseudodiphtheriticum*-treated infant mice than in control mice without bacterial stimulation (**Figure 1**). In general, the effect of the live bacterium was stronger than the elicited by non-viable *C. pseudodiphtheriticum*. In addition, the changes in cytokine levels were more pronounced in BAL (**Figure 1A**) than in serum samples (**Figure 1B**).

Flow cytometry indicated that there were no significant differences between the experimental groups when the numbers of lung antigen presenting cells including dendritic cells ($CD11c^+CD103\text{-}CD11b^{high}$ and $CD11c^+CD103^+CD11b^{low}$ cells) and alveolar macrophages ($CD45^+CD11c^+SiglecF^+$ cells) were compared (**Figure 2**). However, activated lung antigen presenting cells differed in mice nasally treated with *C. pseudodiphtheriticum* (**Figure 2**). For instance, $CD11c^+CD103^+MHCII^+$ and $CD11c^+CD11b^{high}MHCII^+$ populations were significantly greater ($p < 0.05$) in viable or non-viable *C. pseudodiphtheriticum*-treated infant mice than in control mice. In both cases, live bacteria had a stronger influence than non-viable *C. pseudodiphtheriticum* in antigen presenting cells activation. No differences were observed between the groups when total counts of lung $CD3^+CD4^+$ and $CD3^+CD8^+$ T cells were compared (**Figure 3**). Nevertheless, *C. pseudodiphtheriticum* differentially modulated specific IFN-γ producing populations of $CD3^+CD4^+$ and $CD3^+CD8^+$ lymphocytes. Viable bacteria significantly induced higher numbers of IFN-γ specific $CD3^+CD4^+$ T cells, whereas heat-killed *C. pseudodiphtheriticum* increased IFN-γ specific $CD3^+CD8^+$ cells (**Figure 3**). A slight but not significant increase of lung $CD3^+CD4^+IL\text{-}10^+$ T cells was observed in *C. pseudodiphtheriticum*-treated mice.

Corynebacterium pseudodiphtheriticum Modulates Immune Response Triggered by Poly(I:C) and Reduces Lung Injury

After treatment with viable or non-viable *C. pseudodiphtheriticum*, mice were nasally challenged for three consecutive days with poly(I:C). In order to evaluate the extent of lung injury induced by TLR3-triggered inflammation (**Figure 4**), we determined total protein and albumin concentrations, and LDH activity in BAL 2 days after challenge. In addition, we also determined the magnitude of edema by calculating the lung wet:dry ratio. Administration of poly(I:C) resulted in water retention due to the inflammatory response in the lungs in comparison with unchallenged mice. Viable *C. pseudodiphtheriticum* somehow prevented lungs from retaining fluids as it is shown in **Figure 4** reaching levels close to the unchallenged lung wet:dry ratios. Other lung injury parameters, such as protein content, albumin and LDH activity were also significantly ($p < 0.05$) reduced when mice were previously treated with viable or non-viable *C. pseudodiphtheriticum*, being the treatment with live bacteria more effective than heat-killed bacteria.

As we have described previously (Tomosada et al., 2013), nasal challenge with poly(I:C) increased the levels of proinflammatory cytokines and IL-10 (**Figure 5**), and immune cells (**Figure 6**) in the respiratory tract when compared to basal levels. The nasal pretreatments of mice with viable or non-viable *C. pseudodiphtheriticum* differentially modulated the profiles of cytokines measured in BAL. IFN-γ was the most influenced cytokine, showing a significant increase in mice treated with live bacteria in comparison to untreated control mice challenged with poly(I:C), whereas non-viable bacteria slightly increased the levels of IFN-γ (**Figure 5**). To a lesser extent, TNF-α, IL-6, IFN-β, and IL-10 concentrations in BAL were also higher in viable *C. pseudodiphtheriticum*-treated mice. In contrast, only TNF-α and IL-6 were modulated by non-viable bacteria.

The numbers of lung $CD11c^+CD103^+MHCII^+$ and $CD11c^+CD11b^{high}MHCII^+$ dendritic cells were significantly greater ($p < 0.05$) in viable or non-viable *C. pseudodiphtheriticum*-treated infant mice than in control mice (**Figure 6**). In addition, higher numbers of $CD45^+SiglecF^+IFN\text{-}\beta^+$ alveolar macrophages and $CD3^+CD4^+IL\text{-}10^+$ T cells were observed when mice were previously treated with viable *C. pseudodiphtheriticum* in comparison to control mice (**Figure 6**). In contrast, non-viable bacteria did not produce significant changes in the numbers of these immune cells populations. $CD3^+CD4^+IFN\gamma^+$ lymphocyte counts increased in mice which received viable or non-viable *C. pseudodiphtheriticum* before poly(I:C) challenge, being this effect stronger with the viable bacteria (**Figure 6**).

Viable *C. pseudodiphtheriticum* Increases Resistance to Primary RSV Infection

Nasal administration of viable *C. pseudodiphtheriticum* improved health state of infant mice infected with RSV as reflected by the increase in body weight during the studied period (**Figure 7**). Mice treated with non-viable bacteria did not show the improvement of body weight. Virus load was significantly lower in mice treated with viable *C. pseudodiphtheriticum* when compared to those receiving heat-killed bacteria or controls (**Figure 7**). The markers of lung tissue damage in RSV-infected mice showed that the viral infection induced a significant cellular damage and alveolar-capillary barrier alterations (**Figure 7**). Both, BAL LDH and albumin concentrations were significantly lower in infant mice previously treated with viable *C. pseudodiphtheriticum* than in RSV-challenged controls or mice receiving heat-killed bacteria (**Figure 7**).

Viable *C. pseudodiphtheriticum* Increase Resistance to Secondary Pneumococcal Infection

Finally, we addressed whether the nasal treatments with viable and non-viable *C. pseudodiphtheriticum* where able to increase the resistance of infant mice to secondary pneumococcal pneumonia. For that purpose, mice were nasally primed with viable or non-viable bacteria, infected with RSV, and 5 days after virus infection, they were challenged with *S. pneumoniae*. Pneumococcal colonization and bacteremia were evaluated on day 2 post-pneumococcal challenge. In addition, RSV titers as well as lung tissue damage were studied before (day 0) and after (day 2) infection with *S. pneumoniae*. RSV was detected in lungs of infected infant mice before and after pneumococcal infection (**Figure 8**). In

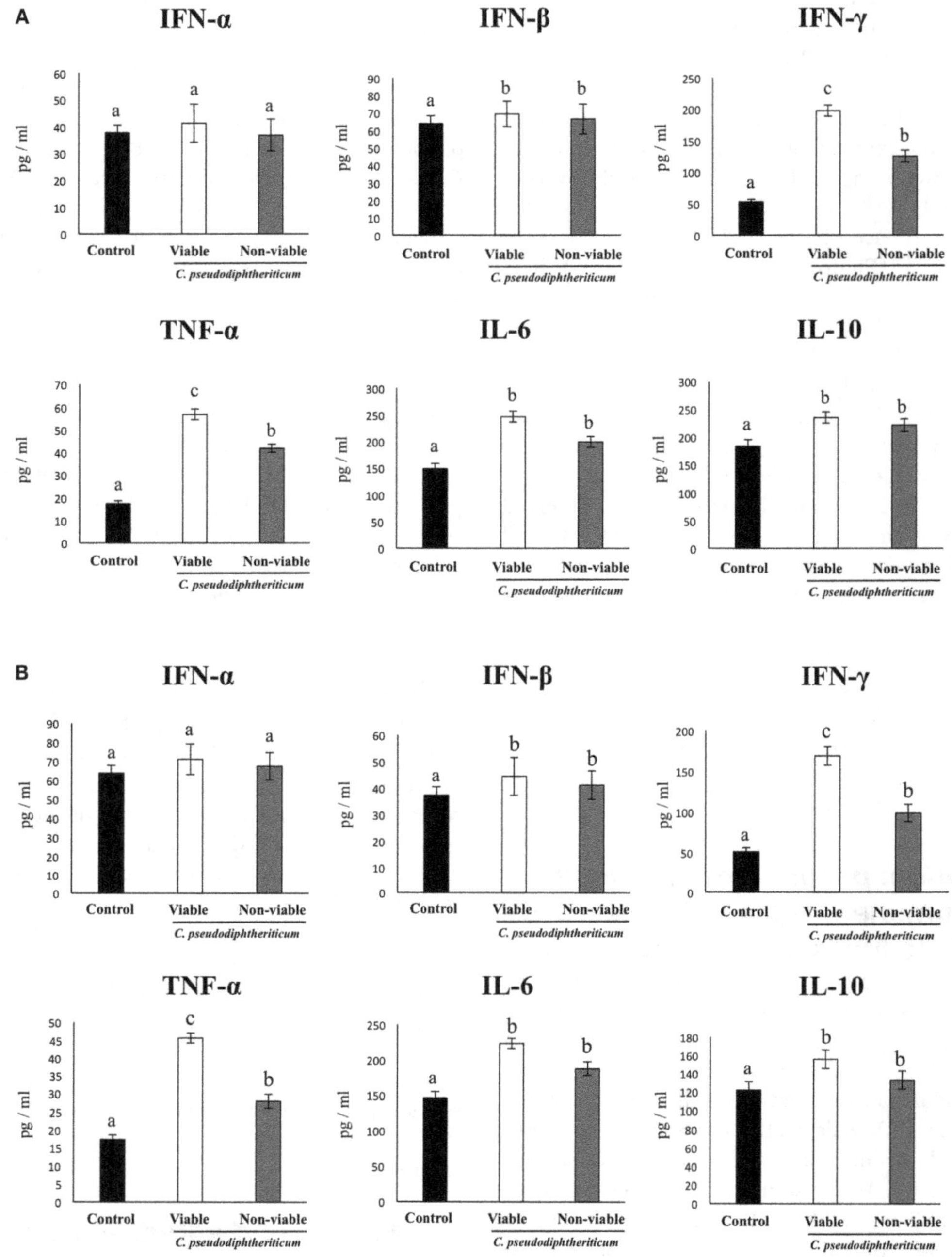

FIGURE 1 | Effect of *Corynebacterium pseudodiphtheriticum* strain 090104 on respiratory and blood cytokines. Viable or non-viable *C. pseudodiphtheriticum* were nasally administered to infant mice during five consecutive days. Non-treated infant mice were used as controls. Levels of tumor necrosis factor (TNF)-α, interferon (IFN)-α, IFN-β, IFN-γ, interleukin (IL)-6, and IL-10 were determined in broncho-alveolar lavages (BAL) **(A)** and serum **(B)**. Experiments were performed with 5–6 mice per group. The results represent data from three independent experiments. Values for bars with different letters were significantly different ($P < 0.05$). Values for bars with shared letters do not differ significantly.

addition, pneumococci were detected in lungs and blood of control infant mice (**Figure 8**). Viable *C. pseudodiphtheriticum* significantly reduced RSV titers as well as lung bacterial cell counts and prevented the dissemination of *S. pneumoniae* into the blood (**Figure 8**). No protective effect was observed for non-viable *C. pseudodiphtheriticum*. When lung injury was studied it was observed that the secondary pneumococcal pneumonia induced a significant increase of the BAL biochemical parameters that evaluate cellular damage and alveolar-capillary barrier alterations (**Figure 8**). Viable *C. pseudodiphtheriticum* significantly reduced pulmonary damage as demonstrated by the lower LDH and albumin content in BAL when compared

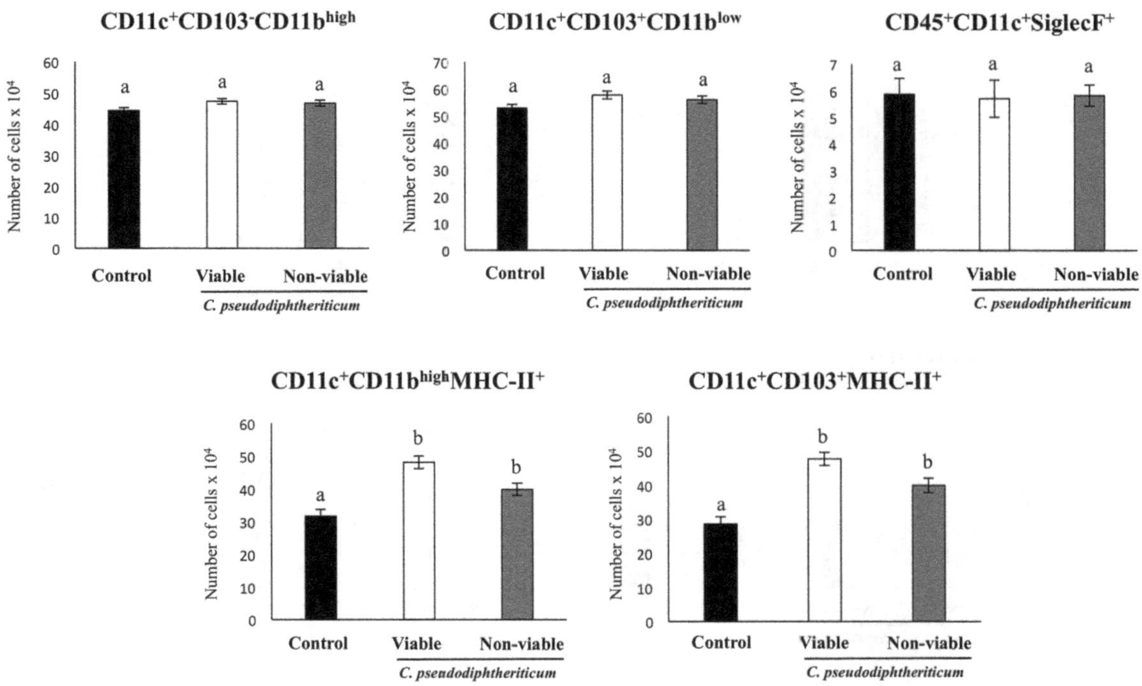

FIGURE 2 | Effect of *Corynebacterium pseudodiphtheriticum* strain 090104 on lung immune cell populations. Viable or non-viable *C. pseudodiphtheriticum* were nasally administered to infant mice during five consecutive days. Non-treated infant mice were used as controls. The numbers of lung antigen presenting cells including MHC-II$^+$CD11c$^+$CD11b^{low}CD103$^+$ and MHC-II$^+$CD11c$^+$CD11b^{high}CD103$^-$ dendritic cells, and CD45$^+$MHC-II$^-$CD11c$^+$SiglecF$^+$ alveolar macrophages were determined by flow cytometry. Experiments were performed with 5–6 mice per group. The results represent data from three independent experiments. Values for bars with different letters were significantly different ($P < 0.05$). Values for bars with shared letters do not differ significantly.

to controls and non-viable bacteria-treated mice (**Figure 8**). Moreover, histological examination of lung of infected infant mice revealed severe inflammatory cell recruitment around alveoli and blood vessels, focal hemorrhage and a significant reduction of gas exchange spaces (**Figure 8**). Lung histology analysis of viable *C. pseudodiphtheriticum*-tretaed mice showed a significant reduction in the alterations of gas exchange spaces, hemorrhage and inflammatory cells infiltration (**Figure 8**) while mice treated with non-viable bacteria were not different from control animals (data not shown).

DISCUSSION

Respiratory viruses are an important cause of fatal pneumonia in children. They also predispose individuals to suffer bacterial infections by disrupting cells, releasing nutrients and reducing ciliary continuity and kinesia. Further, they alter the innate and adaptive immune systems, which may in turn help promoting bacterial infection (Hament et al., 2005; Smith et al., 2014). Therefore, there is a global need for controlling primary respiratory viral infections and secondary bacterial diseases, and beneficial microbes may offer an interesting alternative (Maragkoudakis et al., 2010; Villena et al., 2012; Chiba et al., 2013; Tomosada et al., 2013; Tada et al., 2016).

There is an increasing amount of evidence indicating that respiratory indigenous microbiota contributes to respiratory health by preventing the overgrowth of pathogens and the inflammation they cause (Pettigrew et al., 2012; Bosch et al., 2013). Commensal bacteria may exert health benefits by opposing to bacterial or viral pathogens directly by blocking adhesion sites and/or indirectly by modulating host immune responses in such a way that pathogen clearance is enhanced but inflammation is simultaneously better controlled (Uehara et al., 2000; Pettigrew et al., 2012; Kiryukhina et al., 2013; Liu C. M. et al., 2015). Therefore, respiratory commensal bacteria, if investigated in depth may be a source for developing next generation probiotic preparations for the improvement of respiratory health. In this study, we demonstrated that *C. pseudodiphtheriticum*, a typical commensal of the nasal human mucosa, is a candidate for enhancing respiratory immune responses and protecting against RSV and *S. pneumoniae* infections.

Although there are some safety concerns about *C. pseudodiphtheriticum* because of a few case reports indicating opportunistic infections by this bacterium, it is well accepted that both probiotic and safety properties are strain specific. Genomic analysis revealed the presence of a hemolysin protein in *C. pseudodiphtheriticum* 090104 genome with similar characteristics to the one found in *Bacillus cereus*, which could become a potential risk for health especially in immunocompromised individuals (Karlyshev and Melnikov, 2013). However, the 090104 strain was safe when used in the mouse model studied here, and in clinical trials in healthy volunteers performed before (Uehara et al., 2000; Kiryukhina

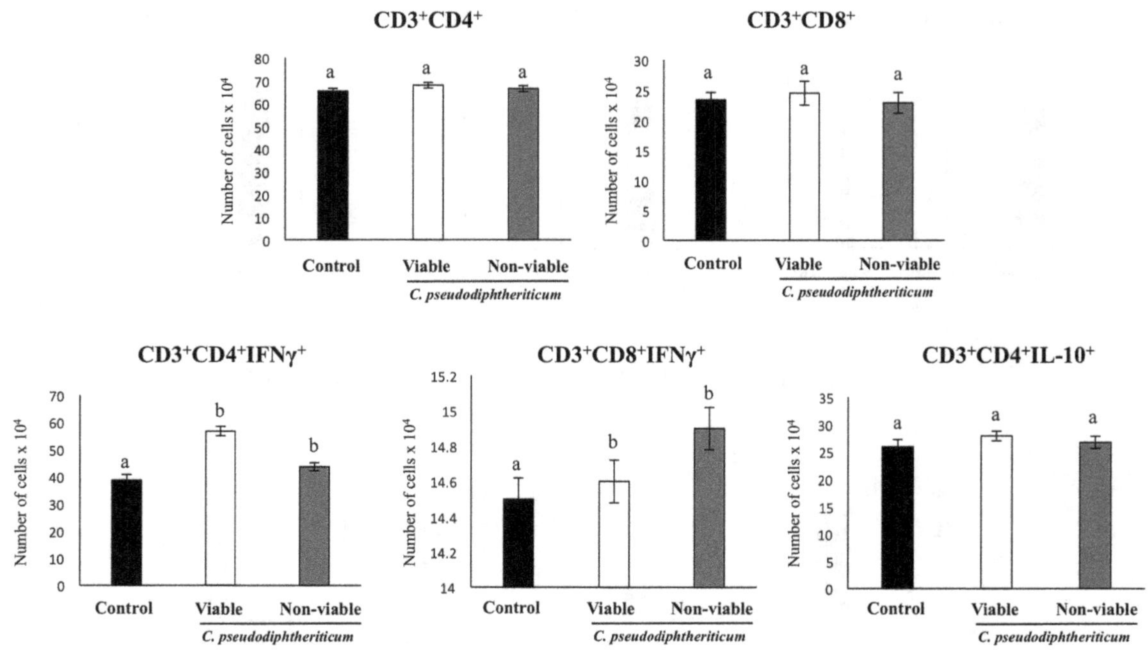

FIGURE 3 | Effect of *Corynebacterium pseudodiphtheriticum* strain 090104 on lung immune cell populations. Viable or non-viable *C. pseudodiphtheriticum* were nasally administered to infant mice during five consecutive days. Non-treated infant mice were used as controls. The numbers of lung T cells including $CD3^+CD4^+IFN\text{-}\gamma^+$, $CD3^+CD4^+IL\text{-}10^+$, and $CD3^+CD8^+IFN\text{-}\gamma^+$ T lymphocytes were determined by flow cytometry. Experiments were performed with 5–6 mice per group. The results represent data from three independent experiments. Values for bars with different letters were significantly different ($P < 0.05$). Values for bars with shared letters do not differ significantly.

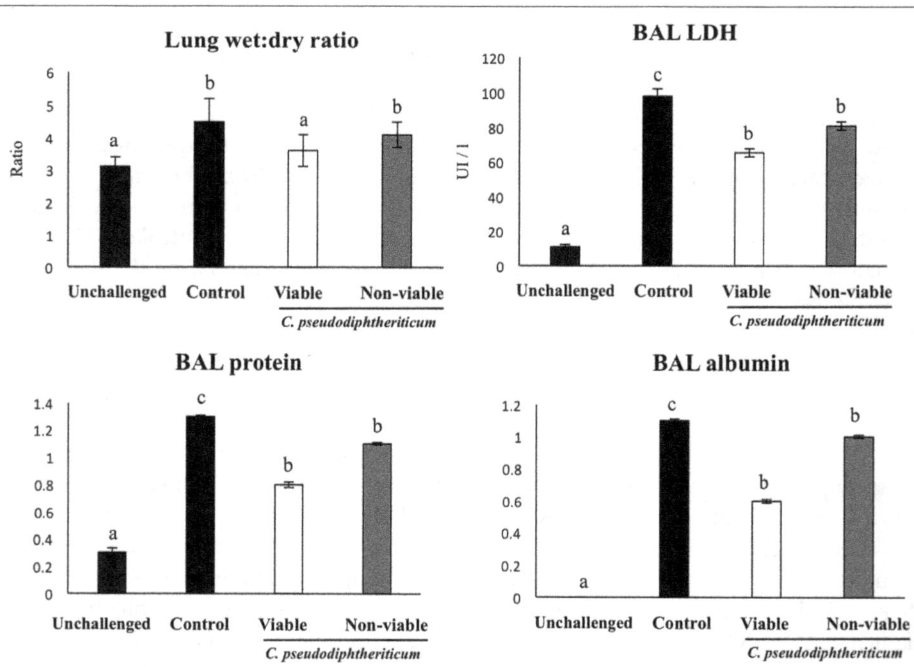

FIGURE 4 | Effect of *Corynebacterium pseudodiphtheriticum* strain 090104 on lung tissue damage induced by the nasal administration of the viral pathogen-associated molecular pattern poly(I:C). Infant mice were nasally primed with viable or non-viable *C. pseudodiphtheriticum* during five consecutive days and then challenged with three once-daily doses of poly(I:C). Non-treated infant mice challenged with poly(I:C) were used as controls. Two days after the last poly(I:C) administration lung wet:dry weight ratio, lactate dehydrogenase (LDH) activity and, albumin and protein concentrations in broncho-alveolar lavages (BAL) were determined. Experiments were performed with 5–6 mice per group. The results represent data from three independent experiments. Values for bars with different letters were significantly different ($P < 0.05$). Values for bars with shared letters do not differ significantly.

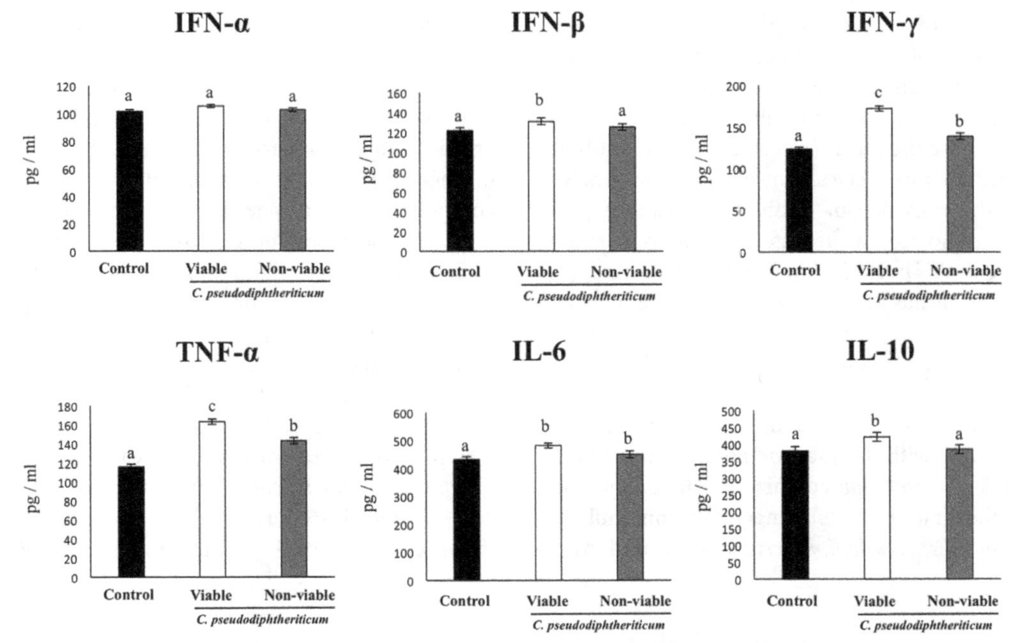

FIGURE 5 | Effect of *Corynebacterium pseudodiphtheriticum* strain 090104 on respiratory cytokines after the nasal administration of the viral pathogen-associated molecular pattern poly(I:C). Infant mice were nasally primed with viable or non-viable *C. pseudodiphtheriticum* during five consecutive days and then challenged with three once-daily doses of poly(I:C). Non-treated infant mice challenged with poly(I:C) were used as controls. Two days after the last poly(I:C) administration the levels of tumor necrosis factor (TNF)-α, interferon (IFN)-α, IFN-β, IFN-γ, interleukin (IL)-6, and IL-10 were determined in broncho-alveolar lavages (BAL). Experiments were performed with 5–6 mice per group. The results represent data from three independent experiments. Values for bars with different letters were significantly different ($P < 0.05$). Values for bars with shared letters do not differ significantly.

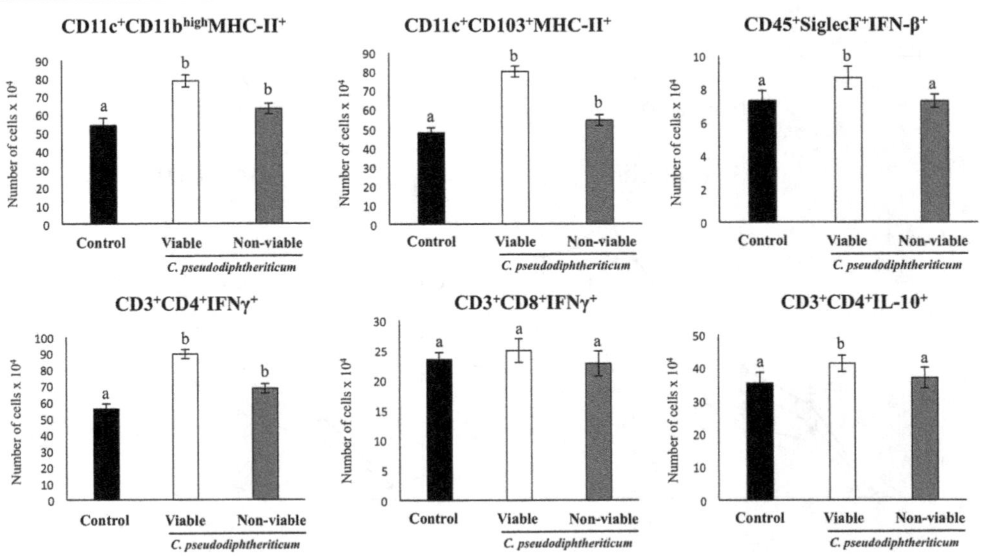

FIGURE 6 | Effect of *Corynebacterium pseudodiphtheriticum* strain 090104 on respiratory immune cell populations after the nasal administration of the viral pathogen-associated molecular pattern poly(I:C). Infant mice were nasally primed with viable or non-viable *C. pseudodiphtheriticum* during five consecutive days and then challenged with three once-daily doses of poly(I:C). Non-treated infant mice challenged with poly(I:C) were used as controls. Two days after the last poly(I:C) administration the numbers of lung T cells including $CD3^+CD4^+IFN\text{-}\gamma^+$, $CD3^+CD4^+IL\text{-}10^+$, and $CD3^+CD8^+IFN\text{-}\gamma^+$ T lymphocytes, as well as antigen presenting cells including $MHC\text{-}II^+CD11c^+CD11b^{low}CD103^+$ and $MHC\text{-}II^+CD11c^+CD11b^{high}CD103^-$ dendritic cells, and $CD45^+MHC\text{-}II^-CD11c^+SiglecF^+$ alveolar macrophages were determined by flow cytometry. Experiments were performed with 5–6 mice per group. The results represent data from three independent experiments. Values for bars with different letters were significantly different ($P < 0.05$). Values for bars with shared letters do not differ significantly.

et al., 2013; Liu C. M. et al., 2015). Our studies evaluating the potential translocation of *C. pseudodiphtheriticum* 090104 in infant mice after its nasal administration showed no adverse effects (data not shown). In addition, *C. pseudodiphtheriticum* 090104 shows resistance to β-lactam antibiotics and macrolides (data not shown) that are the most prevalent acquired antibiotic resistances described for this species. However, genome analysis did not evidence the presence of antibiotic resistance genes acquired by genetic horizontal transfer. Thus, our studies indicate that the use of this bacterium would be safe.

In previous studies, it has been shown that nasal application of *C. pseudodiphtheriticum* allowed the bacteria to colonize the nasal mucosa reducing *S. aureus* infection (Uehara et al., 2000; Kiryukhina et al., 2013; Liu C. M. et al., 2015). In line with these observations, we showed here for the first time that the nasal priming with *C. pseudodiphtheriticum* 090104 reduced RSV and *S. pneumoniae* colonization in infant mice. Moreover, this is the first study showing immunomodulatory properties for viable *C. pseudodiphtheriticum* as well as its capacity to enhance immunity against primary RSV and secondary pneumococcal pneumonia. According to our results, viable *C. pseudodiphtheriticum* was effective in reducing the burden of RSV infection as reflected by the lower viral load, improved body weight, and reduced pulmonary damage. The ameliorated pulmonary injury was related to the modulation of the inflammatory response that is known to be a main component of damage in RSV infections (Rutigliano and Graham, 2004; Bem et al., 2011; Cervantes-Ortiz et al., 2016). Main secreted proinflammatory cytokines in children coursing a natural RSV infection as well as in experimentally RSV inoculated mice are type I IFNs, TNF-α, IL-6, IL-8, MIP-1, RANTES, and MCP-1. Although these cytokines contribute to virus clearance in the early steps of infection, deregulated cytokine response leads to tissue injury (McNamara and Smyth, 2002). In our experiments, pre-treatment of infant mice with *C. pseudodiphtheriticum* enhanced the secretion of IFN-β, TNF-α, and IL-6 but at the same time, it also enhanced the production of IL-10 in response to RSV infection. It

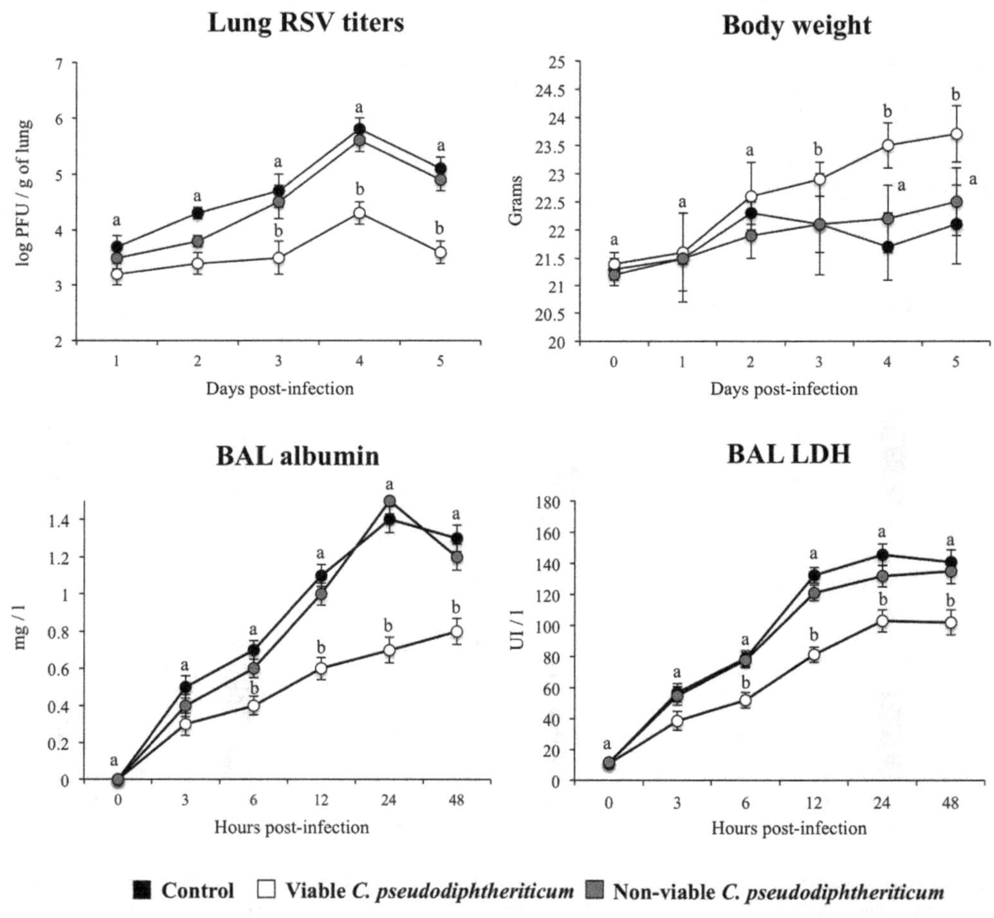

FIGURE 7 | Effect of *Corynebacterium pseudodiphtheriticum* strain 090104 on the resistance to primary Respiratory Syncytial Virus (RSV) infection. Infant mice were nasally primed with viable or non-viable *C. pseudodiphtheriticum* during five consecutive days and then challenged with RSV. Non-treated infant mice challenged with the viral pathogen were used as controls. Lung RSV titers, changes in body weight, and lactate dehydrogenase (LDH) activity and albumin concentrations in broncho-alveolar lavages (BAL) were evaluated on different time points after the viral challenge. Experiments were performed with 5–6 mice per group per each time point. The results represent data from three independent experiments. Values for each time point with different letters were significantly different ($P < 0.05$). Values for each time point with shared letters do not differ significantly.

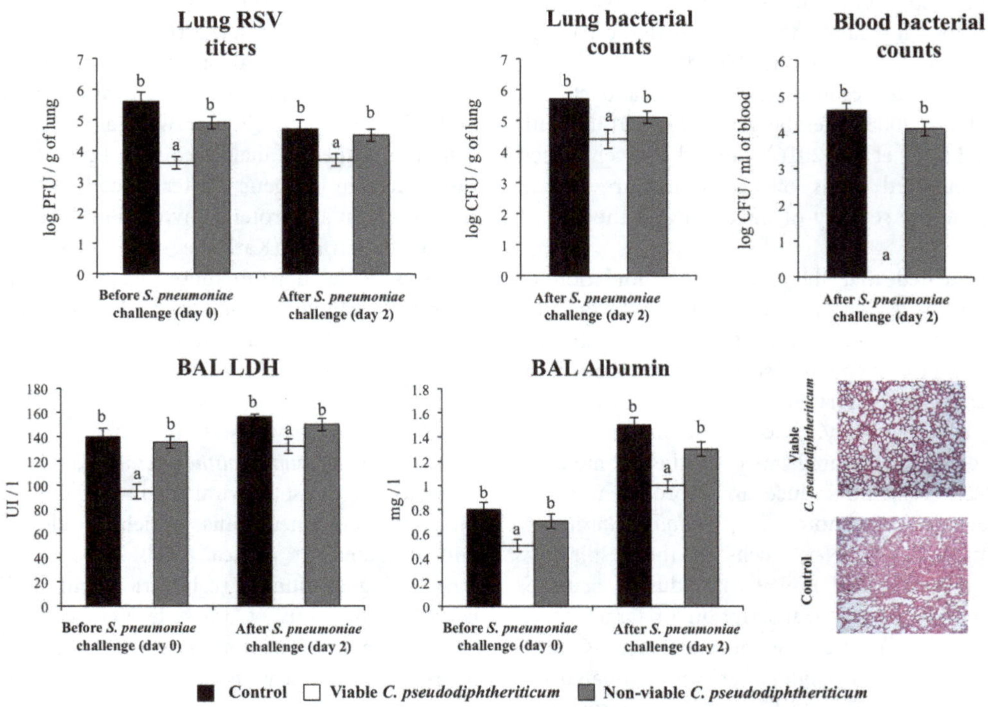

FIGURE 8 | Effect of *Corynebacterium pseudodiphtheriticum* strain 090104 on the resistance to secondary pneumococcal pneumonia after the primary infection with Respiratory Syncytial Virus (RSV). Infant mice were nasally primed with viable or non-viable *C. pseudodiphtheriticum* during five consecutive days, challenged with RSV and, infected with *Streptococcus pneumoniae* 5 days after the viral infection. Non-treated infant mice infected with RSV and challenged with *S. pneumoniae* were used as controls. Lung RSV titers, lung bacterial cells counts, lactate dehydrogenase (LDH) activity and albumin concentrations in broncho-alveolar lavages (BAL), and lung histology were determined on day 2 post-pneumococcal challenge. Lungs histological examination was performed with hematoxylin and eosin stained light micrographs, original magnification ×40. Experiments were performed with 5–6 mice per group. The results represent data from three independent experiments. Values for bars with different letters were significantly different ($P < 0.05$). Values for bars with shared letters do not differ significantly.

was proposed that the most prominent role of IL-10 is its contribution to restrict inflammation during RSV infection, which consequently lowers injury (Stacey et al., 2011; Weiss et al., 2011). The differential regulation of the inflammatory response induced by viable *C. pseudodiphtheriticum* seems to be related to its capacity to modulate TLR3-mediated inflammatory response in the respiratory tract. As others and we demonstrated previously, TLR3 has little effect on RSV clearance but it is necessary to regulate the respiratory immune environment. The absence of an efficient regulation of TLR3 activation significantly contributes to the pulmonary immunopathology associated to RSV infection (reviewed in 42). In fact, respiratory administration of the TLR3 agonist poly(I:C) has been used to mimic the pro-inflammatory and physiopathological consecuences of RSV infections in the lung (Kitazawa and Villena, 2014).

It has also been reported that the exacerbated proinflammatory cytokine/chemokine response is skewed toward a T helper type 2 (Th2) immune response (Cervantes-Ortiz et al., 2016), and that IFN-γ-producing $CD4^+$ and $CD8^+$ T cells contribute to protection during RSV infection (Sun and Lopez, 2016). In our experiments, treatment with viable *C. pseudodiphtheriticum* also increased IFN-γ producing $CD3^+CD4^+$ cells in the lungs of infant mice. The improved numbers of $CD4^+IFN\text{-}\gamma^+$ cells and IFN-γ levels in lung tissue would activate pulmonary macrophages and dendritic cells and induce the enhancement of Th1 cellular response, contributing to the protection induced by *C. pseudodiphtheriticum*.

In line with our previous studies evaluating the effect of beneficial microbes on the susceptibility to viral infections (Villena et al., 2012; Chiba et al., 2013; Tomosada et al., 2013), we found here that the respiratory commensal bacteria *C. pseudodiphtheriticum* improves resistance to RSV infection through the modulation of IFN-β, IFN-γ, and IL-10.

We also demonstrated here that viable *C. pseudodiphtheriticum* significanlty reduced *S. pneumoniae* cell counts in lungs and prevented its dissemination into the blood of infant mice after the primary infection with RSV. The effect of *C. pseudodiphtheriticum* in reducing lung pneumococcal cell counts was modest compared with our own previous studies. We had reported that the nasal administration of viable *Lactococcus lactis* NZ9000 to adult and infant mice reduced in more than two log folds *S. pneumoniae* cell counts in lungs (Medina et al., 2008). Moreover, *C. pseudodiphtheriticum* evaluated in an infant mice model of primary pneumococcal infection also reduced in more than two log folds *S. pneumoniae* cell counts in lungs when compared to untreated controls (data not shown). Despite the modest results obtained here by measuring the burden of the pathogen in the respiratory tract, *C. pseudodiphtheriticum* treatment was able to significantly reduce lung tissue damage and bacterial dissemination into the blood stream. These findings are of importance because experimental and clinical studies (Hament et al., 2005; Weinberger et al., 2013; Smith et al., 2014; Cebey-Lopez et al., 2016) showed that enhanced lung injuries and elevated levels of bacteremia are critical factors that determine the severity of infection and the rate of mortality.

It could be speculated that the beneficial modulation of the inflammatory response during RSV and the reduced lung injuries induced by *C. pseudodiphtheriticum* administration would be related to the improvement of secondary pneumococcal infection. The different respiratory immune environment (such as the levels of IFN-β, IFN-γ, and IL-10 in the lungs) on *C. pseudodiphtheriticum*-treated mice at the moment of pneumococcal infection would induce an improved immune response and protection. Of note, *C. pseudodiphtheriticum* was able to enhance $CD4^+IFN\text{-}\gamma^+$ cells in the respiratory tract. It has been reported that IFN-γ early during acute *S. pneumoniae* pneumonia induces transcription of target genes in the lungs, which are critical for host defense (Gomez et al., 2015). In addition, *C. pseudodiphtheriticu* stimulated the production of IFN-β in $CD45^+SiglecF^+$ alveolar macrophages after poly(I:C) administration. Some studies have showed that IFN-β is involved in the protection against lung tissue injury as well in the control of pneumococcal dissemination into the blood during secondary pneumococcal pneumonia. No significant differences in *S. pneumoniae* counts in the lungs of $IFNAR1^{-/-}$ and $IFNAR1^{+/+}$ mice were observed after pneumococcal challenge. However, pneumococci were observed earlier and at higher numbers in blood samples of $IFNAR1^{-/-}$ mice compared to wild-type animals (LeMessurier et al., 2013). More detailed studies are necessary to fully understand the immune mechanisms involved in the protection against secondary pneumococcal pneumonia induced by *C. pseudodiphtheriticum* 090104.

Interestingly, non-viable bacteria did not have the same protective effect. Non-viable *C. pseudodiphtheriticum* was unable to induce the increase of the numbers of $CD45^+SiglecF^+IFN\text{-}\beta^+$ and $CD4^+IL\text{-}10^+$ cells neither the levels of IFN-β and IL-10 in the respiratory tract. Only increments in $CD4^+IFN\text{-}\gamma^+$ cells and IFN-γ levels were detected but there were significantly lower when compared with those induced by viable bacteria. These results suggest that *C. pseudodiphtheriticum* 090104 colonization of the nasopharynx is indeed needed for reducing RSV infection and secondary bacterial infection. In line with this finding, it has been reported that the presence of viable *Corynebacterium* spp. in the upper respiratory tract is necessary to protect against pathogens since antibiotic perturbations leading to the reduction of beneficial commensal bacteria such as *Dolosigranulum* spp. or *Corynebacterium* spp. increase the risk of respiratory infections of healthy children (Pettigrew et al., 2012; Teo et al., 2015). Genome sequence analysis of the 090104 strain showed that the bacterium has gene clusters encoding fimbrial subunits and sortase A that are proteins involved in the attachment of fimbria to the cell surface (Karlyshev and Melnikov, 2013). To obtain mutants depleted from these genes and study whether these *C. pseudodiphtheriticum* strains lacking attachment proteins are able to beneficially modulate respiratory immunity is an interesting topic that we intend to evaluate in the immediate future.

In conclusion, we present evidence that nasal application of viable *C. pseudodiphtheriticum* could be thought as an alternative to boost antiviral defenses against RSV and secondary pneumococcal pneumonia, which should be further studied and validated in clinical trials. Due to the absence of a long-lasting immunity, re-infection with RSV throughout life is common. Thus, a possible perspective use could be a seasonal application of a nasal next-generation probiotic spray to boost respiratory innate immunity in immunocompetent subjects.

AUTHOR CONTRIBUTIONS

SA, VM, HK, and JV designed the study. MV, HT, HK, and JV wrote the manuscript. PK, PC, MV, and CR did the laboratory work. PK, PC, and JV performed statistical analysis. HT, MV, and JV contributed to data analysis and interpretation. All authors read and approved the manuscript.

ACKNOWLEDGMENTS

This study was supported by a Grant-in-Aid for Scientific Research (B)(2) (No. 16H05019), Challenging Exploratory Research (No. 16K15028) and Open Partnership Joint Projects of JSPS Bilateral Joint Research Projects from the Japan Society for the Promotion of Science (JSPS) to HK and by an ANPCyT–FONCyT Grant PICT-2013 (No. 3219) to JV. This work was also supported by JSPS Core-to-Core Program A (Advanced Research Networks) entitled: "Establishment of international agricultural immunology research-core for a quantum improvement in food safety." This study was also financially supported by grants for "Scientific Research on Innovative Areas" from the Ministry of Education, Culture, Science, Sports and Technology (MEXT) of Japan (Grant numbers: 16H06429, 16K21723, and 16H06435).

REFERENCES

Ahmed, K., Kawakami, K., Watanabe, K., Mitsushima, H., Nagatake, T., and Matsumoto, K. (1995). *Corynebacterium pseudodiphtheriticum*: a respiratory tract pathogen. *Clin. Infect. Dis.* 20, 41–46. doi: 10.1093/clinids/20.1.41

Bem, R. A., Domachowske, J. B., and Rosenberg, H. F. (2011). Animal models of human respiratory syncytial virus disease. *Am. J. Physiol. Lung Cell. Mol. physiol.* 301, L148–L156. doi: 10.1152/ajplung.00065.2011

Bittar, F., Cassagne, C., Bosdure, E., Stremler, N., Dubus, J. C., Sarles, J., et al. (2010). Outbreak of *Corynebacterium pseudodiphtheriticum* infection in cystic fibrosis patients, France. *Emerg. Infect. Dis.* 16, 1231–1236. doi: 10.3201/eid1608.100193

Bosch, A. A., Biesbroek, G., Trzcinski, K., Sanders, E. A., and Bogaert, D. (2013). Viral and bacterial interactions in the upper respiratory tract. *PLoS Pathog.* 9:e1003057. doi: 10.1371/journal.ppat.1003057

Burke, G. J., Malouf, M. A., and Glanville, A. R. (1997). Opportunistic lung infection with *Corynebacterium pseudodiphtheriticum* after lung and heart transplantation. *Med. J. Aust.* 166, 362–364.

Cebey-Lopez, M., Pardo-Seco, J., Gomez- Carballa, A., Martinon-Torres, N., Martinon-Sanchez, J. M., Justicia-Grande, A., et al. (2016). Bacteremia in children hospitalized with respiratory syncytial virus infection. *PLoS ONE* 11:e0146599. doi: 10.1371/journal.pone.0146599

Cervantes-Ortiz, S. L., Zamorano Cuervo, N., and Grandvaux, N. (2016). Respiratory syncytial virus and cellular stress responses: impact on replication and physiopathology. *Viruses* 8:E124. doi: 10.3390/v8050124

Chiba, E., Tomosada, Y., Vizoso-Pinto, M. G., Salva, S., Takahashi, T., Tsukida, K., et al. (2013). Immunobiotic *Lactobacillus rhamnosus* improves resistance of infant mice against respiratory syncytial virus infection. *Int. Immunopharmacol.* 17, 373–382. doi: 10.1016/j.intimp.2013.06.024

Gomez, J. C., Yamada, M., Martin, J. R., Dang, H., Brickey, W. J., Bergmeier, W., et al. (2015). Mechanisms of interferon-γ production by neutrophils and its function during *Streptococcus pneumoniae* pneumonia. *Am. J. Respir Cell Mol. Biol.* 52, 349–364. doi: 10.1165/rcmb.2013-0316OC

Hament, J. M., Aerts, P. C., Fleer, A., van Dijk, H., Harmsen, T., Kimpen, J. L., et al. (2005). Direct binding of respiratory syncytial virus to pneumococci: a phenomenon that enhances both pneumococcal adherence to human epithelial cells and pneumococcal invasiveness in a murine model. *Pediatr. Res.* 58, 1198–1203. doi: 10.1203/01.pdr.0000188699.55279.1b

Hishiki, H., Ishiwada, N., Fukasawa, C., Abe, K., Hoshino, T., Aizawa, J., et al. (2011). Incidence of bacterial coinfection with respiratory syncytial virus bronchopulmonary infection in pediatric inpatients. *J. Inf. Chemother.* 17, 87–90. doi: 10.1007/s10156-010-0097-x

Karlyshev, A. V., and Melnikov, V. G. (2013). Draft genome sequence of *Corynebacterium pseudodiphtheriticum* strain 090104 "Sokolov". *Genome Announc.* 1:e00921-13. doi: 10.1128/genomeA.00921-13

Kiryukhina, N. V., Melnikov, V. G., Suvorov, A. V., Morozova, Y. A., and Ilyin, V. K. (2013). Use of *Corynebacterium pseudodiphtheriticum* for elimination of *Staphylococcus aureus* from the nasal cavity in volunteers exposed to abnormal microclimate and altered gaseous environment. *Probiot. Antimicrob. Proteins* 5, 233–238. doi: 10.1007/s12602-013-9147-x

Kitazawa, H., and Villena, J. (2014). Modulation of respiratory TLR3-anti-viral response by probiotic microorganisms: lessons learned from *Lactobacillus rhamnosus* CRL1505. *Front. Immunol.* 5:201. doi: 10.3389/fimmu.2014.00201

LeMessurier, K. S., Hacker, H., Chi, L., Tuomanen, E., and Redecke, V. (2013). Type I interferon protects against pneumococcal invasive disease by inhibiting bacterial transmigration across the lung. *PLoS Pathog.* 9:e1003727. doi: 10.1371/journal.ppat.1003727

Levine, D. A., Platt, S. L., Dayan, P. S., Macias, C. G., Zorc, J. J., Krief, W., et al. (2004). Risk of serious bacterial infection in young febrile infants with respiratory syncytial virus infections. *Pediatrics* 113, 1728–1734. doi: 10.1542/peds.113.6.1728

Liu, C. M., Price, L. B., Hungate, B. A., Abraham, A. G., Larsen, L. A., Christensen, K., et al. (2015). *Staphylococcus aureus* and the ecology of the nasal microbiome. *Sci. Adv.* 1:e1400216. doi: 10.1126/sciadv.1400216

Liu, L., Johnson, H. L., Cousens, S., Perin, J., Scott, S., Lawn, J. E., et al. (2012). Global, regional, and national causes of child mortality: an updated systematic analysis for 2010 with time trends since 2000. *Lancet* 379, 2151–2161. doi: 10.1016/S0140-6736(12)60560-1

Liu, L., Oza, S., Hogan, D., Perin, J., Rudan, I., Lawn, J. E., et al. (2015). Global, regional, and national causes of child mortality in 2000-13, with projections to inform post-2015 priorities: an updated systematic analysis. *Lancet* 385, 430–440. doi: 10.1016/S0140-6736(14)61698-6

Maragkoudakis, P. A., Chingwaru, W., Gradisnik, L., Tsakalidou, E., and Cencic, A. (2010). Lactic acid bacteria efficiently protect human and animal intestinal epithelial and immune cells from enteric virus infection. *Int. J. Food Microbiol.* 141(Suppl. 1), S91–S97. doi: 10.1016/j.ijfoodmicro.2009.12.024

McNamara, P. S., and Smyth, R. L. (2002). The pathogenesis of respiratory syncytial virus disease in childhood. *Br. Med. Bull.* 61, 13–28. doi: 10.1093/bmb/61.1.13

Medina, M., Villena, J., Salva, S., Vintiñi, E., Langella, P., and Alvarez, S. (2008). Nasal administration of *Lactococcus lactis* improves the local and systemic immune responses against *Streptococcus pneumonia*. *Microbiol. Immunol.* 52, 399–409. doi: 10.1111/j.1348-0421.2008.00050.x

Murawski, M. R., Bowen, G. N., Cerny, A. M., Anderson, L. J., Haynes, L. M., Tripp, R. A., et al. (2009). Respiratory syncytial virus activates innate immunity through Toll-like receptor 2. *J. Virol.* 83, 1492–1500. doi: 10.1128/JVI.00671-08

Olender, A., and Niemcewicz, M. (2010). Macrolide, lincosamide, and streptogramin B-constitutive-type resistance in *Corynebacterium pseudodiphtheriticum* isolated from upper respiratory tract specimens. *Microb. Drug Resist.* 16, 119–122. doi: 10.1089/mdr.2009.0122

Pettigrew, M. M., Laufer, A. S., Gent, J. F., Kong, Y., Fennie, K. P., and Metlay, J. P. (2012). Upper respiratory tract microbial communities, acute otitis media pathogens, and antibiotic use in healthy and sick children. *Appl. Environ. Microbiol.* 78, 6262–6270. doi: 10.1128/AEM.01051-12

Rutigliano, J. A., and Graham, B. S. (2004). Prolonged production of TNF-alpha exacerbates illness during respiratory syncytial virus infection. *J. Immunol.* 173, 3408–3417. doi: 10.4049/jimmunol.173.5.3408

Salva, S., Nunez, M., Villena, J., Ramon, A., Font, G., and Alvarez, S. (2011). Development of a fermented goats' milk containing *Lactobacillus rhamnosus*: *in vivo* study of health benefits. *J. Sci. Food Agric.* 91, 2355–2362. doi: 10.1002/jsfa.4467

Smith, C. M., Sandrini, S., Datta, S., Freestone, P., Shafeeq, S., Radhakrishnan, P., et al. (2014). Respiratory syncytial virus increases the virulence of *Streptococcus pneumoniae* by binding to penicillin binding protein 1a. A new paradigm in respiratory infection. *Am. J. Respir. Crit. Care Med.* 190, 196–207. doi: 10.1164/rccm.201311-2110OC

Stacey, M. A., Marsden, M., Wang, E. C., Wilkinson, G. W., and Humphreys, I. R. (2011). IL-10 restricts activation-induced death of NK cells during acute murine cytomegalovirus infection. *J. Immunol.* 187, 2944–2952. doi: 10.4049/jimmunol.1101021

Sun, Y., and Lopez, C. B. (2016). The innate immune response to RSV: advances in our understanding of critical viral and host factors. *Vaccine* 35, 481–488. doi: 10.1016/j.vaccine.2016.09.030

Tada, A., Zelaya, H., Clua, P., Salva, S., Alvarez, S., Kitazawa, H., et al. (2016). Immunobiotic Lactobacillus strains reduce small intestinal injury induced by intraepithelial lymphocytes after Toll-like receptor 3 activation. *Inflamm. Res.* 65, 771–783. doi: 10.1007/s00011-016-0957-7

Teo, S. M., Mok, D., Pham, K., Kusel, M., Serralha, M., Troy, N., et al. (2015). The infant nasopharyngeal microbiome impacts severity of lower respiratory infection and risk of asthma development. *Cell Host Microbe* 17, 704–715. doi: 10.1016/j.chom.2015.03.008

Tomosada, Y., Chiba, E., Zelaya, H., Takahashi, T., Tsukida, K., Kitazawa, H., et al. (2013). Nasally administered *Lactobacillus rhamnosus* strains differentially modulate respiratory antiviral immune responses and induce protection against respiratory syncytial virus infection. *BMC Immunol.* 14:40. doi: 10.1186/1471-2172-14-40

Uehara, Y., Nakama, H., Agematsu, K., Uchida, M., Kawakami, Y., Abdul Fattah, A. S., et al. (2000). Bacterial interference among nasal inhabitants: eradication of *Staphylococcus aureus* from nasal cavities by artificial implantation of Corynebacterium sp. *J. Hosp. Infect.* 44, 127–133. doi: 10.1053/jhin.1999.0680

Villena, J., Chiba, E., Tomosada, Y., Salva, S., Marranzino, G., Kitazawa, H., et al. (2012). Orally administered *Lactobacillus rhamnosus* modulates the respiratory immune response triggered by the viral pathogen-associated molecular pattern poly(I:C). *BMC Immunol.* 13:53. doi: 10.1186/1471-2172-13-53

Villena, J., Racedo, S., Aguero, G., Bru, E., Medina, M., and Alvarez, S. (2005). *Lactobacillus casei* improves resistance to pneumococcal respiratory infection in malnourished mice. *J. Nutr.* 135, 1462–1469.

Weinberger, D. M., Givon-Lavi, N., Shemer-Avni, Y., Bar-Ziv, J., Alonso, W. J., Greenberg, D., et al. (2013). Influence of pneumococcal vaccines and respiratory syncytial virus on alveolar pneumonia, Israel. *Emerg. Infect. Dis.* 19, 1084–1091. doi: 10.3201/eid1907.121625

Weiss, K. A., Christiaansen, A. F., Fulton, R. B., Meyerholz, D. K., and Varga, S. M. (2011). Multiple CD4+ T cell subsets produce immunomodulatory IL-10 during respiratory syncytial virus infection. *J. Immunol.* 187, 3145–3154. doi: 10.4049/jimmunol.1100764

Zelaya, H., Tada, A., Vizoso-Pinto, M. G., Salva, S., Kanmani, P., Aguero, G., et al. (2015). Nasal priming with immunobiotic *Lactobacillus rhamnosus* modulates inflammation-coagulation interactions and reduces influenza virus-associated pulmonary damage. *Inflamm. Res.* 64, 589–602. doi: 10.1007/s00011-015-0837-6

Zelaya, H., Villena, J., Gramajo Lopez, A., Alvarez, S., and Aguero, G. (2014). Modulation of the inflammation-coagulation interaction during pneumococcal pneumonia by immunobiotic *Lactobacillus rhamnosus* CRL1505: role of toll-like receptor 2. *Microbiol. Immunol.* 58, 416–426. doi: 10.1111/1348-0421.12163

4

Safety Evaluation of a Novel Strain of *Bacteroides fragilis*

Ye Wang[1,2†], Huimin Deng[2,3†], Zhengchao Li[2,3†], Yafang Tan[3], Yanping Han[3], Xiaoyi Wang[3], Zongmin Du[3], Yangyang Liu[4], Ruifu Yang[3], Yang Bai[2*], Yujing Bi[3*] and Fachao Zhi[2*]

[1] Institute of Genetic Engineering, Jinan University, Guangzhou, China, [2] Guangdong Provincial Key Laboratory of Gastroenterology, Department of Gastroenterology, Institute of Gastroenterology, Nanfang Hospital, Southern Medical University, Guangzhou, China, [3] State Key Laboratory of Pathogen and Biosecurity, Beijing Institute of Microbiology and Epidemiology, Beijing, China, [4] Guangzhou ZhiYi biotechnology Co. Ltd., Guangzhou, China

***Correspondence:**
Yang Bai
baiyang1030@hotmail.com
Yujing Bi
byj7801@sina.com
Fachao Zhi
zhifc41532@163.com

† These authors have contributed equally to this work.

Commensal non-toxigenic *Bacteroides fragilis* confers powerful health benefits to the host, and has recently been identified as a promising probiotic candidate. We previously isolated *B. fragilis* strain ZY-312 and identified it as a novel strain based on 16S rRNA sequencing and morphological analyses. We also determined that ZY-312 displayed desirable probiotic properties, including tolerance to simulated digestive fluid, adherence, and *in vitro* safety. In this study, we aim to investigate whether ZY-312 meets the safety criteria required for probiotic bacteria through comprehensive and systematic evaluation. Consequently, the fatty acid profile, metabolite production, and biochemical activity of strain ZY-312 were found to closely resemble descriptions of *B. fragilis* in Bergey's manual. Taxonomic identification of strain ZY-312 based on whole genome sequencing indicated that ZY-312 and ATCC 25285 showed 99.99% similarity. The 33 putative virulence-associated factors identified in ZY-312 mainly encoded structural proteins and proteins with physiological activity, while the lack of *bft* indicated that ZY-312 was non-toxigenic. *In vivo* safety was proven in both normal and immune-deficient mice. The 11 identified antibiotic resistance genes were located on the chromosome rather than on a plasmid, ruling out the risk of plasmid-mediated transfer of antibiotic resistance. *In vitro*, ZY-312 showed resistance to cefepime, kanamycin, and streptomycin. Finally, and notably, ZY-312 exhibited high genetic stability after 100 passages *in vitro*. This study supplements the foundation work on the safety evaluation of ZY-312, and contributes to the development of the first probiotic representative from the dominant Bacteroidetes phylum.

Keywords: *Bacteroides fragilis*, safety evaluation, probiotic, whole genome sequencing, genetic stability

INTRODUCTION

Commensal gut microbiota are important for host health. They contribute to maturation of the immune system, building intestinal commensalism, resisting infectious microbes, digesting indigestible carbohydrates, and producing certain nutrients such as vitamins and short-chain fatty acids (Sekirov et al., 2010; Fijan, 2014). An increasing number of reports have confirmed the link between intestinal flora disorder and disease, especially autoimmune and metabolic diseases (Fijan, 2014; Althani et al., 2016). Although it is not clear who takes the leap and how it happens, dominant members of the intestinal microbiota are now being examined as potential probiotic candidates to assist in the treatment of disease, or become alternatives to antibiotics (McKenney and Pamer, 2015; Miquel et al., 2015).

Approved probiotic products based on intestinal microbiota species mainly include lactic acid bacteria, *Bifidobacterium*, and *Escherichia coli* (Foligne et al., 2013). However, there are currently no probiotic representatives of the phylum Bacteroidetes, the second-largest component of the intestinal flora. Recently, non-toxigenic *Bacteroides fragilis* (NTBF) was shown to have powerful health benefits to the host, and was recommended as a probiotic candidate (Troy and Kasper, 2010; Hsiao et al., 2013; Deng et al., 2016). It is therefore likely that *B. fragilis* will be the first probiotic species from the phylum Bacteroidetes.

We previously isolated a novel *B. fragilis* strain ZY-312, and have carried out basic safety assessments to test its probiotic properties (Deng et al., 2016). Results of 16S rRNA sequence analysis, tolerance to simulated digestive fluid, safety, and adhesion to HT-29 cells suggested *B. fragilis* ZY-312 possessed desirable probiotic properties. However, these results are not sufficient to definitively conclude that ZY-312 is safe for use as a probiotic. According to the framework of evaluations for probiotics from Europe (Miquel et al., 2015) and by the Food and Agriculture Organization of the United Nations and the World Health Organization (FAO/WHO, 2002), thorough characterization of a strain, including examination of the fatty acid profile, metabolite production, and biochemical activity, evaluation of the potential risk of transferable antibiotic resistance and genetic stability, and verification of safety in animals, especially immunodeficient animals, is an integral part of safety assessment (Miquel et al., 2015). Taking advantage of whole genome sequencing technology, we carried out a thorough characterization and systematic evaluation of novel *B. fragilis* strain ZY-312 to determine whether it meets the safety criteria required for probiotics.

MATERIALS AND METHODS

Bacterial Strains and Culture Conditions

Strain ZY-312 was isolated from the feces of a healthy infant, and was previously identified using 16S rRNA gene sequence analysis (Deng et al., 2016). *B. fragilis* strain ATCC 25285 (also known as NCTC 9343) was purchased from the American Type Culture Collection (ATCC). The culture conditions and materials were as described previously for strains ZY-312 and ATCC 25285 (Deng et al., 2016). For the microbial contamination experiment, *E. coli* CBSLAM00087, *Staphylococcus aureus* (*S. aureus*) CMCC(B) 26058, *Salmonella enterica (S. enterica)* serotype Paratyphi B CBSLAM00994, *Pseudomonas aeruginosa* (*P. aeruginosa*) CBSLAM00818, *Candida albicans (C. albicans)* CMCC(F)98001, and *Clostridium sporogenes* (*C. sporogenes*) CMCC(B) 64941 were obtained from the Academy of Military Medical Science, Beijing, China. All strains were verified by PCR amplification of 16S rRNA gene using the universal primers 27 F (5′-AGAGTTTGATCCTGGCTCAG-3′) and 1492 R (5′-GGTTACCTTGTTACGACTT-3′) (Lanes D–J). Amplified products were sequenced (Biomed).

Animals

For acute oral toxicity studies, 6- to 8-week-old female specific pathogen-free (SPF) BALB/c mice and nude mice were procured from the Animal Experiment Center of the Academy of Military Medical Sciences, Beijing, China. The animals had free access to tap water and standard rodent diet. All of the animal experiments were performed in accordance with the approval of the Animal Ethics Committee of the Beijing Institute of Microbiology and Epidemiology, Beijing, China.

Genome Sequencing, Assembly, and Analysis

Total DNA was extracted from all strains using a DNA extraction kit (Qiagen, USA) and the complete genome sequence of strain ZY-312 was determined using an Illumina Hiseq 2000 sequencing system (Xu et al., 2015). A genome sequencing library with an average insert size of 400 bp was generated, and raw short-read sequences were filtered using Seqprep[1] and Sickle[2] software. The genome was then assembled *de novo* using SOAP *de novo* software (Luo et al., 2012). Accuracy of the assembled genome sequence was evaluated by mapping all raw reads onto the scaffolds using SOAPaligner (Cui et al., 2013).

Gene prediction was carried out using Glimmer3.0 software (Xu et al., 2015). Putative antibiotic resistance genes and putative virulence factors were identified by BLAST analysis of the antibiotic resistance genes database (ARDB)[3] (Liu and Pop, 2009) and the virulence factors database (VFDB)[4] (Chen et al., 2005), respectively. A BLAST comparison was performed between the genome sequences of strain ZY-312 and *B. fragilis* strain NCTC 9343 (GenBank accession number NC_003228). A Perl script was written and the average nucleotide identity (ANI) was calculated using BLAST. A neighbor-joining phylogenetic tree was built using treebest based on the ZY-312 complete genome sequence, the complete shotgun sequences of other *B. fragilis* strains, and the complete genome sequences of *B. fragilis* strains NCTC 9343 (GenBank accession number NC_003228), YCH46 (GenBank accession number NC_006347), and *B. fragilis* 638R (GenBank accession number NC_016776).

General Characteristics of ZY-312

ZY-312 was cultured on Eosin methylene blue agar for 24 h at 37°C (*E. coli* as positive control), SS agar for 24 h at 37°C (*S. enterica* serovar Paratyphi B as positive control), Columbia agar containing blood and gentamicin for 48 h at 37°C (*C. sporogenes* as positive control), mannitol sodium chloride agar for 24 h at 37°C (*S. aureus* as positive control), NAC agar

[1] https://github.com/jstjohn/SeqPrep
[2] https://github.com/najoshi/sickle
[3] http://ardb.cbcb.umd.edu/
[4] http://www.mgc.ac.cn/VFs/main.htm

TABLE 1 | Major fatty acids (A) and major metabolites (B) of *Bacteroides fragilis* ZY-312.

Peak name	Percentage (%)
(A)	
$C_{15:0}$ anteiso	32.21
$C_{15:0}$ iso	17.29
$C_{16:0}$	11.66
$C_{16:0}$ 3-OH	11.08
$C_{14:0}$	1.82
$C_{17:0}$ ante 3-OH	1.72
$C_{18:0}$	1.68
$C_{15:0}$	1.63
$C_{18:1}$ CIS 9	1.37
Unable to distinguish	19.55

	ZY-312		ATCC 25285	
	Time (s)	Normalized area	Time (s)	Normalized area
(B)				
Acetic acid	1514	67.24×10^5	1513	27.65×10^5
Butanedioic acid	593	498.29×10^5	592	107.27×10^5
propionic acid	1353	2.65×10^5	1352	5.41×10^5
Phenylacetic acid	2404	1.33×10^5	2403	2.06×10^5
lactic acid	424	556.78×10^5	424	557.94×10^5

for 24 h at 37°C (*P. aeruginosa* as positive control), Sabouraud dextrose agar for 72 h at 28°C (*C. albicans* as positive control), rose bengal agar for 96 h at 28°C (*C. albicans* as positive control), and agar agar for 48 h at 37°C (*S. aureus* as positive control) for excluding microbial contamination. The major fatty acids were analyzed using an HP6890 gas chromatograph (ver. A 5.01), as previously described (Tan et al., 2010). Supernatant from late-logarithmic phase ZY-312 and ATCC 25285 cultures was collected by centrifugation for 10 min at 3000 × *g*, and then analyzed by gas chromatography-mass spectrometry. Carbon-source utilization analyses were carried out using a Biolog AN microPlate test panel (Biolog, USA). Bacterial cells were collected from logarithmic phase ZY-312 and ATCC 25285 cultures and resuspended at a concentration of 1.5×10^8 colony forming units (cfu)/mL, and then inoculated into the test plate. After incubating anaerobically for 16–24 h, test results were read using a microplate reader (SpectraMax, M2), using deionized water as a negative control. To test catalase activity, 3–5 drops (about 100 μL) of 3% hydrogen peroxide (freshly prepared) were dropped onto the center of precipitated bacterial cells on microscope slides. To test gelatin liquefaction activity, bacteria were inoculated into gelatin medium, tryptone soy broth (TSB, OXIOD, UK) solidified with 15% gelatin, using a sterilized needle. Plates were incubated at 37°C for 48 h anaerobically, then placed at 4°C for 3–4 h. To determine hemolytic ability, bacteria were anaerobically cultured on tryptone soy agar (TSA, OXIOD, UK) supplemented with 5% (v/v) goat blood for 48 h at 37°C. To determine motility, bacteria were cultured on semi-solid medium (TSB solidified with 0.5% agar) at 37°C for 48 h anaerobically.

Antibiotic Resistance Testing

Antibiotic resistance testing was performed using the minimum inhibitory concentration (MIC) method as described previously (Fernandez et al., 2005). Test antibiotics were chosen based on the antibiotic resistance genes identified in the annotated genome of ZY-312, with the following antibiotics included in the analysis: cefoxitin, ceftriaxone, cefepime, trimethoprim, clarithromycin, chloromycetin, levofloxacin, streptomycin, kanamycin, tetracycline, vancomycin, and polymyxin B (NIFDC, China). Although *bcrA* was identified in the genome, bacitracin was not used because of high toxicity, while fosmidomycin (*rosA*) is still undergoing testing and was therefore also excluded. Quinupristin/dalfopristin, the targets of the *vatB* gene product are not used in China, and there is no corresponding antibiotic for *ykkC*. ZY-312 was cultivated anaerobically at 37°C for 48 h at a concentration of 10^7 cfu/mL with antibiotics at different concentrations. MIC was determined by measuring optical density at 600 nm (OD_{600}) with a microplate reader (SpectraMax, M2).

Acute Toxicity to Normal Mice and Nude Mice

To assess the acute toxicity of ZY-312, SPF BALB/c mice were randomly assigned into five groups ($n = 5$–8). Each group was administered with ZY-312 in a suspension containing 1×10^9, 5×10^{10}, or 5×10^{11} cfu/day, 0.5 mL/day culture supernatant, or 0.5 mL/day saline via oral gavage for 5 days. General condition and body weight were observed daily for 17–18 days. At the end of the experimental period, blood samples were obtained for hematological and serum biochemistry analyses. Stomach, colon, liver, and spleen were collected, weighed, and prepared for histopathological examination. Nude mice were orally administered with ZY-312 suspension at a dosage of 1×10^9 cfu/day for 3 days. General condition and bodyweight were observed for 7 days.

Genetic Stability

To explore whether genetic variation occurs in ZY-312 during *in vitro* passage, we continuously subcultured ZY-312 for 100 generations. Two parallel tubes were inoculated from an original culture of ZY-312 in TSB supplemented with 5% fetal bovine serum, and then incubated at 37°C in an anaerobic glove box (Bugbox, Ruskin) for 24 h. These initial cultures were designated A_0 and B_0. Subsequent passages were performed by inoculating 1% of each culture into fresh medium every 24 h, until A_{100} and B_{100} were obtained. Genetic variation was evaluated by complete genome sequencing of strains A_{10}, A_{25}, A_{50}, and A_{100}, and B_{10}, B_{25}, B_{50}, and B_{100}, and ANI was calculated for each generation. Morphological variations were observed by colony examination, Gram staining, and scanning electron microscopy (SEM) of A_{100} and B_{100}, with wild-type ZY-312 used for comparison. Growth of ZY-312, A_{100}, and B_{100} under anaerobic conditions was also examined over a 24-h period. Acute toxicity of A_{100} and B_{100} was detected in SPF mice at a dosage of 1×10^9 cfu/day for 3 days, with general condition and bodyweight observed for 7 days.

TABLE 2 | Physiological and biochemical properties of *B. fragilis* ZY-312.

	ZY-312	ATCC		ZY-312	ATCC
(A)					
Water	–	–	Dulcitol	–	–
N-Acetyl-D-galactosamine	+	+	D, L-α-Glycerol phosphate	–	–
N-Acetyl-D-glucosamine	/	+	*N*-Acetyl-β-D-mannosamine	–	–
D-Fructose	+	+	L-Fucose	–	–
Adonitol	–	–	D-Galactose	+	+
Amygdalin	+	+	D-Galacturonic acid	–	–
D-Arabitol	–	–	Gentiobiose	+	+
Arbutin	+	+	D-Gluconic acid	–	–
D-Cellobiose	+	+	D-Glucosaminic acid	–	–
α-Cyclodextrin	+	+	α-D-Glucose	+	+
β-Cyclodextrin	+	+	Glucose-1-phosphate	+	+
Dextrin	+	+	Glucose-6-phosphate	+	+
Glycerol	–	–	α-Methyl-D-galactoside	–	–
i-Erythritol	–	–	β-Methyl-D-galactoside	+	+
m-Inositol	–	–	α-Methyl-D-glucoside	–	–
α-D-Lactose	+	+	β-Methyl-D-glucoside	–	–
Lactulose	+	+	Palatinose	+	+
Maltose	+	+	D-Raffinose	+	+
Maltotriose	+	+	L-Rhamnose	–	–
D-Mannitol	–	–	Salicin	+	–
D-Mannose	+	+	D-Sorbitol	–	–
D-Melezitose	–	–	Stachyose	+	+
D-Melibiose	+	+	Sucrose	+	+
3-Methyl-D-glucose	+	+	D-Trehalose	–	–
Pyruvic acid methyl ester	+	+	D-Lactic acid methyl ester	–	–
Acetic acid	–	–	D-Malic acid	–	–
Formic acid	–	–	L-Malic acid	–	–
Fumaric acid	–	–	Propionic acid	–	–
Glyoxylic acid	–	–	Pyruvic acid	+	+
α-Hydroxybutyric acid	/	/	Turanose	+	+
β-Hydroxybutyric acid	–	–	D-Saccharic acid	–	–
Itaconic acid	–	–	Succinamic acid	–	–
α-Ketobutyric acid	+	+	Succinic acid	–	–
α-Ketovaleric acid	+	+	L-Asparagine	–	–
D,L-Lactic Acid	–	–	m-Tartaric acid	–	–
L-Lactic acid	–	–	Urocanic acid	–	–
L-Alaninamide	–	–	L-Methionine	–	–
L-Alanine	/	+	L-Phenylalanine	–	–
L-Alanyl-L-glutamine	+	/	L-Serine	–	–
L-Alanyl-L-histidine	/	/	L-Threonine	–	–
L-Alanyl-L-threonine	+	+	L-Valine	/	+
Succinic acid monomethyl ester	–	–	L-Valine plus L-aspartic acid	–	–
L-Glutamic acid	–	–	2′-Deoxy adenosine	+	+
L-Glutamine	–	–	Inosine	+	+
Glycyl-L-aspartic acid	+	+	Thymidine	+	+
Glycyl-L-glutamine	–	–	Uridine	+	+
Glycyl-L-methionine	–	–	Glycyl-L-proline	–	–
Thymidine-5′-monophosphate	–	–	Uridine-5′-monophosphate	–	/

	ZY-312	ATCC 25285
(B)		
Catalase assay	Positive	Positive
Gelatin liquefaction test	Weakly positive	Weakly positive
Hemolysis test	Negative	Negative
Dynamic test	Negative	Negative

TABLE 3 | Putative virulence-associated genes identified in the genome of *B. fragilis* ZY-312.

Gene ID	VFDB_ID	Name	Function
YDGL001582	VF0091	Alginate algl	Alginate O-acetyltransferase Algl
YDGL004163	VF0003	Capsule cap8E	Capsular polysaccharide synthesis enzyme Cap8E
YDGL004164	VF0003	Capsule cap8G	Capsular polysaccharide synthesis enzyme Cap8G
YDGL002547	VF0003	Capsule cap8M	Capsular polysaccharide synthesis enzyme Cap8M
YDGL002015	VF0003	Capsule cap8O	Capsular polysaccharide synthesis enzyme Cap8O
YDGL002539	VF0003	Capsule cap8O	Capsular polysaccharide synthesis enzyme Cap8O
YDGL002014	VF0144	Capsule cps4I	UDP-*N*-acetylglucosamine-2-epimerase
YDGL002540	VF0144	Capsule cps4I	UDP-*N*-acetylglucosamine-2-epimerase
YDGL001235	VF0274	Capsule cpsJ	Glycosyl transferase CpsJ(V)
YDGL004140	VF0323	Capsule fcl	Putative fucose syntheses
YDGL002177	VF0323	Capsule glf	UDP-galactopyranose mutase
YDGL001165	VF0072	ClpC clpC	Endopeptidase Clp
YDGL002866	VF0072	ClpC clpC	Endopeptidase Clp
YDGL002842	VF0074	ClpP clpP	ATP-dependent Clp protease
YDGL001133	VF0215	Dispersin aatC	AatC ATB binding protein of ABC transporter
YDGL003303	VF0215	Dispersin aatC	AatC ATB binding protein of ABC transporter
YDGL003305	VF0215	Dispersin aatC	AatC ATB binding protein of ABC transporter
YDGL003564	VF0215	Dispersin aatC	AatC ATB binding protein of ABC transporter
YDGL003567	VF0215	Dispersin aatC	AatC ATB binding protein of ABC transporter
YDGL004218	VF0215	Dispersin aatC	AatC ATB binding protein of ABC transporter
YDGL002299	VF0273	Flagella fleQ	Transcriptional regulator FleQ
YDGL002756	VF0334	HSI-I PA0073	ATP-binding component of ABC transporter
YDGL002122	VF0159	Hsp60 htpB	Hsp60, 60K heat shock protein HtpB
YDGL004141	VF0367	LPS gmd	GDP-mannose 4,6-dehydratase
YDGL001251	VF0106	MgtBC mgtB	Mg^{2+}transport protein
YDGL002018	VF0153	Mip mip	Macrophage infectivity potentiator (Mip)
YDGL003334	VF0298	MprAB mprA	MprB, sensor kinas. MprA, transcriptional factor
YDGL003892	VF0392	*O*-Antigen ddhA	Glucose-1-phosphate cytidylyltransferase
YDGL003891	VF0392	*O*-Antigen ddhB	CDP-glucose 4,6-dehydratase
YDGL003902	VF0392	*O*-Antigen galE	UDP-glucose 4-epimerase
YDGL003150	VF0319	PanC/PanD panD	panD
YDGL003842	VF0169	SodB sodB	Superoxide dismutase
YDGL003057	VF0101	Vi antigen tviB	Vi polysaccharide biosynthesis protein, UDP-glucose/GDP-mannose dehydrogenase

Experimental Replicates and Statistical Methods

All experiments were performed at least in triplicate using independent assays, and values were expressed as the mean ± standard error. An unpaired Student's *t*-test was performed to determine statistically significant differences in the acute toxicity assays. A *p*-value of <0.05 was considered statistically significant.

RESULTS

Morphological Characteristics

Strain ZY-312 only grew under anaerobic conditions (**Supplementary Figure S1**), with no growth observed under aerobic conditions or in 5% CO_2, implying it was an obligate anaerobe. Microbial contamination was excluded by culturing ZY-312 in different culture media under different conditions (**Supplementary Figure S2**). ZY-312 formed circular, low convex, semi-opaque colonies following anaerobic cultivation on blood agar plates (**Supplementary Figure S1**). Cells were Gram-negative, and shown to be rod shaped with rounded ends by scanning electrochemical microscopy (**Supplementary Figure S1**). This morphology matched the descriptions of *B. fragilis* in Bergey's manual (Krieg et al., 2001).

General Characteristics

The major fatty acids of ZY-312 were $C_{15:0}$ anteiso, $C_{15:0}$ iso, $C_{16:0}$, and $C_{16:0}$ 3-OH (**Supplementary Figure S3** and **Table 1A**). The major products in the culture supernatant of ZY-312 were lactic acid, acetic acid, succinic acid, propionic acid, and phenylacetic acid (**Table 1B**). ZY-312 and ATCC 25285 differed in their ability to metabolize L-valine, salicin, L-alanine, L-alanyl-L-glutamine, and *N*-acetyl-D-glucosamine (**Table 2A**). Both strains were positive for catalase activity, weakly positive for gelatin liquefaction, and negative for hemolytic activity and motility

TABLE 4 | Putative antibiotic resistance genes (A) identified in the genome of *Bacteroides fragilis* ZY-312, and minimum inhibitory concentration values (B) for each of the corresponding antibiotics.

Gene ID	Name	Drug
(A)		
YDGL002306	BcrA	Bacitracin
YDGL000449	BL2e_cepa	Cephalosporin
YDGL000258	dfrA22	Trimethoprim
YDGL003477	MefA	Macrolide
YDGL001150	MexF	Chloramphenicol, Fluoroquinolone
YDGL000604	MexY	Aminoglycoside, Glycylcycline
YDGL003440	RosA	Fosmidomycin
YDGL003171	tet37	Tetracycline
YDGL003704	VanRA	Vancomycin, Teicoplanin
YDGL003646	VatB	Streptogramin_A
YDGL000090	YkkC	na_antimicrobials
Antibiotic	**ZY-312**	**ATCC 25285**
(B)		
Cefoxitin	MIC = 2.0	MIC = 1.5
Ceftriaxone	MIC < 64	MIC < 64
Cefepime	MIC > 32	MIC > 32
Trimethoprim	MIC < 16	MIC < 16
Clarithromycin	MIC < 8	MIC < 8
Chloromycetin	MIC < 32	MIC < 32
Levofloxacin	MIC < 8	MIC < 8
Streptomycin	MIC > 1200	MIC > 1200
Kanamycin	MIC > 50	MIC > 50
Tetracycline	MIC < 16	MIC < 16
Vancomycin	4 < MIC < 8	4 < MIC < 8
Polymyxin B	MIC > 8	MIC > 8

Bacitracin was eliminated because of high toxicity. Fosmidomycin is still being researched and was therefore excluded. Quinupristin/dalfopristin are not available in China and were also excluded. No corresponding antibiotic exists for the ykkC gene product.

(**Table 2B**). The physiological and biochemical characteristics of ZY-312 were in accordance with *B. fragilis* as described in Bergey's manual (Krieg et al., 2001).

Genetic Characteristics

The phylogenetic trees generated from the whole genome sequence of ZY-312 and other *B. fragilis* strains are shown in **Supplementary Figures S5, S6**. ZY-312 and ATCC 25285 had an ANI of 99.99%. In total, 33 putative virulence factors (**Table 3**) and 11 antibiotic resistance genes (**Table 4A**) were annotated in the ZY-312 genome based on a minimum of 40% amino acid homology. The complete genome was 4,558,494 bp in length and contained on a single chromosome, with an average GC content of 43.08%, consistent with that of *B. fragilis* (41–44%) (Krieg et al., 2001). All drug-resistance genes were located on the chromosome rather than on plasmids.

Putative Virulence Factors

Through BLAST analysis of the VFDB, a total of 33 virulence factor homologs were identified in the genome of ZY-312 (**Table 3**). Most of these putative virulence genes encoded proteins involved in cellular structure or physiological activities, and none had previously been reported as being related to the pathogenesis of *B. fragilis*. Notably, *bft* was not present in the genome of ZY-312, indicating that it is a non-toxigenic strain.

Antibiotic Resistance

Antibiotic resistance tests were performed based on the antibiotic resistance genes identified in the genome of YZ-312 (**Table 4A**), and results are summarized in **Table 4B**. Based on guidelines for antibiotic resistance breakpoints (Russell and Sambrook, 2002; National Center for Clinical Laboratories, 2006), ZY-312 showed resistance to cefepime, kanamycin, and streptomycin, but was susceptible to ceftriaxone, trimethoprim, clarithromycin, chloramphenicol, tetracycline, and levofloxacin. Without available guidelines for *B. fragilis*, resistance of ZY-312 to vancomycin and polymyxin B could not be confirmed; however, we observed that 4–8 μg/mL vancomycin and >8 μg/mL polymyxin B were sufficient to inhibit ZY-312 growth *in vitro*.

ZY-312 Is Non-pathogenic in Both Normal and Immune-Deficient Mice

To confirm the *in vivo* safety of ZY-312, acute toxicity experiments were performed in both normal SPF BALB/c mice and nude mice. Lacking a thymus and an immune response, nude mice are an ideal animal model for evaluating probiotic safety. No death was observed in the BALB/c mice during the toxicity experiments, no treatment-related toxicity was observed, and no significant difference in body weight was noted between low, medium (**Supplementary Figure S4**), and high (**Figure 1A-1**) dose treatment groups and the control group, respectively. Similarly, no difference was found between the culture supernatant-treated group and the control group (**Figure 1A-2**). In addition, there was no obvious histopathological damage in the stomach, colon, liver, or spleen of BALB/c mice from the high dosage group (**Figure 1B**). There were also no significant differences in blood routine index or hepatorenal function between the high dose and control groups (data not shown). For the immune-deficient mouse toxicity experiments, ZY-312 again had no deleterious effects on body weight (**Figure 1A-3**).

ZY-312 Is Genetically and Phenotypically Stable

To explore whether ZY-312 undergoes major genomic rearrangements during passage, the stability of ZY-312 was examined after 100 generations *in vitro*. A_{100} and B_{100} were morphologically identical to the original ZY-312 strain (**Figure 2A**) based on visual inspection, optical microscopy, and SEM. The growth characteristics of A_{100} and B_{100} (**Figure 2B**) were not significantly different from those of ZY-312. Furthermore, following oral administration of A_{100} or B_{100} at a dose of 1×10^9 cfu/day for 3 days, mice did not show any clinical symptoms or weight loss during the observation period (**Figure 2C**). The calculated ANI values from each generation were at least 99.98% (**Figure 2D**).

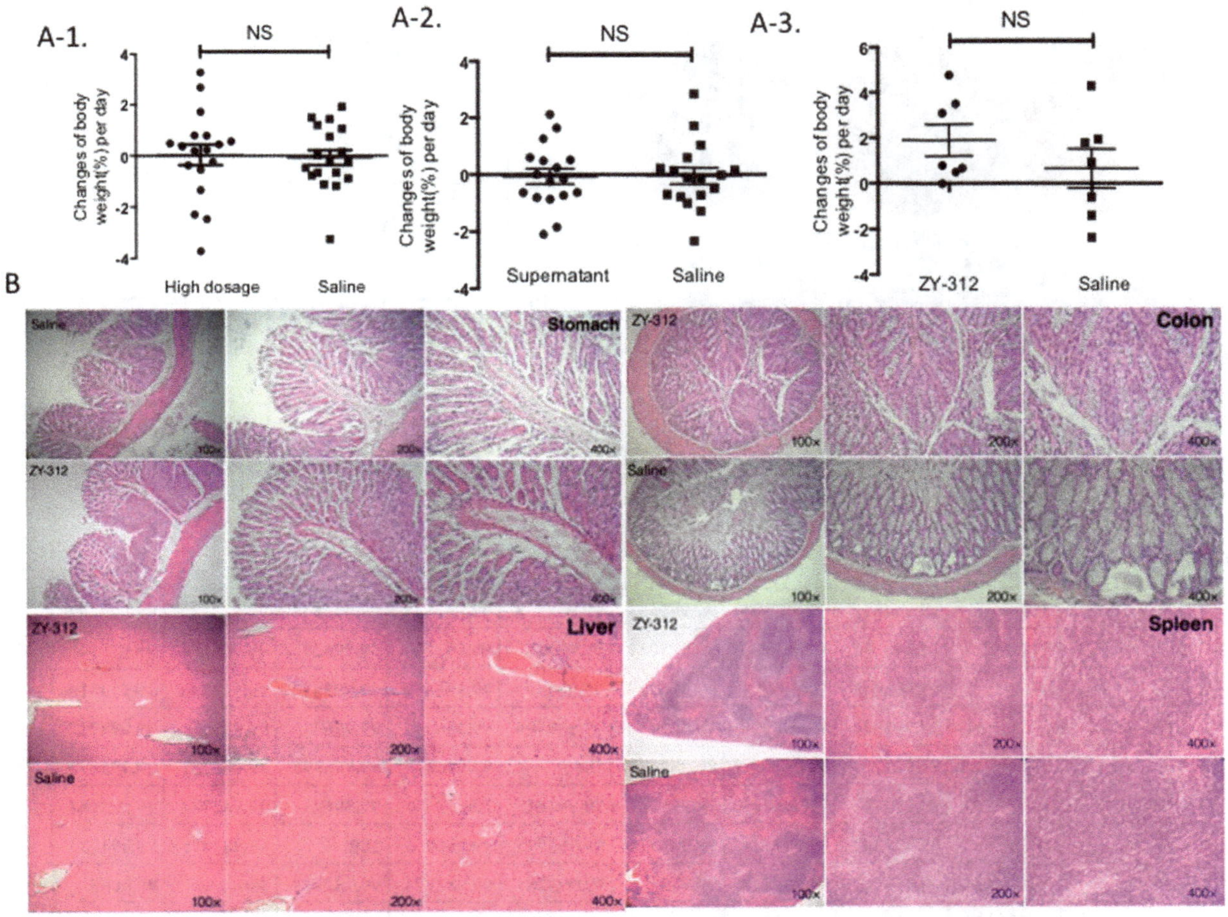

FIGURE 1 | ZY-312 is non-pathogenic in mice. (A) Changes in body weight (%) per day were observed for the experimental and control groups. **(A-1)** Specific pathogen-free (SPF) BALB/c normal mice (n = 8) were treated with 5 × 10^{11} colony forming units (cfu)/day ZY-312 for 5 days and observed for 18 days. A control group was treated with saline. **(A-2)** SPF normal mice (n = 16) were treated with culture supernatant (0.5 mL/day) for 5 days and observed for 17 days. Tryptic soy broth was used for the control group. **(A-3)** Nude mice (n = 5) were treated with ZY-312 at a concentration of 1 × 10^9 cfu/day for 3 days and observed for 7 days. The control group were treated with saline. **(B)** Light micrograph images of the stomach, colon, liver, and spleen from mice belonging to the high dosage group (upper) and control group (lower). No significant lesions were observed (mean ± SE; NS, not significant, t-test).

DISCUSSION

According the recent reports, non-toxic *B. fragilis* now is regarded as a commensal constituent with potential as a probiotic candidate (Hsiao et al., 2013), because of powerful immunoregulatory benefits and health-promoting effects it owns. Although *B. fragilis* makes up a very small part of the human intestinal flora, it plays a unique role in the maturation of the host immune system (Mazmanian et al., 2005; Troy and Kasper, 2010). Mono-colonization of mice with *B. fragilis* was sufficient to correct systemic immune defects in germ-free mice by stimulating maturation of splenic $CD4^+$ T cells (Mazmanian et al., 2005) and rebalancing the Th1/Th2 response. Furthermore, *B. fragilis* can direct an anti-inflammatory response, conferring protection in experimental mouse models of colitis (Mazmanian et al., 2008; Round and Mazmanian, 2010) and of autoimmune encephalomyelitis (Ochoa-Reparaz et al., 2010). Those observed effects were absent in mice treated with a *B. fragilis* PSA-deficient mutant strain. PSA is a dominant member of capsular polysaccharide complex (CPC) at the surface of *B. fragilis*, and contains a zwitterionic motif. *B. fragilis* is associated with clinical anaerobic infection and the CPC, especially PSA plays a key role in arising those diseases (Lindberg et al., 1982; Mazmanian and Kasper, 2006). Nevertheless, the role of PSA plays in intra-abdominal abscess probably is beneficial rather than harmful, since the inflammation aroused by PSA helps limit the spread of other gut bacteria and prevent more serious infection (Mazmanian and Kasper, 2006; Deng et al., 2016). Instead of being recognized as virulence factor, recently, PSA has been reconsidered as a symbiosis factor with health-promoting effect (Mazmanian et al., 2008).

Therefore, under overall considerations about the pros and cons, we believe non-toxic *B. fragilis* is a good choice for probiotic candidate and we decided to isolate a new strain of *B. fragilis* named ZY-312 (Deng et al., 2016) and explore its safety whether

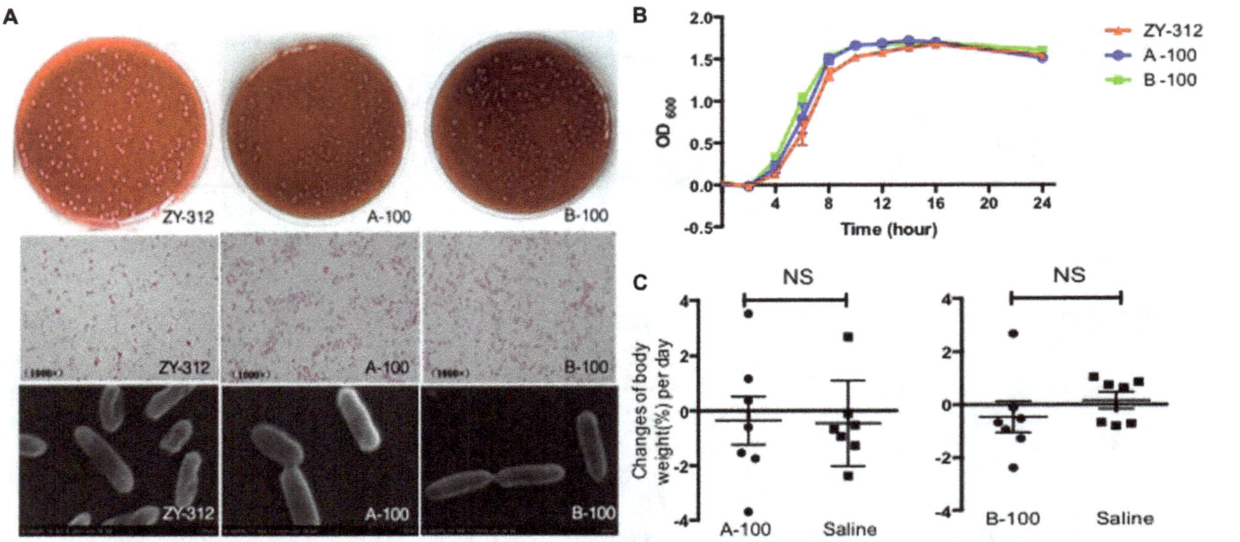

D

	ZY-312	A-10	A-25	A-50	A-100	B-10	B-25	B-50	B-100
ZY-312	100	99.994517	99.997925	99.997651	99.988078	99.995188	99.997648	99.982499	99.996197
A-10	99.994517	100	99.998043	99.998044	99.9892	99.99271	99.998292	99.983112	99.99616
A-25	99.997925	99.998043	100	99.996199	99.9868	99.996659	99.993624	99.979244	99.993318
A-50	99.997651	99.998044	99.996199	100	99.989406	99.996487	99.996375	99.9839	99.994727
A-100	99.988078	99.9892	99.9868	99.989406	100	99.996843	99.996995	99.993781	99.995896
B-10	99.995188	99.99271	99.996659	99.996487	99.996843	100	99.996933	99.982974	99.995984
B-25	99.997648	99.998292	99.993624	99.996375	99.996995	99.996933	100	99.982475	99.994383
B-50	99.982499	99.983112	99.979244	99.9839	99.993781	99.982974	99.982475	100	99.9955
B-100	99.996197	99.99616	99.993318	99.994727	99.995896	99.995984	99.994383	99.9955	100

FIGURE 2 | ZY-312 is genetically stable. (A) Gram-stained ZY-312, A_{100}, and B_{100} cells following anaerobic culture on tryptic soy agar (5% sheep blood) for 48 h at 37°C. Observation were made using a light microscope (4000×) and a scanning electron microscope (30000×). **(B)** Growth curves of ZY-312, A_{100}, and B_{100} cultured anaerobically for 24 h. **(C)** SPF BALB/c normal mice (n = 8) were treated with A_{100} or B_{100} at a concentration of 1×10^9 cfu/day for 3 days and observed for 7 days. A control group was treated with saline. **(D)** Average nucleotide identities were calculated between each generation.

satisfy the criteria required for probiotic bacteria. Although the health benefits of *B. fragilis* are generally recognized, much work still needs to be done to obtain certification of this species as a probiotic. Probiotics are defined as non-pathogenic live microorganisms that confer health benefits to the host when administered in adequate amounts (FAO/WHO, 2002). As living microorganisms with the potential for infection or *in situ* toxin production, probiotics should fulfill health and safety claims before entering the market. Safety assessment is the chief task for certifying a probiotic, as any adverse effects should be predicted in advance. Accordingly (FAO/WHO, 2002; Miquel et al., 2015), correct identification, sufficient characterization, and evaluation of potential risk and probiotic properties are integral for evaluation of a new probiotic.

Previously, we demonstrated that novel strain ZY-312, isolated from the feces of a healthy breast-fed infant, possessed similar morphological and growth characteristics to typical *B. fragilis* strains, as well as exhibiting desirable probiotic properties, including tolerance to air, simulated gastric fluid (pH 3.0), simulated intestinal fluid and ox bile (pH 6.8), adhesion, and *in vitro* safety in colon cells (Deng et al., 2016). Based on these results, we carried out a more thorough characterization and systemic evaluation of ZY-312 in the current study. As recommended (FAO/WHO, 2002), phenotypic testing, fatty acid analysis, metabolite production, biochemical activity, and *in vivo* toxicity testing, in combination with genetic analysis, taxonomic identification, and putative virulence and antibiotic resistance gene identification analysis, were performed to determine whether ZY-312 is safe for use as a probiotic. The major fatty acids and metabolic products of ZY-312 closely resemble descriptions of *B. fragilis* in Bergey's manual, as do the results of biochemical activity testing. Our previous work showed that the 16S rRNA sequence of ZY-312 was 99% identical to that of *B. fragilis* strain ATCC 28285. However, 16S rRNA sequence analysis has potential drawbacks for separating closely related species because of low taxonomic resolution. Whole genome sequencing identifies taxa with higher taxonomic resolution, and provides more information about gene function, such as putative virulence factors and antibiotic resistance genes (Rijkers et al., 2011; Miquel et al., 2015). Taking advantage of whole genome sequencing technology in the current study, we showed that ZY-312 and ATCC 25285 shared 99.99% ANI, and were derived from the same origin (**Supplementary Figure S5**), consistent with previous results. Furthermore, a total of 33 putative virulence factors and 11 antibiotic resistance genes were annotated in the genome of ZY-312 through comparative analysis with the VFDB and the ARDB, respectively. The putative virulence factors consisted of structural proteins and proteins with physiological activity, and none had previously been reported in association with the pathogenesis of *B. fragilis*. Because of the absence of *bft*, ZY-312 was identified as a NTBF strain.

There are many reports claiming probiotic safety based on an assessed lack of infectivity in normal animals (Bernardeau et al., 2002; Shokryazdan et al., 2016). However, confidence would be increased if assessment could be performed in immunodeficient animals (FAO/WHO, 2002). Therefore, we examined the safety of ZY-312 in both normal and immunodeficient mice. The SPF normal mice treated with high doses or supernatant of ZY-312 did not display any significant strain-related toxigenic symptoms, based on the assessment of body weight changes, histopathological examination, blood routine index, and hepatorenal function. Notably, ZY-312 also proved safe in nude mice (**Figure 1A-3**).

The FAO/WHO recommends that probiotic strains should be fully characterized, including determination of antibiotic resistance patterns, and should have no risk of transferring antibiotic resistance (FAO/WHO, 2002). Theoretically, consumption of probiotics with transferrable antibiotic resistance genes might lead to refractory infections if multiple antibiotic resistance genes are transferred to a pathogen (Borchers et al., 2009; Sanders et al., 2010). We demonstrated that there is no risk of ZY-312 spreading antibiotic resistance because all identified drug-resistance genes (**Table 4A**) were located in the chromosome rather than on a plasmid. Moreover, we verified the antibiotic resistance phenotype of ZY-312, and discovered that it is resistant to cefepime, kanamycin, and streptomycin, but susceptible to ceftriaxone, trimethoprim, clarithromycin, chloramphenicol, tetracycline, and levofloxacin. The MICs of vancomycin and polymyxin B for ZY-312 were also identified (**Table 4B**). The inconsistencies between genotype and observed phenotype might stem from the fact that putative antibiotic resistance genes were annotated based on 40% amino acid homology, meaning that some genes were incorrectly identified in the genome of ZY-312, and are likely not present.

As potential genetic variation might lead to unpredictable risk, genetic stability should also be confirmed prior to starting large-scale production of ZY-312-based probiotics (Sanders et al., 2010). We confirmed that following *in vitro* passage of 100 generations from the original strain of ZY-312, there was no significant difference between A_{100}, B_{100}, and the parental strain with respect to morphological characteristics and growth features. No *in vivo* toxicity was observed for A_{100} or B_{100}, and the ANI between each generation was at least 99.98%, demonstrating that ZY-312 has a high degree of genetic stability.

CONCLUSION

We confirmed that ZY-312 is a NTBF strain, without potential virulence factors or risk of spreading antibiotic resistance genes. As well as having desirable probiotic properties (Deng et al., 2016), ZY-312 has a high degree of genetic stability and is non-pathogenic, even to immune-deficient mice. Therefore, ZY-312 is most likely safe for use in future probiotic applications. This study supplements the initial safety assessment work already carried out for ZY-312, and contributes to the development of the first probiotic representative from the dominant Bacteroidetes phylum.

AUTHOR CONTRIBUTIONS

YW did the experiments with DNA and bacteria, analyzed data, and contributed to revising the manuscript; HD did the experiments with bacteria and mice, analyzed data, and wrote the manuscript; ZL did the experiments with mice, analyzed data, and contributed to revising the manuscript; YT, YH, XW, and ZD analyzed data; YL and RY designed the experiments and contributed to revising the manuscript; YjB designed experiments, analyzed data, and provided overall direction, YB and FZ provided overall directions and contributed to revising the manuscript.

ACKNOWLEDGMENTS

This work was supported by National High Technology Research and Development Program 863 (No. 2015AA020702) and Science and Technology Program of Guangdong, China (Nos. 2015A010101345 & 2016B090918064 & 2016A020217010).

SUPPLEMENTARY MATERIAL

FIGURE S1 | (A) Colonies of ZY-312 on tryptone soy agar (5% sheep blood) following culture in 5% CO_2 **(A-A)**, air **(A-B)**, or anaerobically **(A-C)** for 48 h at 37°C. **(B)** Cells observed under light microscope following Gram staining (4000×). **(C)** Cells observed under scanning electron microscope (5000×).

FIGURE S2 | Confirmation of no microbial contamination. (A) *Escherichia coli* and ZY-312 cultured on Eosin methylene blue agar for 24 h at 37°C. **(B)** *Salmonella enterica* serovar Paratyphi B and ZY-312 cultured on SS agar for 24 h at 37°C. **(C)** *Clostridium sporogenes* and ZY-312 cultured anaerobically on Columbia agar containing blood and gentamicin for 48 h at 37°C. **(D)** *Staphylococcus aureus* and ZY-312 cultured on mannitol sodium chloride agar for 24 h at 37°C. **(E)** *Pseudomonas aeruginosa* and ZY-312 cultured on NAC agar for 24 h at 37°C. **(F)** *Candida albicans* and ZY-312 cultured on Sabouraud dextrose agar for 72 h at 28°C. **(G)** *S. aureus* and ZY-312 cultured on agar agar for 48 h at 37°C. **(H)** *C. albicans* and ZY-312 cultured on rose bengal agar for 96 h at 28°C.

FIGURE S3 | The major fatty acids of ZY-312 as identified by gas chromatography.

FIGURE S4 | Acute toxicity of ZY-312 to mice. Changes in body weight (%) per day were observed for the experimental and control groups. (A) Specific pathogen-free (SPF) BALB/c normal mice ($n = 5$) were treated with ZY-312 at a concentration of 1×10^9 cfu/day for 5 days and observed for 15 days. The control group mice were treated with saline. **(B)** SPF normal mice ($n = 5$) were treated with ZY-312 at a concentration of 5×10^{10} cfu/day for 5 days and observed for 18 days. Tryptic soy broth was used to treat the control group. No significant weight loss was observed in any of the animals (mean ± SE; NS, not significant, *t*-test).

FIGURE S5 | Phylogenetic tree based on complete shotgun sequences showing the relationship between *Bacteroides fragilis* ZY-312 and closely related species. The tree was constructed using the neighbor-joining method.

FIGURE S6 | Phylogenetic tree based on complete genome sequences showing the relationship between *B. fragilis* strain ZY-312, *B. fragilis* NCTC 9343, *B. fragilis* YCH46, and *B. fragilis* 638R. The tree was constructed using the neighbor-joining method.

REFERENCES

Althani, A. A., Marei, H. E., Hamdi, W. S., Nasrallah, G. K., El Zowalaty, M. E., Al Khodor, S., et al. (2016). Human microbiome and its association with health and diseases. *J. Cell. Physiol.* 231, 1688–1694. doi: 10.1002/jcp.25284

Bernardeau, M., Vernoux, J. P., and Gueguen, M. (2002). Safety and efficacy of probiotic lactobacilli in promoting growth in post-weaning Swiss mice. *Int. J. Food Microbiol.* 77, 19–27.

Borchers, A. T., Selmi, C., Meyers, F. J., Keen, C. L., and Gershwin, M. E. (2009). Probiotics and immunity. *J. Gastroenterol.* 44, 26–46. doi: 10.1007/s00535-008-2296-0

Chen, L., Yang, J., Yu, J., Yao, Z., Sun, L., Shen, Y., et al. (2005). VFDB: a reference database for bacterial virulence factors. *Nucleic Acids Res.* 33, D325–D328. doi: 10.1093/nar/gki008

Cui, Y., Yu, C., Yan, Y., Li, D., Li, Y., Jombart, T., et al. (2013). Historical variations in mutation rate in an epidemic pathogen, *Yersinia pestis*. *Proc. Natl. Acad. Sci. U.S.A.* 110, 577–582. doi: 10.1073/pnas.1205750110

Deng, H., Li, Z., Tan, Y., Guo, Z., Liu, Y., Wang, Y., et al. (2016). A novel strain of *Bacteroides fragilis* enhances phagocytosis and polarises M1 macrophages. *Sci. Rep.* 6:29401. doi: 10.1038/srep29401

FAO/WHO (2002). *Guidelines for the Evaluation of Probiotics in Food: Joint FAO/WHO Working Group on Drafting Guidelines for the Evaluation of Probiotics in Food.* Geneva: World Health Organization.

Fernandez, M. F., Boris, S., and Barbes, C. (2005). Safety evaluation of *Lactobacillus delbrueckii* subsp. *lactis* UO 004, a probiotic bacterium. *Res. Microbiol.* 156, 154–160. doi: 10.1016/j.resmic.2004.09.006

Fijan, S. (2014). Microorganisms with claimed probiotic properties: an overview of recent literature. *Int. J. Environ. Res. Public Health* 11, 4745–4767. doi: 10.3390/ijerph110504745

Foligne, B., Daniel, C., and Pot, B. (2013). Probiotics from research to market: the possibilities, risks and challenges. *Curr. Opin. Microbiol.* 16, 284–292. doi: 10.1016/j.mib.2013.06.008

Hsiao, E. Y., McBride, S. W., Hsien, S., Sharon, G., Hyde, E. R., McCue, T., et al. (2013). Microbiota modulate behavioral and physiological abnormalities associated with neurodevelopmental disorders. *Cell* 155, 1451–1463. doi: 10.1016/j.cell.2013.11.024

Krieg, N. R., Ludwig, W., Euzéby, J., and Whitman, W. B. (2001). *Bergey's Manual of Systematic Bacteriology*, 2nd Edn, Vol. 1. New York, NY: Springer.

Lindberg, A. A., Weintraub, A., Kasper, D. L., and Lonngren, J. (1982). Virulence factors in infections with *Bacteroides fragilis*: isolation and characterization of capsular polysaccharide and lipopolysaccharide. *Scand. J. Infect. Dis. Suppl.* 35, 45–52.

Liu, B., and Pop, M. (2009). ARDB–antibiotic resistance genes database. *Nucleic Acids Res.* 37, D443–D447. doi: 10.1093/nar/gkn656

Luo, R., Liu, B., Xie, Y., Li, Z., Huang, W., Yuan, J., et al. (2012). SOAPdenovo2: an empirically improved memory-efficient short-read de novo assembler. *Gigascience* 1:18. doi: 10.1186/2047-217X-1-18

Mazmanian, S. K., and Kasper, D. L. (2006). The love-hate relationship between bacterial polysaccharides and the host immune system. *Nat. Rev. Immunol.* 6, 849–858. doi: 10.1038/nri1956

Mazmanian, S. K., Liu, C. H., Tzianabos, A. O., and Kasper, D. L. (2005). An immunomodulatory molecule of symbiotic bacteria directs maturation of the host immune system. *Cell* 122, 107–118. doi: 10.1016/j.cell.2005.05.007

Mazmanian, S. K., Round, J. L., and Kasper, D. L. (2008). A microbial symbiosis factor prevents intestinal inflammatory disease. *Nature* 453, 620–625. doi: 10.1038/nature07008

McKenney, P. T., and Pamer, E. G. (2015). From hype to hope: the gut microbiota in enteric infectious disease. *Cell* 163, 1326–1332. doi: 10.1016/j.cell.2015.11.032

Miquel, S., Beaumont, M., Martin, R., Langella, P., Braesco, V., and Thomas, M. (2015). A proposed framework for an appropriate evaluation scheme for microorganisms as novel foods with a health claim in Europe. *Microb. Cell Fact.* 14:48. doi: 10.1186/s12934-015-0229-1

National Center for Clinical Laboratories (2006). *The National Clinical Test Regulation of Operation*, 3rd Edn. Nanjing: Southeast University Press.

Ochoa-Reparaz, J., Mielcarz, D. W., Ditrio, L. E., Burroughs, A. R., Begum-Haque, S., Dasgupta, S., et al. (2010). Central nervous system demyelinating disease protection by the human commensal *Bacteroides fragilis* depends on polysaccharide A expression. *J. Immunol.* 185, 4101–4108. doi: 10.4049/jimmunol.1001443

Rijkers, G. T., de Vos, W. M., Brummer, R. J., Morelli, L., Corthier, G., and Marteau, P. (2011). Health benefits and health claims of probiotics: bridging science and marketing. *Br. J. Nutr.* 106, 1291–1296. doi: 10.1017/S000711451100287X

Round, J. L., and Mazmanian, S. K. (2010). Inducible Foxp3+ regulatory T-cell development by a commensal bacterium of the intestinal microbiota. *Proc. Natl. Acad. Sci. U.S.A.* 107, 12204–12209. doi: 10.1073/pnas.0909122107

Russell, D. W., and Sambrook, J. (2002). *Molecular Cloning*. Beijing: Science Press.

Sanders, M. E., Akkermans, L. M., Haller, D., Hammerman, C., Heimbach, J., Hormannsperger, G., et al. (2010). Safety assessment of probiotics for human use. *Gut Microbes* 1, 164–185. doi: 10.4161/gmic.1.3.12127

Sekirov, I., Russell, S. L., Antunes, L. C., and Finlay, B. B. (2010). Gut microbiota in health and disease. *Physiol. Rev.* 90, 859–904. doi: 10.1152/physrev.00045.2009

Shokryazdan, P., Faseleh Jahromi, M., Liang, J. B., Kalavathy, R., Sieo, C. C., and Ho, Y. W. (2016). Safety assessment of two new *Lactobacillus* strains as probiotic for human using a rat model. *PLoS ONE* 11:e0159851. doi: 10.1371/journal.pone.0159851

Tan, Y., Wu, M., Liu, H., Dong, X., Guo, Z., Song, Z., et al. (2010). Cellular fatty acids as chemical markers for differentiation of *Yersinia pestis* and *Yersinia pseudotuberculosis*. *Lett. Appl. Microbiol.* 50, 104–111. doi: 10.1111/j.1472-765X.2009.02762.x

Troy, E. B., and Kasper, D. L. (2010). Beneficial effects of *Bacteroides fragilis* polysaccharides on the immune system. *Front. Biosci. (Landmark Ed.)* 15, 25–34.

Xu, T., Yu, M., Lin, H., Zhang, Z., Liu, J., and Zhang, X. H. (2015). Genomic insight into *Aquimarina longa* SW024^T: its ultra-oligotrophic adapting mechanisms and biogeochemical functions. *BMC Genomics* 16:772. doi: 10.1186/s12864-015-2005-3

5

Characterization of Bile Salt Hydrolase from *Lactobacillus gasseri* FR4 and Demonstration of its Substrate Specificity and Inhibitory Mechanism Using Molecular Docking Analysis

*Rizwana Parveen Rani[1], Marimuthu Anandharaj[2] and Abraham David Ravindran[1]**

[1] Department of Biology, The Gandhigram Rural Institute – Deemed University, Gandhigram, India, [2] Biodiversity Research Center, Academia Sinica, Taipei, Taiwan

Correspondence:
Abraham David Ravindran
david_gribiology@rediffmail.com

Probiotic bacteria are beneficial to the health of poultry animals, thus are used as alternative candidates for antibiotics used as growth promoters (AGPs). However, they also reduce the body weight gain due to innate bile salt hydrolase (BSH) activity. Hence, the addition of a suitable BSH inhibitor along with the probiotic feed can decrease the BSH activity. In this study, a BSH gene (981 bp) encoding 326-amino acids was identified from the genome of *Lactobacillus gasseri* FR4 (*Lg*BSH). The *Lg*BSH-encoding gene was cloned and purified using an *Escherichia coli* BL21 (DE3) expression system, and its molecular weight (37 kDa) was confirmed by SDS–PAGE and a Western blot analysis. *Lg*BSH exhibited greater hydrolysis toward glyco-conjugated bile salts compared to tauro-conjugated bile salts. *Lg*BSH displayed optimal activity at 52°C at a pH of 5.5, and activity was further increased by several reducing agents (DTT), surfactants (Triton X-100 and Tween 80), and organic solvents (isopropanol, butanol, and acetone). Riboflavin and penicillin V, respectively, inhibited *Lg*BSH activity by 98.31 and 97.84%. A homology model of *Lg*BSH was predicted using *Ef*BSH (4WL3) as a template. Molecular docking analysis revealed that the glycocholic acid had lowest binding energy of −8.46 kcal/mol; on the other hand, inhibitors, i.e., riboflavin and penicillin V, had relatively higher binding energies of −6.25 and −7.38 kcal/mol, respectively. Our results suggest that *L. gasseri* FR4 along with riboflavin might be a potential alternative to AGPs for poultry animals.

Keywords: bile salt hydrolase, *Lactobacillus gasseri* FR4, antibiotics used as growth promoters, homology modeling, docking analysis

INTRODUCTION

In recent years, probiotics have been considered as alternative candidates for antibiotics used as growth promoters (AGPs). Basically, AGPs are group of antibiotics (i.e., bambermycin, lincomycin, tylosin, etc.) used in animal feed at sub-therapeutic levels to improve the growth performance and average body mass gain of food animals (Wang et al., 2012). However, negative impacts of AGPs include the emergence of antibiotic-resistant bacteria which may be transmitted to humans and cause food safety threats and public health issues (Marshall and Levy, 2011; Lin, 2014). European Union member countries have banned use of all AGPs for food animals (Marshall and Levy, 2011). However, banning AGPs has severely affected the health and productivity of poultry animals in several countries (Casewell et al., 2003). Hence, the use of probiotics has emerged as an alternative for AGPs and several health-promoting effects were observed (Lin, 2011). Although probiotic feed supplements improve the growth performance of poultry animals, substantial losses or no significant increases in body weight were observed in probiotic (especially *Lactobacillus* strains) treated animals (Million et al., 2012; Angelakis et al., 2013). This is due to the production of higher amounts of bile salt hydrolase (BSH) enzymes. Generally, BSH activity is considered as a functional probiotic biomarker due to its health-protective effects (i.e., cholesterol reduction, bile tolerance, antimicrobial activity, etc.) (Miremadi et al., 2014). BSH activities may contribute to microbial bile resistance, colonization of the gastrointestinal tract (GIT), host metabolism and energy harvest (Begley et al., 2006; Lin et al., 2014). Probiotic microorganisms have the ability to transform bile salts to a great extent through a bile salt deconjugation mechanism. Bile salts are synthesized from cholesterol, conjugated with glycine or taurine in the liver, stored in the gall bladder and secreted into the small intestine (Kim and Lee, 2005). Bile salts play a significant role in lipid digestion and act as a biological detergent (Hofmann and Eckmann, 2006). The BSH enzyme has the ability to hydrolyze conjugated bile salts into a deconjugated form and release free amino acids. Deconjugated bile salts are much less soluble, hence are not absorbed by intestinal cells and are excreted in feces. This mechanism results in higher utilization of cholesterol for the *de novo* synthesis of bile acids, thereby lowering the serum cholesterol levels (Begley et al., 2006).

To be used as an alternative for AGPs, BSH activities of probiotic bacteria should be inhibited by a specific inhibitor, which could be supplemented along with the probiotic feed. This will dramatically decrease the BSH activity and increase fat deposition in poultry animals (Joyce and Gahan, 2014). Recently several researchers have identified potential BSH inhibitors including gossypetin, caffeic acid phenethyl ester (CAPE), epicatechin monogallate, riboflavin and demonstrated the inhibition of BSH enzyme activity (Lin et al., 2014; Smith et al., 2014). However, BSHs of different microorganism have different protein structures and substrate specificities. Identification of potential BSH inhibitors relies on the availability of defined crystal structures of BSH enzymes (Smith et al., 2014). Hence modern computational strategies, such as homology modeling and molecular docking studies can be used to identify safe, potent and cost-effective BSH inhibitors using *in silico* analysis. The identified novel BSH inhibitors can then be used alongside BSH-positive probiotic microorganisms to decrease host fat digestion in food animals and in turn enhance the profitability of feed-additive industries (Knarreborg et al., 2004; Wang et al., 2012; Lin, 2014). In our previous study, a probiotic *Lactobacillus gasseri* FR4 from the GIT of free-range chickens (*Gallus gallus* subsp. *domesticus*) was isolated and efficiently hydrolyzed taurodeoxycholate (TDC) to deoxycholate on de Man Rogosa Sharpe (MRS)-TDC agar plate (Parveen Rani et al., 2016). We hypothesize that this hydrolysis activity is due to the production of a BSH enzyme. To use this probiotic bacteria as an alternative for AGPs, this BSH enzyme activity should be inhibited. Therefore, we sought to find a potential candidate to inhibit BSH activity.

In this study, we have identified a gene responsible for BSH activity of the probiotic *L. gasseri* FR4, which was cloned and the enzyme overexpressed, purified and characterized. Several compounds were screened to identify a potential BSH inhibitors and riboflavin exhibited higher percentage of inhibition. The protein structure of newly identified BSH enzyme was modeled using homology modeling. Molecular docking analysis was performed to identify the substrate specificity and inhibitory mechanism of identified inhibitors.

MATERIALS AND METHODS

Bacterial Strains and Plasmids

The probiotic *L. gasseri* FR4 was previously isolated from the GIT of free-range chickens (Parveen Rani et al., 2016). The strain was routinely subcultured in MRS media at 37°C under anaerobic conditions. *Escherichia coli* DH5α and BL21 (DE3) strains were, respectively, used for the cloning and expression of the BSH enzyme. The *E. coli* expression vector, pET21b (+), was used for expression of His-tagged (6x) recombinant BSH. The cloning and expression hosts were maintained in Luria-Bertani (LB) broth supplemented with ampicillin (100 μg/ml) at 37°C under aerobic conditions.

Identification of the BSH Gene

To identify the putative BSH gene, we mined the available whole-genome sequence of *L. gasseri* ATCC 33323 = JCM 1131 (NC_008530.1) using the Basic Local Alignment Search Tool (BLAST) algorithm from the National Center for Biotechnology Information (NCBI)[1]. The putative BSH gene was aligned with other bacterial BSHs using the Clustal omega multiple sequence alignment tool[2], and the secondary structure was predicted using ESpript 3.0[3] (Robert and Gouet, 2014). The phylogenetic relationship of the identified putative BSH of *L. gasseri* FR4 was confirmed by an unweighted pair group method with arithmetic mean (UPGMA) phylogenetic tree using MEGA6 software (Tamura et al., 2013).

Genomic DNA Extraction and Cloning of the BSH Gene

Genomic DNA of *L. gasseri* FR4 was extracted using a DNeasy Blood & Tissue Kits (Qiagen, Germany) according to the manufacturer's instructions. The putative BSH gene (975 bp) was amplified from the purified genomic DNA using *Lg*BSH-F

[1] http://www.ncbi.nlm.nih.gov/

[2] http://www.ebi.ac.uk/Tools/msa/clustalo/

[3] http://espript.ibcp.fr/ESPript/ESPript/

(5′-gcgGGATCCTGTACCTCAATTATTT-3′) and *Lg*BSH-R (5′-gagCTCGAGATTTTGATAGTTAATATG-3′) primer pairs, respectively, flanked with *Bam*HI and *Xho*I (the underlined sequences) (Supplementary Figure S1). The amplified polymerase chain reaction (PCR) product was purified using a QIAquick PCR purification kit (Qiagen, Germany). pET21b (+) vector DNA and the amplified *Lg*BSH-encoding gene were digested with *Bam*HI and *Xho*I (New England Biolabs), resolved in a 1% agarose gel, extracted from the gel and ligated using T4 DNA ligase (ThermoFisher Scientific). The resulting plasmid was transformed into *E. coli* DH5α-competent cells and plated on LB agar plates with ampicillin (100 μg/ml). The plasmid was extracted and sequenced using T7-F and T7-R universal primers and no mutations in the coding sequence of *Lg*BSH-encoding gene were detected (Supplementary Figure S2).

Expression and Purification of Recombinant *Lg*BSH

To express the recombinant *Lg*BSH, the pET21b-BSH plasmid was purified from *E. coli* DH5α and transformed into the expression host *E. coli* BL21 (DE3). Protein expression and purification was performed as described in Kumar et al. (2013). Briefly, *E. coli* BL21 (DE3) cells harboring the pET21b-BSH plasmid were cultured overnight and cells with an optical density (OD) of 0.15 were inoculated into 50 ml of LB broth with ampicillin. When the culture reached 0.6 OD, 500 μl of 100 mM isopropyl-β-d-thiogalactopyranoside (IPTG) was added and incubated for 3 h to allow protein expression. Then, centrifugation was performed at 8000 rpm for 10 min at 4°C. Cells were resuspended in lysis buffer containing 50 mM Tris-HCl (pH 7.5), 100 mM NaCl, 1 mM dithiothreitol (DTT), and 1x SIGMAFAST™ protease inhibitor cocktail (Sigma-Aldrich, St. Louis, MO, United States). Then, sonication was performed at six cycles of 20 s on/off with a 60% amplitude and 50% duty cycle on ice using a 3-mm probe (Sonics Vibracell-VCX130, United States). Sonicated cells were centrifuged at 8000 rpm for 10 min (at 4°C) and the cell pellets and lysate were separated. *Lg*BSH from the cell lysate was purified using a Ni^{2+}-NTA agarose column, and the purity was analyzed using 12% (wt/vol) sodium dodecylsulfate (SDS)–polyacrylamide gel electrophoresis (PAGE). The molecular weight of purified *Lg*BSH was further confirmed by a Western blot analysis, using a primary antibody against His-Tag (1:5000) and a horseradish peroxidase (HRP)-conjugated anti-mouse secondary antibody (1:10000). The protein concentration was estimated using the Bradford method (Protein Assay Kit, Bio-Rad).

BSH Activity

Bile salt hydrolase activity was measured by the method described in Wang et al. (2012) with some modifications. Briefly, a 200-μl reaction mixture containing 178 μl of sodium-phosphate buffer (0.1 M, pH 6.0), 10 μl of purified recombinant *Lg*BSH, 2 μl of 1 M DTT, and 10 μl of 100 mM conjugated bile acid were mixed and incubated 37°C for 30 min. The reaction was terminated by mixing of 50 μl of the reaction mixture with an equal volume of 15% (w/v) trichloroacetic acid, and subsequently the precipitates were removed by centrifugation at 13,000 × *g* for 10 min. To estimate concentrations of the liberated amino acids (glycine or taurine) from the conjugated bile acids, 50 μl of the above supernatant was mixed with 950 μl of Ninhydrin reagent and 100 μl of sodium-citrate buffer (0.5 M, pH 5.5). The mixture was kept in a water bath for 15 min and cooled in ice. Absorbance was measured at 570 nm and the amino acid concentration was estimated using a standard curve of either glycine or taurine based on the conjugated bile salts used. The enzyme activity was expressed as micromoles of amino acid released per minute per milligram of BSH. All experiments were performed in triplicate.

Biochemical Characterization of *Lg*BSH

Substrate Specificity of *Lg*BSH

The substrate specificity of purified recombinant *Lg*BSH was determined using different glyco- or tauro-conjugated bile salts [glycocholic acid (GCA), glycodeoxycholic acid (GDCA), taurocholic acid (TCA), and taurodeoxycholic acid (TDCA)] as well as non-substrate compounds (penicillin V and ampicillin) as a substrate. The assay was performed as described above.

Effect of pH and Temperature on *Lg*BSH Activity

To identity the optimum temperature for *Lg*BSH activity, a standard reaction mixture (200 μl) was incubated at different temperature ranges (20–90°C). Similarly, a suitable pH was optimized by performing the enzyme assay at various pH values (pH 3–9). The pH was adjusted by replacing the buffer in the reaction mixture, i.e., sodium acetate buffer (pH 3–6), phosphate buffer (pH 7), and glycine-NaOH buffer (pH 8 and 9). Each experiment was performed in triplicate.

Effects of Reducing Agents, Surfactants, Solvents, and Enzymes on *Lg*BSH Activity

The effects of various reducing agents (DTT, β-ME, and EDTA; 10 mM each), surfactants (Triton X-100 and SDS; 10 mM each and 0.5% Tween 80), and solvents (chloroform, ethanol, acetone, methanol, isopropanol, and butanol; 10% v/v each) on *Lg*BSH activity were demonstrated. Briefly, 200 μl of the reaction mixture was separately added to various reducing agents, surfactants, and solvents and incubated for 30 min at 25°C. After incubation, an enzyme assay was performed using GCA as a substrate, and each experiment was performed in triplicate.

The effects of different enzymes (i.e., lysozyme, proteinase K, pepsin, α-amylase, lipase, and catalase) on *Lg*BSH activity were studied. The reaction mixture (200 μl) was treated with 2 mg/ml of each enzyme and incubated for 30 min at 25°C. The enzyme activity was evaluated after incubation as described earlier and untreated *Lg*BSH served as a control. Each experiment was performed in triplicate.

Inhibitory Effects of Feed Additives on *Lg*BSH Activity

To identify suitable candidates for a BSH inhibitor, various commonly used animal feed additives were screened, which including metal ions, AGPs, and other recently identified BSH inhibitors. *Lg*BSH was pre-incubated with various metal ions (i.e., $CuCl_2$, $CuSO_4$, $MnCl_2$, $MnSO_4$, $MgCl_2$, $MgSO_4$, $ZnCl_2$, $ZnSO_4$, $CaCl_2$, $NaHIO_3$, and KIO_3) at a concentration of 5 mM for 30 min at 37°C (Wang et al., 2012). Similarly, AGPs, including penicillin V, ampicillin, oxytetracycline, doxycycline hydrochloride, neomycin, erythromycin, and lincomycin, were used at a concentration of 5 mM (Wang et al., 2012; Smith et al., 2014). Apart from these feed additives, several other compounds were also recently screened as BSH inhibitors which included riboflavin (Smith et al., 2014) and ascorbic acid; hence we also tested their inhibitory efficiencies against *Lg*BSH at the concentration of 5 mM. The inhibitory efficiency of inhibitors on *Lg*BSH activity was tested and calculated by dividing the mean activity of the control (without inhibitor) by the treatment group (with inhibitor).

Homology Modeling of *Lg*BSH

To determine the 3D structure of *Lg*BSH, the protein sequence was blasted against the protein data bank (PDB) database. The online software, Protein Homology/analogY Recognition Engine V 2.0[4] (Phyre2), was used to predict the homologous structure of *Lg*BSH using the intensive mode (Kelley et al., 2015). Bumps were removed from the modeled protein and missing side chain atoms were added using the 'WHAT IF Web Interface.'[5] The predicted protein structure was validated using protein structure validation (PSVS) tool[6]. Ramachandran plot was used to analyze the structure quality. The modeled *Lg*BSH protein structures were visualized, and images were rendered using UCSF-Chimera software (Pettersen et al., 2004). Residues involved in substrate binding were identified using the computed atlas of the surface topography of proteins (CASTP) (Dundas et al., 2006) and the SiteHound-web server[7] (Hernandez et al., 2009). Then, predicted residues were compared with the templates. These residues were used to predict putative binding sites for ligands during the docking analysis.

Docking Analysis

To perform the molecular docking studies, SwissDock, a small protein molecule docking web service based on EADock DSS (Fast docking using the CHARMM force field with EADock DSS) was used (Grosdidier et al., 2011). Ligands including GCA ($C_{26}H_{43}NO_6$), GDCA ($C_{26}H_{43}NO_5$), TCA ($C_{26}H_{45}NO_7S$), penicillin V (PenV: $C_{16}H_{18}N_2O_5S$), and riboflavin ($C_{17}H_{20}N_4O_6$) were obtained from the ZINC database[8] and were used in the docking analysis. Ligand structures are shown in Supplementary Figure S3. The root mean square deviation (RMSD) was used to identify the best docked complexes. The predicted docking clusters were analyzed using UCSF-Chimera.

[4]http://www.sbg.bio.ic.ac.uk/phyre2

[5]http://swift.cmbi.ru.nl/servers/html/index.html

[6]http://psvs-1_5-dev.nesg.org

[7]http://sitehound.sanchezlab.org

[8]http://zinc.docking.org/

RESULTS

Identification of the BSH Gene from *L. gasseri* FR4

In our previous study, BSH activity of *L. gasseri* FR4 was demonstrated using a direct plate assay method which exhibited halos of precipitated deoxycholate on MRS-TDC agar due to the hydrolysis of TDC (Parveen Rani et al., 2016). Based on the BLAST results, a putative BSH gene (981 bp) encoding a 326-amino acid (aa) choloylglycine hydrolase family (EC 3.5.1.24) protein was identified from the genome of *L. gasseri* (NC_008530.1). The theoretical molecular weight and isoelectric point of the putative BSH were, respectively, estimated to be 36.69 kDa and 5.18 using the ExPASy analysis tool[9]. The deduced amino acid sequence of the putative *Lg*BSH was aligned with amino acid sequences of available BSH crystal structure sequences from different bacterial species. *Lg*BSH shared a sequence identity of 54% with *Enterococcus faecalis* BSH (*Ef*BSH; 4WL3), 47% with *L. salivarius* BSH (*Ls*BSH; 5HKE), 38% with *Clostridium perfringens* BSH (*Cp*BSH; 2RLC), and 37% with *Bifidobacterium longum* BSH (*Bl*BSH; 2HEZ). *Lg*BSH also shared the lowest identity of 30% with penicillin V acylase (PVA) of *Lysinibacillus sphaericus* (2PVA), since though both enzymes belong to the choloylglycine hydrolase family.

The multiple sequence alignment results revealed similarities of conserved amino acid residues among all of the selected BSHs, which included a catalytic nucleophile residue, Cys1, and other conserved amino acids, such as Arg16, Asp19, Asn79, Asn171, and Arg224 (amino acids were numbered from cysteine) (**Figure 1**). Rossocha et al. (2005), Kumar et al. (2006), and Xu et al. (2016) reported that Cys1 plays an important role in the activity of BSH. This further confirmed that the identified gene belonged to BSH.

The evolutionary relationship of *Lg*BSH with other bacterial choloylglycine hydrolase family proteins (BSH/PVA) was inferred using a UPGMA phylogenetic analysis. Evolutionary distances were computed using the Poisson correction method and are in units of the number of amino acid substitutions per site. The analysis involved 37 aa sequences of BSH and PVA from various bacterial taxa. All positions containing gaps and missing data were eliminated. There were 266 positions in total in the final dataset. The phylogenetic tree showed that BSHs of *Lactobacillus* spp. were distinct from the PVA, which has an evolutionary relationship with BSH. *Lg*BSH was closely related to BSHs of *E. faecalis, C. perfringens,* and *L. salivarius* (Supplementary Figure S4).

Expression and Purification of Recombinant *Lg*BSH

The expression vector pET21b (+) harboring the *Lg*BSH-encoding gene was transformed into *E. coli* BL21 (DE3) to overexpress *Lg*BSH. A recombinant *Lg*BSH protein band was observed after IPTG induction on SDS–PAGE at

[9]http://web.expasy.org/compute_pi

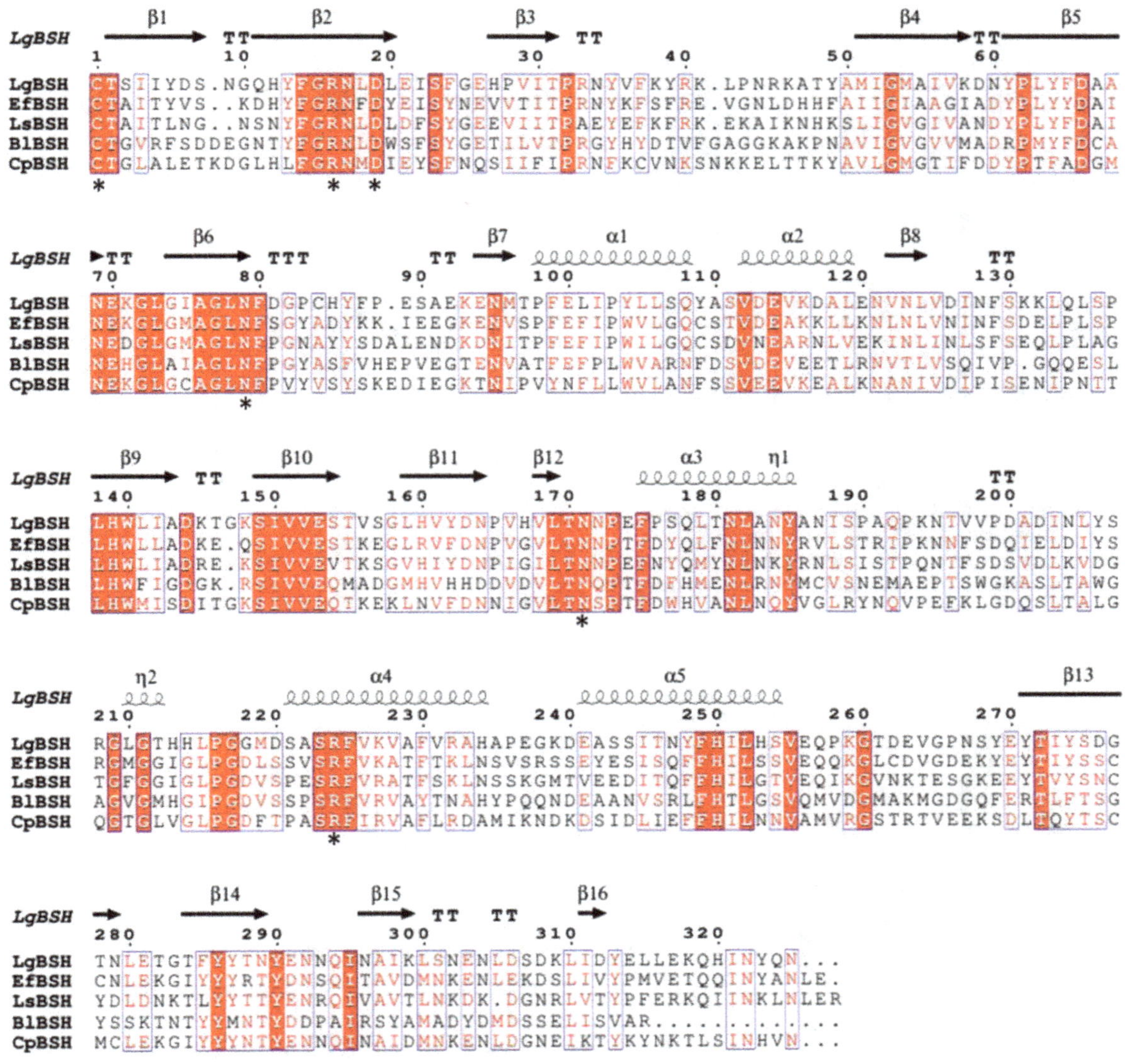

FIGURE 1 | Multiple sequence alignment of bile salt hydrolase (BSH) amino acid sequences from different bacterial species. The protein sequences were aligned with Clustal Omega (http://www.ebi.ac.uk/Tools/msa/clustalo/) software and identical residues were identified by ESPript 3.0 (http://espript.ibcp.fr/ESPript/ESPript/). The identical residues are shown in red background and the similar residues are shown as red color. The conserved residues (Cys-1, Arg-16, Asp-19, Asn-79, Asn-171, and Arg-224) were marked as black asterisk (*).

around 37 kDa, which is the calculated molecular mass of *Lg*BSH (**Figure 2A**, lane 3). A single band was observed at 37 kDa after purification with Ni^{2+}-NTA agarose column, thus confirming the homogeneity and purity of *Lg*BSH (**Figure 2A**, lane 4). The Western blot analysis using anti-His antibodies also confirmed the molecular weight of purified *Lg*BSH (**Figure 2B**).

Biochemical Characterization of *Lg*BSH

Substrate Specificity of *Lg*BSH

To determine the substrate specificity of purified *Lg*BSH, four major glyco- or tauro-conjugated bile salts were used along with two non-substrate compounds (i.e., penicillin V and ampicillin). The highest *Lg*BSH activity was observed with GDCA as a substrate and was set as 100% activity. *Lg*BSH showed greater hydrolysis toward glyco-conjugated bile salts (GCA and GDCA) than to tauro-conjugated (TCA and TDCA) bile salts (**Figure 3**). However, very weak activity (4.78%) was observed when using penicillin V as a substrate, and no activity was detected with ampicillin (**Figure 3**). These results further confirmed that the identified *Lg*BSH was not PVA.

Effects of pH and Temperature on *Lg*BSH Activity

To determine the optimal pH for maximal *Lg*BSH activity, various pH values (pH 3–9) were used and optimal *Lg*BSH activity was observed in the range of pH 5.5–6.5. The maximal BSH activity (18.68 ± 1.15 μmol/min/mg) was observed at pH 5.5. Activities decreased at lower and higher pH values (**Figure 4A**). The optimal temperature for *Lg*BSH activity was determined using various temperature values (20–90°C). The

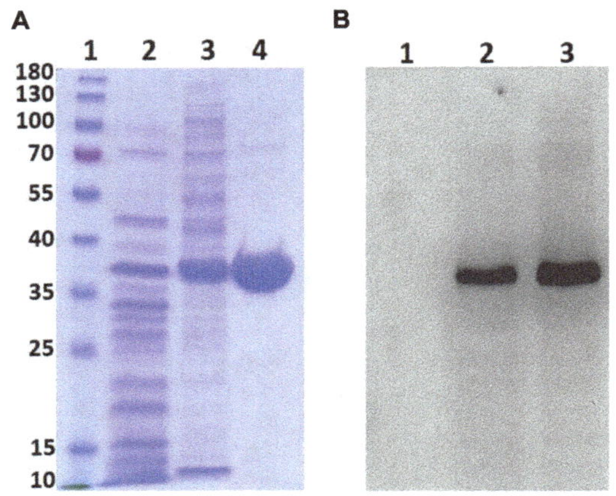

FIGURE 2 | Expression and purification of *Lg*BSH. SDS–PAGE analysis of *Lg*BSH **(A)**. Lane1: Marker (PageRuler™ Prestained Protein Ladder, 10–180 kDa), Lane2: cell lysate of *Escherichia coli* BL21 wild type, Lane3: cell lysate of *E. coli* BL21 expressing *Lg*BSH, Lane4: purified *Lg*BSH. Western blotting analysis of *Lg*BSH using anti-His antibody **(B)**. Lane1: cell lysate of *E. coli* BL21 wild type, Lane2: cell lysate of *E. coli* BL21 expressing *Lg*BSH, Lane3: purified *Lg*BSH.

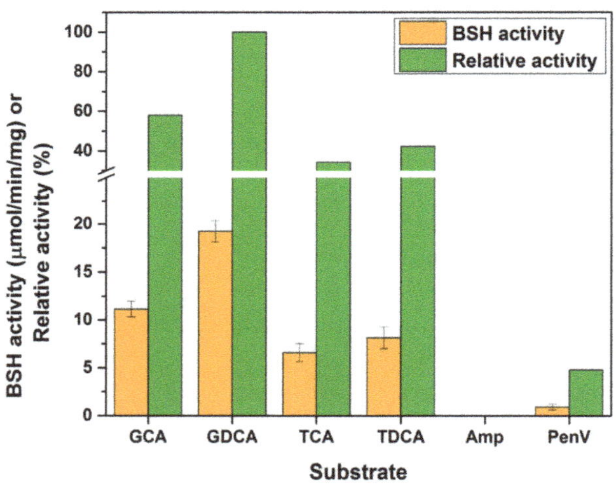

FIGURE 3 | Determining the substrate specificity of *Lg*BSH using various bile salts as well as non-substrate compounds. The BSH activity was expressed as the µmol/min/mg. All the experiments were performed in triplicate and mean ± SD values are represented.

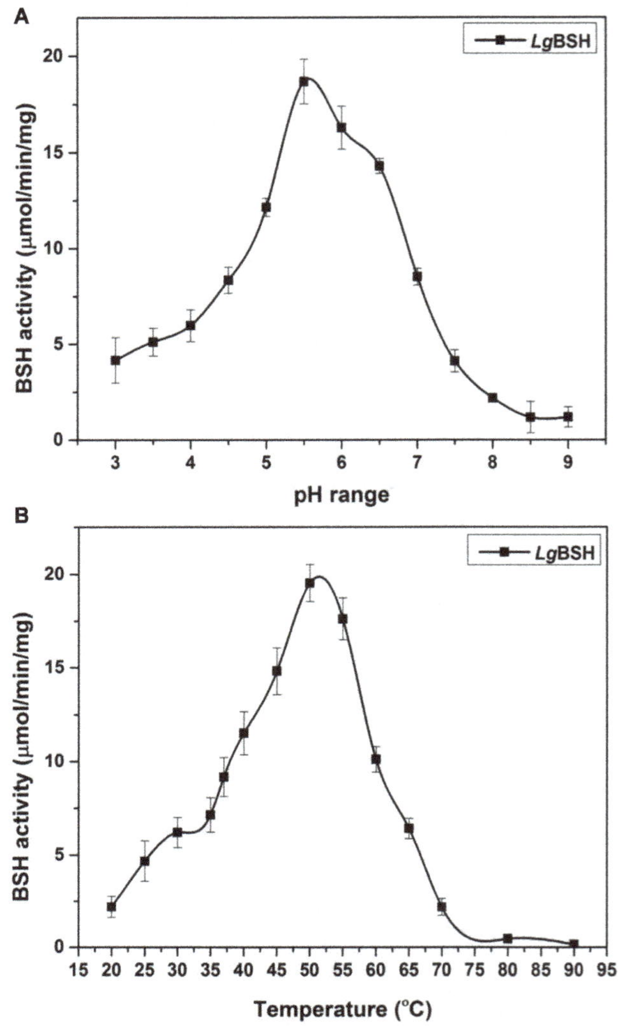

FIGURE 4 | Effect of various pH **(A)** and temperature **(B)** on *Lg*BSH activity. The assay was performed using glycocholic acid (GCA) as a substrate and activity was expressed as the µmol/min/mg. All the experiments were performed in triplicate and mean ± SD values are represented.

maximal BSH activity was observed at 52°C and enzyme activity sharply declined with increasing temperatures (**Figure 4B**).

Effects of Various Reducing Agents, Surfactants, Solvents, and Enzymes on *Lg*BSH Activity

The effects of various reducing agents on *Lg*BSH were analyzed. *Lg*BSH activity increased by about 18% when the enzyme was treated with 10 mM DTT (118.06%). However, the activity reduced by 2 and 4%, when treated with β-mercaptoethanol (98.18%) and EDTA (96.14%), respectively (**Table 1**). Surfactants such as Triton X-100 and Tween 80 significantly increased *Lg*BSH activity by 43 and 28%, respectively. Generally, surfactants or detergents possibly interact with the surfaces of enzymes, thereby enhancing the solubility and stability of proteins (Avinash et al., 2015). On the other hand, SDS dramatically reduced BSH activity by 93% at a concentration of 10 mM.

Organic solvents such as isopropanol, butanol, and acetone, respectively, enhanced *Lg*BSH activities by 41, 18, and 8% when the enzyme was treated with a 10% (v/v) concentration. Several solvents such as methanol, ethanol, and chloroform significantly decreased the enzyme activity. Among them, treatment with methanol drastically decreased the enzyme activity by 31% (**Table 1**).

The influences of various enzymes on *Lg*BSH activity was investigated by treating BSH with appropriate enzymes. Proteinase K and pepsin, respectively, decreased *Lg*BSH activity by 97 and 85%, thus confirming that proteinase K might degrade the BSH enzyme. However, enzymes like lysozyme, α-amylase,

TABLE 1 | Effects of various reducing agents, surfactants, solvents, and enzymes on purified *Lactobacillus gasseri* bile salt hydrolase (*Lg*BSH) activity.

Treatment	Compound	Relative activity (%)[a]
Control		100%
Reducing agents	DTT[b]	118.06 ± 0.31
(10 mM)	β-Mercaptoethanol	98.18 ± 0.83
	EDTA[b]	96.14 ± 1.16
Surfactants	Triton X-100	143.12 ± 1.47
(10 mM or 0.5%)	Tween 80	128.19 ± 0.82
	SDS[b]	2.86 ± 0.19
Solvents	Chloroform	98.91 ± 1.16
(10% [vol/vol])	Ethanol	86.16 ± 1.67
	Acetone	108.71 ± 1.05
	Methanol	69.15 ± 2.15
	Isopropanol	141.21 ± 1.26
	Butanol	118.20 ± 2.19
Enzymes	Lysozyme	91.35 ± 0.92
	Proteinase K	3.49 ± 0.19
	Pepsin	15.16 ± 1.68
	α-Amylase	98.41 ± 1.24
	Lipase	101.19 ± 0.62
	Catalase	98.13 ± 0.53

[a]*The relative activity percentage was calculated based on the control with no treatment, and the assay was performed using glycocholic acid as a substrate.*
[b]*DTT, dithiothreitol; EDTA, ethylenediaminetetraacetic acid; SDS, sodium dodecylsulfate.*

TABLE 2 | Inhibitory effects of various compounds on *L. gasseri* bile salt hydrolase (*Lg*BSH) activity.

Compound type	Compound name	Inhibition %[a]
Metal ion or feed additive	$CuCl_2$	98.13
	$CuSO_4$	94.36
	$MnCl_2$	76.42
	$MnSO_4$	73.98
	$MgCl_2$	36.14
	$MgSO_4$	32.69
	$ZnCl_2$	54.21
	$ZnSO_4$	39.64
	$CaCl_2$	18.64
	$NaHIO_3$	98.26
	KIO_3	97.64
Antibiotics used as growth promoters (AGPs)	Penicillin V	97.84
	Ampicillin	96.39
	Oxytetracycline	95.97
	Doxycycline hydrochloride	97.51
	Neomycin	82.93
	Erythromycin	41.62
	Lincomycin	18.58
Potential inhibitors	Riboflavin	98.31
	Ascorbic acid	32.96

[a]*The inhibition percentage was calculated by dividing the mean activity of the control (without an inhibitor) and treatment (with an inhibitor). The assay was performed with 5 mM of each inhibitor, and glycocholic acid was used as a substrate.*

lipase, and catalase did not affect *Lg*BSH activity. This was due to the inefficiencies of these enzymes on *Lg*BSH (**Table 1**).

Inhibitory Effects of Feed Additives on *Lg*BSH Activity

Various commonly used feed additives and AGPs were screened to identify a suitable *Lg*BSH inhibitor. Among the tested compounds, more than 95% inhibition was observed with riboflavin, $NaHIO_3$, $CuCl_2$, penicillin V, KIO_3, doxycycline hydrochloride, ampicillin, and oxytetracycline (**Table 2**). The lowest inhibitory percentage (<50%) was observed with erythromycin, $ZnSO_4$, $MgCl_2$, ascorbic acid, $MgSO_4$, $CuCl_2$, and lincomycin. Among all of the tested inhibitors, riboflavin might be a good candidate for application in animal feed.

Homology Modeling of *Lg*BSH

Protein BLAST search of *Lg*BSH showed highest identity of about 54% with the BSH of *E. faecalis* (4WL3), and 47% identity with the BSH of *L. salivarius* (5HKE). The homology model of *Lg*BSH was predicted with the Phyre2 algorithm using *Ef*BSH (4WL3) as a template (**Figure 5A**), since it had a 100% confidence level (Supplementary Figure S5). The superimposed structure of *Ef*BSH, *Ls*BSH with the *Lg*BSH revealed similarities among their structures and their catalytic active sites contains nucleophile residue (Cys1) (**Figure 5B**). Residues involved in catalysis were identified based on the superimposed structure, including Cys1, Arg16, Asp19, Asn79, Asn171, and Arg224. However, residues in the substrate-binding pocket were conservatively replaced. Two loops were identified near the substrate-binding pockets: loop I contained 8 aa from 20 to 27 (LEISFGEH), and loop II contained 15 aa from 124 to 138 (LVDINFSKKLQLSPL). The secondary structure prediction of *Lg*BSH using PSIPRED V 3.3 revealed that *Lg*BSH contains 14.11% of α-helix, 60.12% of random coil, and 25.76% of extended strand (Supplementary Figure S6). The secondary structural pattern of *Lg*BSH was similar to *Ef*BSH.

The PSVS analysis results of predicted *Lg*BSH structure suggested that the model was of a good quality. The Ramachandran plot analysis showed that 91.6% of residues lies in the most favored regions; 8.1 and 0.4% of residues lies in allowed and disallowed regions, respectively (Supplementary Figure S7). The Procheck G-factor (all dihedral angles) was found to be −0.19, and the VERIFY-3D results showed that 85.54% of residues had an average 3D-1D score of >0.2, thus confirming that the predicted *Lg*BSH structure contained no conformational errors (Supplementary Figure S8). The overall *Z*-score of the ProSA analysis was −6.57 (Supplementary Figure S9), which is in the range of scores typically found for native proteins of similar sizes (Wiederstein and Sippl, 2007). The overall quality factor of the predicted *Lg*BSH model was calculated by ERRAT, and results showed 90.033, which further confirmed the quality of the predicted structure (Supplementary Figure S10). The RMSDs of bond angles and bond lengths were 2.2° and 0.019 Å, respectively. The modeled *Lg*BSH protein structure was submitted to Protein Model Data Base[10] (PMDB) with the model id PM0080976.

[10]https://bioinformatics.cineca.it/PMDB/

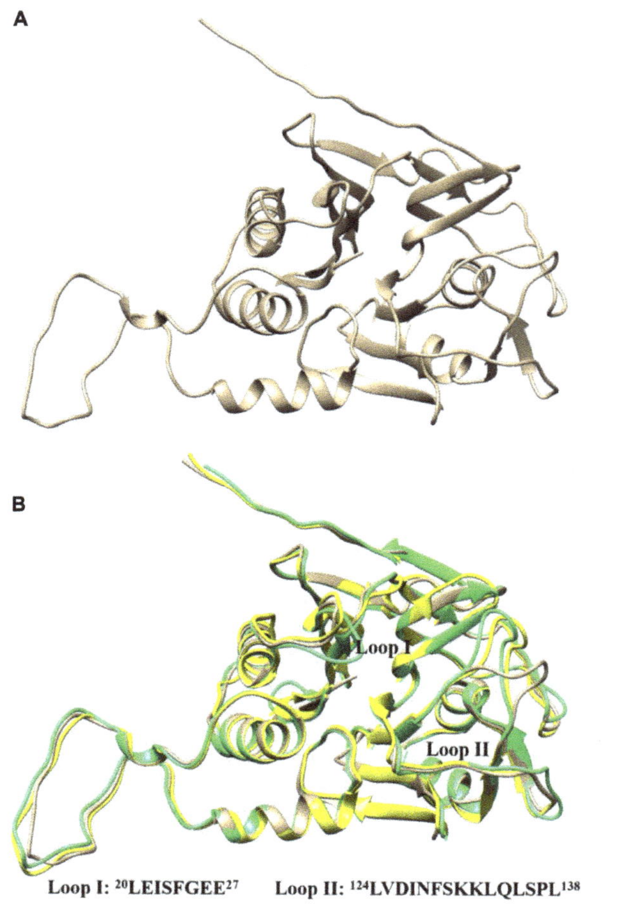

FIGURE 5 | Three-dimensional structure of *Lg*BSH predicted by homology modeling using *Enterococcus faecalis* BSH (4WL3) as template **(A)**. Three-dimensional superimposed structures of *Lg*BSH (tan) with their closest homology structures *Ef*BSH (4WL3) (yellow) and *Ls*BSH (5HKE) (spring green) using UCSF-Chimera. The sequences of loops (I and II) present in the substrate-binding pockets were represented in the figure **(B)**.

The CASTp analysis revealed residues involved in substrate binding. On the whole, 19 possible residues were identified and compared to binding pocket residues of the template protein (Supplementary Figure S11). The approximate binding site volume of *Lg*BSH was found to be 551.7 Å^3. The SiteHound analysis revealed that the total interaction energy (TIE) of the substrate-binding pocket was −480.02 kcal/mol with the lowest and highest interaction energies of −22.34 and −8.96 kcal/mol, respectively.

Molecular Docking Studies to Identify the Substrate Specificity and Inhibitors

*Lg*BSH had a substrate preference toward glyco-conjugated bile salts (GCA and GDCA), compared to tauro-conjugated bile salts. Hence, to demonstrate the substrate specificity, GCA, GDCA, and TCA were docked with *Lg*BSH, and their hydrogen bonding interactions with the enzyme were identified (**Figure 6**). Cys2 and Lys59 (amino acids were numbered from methionine) residues in the substrate-binding pocket of *Lg*BSH formed hydrogen bonds with GCA, with respective bond lengths of 2.637 and 2.252 Å (**Figures 6A,B**). Similarly, Cys2, Phe25, and Lys59 interacted with GDCA via hydrogen bonding with respective bond lengths of 2.384, 1.864, and 2.031 Å (**Figures 6C,D**). On the other hand, TCA formed hydrogen bonds with Lys59 and Gln135 with respective bond lengths of 2.224 and 2.123 Å, (**Figures 6E,F**). However, the binding energy of GCA was found to be lower (−8.46 kcal/mol) than that of GDCA (−6.81 kcal/mol) and TCA (−7.91 kcal/mol), thus further confirming the binding strength of GCA over other substrates.

Based on previous experimental data, we found that riboflavin and penicillin V, respectively, inhibited *Lg*BSH activity by 98.31 and 97.84%. To further investigate the mechanism behind this inhibition and support our experimental data, both substrate (GCA) and inhibitors (riboflavin and penicillin V) were docked with the modeled protein structure using the SwissDock algorithm. All ligands showed favorable binding energies, among which the substrate GCA had the lowest binding energy of −8.46 kcal/mol, while on the other hand, inhibitors, i.e., penicillin V and riboflavin, had relatively higher binding energies of −7.38 and −6.25 kcal/mol, respectively (**Figure 7**).

DISCUSSION

Bile salt hydrolase enzymes of several LAB species play a central role in the lipid metabolism of hosts. During the past several decades, probiotic bacteria with BSH activity were used to alleviate cholesterol levels in humans and animals (Jones et al., 2004). Several authors have previously identified and crystallized BSH enzymes from various bacterial species including *C. perfringens* (Rossocha et al., 2005), *B. longum* (Kumar et al., 2006), *L. salivarius* (Xu et al., 2016), and *E. faecalis.* Kumar et al. (2013) identified and cloned a gene encoding the BSH enzyme from *L. fermentum* NCDO394. The nucleotide sequence of the putative BSH gene contained an open reading frame (ORF) of 978 nucleotides encoding a predicted protein of 325 aa. They reported that the deduced BSH protein had significant similarity to the penicillin V amidases of other *Lactobacillus* spp. Wang et al. (2012) identified a BSH gene from the genome of *L. salivarius* NRRL B-30514, a chicken isolate. Similarly, we have identified a putative BSH gene (981 bp) encoding 326 aa from the genome of *L. gasseri* FR4. The molecular mass of purified *Lg*BSH was found to be 37 kDa on SDS–PAGE and was further confirmed by a Western blot analysis (**Figures 2A,B**). This result is further supported by several publications, where the molecular mass of the BSH enzyme was reported as 37 kDa on SDS–PAGE (Wang et al., 2012; Kumar et al., 2013; Jayashree et al., 2014).

Generally, BSH enzymes have a broad range of substrate specificity toward glyco- and tauro-conjugated bile salts (Lambert et al., 2008; Oh et al., 2008). Purified *Lg*BSH exhibited substrate specificity toward glycine-conjugated bile salts (GCA and GDCA) and in particular, maximal activity was observed on GDCA (**Figure 3**). However, the activity was inhibited when using non-substrate compounds (i.e., ampicillin and

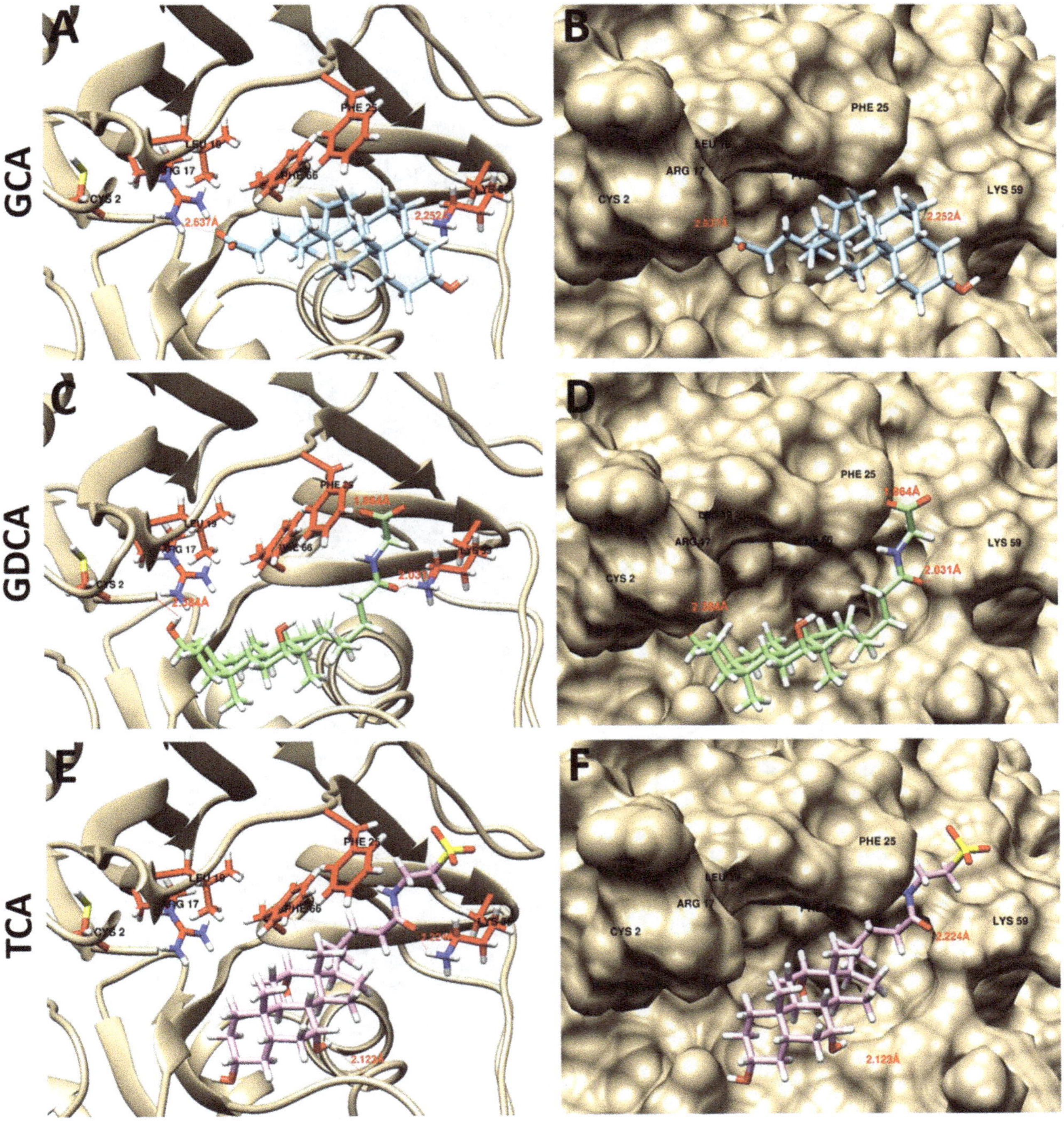

FIGURE 6 | Docking analysis of GCA **(A,B)**, glycodeoxycholic acid (GDCA) **(C,D)**, and taurocholic acid (TCA) **(E,F)** with *Lg*BSH to determine the substrate specificity and identify the hydrogen bonding between enzyme and substrate. Docking was performed using SwissDock and the outputs were analyzed using UCSF-Chimera.

penicillin V) as a substrate. Kumar et al. (2013) studied the characteristics of recombinant (r) BSH of *L. fermentum* NCDO394 and identified that purified rBSH enzyme hydrolyzed six major bile substrates, with a special preference toward glycine-conjugated bile salts and exhibited maximal activity against GCA. Previous studies also confirmed that BSHs from *Lactobacillus* spp., including *L. salivarius* (Wang et al., 2012), *L. plantarum* CGMCC 8198 (Gu et al., 2014), and BSH-C of *L. johnsonii* PF01 (Chae et al., 2013), had a substrate specificity toward glyco-conjugated bile salts. Biochemical characterization studies revealed that the pH and temperature optima of *Lg*BSH were, respectively, found to be 5.5 and 52°C. Our results are in accordance with the results of Wang et al. (2012), in which the BSH from *L. salivarius* showed maximal activity

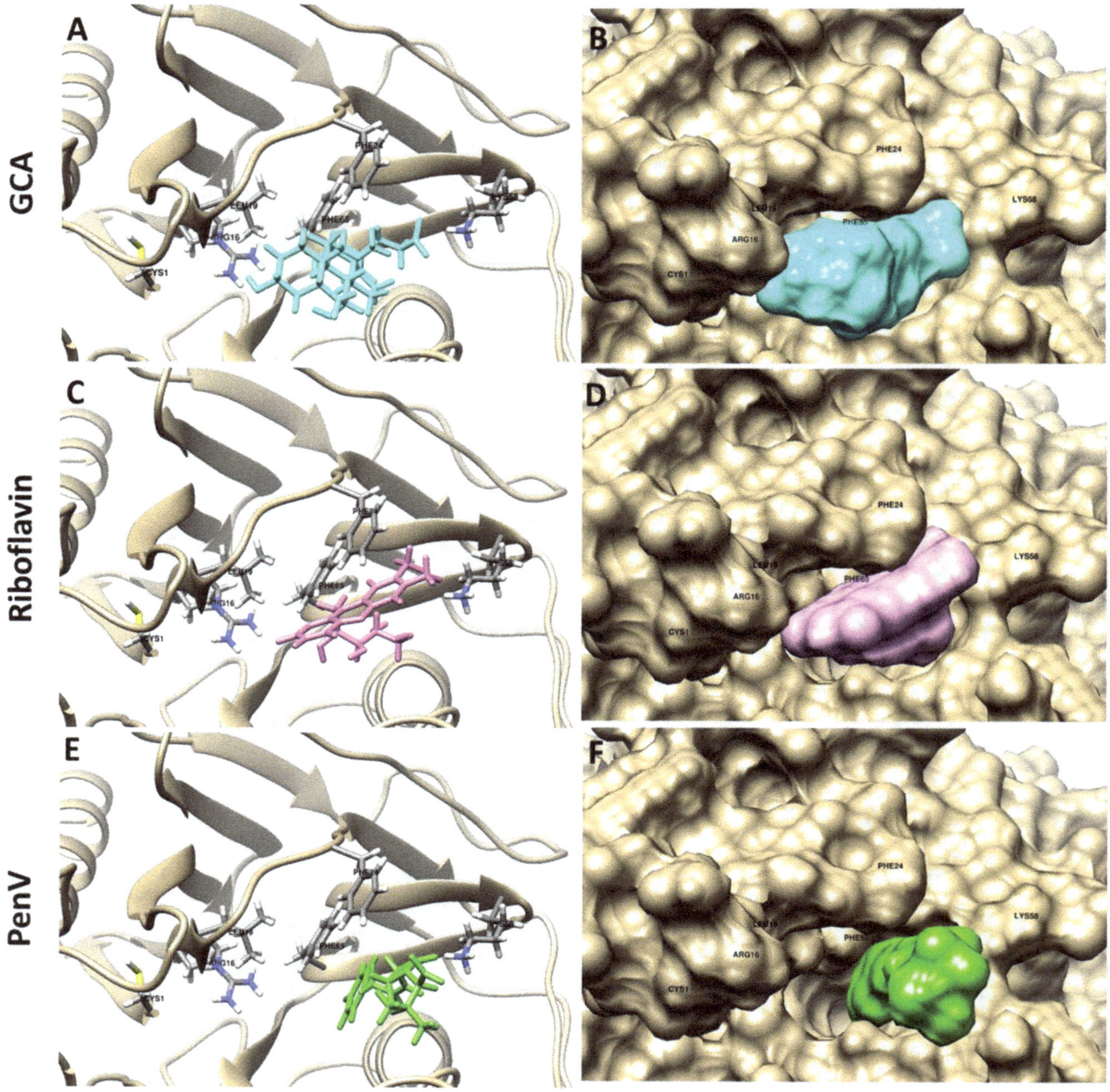

FIGURE 7 | Docking analysis of GCA (**A,B**: cyan), riboflavin (**C,D**: pink), and penicillin V (**E,F**: green) with *Lg*BSH to determine the inhibitory effects. Docking was performed using SwissDock and the outputs were analyzed using UCSF-Chimera.

at 41°C and pH 5.4. Kumar et al. (2013) also found that the optimal pH and temperature for enzymatic activity of BSH from *L. fermentum* NCDO394 were pH 6.0 and 37°C, respectively.

The evolution of protein structures is relatively slower than the evolution of nucleic acids, thus providing stability to protein structures. Proteins with similar sequences have retained identical structure during evolution, and proteins from distantly related organisms with less sequence similarity also have similar protein structures and retain similar functions (Kaczanowski and Zielenkiewicz, 2010; Chae et al., 2013). Although BSHs of various species had the highest sequence divergence, the protein structures were still very similar. Hence, homology modeling is an ideal approach to obtain the putative structure of the identified BSH enzyme, thus helps to understand the characteristics of the substrate-binding pocket and other functions of the enzyme. Superimposing the structure of *Lg*BSH onto that of *Ef*BSH revealed similarities of protein structures and binding pockets. Since BSH and PVA evolved from the same origin, both enzymes have the same catalytically important active site residues (Cys1, Arg16, Asp19, Asn79, Asn171, and Arg224) except for Asn79, where PVA uses tyrosine instead of asparagine (Rossocha et al., 2005). Recently, Xu et al. (2016) resolved the crystal structure of the BSH enzyme from *L. salivarius,* which had 47% sequence similarity with *Lg*BSH. Hence, we used this crystal structure to characterize our *Lg*BSH. Two loops (loops I and II) were identified from the substrate-binding pocket of *Lg*BSH. According to Xu et al. (2016), residues Leu133 (Leu133 in *Ls*BSH and Leu132 in *Ef*BSH) and Phe129 (Phe129 in *Ls*BSH and Phe128 in *Ef*BSH) in loop II might contribute to limiting the spatial configuration via condensing the entrance of the substrate-binding pocket. Similarly, the Phe24 (Tyr23 in *Ls*BSH and Tyr23 in *Ef*BSH) residue in loop I along with the Phe64 (Phe64 in *Ls*BSH and Phe64 in *Ef*BSH) residue might allow the substrate to intensely dock into the substrate-binding pocket, and thus may also be involved in enzyme–substrate interactions (Rossocha et al., 2005; Xu et al., 2016). The mode of substrate binding is dependent on the loops surrounding the active site, which also define the volume of the site (**Figure 5B**). Polar complementarity toward conjugated bile acids was also proposed as an important facet of substrate specificity (Chand et al., 2017). *Lg*BSH exhibited substrate specificity toward glyco-conjugated bile salts and had the lowest binding energy. Similarly, BSHs from most bacterial species had substrate preferences toward glyco-conjugated bile salts rather than tauro-conjugated ones. The major reasons for these phenomena include, steric hindrance caused by a sulfur atom of taurine and an abundance of glyco-conjugated bile salts in nature (Chand et al., 2017).

Recent epidemiological studies suggests that the use of AGPs is related to the emergence of antibiotic-resistant bacteria which may be transmitted to humans and cause significant threats to food safety and public health (Lin, 2014). However, a ban on AGP usage would create challenges for the animal feed and feed-additive industries. Several products, viz., probiotics, prebiotics, and organic acids, are used to change the intestinal microbiota to improve animal health and production. Studies using swine and poultry fostered understanding of the relationships between AGP supplementation and GIT bacterial compositions. Results of several studies proved that AGPs have created bacterial shifts, have altered the microbial diversity of the intestines, and suggested that certain GIT populations might be more related to animal growth (Danzeisen et al., 2011; Kim et al., 2012; Lin, 2014). However, probiotic feed supplements lead to decreased body mass gains in treated animals. This can be overcome by feeding animals with suitable BSH inhibitors along with the probiotic feed. A high purity of BSH enzymes is necessary to screen BSH inhibitors and study the substrate specificity of the enzyme. Hence, we have purified the BSH enzyme using His tag and used screened various compounds to identify potential BSH inhibitors. The results suggested that $CuCl_2$ decreased BSH activity by 98.13% among all of the tested metal ions (**Table 2**). Wang et al. (2012) demonstrated that copper ($CuCl_2$) and zinc ($ZnSO_4$) inhibited BSH activities by 98.1 and 89.5%, respectively. Conversely, we found that inhibition of *Lg*BSH activity by zinc ($ZnCl_2$ or $ZnSO_4$) was not significant. We also tested the inhibitory effects of currently used AGPs and found that all tested antibiotics (except erythromycin and lincomycin) had significant inhibitory effects on *Lg*BSH. However, the long-term use of these metal ions and AGPs might affect animal health, increase production costs and accumulation of metal ions in treated animals. Recently, Smith et al. (2014) performed high-throughput screening (HTS) to identify safe and cost-effective BSH inhibitors and reported that riboflavin and phenethyl caffeate can act as potential BSH inhibitors. These results were further supported by Lin et al. (2014), who reported that riboflavin and CAPE could inhibit BSH activity. Hence, we used riboflavin as a novel inhibitor and found that *Lg*BSH activity was reduced by up to 98.31% (**Table 2**). Riboflavin (or vitamin B2) play key roles in various intracellular (i.e., energy metabolism) and extracellular (i.e., quorum sensing and extracellular electron transfer) processes in bacteria. Hence, riboflavin has been used as a feed additive for several animals to overcome vitamin B2 deficiencies (Smith et al., 2014; Gutiérrez-Preciado et al., 2015). The Food and Drug Administration (FDA) of United States of America (USA) has already approved riboflavin as a feed additive, since it has well-known metabolic functions (Smith et al., 2014). The addition of riboflavin along with the probiotic *L. gasseri* FR4 can serve as a BSH inhibitor and also increase survival rates of probiotic bacteria. Gutiérrez-Preciado et al. (2015) performed extensive analyses on riboflavin transporters across all bacterial strains and found that *L. gasseri* has its unique transporter for riboflavin. Stahly et al. (2007) conducted a swine study and reported that dietary supplementation with riboflavin (20 mg/kg feed) significantly enhanced the body weight and feed efficiency in pigs. The current studies suggested this might be due to inhibition of the BSH enzyme produced by probiotic microorganisms present in the swine's intestines. To further unravel the mechanism behind the inhibitory effect of riboflavin, we performed a molecular docking analysis using the predicted *Lg*BSH structure. Results showed that both substrate and inhibitors (riboflavin and penicillin V) could bind to the substrate-binding pocket of *Lg*BSH with almost the same binding affinity/energy (**Figure 7**). This might have been due to the inverse mode of binding of riboflavin and penicillin V. This study provides some new insights into the inhibitory effects of several potential BSH inhibitors, and these might serve as alternatives for AGPs.

CONCLUSION

In this study, we identified and characterized a novel BSH enzyme from probiotic *L. gasseri* FR4. *Lg*BSH showed greater hydrolysis toward glyco-conjugated bile salts than to tauro-conjugated bile salts, and no hydrolysis was observed on penicillin V. The homology modeling studies revealed the 3D structure of *Lg*BSH, which has a structural similarity with previously identified BSH enzymes. *Lg*BSH activity was dramatically inhibited by riboflavin and confirmed by molecular docking analysis. Riboflavin had almost the same binding energy as GCA, thus helping in the inhibition of *Lg*BSH. Hence, supplementation of *L. gasseri* FR4 along with riboflavin might be used as an alternative for AGPs for poultry animals. However, detailed animal studies are necessary to further confirm the efficiency of BSH inhibitors on animal growth and performance.

AUTHOR CONTRIBUTIONS

AR, RR, and MA contributed with the conception and experimental design. RR, carried out all experiments. MA and RR performed the homology modeling and docking analysis. MA and RR analyzed and interpreted the results. RR written the manuscript and corrected by AR and MA. All authors performed a critical revision of the manuscript and approved the final version.

ACKNOWLEDGMENTS

The authors are thankful to Department of Biology, The Gandhigram Rural Institute-Deemed University for providing laboratory facility to carry out the entire research. Author RR is thankful to Department of Science and Technology (DST), Ministry of Science and Technology, India for providing fellowship under DST-INSPIRE (IF140278) fellowship. The authors are thankful to Mr. Narendrakumar Ravivaradharajulu for English revision.

REFERENCES

Angelakis, E., Merhej, V., and Raoult, D. (2013). Related actions of probiotics and antibiotics on gut microbiota and weight modification. *Lancet Infect. Dis.* 13, 889–899. doi: 10.1016/S1473-3099(13)70179-8

Avinash, V. S., Ramasamy, S., Suresh, C. G., and Pundle, A. (2015). Penicillin V acylase from *Pectobacterium atrosepticum* exhibits high specific activity and unique kinetics. *Int. J. Biol. Macromol.* 79, 1–7. doi: 10.1016/j.ijbiomac.2015.04.036

Begley, M., Hill, C., and Gahan, C. G. (2006). Bile salt hydrolase activity in probiotics. *Appl. Environ. Microbiol.* 72, 1729–1738. doi: 10.1128/AEM.72.3.1729-1738.2006

Casewell, M., Friis, C., Marco, E., McMullin, P., and Phillips, I. (2003). The European ban on growth-promoting antibiotics and emerging consequences for human and animal health. *J. Antimicrob. Chemother.* 52, 159–161. doi: 10.1093/jac/dkg313

Chae, J. P., Valeriano, V. D., Kim, G. B., and Kang, D. K. (2013). Molecular cloning, characterization and comparison of bile salt hydrolases from *Lactobacillus johnsonii* PF01. *J. Appl. Microbiol.* 114, 121–133. doi: 10.1111/jam.12027

Chand, D., Avinash, V. S., Yadav, Y., Pundle, A. V., Suresh, C. G., and Ramasamy, S. (2017). Molecular features of bile salt hydrolases and relevance in human health. *Biochim. Biophys. Acta* 1861(1 Pt A), 2981–2991. doi: 10.1016/j.bbagen.2016.09.024

Danzeisen, J. L., Kim, H. B., Isaacson, R. E., Tu, Z. J., and Johnson, T. J. (2011). Modulations of the chicken cecal microbiome and metagenome in response to anticoccidial and growth promoter treatment. *PLoS ONE* 6:e27949. doi: 10.1371/journal.pone.0027949

Dundas, J., Ouyang, Z., Tseng, J., Binkowski, A., Turpaz, Y., and Liang, J. (2006). CASTp: computed atlas of surface topography of proteins with structural and topographical mapping of functionally annotated residues. *Nucleic Acids Res.* 34(Suppl. 2), W116–W118. doi: 10.1093/nar/gkl282

Grosdidier, A., Zoete, V., and Michielin, O. (2011). SwissDock, a protein-small molecule docking web service based on EADock DSS. *Nucleic Acids Res.* 39(Suppl. 2), W270–W277. doi: 10.1093/nar/gkr366

Gu, X.-C., Luo, X.-G., Wang, C.-X., Ma, D.-Y., Wang, Y., He, Y.-Y., et al. (2014). Cloning and analysis of bile salt hydrolase genes from *Lactobacillus plantarum* CGMCC No. 8198. *Biotechnol. Lett.* 36, 975–983. doi: 10.1007/s10529-013-1434-9

Gutiérrez-Preciado, A., Torres, A. G., Merino, E., Bonomi, H. R., Goldbaum, F. A., and García-Angulo, V. A. (2015). Extensive identification of bacterial riboflavin transporters and their distribution across bacterial species. *PLoS ONE* 10:e0126124. doi: 10.1371/journal.pone.0126124

Hernandez, M., Ghersi, D., and Sanchez, R. (2009). SITEHOUND-web: a server for ligand binding site identification in protein structures. *Nucleic Acids Res.* 37(Suppl. 2), W413–W416. doi: 10.1093/nar/gkp281

Hofmann, A. F., and Eckmann, L. (2006). How bile acids confer gut mucosal protection against bacteria. *Proc. Natl. Acad. Sci. U.S.A.* 103, 4333–4334. doi: 10.1073/pnas.0600780103

Jayashree, S., Pooja, S., Pushpanathan, M., Rajendhran, J., and Gunasekaran, P. (2014). Identification and characterization of bile salt hydrolase genes from the genome of *Lactobacillus fermentum* MTCC 8711. *Appl. Biochem. Biotechnol.* 174, 855–866. doi: 10.1007/s12010-014-1118-5

Jones, M. L., Chen, H., Ouyang, W., Metz, T., and Prakash, S. (2004). Microencapsulated genetically engineered *Lactobacillus plantarum* 80 (pCBH1) for bile acid deconjugation and its implication in lowering cholesterol. *J. Biomed. Biotechnol.* 2004, 61–69. doi: 10.1155/S1110724304307011

Joyce, S. A., and Gahan, C. G. (2014). The gut microbiota and the metabolic health of the host. *Curr. Opin. Gastroenterol.* 30, 120–127. doi: 10.1097/MOG.0000000000000039

Kaczanowski, S., and Zielenkiewicz, P. (2010). Why similar protein sequences encode similar three-dimensional structures? *Theor. Chem. Acc.* 125, 643–650. doi: 10.1007/s00214-009-0656-3

Kelley, L. A., Mezulis, S., Yates, C. M., Wass, M. N., and Sternberg, M. J. E. (2015). The Phyre2 web portal for protein modeling, prediction and analysis. *Nat. Protoc.* 10, 845–858. doi: 10.1038/nprot.2015.053

Kim, G.-B., and Lee, B. H. (2005). Biochemical and molecular insights into bile salt hydrolase in the gastrointestinal microflora - a review. *Asian Australas. J. Anim. Sci.* 18, 1505–1512. doi: 10.5713/ajas.2005.1505

Kim, H. B., Borewicz, K., White, B. A., Singer, R. S., Sreevatsan, S., Tu, Z. J., et al. (2012). Microbial shifts in the swine distal gut in response to the treatment with antimicrobial growth promoter, tylosin. *Proc. Natl. Acad. Sci. U.S.A.* 109, 15485–15490. doi: 10.1073/pnas.1205147109

Knarreborg, A., Lauridsen, C., Engberg, R. M., and Jensen, S. K. (2004). Dietary antibiotic growth promoters enhance the bioavailability of α-tocopheryl acetate in broilers by altering lipid absorption. *J. Nutr.* 134, 1487–1492.

Kumar, R., Rajkumar, H., Kumar, M., Varikuti, S. R., Athimamula, R., Shujauddin, M., et al. (2013). Molecular cloning, characterization and heterologous expression of bile salt hydrolase (Bsh) from *Lactobacillus fermentum* NCDO394. *Mol. Biol. Rep.* 40, 5057–5066. doi: 10.1007/s11033-013-2607-2

Kumar, R. S., Brannigan, J. A., Prabhune, A. A., Pundle, A. V., Dodson, G. G., Dodson, E. J., et al. (2006). Structural and functional analysis of a conjugated bile salt hydrolase from *Bifidobacterium longum* reveals an evolutionary relationship with penicillin V acylase. *J. Biol. Chem.* 281, 32516–32525. doi: 10.1074/jbc.M604172200

Lambert, J. M., Bongers, R. S., de Vos, W. M., and Kleerebezem, M. (2008). Functional analysis of four bile salt hydrolase and penicillin acylase family members in *Lactobacillus plantarum* WCFS1. *Appl. Environ. Microbiol.* 74, 4719–4726. doi: 10.1128/aem.00137-08

Lin, J. (2011). Effect of antibiotic growth promoters on intestinal microbiota in food animals: a novel model for studying the relationship between gut microbiota and human obesity? *Front. Microbiol.* 2:53. doi: 10.3389/fmicb.2011.00053

Lin, J. (2014). Antibiotic growth promoters enhance animal production by targeting intestinal bile salt hydrolase and its producers. *Front. Microbiol.* 5:33. doi: 10.3389/fmicb.2014.00033

Lin, J., Negga, R., Zeng, X., and Smith, K. (2014). Effect of bile salt hydrolase inhibitors on a bile salt hydrolase from *Lactobacillus acidophilus*. *Pathogens* 3, 947–956. doi: 10.3390/pathogens3040947

Marshall, B. M., and Levy, S. B. (2011). Food animals and antimicrobials: impacts on human health. *Clin. Microbiol. Rev.* 24, 718–733. doi: 10.1128/cmr.00002-11

Million, M., Angelakis, E., Paul, M., Armougom, F., Leibovici, L., and Raoult, D. (2012). Comparative meta-analysis of the effect of *Lactobacillus* species on weight gain in humans and animals. *Microb. Pathog.* 53, 100–108. doi: 10.1016/j.micpath.2012.05.007

Miremadi, F., Ayyash, M., Sherkat, F., and Stojanovska, L. (2014). Cholesterol reduction mechanisms and fatty acid composition of cellular membranes of probiotic Lactobacilli and Bifidobacteria. *J. Funct. Foods* 9, 295–305. doi: 10.1016/j.jff.2014.05.002

Oh, H. K., Lee, J. Y., Lim, S. J., Kim, M. J., Kim, G. B., Kim, J. H., et al. (2008). Molecular cloning and characterization of a bile salt hydrolase from *Lactobacillus acidophilus* PF01. *J. Microbiol. Biotechnol.* 18, 449–456.

Parveen Rani, R., Anandharaj, M., Hema, S., Deepika, R., and David Ravindran, A. (2016). Purification of antilisterial peptide (subtilosin A) from novel *Bacillus tequilensis* FR9 and demonstrate their pathogen invasion protection ability using human carcinoma cell line. *Front. Microbiol.* 7:1910. doi: 10.3389/fmicb.2016.01910

Pettersen, E. F., Goddard, T. D., Huang, C. C., Couch, G. S., Greenblatt, D. M., Meng, E. C., et al. (2004). UCSF Chimera–a visualization system for exploratory research and analysis. *J. Comput. Chem.* 25, 1605–1612. doi: 10.1002/jcc.20084

Robert, X., and Gouet, P. (2014). Deciphering key features in protein structures with the new ENDscript server. *Nucleic Acids Res.* 42, W320–W324. doi: 10.1093/nar/gku316

Rossocha, M., Schultz-Heienbrok, R., von Moeller, H., Coleman, J. P., and Saenger, W. (2005). Conjugated bile acid hydrolase is a tetrameric N-terminal thiol hydrolase with specific recognition of its cholyl but not of its tauryl product. *Biochemistry* 44, 5739–5748. doi: 10.1021/bi0473206

Smith, K., Zeng, X., and Lin, J. (2014). Discovery of bile salt hydrolase inhibitors using an efficient high-throughput screening system. *PLoS ONE* 9:e85344. doi: 10.1371/journal.pone.0085344

Stahly, T. S., Williams, N. H., Lutz, T. R., Ewan, R. C., and Swenson, S. G. (2007). Dietary B vitamin needs of strains of pigs with high and moderate lean growth12. *J. Anim. Sci.* 85, 188–195. doi: 10.2527/jas.2006-086

Tamura, K., Stecher, G., Peterson, D., Filipski, A., and Kumar, S. (2013). MEGA6: molecular evolutionary genetics analysis version 6.0. *Mol. Biol. Evol.* 30, 2725–2729. doi: 10.1093/molbev/mst197

Wang, Z., Zeng, X., Mo, Y., Smith, K., Guo, Y., and Lin, J. (2012). Identification and characterization of a bile salt hydrolase from *Lactobacillus salivarius* for development of novel alternatives to antibiotic growth promoters. *Appl. Environ. Microbiol.* 78, 8795–8802. doi: 10.1128/AEM.02519-12

Wiederstein, M., and Sippl, M. J. (2007). ProSA-web: interactive web service for the recognition of errors in three-dimensional structures of proteins. *Nucleic Acids Res.* 35(Suppl. 2), W407–W410. doi: 10.1093/nar/gkm290

Xu, F., Guo, F., Hu, X.-J., and Lin, J. (2016). Crystal structure of bile salt hydrolase from *Lactobacillus salivarius*. *Acta Crystallogr. Sect. F* 72, 376–381. doi: 10.1107/S2053230X16005707

6

Emerging Trends in "Smart Probiotics": Functional Consideration for the Development of Novel Health and Industrial Applications

Racha El Hage, Emma Hernandez-Sanabria and Tom Van de Wiele*

Center for Microbial Ecology and Technology, Faculty of Bioscience Engineering, Ghent University, Ghent, Belgium

***Correspondence:**
Tom Van de Wiele
tom.vandewiele@ugent.be

The link between gut microbiota and human health is well-recognized and described. This ultimate impact on the host has contributed to explain the mutual dependence between humans and their gut bacteria. Gut microbiota can be manipulated through passive or active strategies. The former includes diet, lifestyle, and environment, while the latter comprise antibiotics, pre- and probiotics. Historically, conventional probiotic strategies included a phylogenetically limited diversity of bacteria and some yeast strains. However, biotherapeutic strategies evolved in the last years with the advent of fecal microbiota transplant (FMT), successfully applied for treating CDI, IBD, and other diseases. Despite the positive outcomes, long-term effects resulting from the uncharacterized nature of FMT are not sufficiently studied. Thus, developing strategies to simulate the FMT, using characterized gut colonizers with identified phylogenetic diversity, may be a promising alternative. As the definition of probiotics states that the microorganism should have beneficial effects on the host, several bacterial species with proven efficacy have been considered next generation probiotics. Non-conventional candidate strains include *Akkermansia muciniphila*, *Faecalibacterium prausnitzii*, *Bacteroides fragilis*, and members of the Clostridia clusters IV, XIVa, and XVIII. However, viable intestinal delivery is one of the current challenges, due to their stringent survival conditions. In this review, we will cover current perspectives on the development and assessment of next generation probiotics and the approaches that industry and stakeholders must consider for a successful outcome.

Keywords: FMT, next generation probiotics, bacterial consortium, synthetic community, CDI

INTRODUCTION

The gut microbiota plays a significant role in human health, participating in several functions beneficial to the host (Patel and DuPont, 2015; Kristensen et al., 2016). It has been implicated in preventing pathogen colonization (Hand, 2016), shaping our immune system (Round and Mazmanian, 2009; Patel and DuPont, 2015; Macpherson et al., 2017), stimulating the production of gastrointestinal hormones (Saulnier et al., 2013), and regulating brain behavior (De Palma et al., 2014, 2017) through production of neuroactive substances (Steenbergen et al., 2015; Kristensen et al., 2016).

Additionally, the gut microbiota has been involved in the fermentation of non-digestible carbohydrates reaching the colon. This process leads to the production of short chain fatty acids (SCFAs), which elicit health benefits (den Besten et al., 2013). The human gut microbiota can be manipulated through either passive or active processes. Passive factors include hygiene, lifestyle, and diet. For instance, primary colonizers of the gut involved in the immune development are shifted by sanitary practices (Zhou, 2016). In addition, dietary constituents can promote phylogenetic variations in the microbiota (Graf et al., 2015). In this context, prebiotics are defined as "a substrate that is selectively utilized by host microorganisms conferring a health benefit" (Gibson et al., 2017). Prebiotics act as growth substrates (Patrascu et al., 2017) to enhance the activity of bacterial genera (Scott et al., 2015) such as bifidobacteria and butyrate-producing clostridia (Rivière et al., 2016). SCFA and vitamins resulting from the fermentation of these components are crucial for human health (Graf et al., 2015). In terms of lifestyle factors, physical activity is known to positively impact the diversity of gut microbiota. In fact, gut microbiota of athletes is more diverse than that of non-athletic subjects (Clarke et al., 2014). Amongst the active processes manipulating microbiota composition are antibiotics and probiotics. Antibiotic use has been linked to dysbiosis (Langdon et al., 2016), even leading to low diversity, evenness, and taxonomic richness (Dethlefsen and Relman, 2010; Francino, 2016). Moreover, presence and expression of microbial genes are altered following antibiotic therapy (Reijnders et al., 2016). These detrimental outcomes may lead to decreased SCFA, glycolysis, vitamin production, homeostasis of the immune system, and impaired protection against pathogens (Guarner and Malagelada, 2003). As a result, antibiotic associated diarrhea (AAD) and recurrent infectious diseases like *Clostridium difficile* infection (CDI) may occur (Francino, 2016).

On the other side of the spectrum are probiotics, which can affect the host either directly or through their products, or even influence the activity of resident bacteria in the host (Scott et al., 2015). Probiotics are defined as "live microorganisms which when administered in adequate amounts confer a health benefit on the host" (WHO/FAO, 2006; Hill et al., 2014). The effect of probiotics in preventing metabolic syndromes such as obesity, type 2 diabetes (Kasińska and Drzewoski, 2015), and dyslipidemia has been reported (Asemi et al., 2013). For instance, administration of *Bifidobacterium* (Yin, 2010; Chen et al., 2011; Plaza-Diaz et al., 2014; Reichold et al., 2014; Savcheniuk et al., 2014; Wang et al., 2014) and *Lactobacillus* species reduced body weight gain and adipose tissue in mice fed high-fat diet through stimulation of adiponectin production (Kim et al., 2013; Kobyliak et al., 2016). In addition, lactobacilli have been proven to have therapeutic effects in different pathologies (Di Cerbo et al., 2016). Moreover, probiotics regulate the mucosal immune response (Klaenhammer et al., 2012), improving the activity of macrophages (Sang, 2010) and changing the expression of the genes associated. Even though these outcomes depend on specific bacteria and strains, probiotics may interact with TLR and downregulate the expression of NF-κB and pro-inflammatory cytokines (Ng et al., 2009; Plaza-Diaz, 2014). For instance, peptides of microbial anti-inflammatory molecules (MAMs) that are found in the *Faecalibacterium prausnitzii* supernatant inhibit the NF-κB pathway *in vitro* and *in vivo* (Breyner et al., 2017), confirming the anti-inflammatory and therapeutic properties of *F. prausnitzii* (Martín et al., 2014). These properties and protective effects of *F. prausnitzii* were identified in different models such as dinitrobenzene sulfate (DNBS)-induced colitis model, dextran sodium sulfate (DSS)-induced colitis (Breyner et al., 2017), and 2,4,6-trinitrobenzenesulfonic acid (TNBS)-induced acute colitis in mice (Miquel et al., 2015). Additionally, levels of anti-inflammatory cytokines and immunoglobulins, immune cell proliferation, and production of proinflammatory cytokines produced by the T cells may be modulated following probiotic supplementation (Miettinen et al., 1996; Nazemian et al., 2016). Furthermore, probiotics can be alternative strategies for inflammatory disorders, as they upregulate the production of CD4+Foxp3+ regulatory T cells (T_{regs}) (Kwon et al., 2010; Yan and Polk, 2011).

Different effects on the immune function may be species- and strain-related (Klaenhammer et al., 2012). It has been reported that probiotics have therapeutic effect on the central nervous system by reducing the intestinal inflammation. In this way, the regulation of HPA axis and the activity of the neurotransmitters may be improved (Wallace and Milev, 2017). Probiotics from *Bifidobacterium* and *Lactobacillus* genera are usually delivered through fermented products such as yogurts, milk, and cheeses, or they can be delivered as food supplements (Besseling-van der Vaart et al., 2016).

MONOSTRAIN AND MULTISTRAIN PROBIOTICS

Probiotics have been categorized into monostrain or multistrain/multispecies products (Timmerman et al., 2004). Different studies have confirmed positive effects on health when multistrain probiotics are used, due to the symbiosis among strains (Timmerman et al., 2004). Strains in multispecies probiotics can be from different genera. For instance, the efficacy of the multispecies probiotic consortium VSL#3 (*Streptococcus thermophilus*, *Eubacterium faecium*, *Bifidobacterium breve*, *Bifidobacterium infantis*, *Bifidobacterium longum*, *Lactobacillus acidophilus*, *Lactobacillus plantarum*, *Lactobacillus casei*, and *Lactobacillus delbrueckii* subspecies *bulgaricus*) was proven for the treatment of ulcerative colitis (Venturi et al., 1999; Timmerman et al., 2004). Besides, VSL#3 supplementation in women with gestational diabetes mellitus (GDM) may help regulate inflammatory markers and positively influence glycemic control (Jafarnejad et al., 2016). In addition, Chapman et al. (2011) described that probiotic mixtures were more effective than single-strain probiotics in inhibiting pathogen growth and atopic dermatitis, suggesting further application on other diseases like IBD. Another multispecies probiotic called Ecologic®Tolerance/Syngut™ was developed using four different probiotic strains (*Bifidobacterium lactis* W51,

L. acidophilus W22, *L. plantarum* W21, and *Lactococcus lactis* W19). Strains of this consortium have been proven to strengthen the gut barrier function, have beneficial effects on post-immunological induced stress, inhibit Th2, and stimulate IL-10 levels, thus providing beneficial effects in patients with food intolerance (Besseling-van der Vaart et al., 2016). Moreover, a multispecies probiotic consortium, Ecologic AAD (*B. bifidum* W23, *B. lactis* W18, *B. longum* W51, *E. faecium* W54, *L. acidophilus* W37 and W55, *L. paracasei* W72, *L. plantarum* W62, *L. rhamnosus* W71, and *L. salivarius* W24), reduced diarrhea-like bowel movements when administered in healthy volunteers taking amoxicillin (Koning et al., 2008). Multispecies probiotics also prevented rise in fasting plasma glucose (FPG), to decrease high sensitivity C-reactive protein (hs-CRP), and to increase plasma glutathione (GSH) in diabetic patients (Asemi et al., 2013). van Minnen et al. (2007) provided evidence that manipulation of the intestinal flora with multispecies probiotics reduced bacterial translocation, morbidity and mortality in a rat model of acute pancreatitis. Furthermore, multispecies probiotics rapidly relieved IBS symptoms and shifted the microbiota composition (Yoon et al., 2013). According to these results, combining specific probiotic effects from diverse strains can lead to an additive and more synergetic multispecies probiotic consortium (Timmerman et al., 2007).

However, the phylogenetic origin of probiotics is currently limited to conventional formulations of *Bifidobacterium*, *Lactobacillus* species and other lactic acid bacteria (LAB) (Govender et al., 2013) or yeast strains. This may decrease the probiotic effectiveness in the prevention or therapy of diseases entailing severe dysbiosis. Hence, a functionally and phylogenetically diverse probiotic product may be desirable when alterations in the gut microbiota composition are present (Marotz and Zarrinpar, 2016). For instance, CDI and recurrent CDI are major medical conditions that need urgent treatment when conventional antibiotics fail. As a result, development of complex communities with targeted functions is needed.

THE DILEMMA OF FECAL MICROBIOTA TRANSPLANT (FMT)

Fecal microbiota transplant (FMT) or fecal bacteriotherapy is an alternative strategy successfully used for the treatment of CDI (Kelly, 2013). Severe antibiotic therapy and CDI trigger dysbiosis, reducing diversity and functionality of the gut endogenous microbiota (Brandt, 2012). In this case, *C. difficile* spores can germinate, colonize, and thrive in the gut. Treatment of CDI requires additional antibiotics, increasing the risk of recurrent CDI (rCDI) after cessation of treatment, as a result of the dysbiosis caused by antibiotic therapy (Becattini et al., 2016; Francino, 2016), due to infection with the original strain (Barbut et al., 2000; Marsh et al., 2012) or re-infection caused by a different strain (Johnson et al., 1989; Kelly, 2009; Figueroa et al., 2012).

Poor colonization resistance from the gut microbiota and the patient's poor immune response further contribute to CDI risk (Pérez-Cobas et al., 2015). Recurrent CDI risk is 10–20% after initial CDI (Surawicz et al., 2013), and it increases to 45% after a first relapse, and to 60% for those with two or more recurrences (Bartlett, 1990). However, FMT can resolve both CDI and rCDI (Bakken, 2009), with a success rate of 90% when further antibiotic treatments fail (Youngster et al., 2014; Rao and Safdar, 2015). Given the success of FMT, it is now being considered as potential treatment for disorders such as ulcerative colitis (Shi et al., 2016), irritable bowel syndrome (Distrutti et al., 2016), and metabolic syndrome (Hartstra et al., 2015). For instance, FMT induced remission in patients with active ulcerative colitis (Moayyedi et al., 2015), potentially as a result of the introduction of normal flora and the subsequent correction of the imbalance in the microbiota caused by the disease (Bakken et al., 2011). The complexity of the fecal sample can be the key factor behind the positive shift in the microbiota composition generated by the FMT (Marotz and Zarrinpar, 2016). Thus, diversity of the donor microbiome may be crucial (Leszczyszyn et al., 2016). Indeed, some patients do not respond to FMT, probably because only specific bacterial phylotypes can be therapeutic when effectively transferred (Vermeire et al., 2015). Hence, FMT efficacy for treating gastrointestinal disorders is controversial (Sbahi and Di Palma, 2016). Adverse effects after FMT include nausea, vomit, fever, abdominal pain, and diarrhea (Vermeire et al., 2015; Pigneur and Sokol, 2016). Data for long-term effects of FMT is lacking, but theoretically, any disease phenotype from the donor can be transferred to the patient (Sbahi and Di Palma, 2016). This could be expected, as the uncharacterized nature of FMT may result in undetected or unmonitored risk factors such as viruses, pathogens or even allergens being passed to the FMT recipient, causing disease. To overcome this problem, Petrof et al. (2013) developed a synthetic bacteria cocktail with characterized nature to substitute FMT. Alternatively, a thorough pre-screening should be performed on the donor before the actual procedure of the FMT. Thus, the French Group of Fecal microbiota Transplantation (FGFT) was created to secure and evaluate the practice in this field (Sokol et al., 2016). Despite having experience treating CDI, FMT is not yet the top treatment choice of physicians (Zipursky et al., 2014). However, the majority of gastroenterologists and physicians in metropolitan areas were supportive to the idea of creating a fecal transplantation center, and a high percentage of the physicians would refer their patients to those centers (Jiang et al., 2013).

ALTERNATIVES FOR FECAL MICROBIOTA TRANSPLANT (FMT)

Additional microbiome therapeutics using characterized microbial communities of selected fecal bacteria could be developed to replace FMT, and yield the desired outcome (Sbahi and Di Palma, 2016). For instance, Petrof et al. (2013) described a stool substitute constituted by 33 different purified

TABLE 1 | Strains composing the RePOOPulate consortium.

Composition of Stool Substitute (RePOOPulate)
Acidaminococcus intestinalis
Bacteroides ovatus
Bifidobacterium adolescentis (two different strains)
Bifidobacterium longum (two different strains)
Blautia producta
Clostridium cocleatum
Collinsella aerofaciens
Dorea longicatena (two different strains)
Escherichia coli
Eubacterium desmolans
Eubacterium eligens
Eubacterium limosum
Eubacterium rectale (four different strains)
Eubacterium ventriosum
Faecalibacterium prausnitzii
Lachnospira pectinoshiza
Lactobacillus casei/paracasei
Lactobacillus casei
Parabacteroides distasonis
Raoultella sp.
Roseburia faecalis
Roseburia intestinalis
Ruminococcus torques (two different strains)
Ruminococcus obeum (two different strains)
Streptococcus mitis

intestinal bacteria isolated from a healthy donor (**Table 1**), to treat rCDI. In this study, the synthetic bacterial mixture was infused through the colon of the infected patient causing a change in the stool microbial profile. Major shifts reflecting the isolates of the synthetic mixture were still detectable 6 months after treatment. Thus, the concept of "RePOOPulate" the gut microbiome was coined. Authors of the study suggested that using a synthetic stool substitute may be an effective method to replace the use of FMT for treating rCDI. Although further validation is needed, complete resolution of the infection was achieved. Several advantages of this synthetic stool substitute can be highlighted. The composition of the administered bacterial cocktail is accurately characterized, facilitating registration. Further, assembly of the synthetic bacterial cocktail is highly reproducible enabling standardization and upscaling. In addition, patient safety can be guaranteed, because the bacterial mixture can be rendered pathogen- and virus-free (Petrof et al., 2013). These data suggest that a multi-species community such as that in the RePOOPulate study, can be more effective than single-strain probiotics or mixed cultures of probiotic species. This can be because the RePOOPulate community preserved its structure and thus successfully colonized a new environment (Petrof et al., 2013). Moreover, RePOOPulate consisted of a more phylogenetically diverse community including strains with beneficial health effects that can be candidates for next generation probiotics.

NEXT GENERATION PROBIOTICS

Looking at its internationally recognized definition, probiotics are live microorganisms that, when administered in adequate numbers, confer health benefits on the host. Probiotics are usually isolated from our commensal gut bacteria, but cannot be given the definition of probiotics until their stability, content, and health effect are characterized (Sanders, 2008). Probiotics are thought to improve the balance in the host, prevent disturbances, and decrease the risk of pathogen colonization (Goldenberg et al., 2013). They have been referred to as functional foods or beneficial bacteria, and they have been considered for the prevention and treatment of *C. difficile*-associated diarrhea (CDAD) (Goldenberg et al., 2013). Probiotics can be found as capsules or food supplements in health food stores and supermarkets (Goldenberg et al., 2013). Pattani et al. (2013) reported that *Lactobacillus*-based formulations combined with antibiotics reduced the risk of AAD and CDI. They however, suggested that larger studies are needed to decide on the use of probiotic/antibiotic combination as a therapy over the single species probiotic (Pattani et al., 2013). Furthermore, findings from randomized control trials (RCTs) and meta analyses suggest that there is moderate evidence on the ability of probiotics to prevent primary CDI (people at risk of CDI), but there is no enough evidence suggesting the probiotics can prevent secondary CDI (recurrent CDI) (Evans and Johnson, 2015). There are still some evidence gaps for the use of probiotics in the prevention of CDI such as the interaction between specific classes of antibiotics with the probiotics used on CDI risk, the bacterial taxa that provides the best efficacy in the prevention of CDI, and the use of probiotics in immunocompromised or critically ill patients (Rao and Young, 2017). Hence, future RCT should consider these different concerns (Rao and Young, 2017). Besides, probiotics impact the gut-brain axis.

For example, *Bifidobacterium longum* NC3001 had beneficial effects on psychiatric comorbidities, which in turn could temporarily improve the quality of life in IBS patients, indicating that this probiotic reduces limbic reactivity (Pinto-Sanchez et al., 2017).

Overall, classical probiotics show limited effects on the human gut microbiota seeking the need for a better selection and formulation of bacterial strains (Neef and Sanz, 2013). Results from previous studies show promising outcomes in the treatment or prevention of diverse metabolic and inflammatory diseases by specific bacteria (Neef and Sanz, 2013). Those probiotics encompass species different from *Lactobacillus* and *Bifidobacterium* (Cani and Van Hul, 2015; Patel and DuPont, 2015). Nevertheless, the gut microbiome is a complex community, which makes it difficult to define the host–microbe interaction.

The United Nations Food and Agriculture organization (FAO) definition of probiotics is broad, allowing flexibility in terms of the phylogenetic origin of probiotics. Information generated from previous studies assisted in the selection of next generation probiotics, which include members from *Clostridium* clusters IV, XIVa and XVIII, *F. prausnitzii, Akkermansia muciniphila, Bacteroides uniformis* (Neef and Sanz, 2013; Patel and DuPont, 2015), *Bacteroides fragilis* (Round et al., 2011), and *Eubacterium hallii* (Udayappan et al., 2016). These next generation probiotics were evaluated in preclinical trials and yielded positive outcomes for inflammatory and metabolic disorders (Neef and Sanz, 2013; Patel and DuPont, 2015). In addition, new techniques are required for the development of new probiotic products containing strains from human origin. This is to say, these strains must come from the major groups of the intestinal microbiota, they have to be defined to have a safe status and proven to have potential beneficial effects (Martín et al., 2017). In the following sections, we will discuss some of the most promising bacterial species that are currently under consideration for being used as next-generation probiotics.

Faecalibacterium prausnitzii

Faecalibacterium prausnitzii is an extreme oxygen sensitive (EOS) bacterium (Martín et al., 2017) belonging to the *Clostridium* cluster IV, and it accounts for 3–5% of the total fecal bacteria, and it is one of the predominant groups in the human feces (Breyner et al., 2017). Quévrain et al. (2016) reported low proportions of this species in the fecal and mucosa-associated microbiome in Crohn's disease (CD). *F. prausnitzii* may possess *in vivo* and *in vitro* anti-inflammatory effects. *F. prausnitzii* may possess *in vivo* and *in vitro* anti-inflammatory effects. Breyner et al. (2017) confirmed the anti-inflammatory properties of MAM, and their ability to reduce Th1 and Th17 pro-inflammatory cytokines in Mesenteric Lymphatic Node (MLN) and colon tissues in both DNBS and DSS colitis model. MAM was also able to improve TGFβ cytokine which affects NF-κB activation in DNBS model thus protecting the host and decreasing intestinal inflammation (Breyner et al., 2017). In addition, *F. prausnitzii* can induce the *Clostridium*-specific IL-10-secreting regulatory T cell subset, present in several human colonic cells. Its capacity for lowering IL-12 and IFNγ production indicates that the interaction between *F. prausnitzii* and the host shape and maintain the gut barrier immune function (Quévrain et al., 2016). In this way, anti-inflammatory molecules from *F. prausnitzii* may be used as targeted anti-inflammatory drugs for CD. Moreover, MAM could function as a CD biomarker, predicting loss of *F. prausnitzii* functionality. However, further research should be conducted to elucidate the MAM production mechanisms, before considering it for CD management. Sokol colleagues reported that low proportions of *F. prausnitzii* on a resected ileal Crohn's mucosa were associated with CD recurrence after 6 months. In addition, the oral administration of live *F. prausnitzii* or its supernatant in mice could reduce the severity of trinitrobenzene sulfonic acid (TNBS) colitis and correct the associated dysbiosis (Sokol et al., 2008). The results from this study suggest that *F. prausnitzii* can be considered as a promising probiotic candidate for the treatment of pathologies characterized by chronic gut inflammation (Sokol et al., 2008). Besides, all *F. prausnitzii* strains have proven anti-inflammatory properties, which allows them to further be tested in murine models to determine their beneficial effects before moving to human trials (Martín et al., 2017).

Akkermansia muciniphila

Recent evidence shows that there is a link between the altered gut microbiota and metabolic diseases like obesity, diabetes mellitus, and cardiovascular disease (Schneeberger et al., 2015; Dao et al., 2016; Li et al., 2016). Higher abundance of *A. muciniphila*, a mucin degrading microbe, was associated with healthier metabolic status. Everard et al. (2014) and Schneeberger et al. (2015) studied the effects of high fat diet on metabolic parameters and the gut microbiota composition over time, and they found that *A. muciniphila* was decreased. The negative impact on *A. muciniphila* was associated with expression of lipid metabolism, inflammatory markers in adipose tissue, and different parameters like increased blood glucose, insulin resistance and plasma triglycerides (Schneeberger et al., 2015). This prompted the research toward investigating the putatively positive role of *A. muciniphila* in adipose tissue homeostasis and metabolism. Dao et al. (2016) assessed clinical parameters and *A. muciniphila* abundance before and after a 6-week calorie restriction period, followed by stabilization diet. The results of this intervention study indicate that the higher abundance of *A. muciniphila* at baseline was associated with improvement in blood glucose homeostasis, lipid profile, and body fat distribution after the intervention. Thus, *A. muciniphila* can be used as a prognostic tool for the success of diet interventions (Dao et al., 2016). Moreover, Li et al. (2016) reported that administration of *A. muciniphila* could reverse the atherosclerotic lesions, improve metabolic endotoxemia-induced inflammation, and ultimately restore the gut barrier.

Bacteroides fragilis and *Bacteroides uniformis*

Bacteroides species are commensal bacteria that represent 25% of our gut bacterial population. They are gram negative, anaerobic, bile resistant, and non-spore forming bacteria. *Bacteroides* can be passed from the mother to the child during vaginal delivery, thus becoming primary colonizers of the gut. When retained in the gut, *Bacteroides* act as commensals and can be beneficial for the host (Wexler, 2007). The most common isolate from the clinical specimens is *B. fragilis*, which is the most virulent *Bacteroides* species (Wexler, 2007).

Bacterial colonization of the gut can greatly affect the immune system, either through the direct host–bacteria interaction, or by molecules produced by our commensal bacteria. *B. fragilis* produces polysaccharide A (PSA), which is an immunomodulatory molecule that activates the T-cell dependent immune responses (Troy and Kasper, 2010). Those responses are involved in the development and homeostasis of the host immune system (Troy and Kasper, 2010). Furthermore, Round et al. (2011) demonstrated that *B. fragilis* activates Toll-like receptor (TLR) pathways. This occurs because

PSA signals through TLR2 on Foxp3+ (forkhead box P3) regulatory T cells to boost immunologic tolerance. As a result, PSA can be considered as a model symbiosis factor, because it preserves the balance between T cell types and maintains the immune system homeostasis (Round et al., 2011).

As for *Bacteroides uniformis* (*B. uniformis*) CECT 7771, it is considered a potential probiotic strain originally isolated from the feces of healthy breastfed infants. Oral administration of this specific strain in high fat diet-fed mice improved lipid profile, reduced glucose insulin and leptin levels, increased TNF-α production by dendritic cells (DCs) in response to LPS stimulation, and increased phagocytosis (Gauffin Cano et al., 2012). Thus, administration of *B. uniformis* CECT 7771 can ameliorate metabolic disorder and immunological dysfunction related to intestinal dysbiosis in obese mice (Gauffin Cano et al., 2012; Yang et al., 2016). Furthermore, acute administration of this strain to mice did not promote adverse effects on health status or food intake, and there was no bacteria translocation to blood, liver, or lymph nodes. This indicates that there are no safety concerns for this strain in mice, but further investigation should be completed in humans (Fernández-Murga and Sanz, 2016).

Eubacterium hallii

Eubacterium hallii is an important anaerobic butyrate-producer resident in our gut, which influences the intestinal metabolic balance (Engels et al., 2016). Butyrate has been proposed to lower mucosal inflammation and oxidative status, strengthen the epithelial barrier function, and modulate intestinal motility in addition to being an energy source for colonocytes (Canani et al., 2011). *E. hallii* can yield propionate from a broad range of substrates. This versatility may enhance the host–gut microbiota homeostasis (Engels et al., 2016). Moreover, administration of *E. hallii* in obese and diabetic db/db mice increased energy metabolism and improved insulin sensitivity. However, increasing dosage of *E. hallii* did not impact body weight or food intake, indicating that this strain can a safe and effective alternative for insulin sensitivity (Udayappan et al., 2016).

COCKTAILS OF *Clostridium* CLUSTER IV AND XIVA MEMBERS

As previously described, T_{regs} can regulate immune homeostasis and serve as a therapeutic target for different gut inflammatory disorders. Induction of the colonic T_{regs} is dependent on special properties of our commensal bacteria. *Clostridium* spp. belonging to clusters IV and XIVa (also known as *Clostridium leptum* and *coccoides* groups, respectively) are exceptional inducers of T_{regs} in the colon and can be considered as therapeutic options for IBD and allergies (Atarashi et al., 2011). Previous work indicated that a cocktail of strains isolated for the human gut microbiota can be more effective than a single strain in preventing or treating disease. Thus, Atarashi et al. (2013) isolated 17 strains belonging to Clostridia clusters XIVa, IV, and XVIII from a human fecal sample, which were effective in T_{reg} cell differentiation and accumulation in mouse colon. Authors proposed that the SCFAs produced by this community influenced the expression of *Foxp3*, a key gene controlling T_{reg} cell development (Atarashi et al., 2013). Incidentally, Clostridia clusters XIVa and IV are decreased in fecal samples from patients with inflammatory bowel disease (IBD), and thus the cocktail of the 17 strains could potentially reverse this dysbiosis (Atarashi et al., 2013).

INDUSTRIAL APPLICATIONS AND INTERESTS

Current Developments

Since the manipulation of the gut microbiota has been proven to be promising to prevent and treat different diseases, pharmaceutical and food industries would be interested in the potential therapeutic approaches described before. For instance, Seres health and Rebiotix companies are working on developing a defined microbial cocktail and a standardized commercially prepared FMT, respectively. These therapeutic approaches are intended to treat CDI, and that can be used as an alternative for FMT. Synthetic microbial communities designed for transplants are expected to meet production, mode of action and safety standards (Orenstein et al., 2015; van der Lelie et al., 2017). For instance, Seres health developed SER-109, a novel biological agent proposed to restore the balance in the gut microbiome, promoting resistance to pathogenic invaders like *C. difficile* (Khanna et al., 2016). Seres health also developed SER-287 for the treatment of IBD and in specific ulcerative colitis (Inflammatory Bowel Disease | Seres Therapeutics, 2017). Rebiotix commercially developed RBX2660, a mix of live human microbes for effective treatment of recurrent CDI (Ramesh et al., 2016). Moreover, other formulations including strains belonging to Clostridia classes IV and XIVa were designed to modulate the immune response (Atarashi et al., 2013). The original community of 17 strains (VE202) was developed by Vendanta Biosciences and Johnson and Johnson, and has provided an effective treatment for autoimmune disorders (Reardon, 2014; Ratner, 2015; van der Lelie et al., 2017).

Technical Challenges

Several challenges concerning the stability of the probiotic during the probiotic production are still unsolved. Microorganisms require strict conditions to grow, such as specific nutritional media and environmental conditions (suitable temperature, pH, water activity, oxygen content, among others). The product manufacturing and storage processes may impact the viability of the bacterial strains, influencing probiotic stability and properties. In addition, it is fundamental to consider the viability of the probiotics after consumption. Bacterial strains should remain viable at sufficient numbers through the gastrointestinal tract (GIT) passage. Therefore, the selection of optimal culture medium and cell protectants is crucial to enhance the efficacy of the probiotic product. Moreover, as most probiotic strains are strict anaerobes or facultative anaerobes, oxygen permeation into carriers should be reduced, or oxygen scavengers should be introduced to reduce the redox potential (Shah et al., 2010). Probiotic bacteria can also be protected by microencapsulation, which has been proposed to improve the stability of the strains and can adapt to the GIT conditions (Heidebach et al., 2012). Nowadays, yogurts and fermented milk are the best-established vehicles for probiotics in the market. However, some probiotic strains are sensitive to the different conditions in fermented products, like oxygen and pH, which can, in turn, affect the stability of probiotics through post-acidification during their storage in the fridge. To minimize this phenomenon, strains that lack the ability to post-acidify should be selected (Damin et al., 2008). As a result, this can cause an economic burden for manufacturers, limiting the addition of probiotics in different products (Gueimonde and Sánchez, 2012). Furthermore, manufacturing the probiotic product in a reproducible manner is a critical aspect (Paulo Sousa e Silva and Freitas, 2014). Several attempts to fix the number of viable probiotic strains throughout the products (Shah et al., 2010) have been attempted, to no avail.

Regulatory Challenges

Probiotics are classified in different categories across countries. Their names and use as functional foods may vary according to different systems. For instance, probiotics fall in the Qualified Presumption of Safety (QPS) list provided by the European Food Safety Authority (EFSA) and referred to as functional foods since there was no legal definition for probiotics. The market for probiotics as functional foods expanded, as a result of probiotic food products like yogurts and fermented milk (Baldi and Arora, 2015), containing conventional LAB. The QPS list is periodically updated according to the safety assessment of the biological products recommended to be added, and not all can be approved (Scientific Opinion on The Maintenance of The List of QPS Biological Agents Intentionally Added to EFSA Panel on Biological Hazards (BIOHAZ), 2013; Ricci et al., 2017). A similar system applies in the United States as Generally Recognized as Safe (GRAS) products should be approved by the FDA. However, if a probiotic is used as a dietary supplement in the United States, then it is considered as "food" and should be regulated by the Dietary Supplement Health and Education Act (DSHEA). If the probiotic was considered to have therapeutic purpose, the probiotic drug should be proven to be safe and effective to be approved by the FDA. Nevertheless, for both the FDA and EFSA, probiotics cannot be used in health claims. On the other hand, Japan acts as a global market leader, where probiotics are considered as both foods and drugs. According to the Japanese regulations, probiotic products are in different category than foods and Foods for Specific Health Uses (FOSHU). Efficacy claims for probiotic products are prohibited on the labeling until the product gets the permission from the Ministry of Health and Welfare (MHLW) to be considered FOSHU, for which efficacy and safety validation is mandatory. FOSHU categorizes the food claims according to the scientific evidence and the strength of the supporting data provided. The government then divided the FOSHU health claims into subcategories, in which their effect could be in GIT, metabolism, cholesterol moderation, or bone health. Japanese regulations also approve new health claims on a regular basis (Baldi and Arora, 2015).

As the definition and classification of probiotics by regulatory agents throughout the world is different, the status of probiotic products is still uncertain. Thus, reservations about probiotic products claims may arise among regulatory bodies, producers, and consumers. Since the probiotic concept is invading the world, further investigation for probiotic traits is needed. Moreover, most probiotics only include LAB, which possess limited phylogenetic diversity and functionality. Hence, critical update of the screenings required by regulatory agents is urgently needed.

Medical Application

Despite the different studies and outcomes of FMT, FDA approval in North America has not been granted. At the beginning, FMT was considered as investigational new drugs (INDs), and FDA authorization was mandatory. Currently, patients unresponsive to standard antibiotic CDI therapies can opt for FMT after completing an informed consent, where they are notified that FMT is still under investigation. However, SERES 109 and RBX2660 have been granted the Orphan Drug designation by the FDA (Rebiotix Media, 2015; Seres Therapeutics, 2015). As for the EMA in Europe, the use of FMT for the treatment of CDI has not been yet regulated (van Nood et al., 2014; Lowes, 2016). Yet, FMT is regularly applied to curb infections across Europe, and it is considered in clinical trials for many other pathologies. In the search for safe FMT alternatives, research on microbiotic medicinal products (MMP) is in full development and novel applications are continuously being considered. These MMP developments require novel views and strategies from the scientific world, the industry, the medical field, and the regulatory bodies. In this context, platforms like the Pharmabiotic Research Institute have been created, to facilitate discussion between different stakeholders (Pharmabiotic Research Institute, 2017). Overall, additional research needs to be conducted before using FMT alternatives containing characterized microbial communities and next generation probiotics, to guarantee their safety and reproducible efficacy.

CONCLUSION

FMT may be replaced with a characterized multispecies bacterial mixture that can be safer, free of allergens or viruses, and capable of treating CDI. With the current *in vitro* and *in vivo* data, next generation probiotics hold promise to treat diverse medical conditions, and they can be more effective than single or multi strains of the commercial probiotics. Moreover, several different strains with proven health benefits can also be considered candidates for next generation probiotics and other microbiota-based drugs. However, additional research is required for an increased understanding of the interactions among those strains, aiming at producing a successful therapeutic formulation. Research should be conducted to demonstrate whether these probiotics can be applicable to humans, as safety assessments have only been completed in animals. Effective carriage of bacterial strains in food matrices is critical for survival. Thus, optimisation of the growing conditions, and even encapsulation must be considered to promote delivery and release of the live product in the colon. The development of next generation probiotics and MMPs hold promise for innovation in both the food/feed sector and the pharmaceutical industry. A close interaction between academia, industry and regulatory agencies is essential for developing safe and health-promoting products, as both prophylactic and therapeutic strategies.

AUTHOR CONTRIBUTIONS

Conceived and designed the review: REH, EH-S, and TVW. Funding acquisition: TVW. Wrote the paper: REH. Reviewed the manuscript: REH, EH-S, and TVW.

ACKNOWLEDGMENT

The research leading to these results has received funding from the People Program (Marie Curie Actions) of the European Union's Seventh Framework Program FP7/2007–2013/under REA grant agreement n° 606713.

REFERENCES

Asemi, Z., Zare, Z., Shakeri, H., Sabihi, S.-S., and Esmaillzadeh, A. (2013). Effect of multispecies probiotic supplements on metabolic profiles, Hs-CRP, and oxidative stress in patients with Type 2 diabetes. *Ann. Nutr. Metab.* 63, 1–9. doi: 10.1159/000349922

Atarashi, K., Tanoue, T., Oshima, K., Suda, W., Nagano, Y., Nishikawa, H., et al. (2013). Treg induction by a rationally selected mixture of Clostridia strains from the human microbiota. *Nature* 500, 232–236. doi: 10.1038/nature12331

Atarashi, K., Tanoue, T., Shima, T., Imaoka, A., Kuwahara, T., Momose, Y., et al. (2011). Induction of colonic regulatory T cells by indigenous *Clostridium* species. *Science* 331, 337–341. doi: 10.1126/science.1198469

Bakken, J. S. (2009). Fecal bacteriotherapy for recurrent *Clostridium difficile* infection. *Anaerobe* 15, 285–289. doi: 10.1016/j.anaerobe.2009.09.007

Bakken, J. S., Borody, T., Brandt, L. J., Brill, J. V., Demarco, D. C., Franzos, M. A., et al. (2011). Treating *Clostridium difficile* infection with fecal microbiota transplantation. *Clin. Gastroenterol. Hepatol.* 9, 1044–1049. doi: 10.1016/j.cgh.2011.08.014

Baldi, A., and Arora, M. (2015). Regulatory categories of probiotics across the globe: a review representing existing and recommended categorization. *Indian J. Med. Microbiol.* 33(Suppl.), 2–10. doi: 10.4103/0255-0857.150868

Barbut, F., Richard, A., Hamadi, K., Chomette, V., Burghoffer, B., and Petit, J.-C. (2000). Epidemiology of recurrences or reinfections of *Clostridium difficile*-associated diarrhea. *J. Clin. Microbiol.* 38, 2386–2388.

Bartlett, J. G. (1990). *Clostridium difficile*: clinical considerations. *Clin. Infect. Dis.* 12(Suppl. 2), S243–S251. doi: 10.1093/clinids/12.supplement_2.s243

Becattini, S., Taur, Y., and Pamer, E. G. (2016). Antibiotic-induced changes in the intestinal microbiota and disease. *Trends Mol. Med.* 22, 458–478. doi: 10.1016/j.molmed.2016.04.003

Besseling-van der Vaart, I., Heath, M. D., Guagnini, F., and Kramer, M. F. (2016). In vitro evidence for efficacy in food intolerance for the multispecies probiotic formulation Ecologic® Tolerance (Syngut™). *Benef. Microbes* 7, 111–118. doi: 10.3920/bm2015.0051

Brandt, L. J. (2012). Fecal transplantation for the treatment of *Clostridium difficile* infection. *Gastroenterol. Hepatol.* 8, 191–194.

Breyner, N. M., Michon, C., de Sousa, C. S., Vilas Boas, P. B., Chain, F., Azevedo, V. A., et al. (2017). Microbial anti-inflammatory molecule (MAM) from *Faecalibacterium prausnitzii* shows a protective effect on DNBS and DSS-induced colitis model in mice through inhibition of NF-κB pathway. *Front. Microbiol.* 8:114. doi: 10.3389/fmicb.2017.00114

Canani, R. B., Costanzo, M. D., Leone, L., Pedata, M., Meli, R., and Calignano, A. (2011). Potential beneficial effects of butyrate in intestinal and extraintestinal diseases. *World J. Gastroenterol.* 17, 1519–1528. doi: 10.3748/wjg.v17.i12.1519

Cani, P. D., and Van Hul, M. (2015). Novel opportunities for next-generation probiotics targeting metabolic syndrome. *Curr. Opin. Biotechnol.* 32, 21–27. doi: 10.1016/j.copbio.2014.10.006

Chapman, C., Gibson, G., and Rowland, I. (2011). Health benefits of probiotics: are mixtures more effective than single strains? *Eur. J. Nutr.* 50, 1–17. doi: 10.1007/s00394-010-0166-z

Chen, J., Wang, R., Li, X.-F., and Wang, R.-L. (2011). *Bifidobacterium adolescentis* supplementation ameliorates visceral fat accumulation and insulin sensitivity in an experimental model of the metabolic syndrome. *Br. J. Nutr.* 107, 1429–1434. doi: 10.1017/s0007114511004491

Clarke, S. F., Murphy, E. F., O'Sullivan, O., Lucey, A. J., Humphreys, M., Hogan, A., et al. (2014). Exercise and associated dietary extremes impact on gut microbial diversity. *Gut* 63, 1913–1920. doi: 10.1136/gutjnl-2013-306541

Damin, M. R., Minowa, E., Alcântara, M. R., and Oliveira, M. N. (2008). Effect of cold storage on culture viability and some rheological properties of fermented milk prepared with yogurt and probiotic bacteria. *J. Texture Stud.* 39, 40–55. doi: 10.1111/j.1745-4603.2007.00129.x

Dao, M. C., Everard, A., Aron-Wisnewsky, J., Sokolovska, N., Prifti, E., Verger, E. O., et al. (2016). *Akkermansia muciniphila* and improved metabolic health during a dietary intervention in obesity: relationship with gut microbiome richness and ecology. *Gut* 65, 426–436. doi: 10.1136/gutjnl-2014-308778

De Palma, G., Collins, S. M., and Bercik, P. (2014). The microbiota-gut-brain axis in functional gastrointestinal disorders. *Gut Microbes* 5, 419–429. doi: 10.4161/gmic.29417

De Palma, G., Lynch, M. D. J., Lu, J., Dang, V. T., Deng, Y., Jury, J., et al. (2017). Transplantation of fecal microbiota from patients with irritable bowel syndrome alters gut function and behavior in recipient mice. *Sci. Transl. Med.* 9:eaaf6397. doi: 10.1126/scitranslmed.aaf6397

den Besten, G., van Eunen, K., Groen, A. K., Venema, K., Reijngoud, D.-J., and Bakker, B. M. (2013). The role of short-chain fatty acids in the interplay between diet, gut microbiota, and host energy metabolism. *J. Lipid Res.* 54, 2325–2340. doi: 10.1194/jlr.r036012

Dethlefsen, L., and Relman, D. A. (2010). Incomplete recovery and individualized responses of the human distal gut microbiota to repeated antibiotic perturbation. *Proc. Natl. Acad. Sci. U.S.A.* 108(Suppl. 1), 4554–4561. doi: 10.1073/pnas.1000087107

Di Cerbo, A., Palmieri, B., Aponte, M., Morales-Medina, J. C., and Iannitti, T. (2016). Mechanisms and therapeutic effectiveness of lactobacilli. *J. Clin. Pathol.* 69, 187–203. doi: 10.1136/jclinpath-2015-202976

Distrutti, E., Monaldi, L., Ricci, P., and Fiorucci, S. (2016). Gut microbiota role in irritable bowel syndrome: new therapeutic strategies. *World J. Gastroenterol.* 22, 2219–2241. doi: 10.3748/wjg.v22.i7.2219

EFSA Panel on Biological Hazards (BIOHAZ) (2013). Scientific opinion on the maintenance of the list of QPS biological agents intentionally added to food and feed (2013 update). *EFSA J.* 11:3449. doi: 10.2903/j.efsa.2013.3449

Engels, C., Ruscheweyh, H.-J., Beerenwinkel, N., Lacroix, C., and Schwab, C. (2016). The common gut microbe *Eubacterium hallii* also contributes to intestinal propionate formation. *Front. Microbiol.* 7:713. doi: 10.3389/fmicb.2016.00713

Evans, C. T., and Johnson, S. (2015). Prevention of *Clostridium difficile* infection with probiotics. *Clin. Infect. Dis.* 60(Suppl. 2), S122–S128. doi: 10.1093/cid/civ138

Everard, A., Lazarevic, V., Gaïa, N., Johansson, M., Ståhlman, M., Backhed, F., et al. (2014). Microbiome of prebiotic-treated mice reveals novel targets involved in host response during obesity. *ISME J.* 8, 2116–2130. doi: 10.1038/ismej.2014.45

Fernández-Murga, M. L., and Sanz, Y. (2016). Safety assessment of *Bacteroides uniformis* CECT 7771 isolated from stools of healthy breast-fed infants. *PLOS ONE* 11:e0145503. doi: 10.1371/journal.pone.0145503

Figueroa, I., Johnson, S., Sambol, S. P., Goldstein, E. J. C., Citron, D. M., and Gerding, D. N. (2012). Relapse versus reinfection: recurrent *Clostridium difficile* infection following treatment with fidaxomicin or vancomycin. *Clin. Infect. Dis.* 55(Suppl. 2), S104–S109. doi: 10.1093/cid/cis357

Francino, M. P. (2016). Antibiotics and the human gut microbiome: dysbioses and accumulation of resistances. *Front. Microbiol.* 6:1543. doi: 10.3389/fmicb.2015.01543

Gauffin Cano, P., Santacruz, A., Moya, Á., and Sanz, Y. (2012). *Bacteroides uniformis* CECT 7771 ameliorates metabolic and immunological dysfunction in mice with high-fat-diet induced obesity. *PLOS ONE* 7:e41079. doi: 10.1371/journal.pone.0041079

Gibson, G. R., Hutkins, R., Sanders, M. E., Prescott, S. L., Reimer, R. A., Salminen, S. J., et al. (2017). Expert consensus document: the international scientific association for probiotics and prebiotics (ISAPP) consensus statement on the definition and scope of prebiotics. *Nat. Rev. Gastroenterol. Hepatol.* 14, 491–502. doi: 10.1038/nrgastro.2017.75

Goldenberg, J. Z., Ma, S. S. Y., Saxton, J. D., Martzen, M. R., Vandvik, P. O., Thorlund, K., et al. (2013). Probiotics for the prevention of *Clostridium difficile*-associated diarrhea in adults and children. *Cochrane Database Syst. Rev.* doi: 10.1002/14651858.CD006095.pub3

Govender, M., Choonara, Y. E., Kumar, P., du Toit, L. C., van Vuuren, S., and Pillay, V. (2013). A review of the advancements in probiotic delivery: conventional vs. non-conventional formulations for intestinal flora supplementation. *AAPS PharmsciTech* 15, 29–43. doi: 10.1208/s12249-013-0027-1

Graf, D., Di Cagno, R., Fåk, F., Flint, H. J., Nyman, M., Saarela, M., et al. (2015). Contribution Of diet to the composition of the human gut microbiota. *Microb. Ecol. Health Dis.* 26:26164. doi: 10.3402/mehd.v26.26164

Guarner, F., and Malagelada, J.-R. (2003). Gut flora in health and disease. *Lancet* 361, 512–519. doi: 10.1016/s0140-6736(03)12489-0

Gueimonde, M., and Sánchez, B. (2012). Enhancing probiotic stability in industrial processes. *Microb. Ecol. Health Dis.* 23:18562. doi: 10.3402/mehd.v23i0.18562

Hand, T. W. (2016). The role of the microbiota in shaping infectious immunity. *Trends Immunol.* 37, 647–658. doi: 10.1016/j.it.2016.08.007

Hartstra, A. V., Bouter, K. E. C., Bäckhed, F., and Nieuwdorp, M. (2015). Insights into the role of the microbiome in obesity and type 2 diabetes. *Diabetes Care* 38, 159–165. doi: 10.2337/dc14-0769

Heidebach, T., Först, P., and Kulozik, U. (2012). Microencapsulation of probiotic cells for food applications. *Crit. Rev. Food Sci. Nutr.* 52, 291–311. doi: 10.1080/10408398.2010.499801

Hill, C., Guarner, F., Reid, G., Gibson, G. R., Merenstein, D. J., Pot, B., et al. (2014). Expert consensus document: the international scientific association for probiotics and prebiotics consensus statement on the scope and appropriate use of the term probiotic. *Nat. Rev. Gastroenterol. Hepatol.* 11, 506–514. doi: 10.1038/nrgastro.2014.66

Jafarnejad, S., Saremi, S., Jafarnejad, F., and Arab, A. (2016). Effects of a multispecies probiotic mixture on glycemic control and inflammatory status in women with gestational diabetes: a randomized controlled clinical trial. *J. Nutr. Metab.* 2016:5190846. doi: 10.1155/2016/5190846

Jiang, Z.-D., Hoang, L. N., Lasco, T. M., Garey, K. W., and DuPont, H. L. (2013). Physician attitudes toward the use of fecal transplantation for recurrent *Clostridium difficile* infection in a metropolitan area. *Clin. Infect. Dis.* 56, 1059–1060. doi: 10.1093/cid/cis1025

Johnson, S., Adelmann, A., Clabots, C. R., Peterson, L. R., and Gerding, D. N. (1989). Recurrences of *Clostridium difficile* diarrhea not caused by the original infecting organism. *J. Infect. Dis.* 159, 340–343. doi: 10.1093/infdis/159.2.340

Kasińska, M. A., and Drzewoski, J. (2015). Effectiveness of probiotics in Type 2 diabetes: a meta-analysis. *Pol. Arch. Intern. Med.* 125, 803–813. doi: 10.20452/pamw.3156

Kelly, C. P. (2009). A 76-year-old man with recurrent *Clostridium difficile*-associated diarrhea. *JAMA* 301, 954–962. doi: 10.1001/jama.2009.171

Kelly, C. P. (2013). Fecal microbiota transplantation—an old therapy comes of age. *N. Engl. J. Med.* 368, 474–475. doi: 10.1056/nejme1214816

Khanna, S., Pardi, D. S., Kelly, C. R., Kraft, C. S., Dhere, T., Henn, M. R., et al. (2016). A novel microbiome therapeutic increases gut microbial diversity and prevents recurrent *Clostridium difficile* infection. *J. Infect. Dis.* 214, 173–181. doi: 10.1093/infdis/jiv766

Kim, S.-W., Park, K.-Y., Kim, B., Kim, E., and Hyun, C.-K. (2013). *Lactobacillus rhamnosus* GG improves insulin sensitivity and reduces adiposity in high-fat diet-fed mice through enhancement of adiponectin production. *Biochem. Biophys. Res. Commun.* 431, 258–263. doi: 10.1016/j.bbrc.2012.12.121

Klaenhammer, T. R., Kleerebezem, M., Kopp, M. V., and Rescigno, M. (2012). The impact of probiotics and prebiotics on the immune system. *Nat. Rev. Immunol.* 12, 728–734. doi: 10.1038/nri3312

Kobyliak, N., Conte, C., Cammarota, G., Haley, A. P., Styriak, I., Gaspar, L., et al. (2016). Probiotics in prevention and treatment of obesity: a critical view. *Nutr. Metab.* 13, 14. doi: 10.1186/s12986-016-0067-0

Koning, C. J., Jonkers, D. M., Stobberingh, E. E., Mulder, L., Rombouts, F. M., and Stockbrügger, R. W. (2008). The effect of a multispecies probiotic on the intestinal microbiota and bowel movements in healthy volunteers taking the antibiotic amoxycillin. *Am. J. Gastroenterol.* 103, 178–189. doi: 10.1111/j.1572-0241.2007.01547.x

Kristensen, N. B., Bryrup, T., Allin, K. H., Nielsen, T., Hansen, T. H., and Pedersen, O. (2016). Alterations in fecal microbiota composition by probiotic supplementation in healthy adults: a systematic review of randomized controlled trials. *Genome Med.* 8, 52. doi: 10.1186/s13073-016-0300-5

Kwon, H.-K., Lee, C.-G., So, J.-S., Chae, C.-S., Hwang, J.-S., Sahoo, A., et al. (2010). Generation of regulatory dendritic cells and $CD4^{+}Foxp3^{+}$ T cells by probiotics administration suppresses immune disorders. *Proc. Natl. Acad. Sci. U.S.A.* 107, 2159–2164. doi: 10.1073/pnas.0904055107

Langdon, A., Crook, N., and Dantas, G. (2016). The effects of antibiotics on the microbiome throughout development and alternative approaches for therapeutic modulation. *Genome Med.* 8:39. doi: 10.1186/s13073-016-0294-z

Leszczyszyn, J. J., Radomski, M., and Leszczyszyn, A. M. (2016). Intestinal microbiota transplant – current state of knowledge. *Reumatologia* 54, 24–28. doi: 10.5114/reum.2016.58758

Li, J., Lin, S., Vanhoutte, P. M., Woo, C. W., and Xu, A. (2016). *Akkermansia muciniphila* protects against atherosclerosis by preventing metabolic endotoxemia-induced inflammation in apoe-/-mice clinical. *Circulation* 133, 2434–2446. doi: 10.1161/circulationaha.115.019645

Lowes, R. (2016). *FDA Proposes Tighter Rules For Fecal Transplants.* New York, NY: Medscape.

Macpherson, A. J., de Agüero, M. G., and Ganal-Vonarburg, S. C. (2017). How nutrition and the maternal microbiota shape the neonatal immune system. *Nat. Rev. Immunol.* 17, 508–517. doi: 10.1038/nri.2017.58

Marotz, C. A., and Zarrinpar, A. (2016). Treating obesity and metabolic syndrome with fecal microbiota transplantation. *Yale J. Biol. Med.* 89, 383–388.

Marsh, J. W., Arora, R., Schlackman, J. L., Shutt, K. A., Curry, S. R., and Harrison, L. H. (2012). Association of relapse of *Clostridium difficile* disease with BI/NAP1/027. *J. Clin. Microbiol.* 50, 4078–4082. doi: 10.1128/jcm.02291-12

Martín, R., Chain, F., Miquel, S., Lu, J., Gratadoux, J.-J., Sokol, H., et al. (2014). The commensal bacterium *Faecalibacterium prausnitzii* is protective in DNBS-induced chronic moderate and severe colitis models. *Inflamm. Bowel Dis.* 20, 417–430. doi: 10.1097/01.mib.0000440815.76627.64

Martín, R., Miquel, S., Benevides, L., Bridonneau, C., Robert, V., Hudault, S., et al. (2017). Functional characterization of novel *Faecalibacterium prausnitzii* strains isolated from healthy volunteers: a step forward in the use of *F. prausnitzii* as a next-generation probiotic. *Front. Microbiol.* 8:1226. doi: 10.3389/fmicb.2017.01226

Miettinen, M., Vuopio-Varkila, J., and Varkila, K. (1996). Production of human tumor necrosis factor alpha, interleukin-6, and interleukin-10 is induced by lactic acid bacteria. *Infect. Immun.* 64, 5403–5405.

Miquel, S., Leclerc, M., Martin, R., Chain, F., Lenoir, M., Raguideau, S., et al. (2015). Identification of metabolic signatures linked to anti-inflammatory effects of *Faecalibacterium prausnitzii*. *mBio* 6:e00300-15. doi: 10.1128/mbio.00300-15

Moayyedi, P., Surette, M. G., Kim, P. T., Libertucci, J., Wolfe, M., Onischi, C., et al. (2015). Fecal microbiota transplantation induces remission in patients with active ulcerative colitis in a randomized controlled trial. *Gastroenterology* 149, 102.e6–109.e6. doi: 10.1053/j.gastro.2015.04.001

Nazemian, V., Shadnoush, M., Manaheji, H., and Zaringhalam, J. (2016). Probiotics and inflammatory pain: a literature review study. *Middle East J. Rehabil. Health Stud.* 3:e36087. doi: 10.17795/mejrh-36087

Neef, A., and Sanz, Y. (2013). Future for probiotic science in functional food and dietary supplement development. *Curr. Opin. Clin. Nutr. Metab. Care* 16, 679–687. doi: 10.1097/mco.0b013e328365c258

Ng, S. C., Hart, A. L., Kamm, M. A., Stagg, A. J., and Knight, S. C. (2009). Mechanisms of action of probiotics: recent advances. *Inflamm. Bowel Dis.* 15, 300–310. doi: 10.1002/ibd.20602

Orenstein, R., Dubberke, E., Hardi, R., Ray, A., Mullane, K., Pardi, D. S., et al. (2015). Safety and durability of RBX2660 (microbiota suspension) for recurrent *Clostridium difficile* infection: results of the PUNCH CD study. *Clin. Infect. Dis.* 62, 596–602. doi: 10.1093/cid/civ938

Patel, R., and DuPont, H. L. (2015). New approaches for bacteriotherapy: prebiotics, new-generation probiotics, and synbiotics. *Clin. Infect. Dis.* 60(Suppl. 2), S108–S121. doi: 10.1093/cid/civ177

Patrascu, O., Béguet-Crespel, F., Marinelli, L., Le Chatelier, E., Abraham, A. L., Leclerc, M., et al. (2017). A fibrolytic potential in the human ileum mucosal microbiota revealed by functional metagenomic. *Sci. Rep.* 7:40248. doi: 10.1038/srep40248

Pattani, R., Palda, V. A., Hwang, S. W., and Shah, P. S. (2013). Probiotics for the prevention of antibiotic-associated diarrhea and *Clostridium difficile* infection among hospitalized patients: systematic review and meta-analysis. *Open Med.* 7, 56–67.

Paulo Sousa e Silva, J., and Freitas, A. C. (2014). *Probiotic Bacteria*, 1st Edn. Singapore: Pan Stanford Publishing.

Pérez-Cobas, A., Moya, A., Gosalbes, M., and Latorre, A. (2015). Colonization resistance of the gut microbiota against *Clostridium difficile. Antibiotics* 4, 337–357. doi: 10.3390/antibiotics4030337

Petrof, E. O., Gloor, G. B., Vanner, S. J., Weese, S. J., Carter, D., Daigneault, M. C., et al. (2013). Stool substitute transplant therapy for the eradication of *Clostridium difficile* infection: 'RePOOPulating' the gut. *Microbiome* 1:3. doi: 10.1186/2049-2618-1-3

Pharmabiotic Research Institute (2017). *PRI: Microbiotic Medicinal Products.* Available at: http://www.pharmabiotic.org/

Pigneur, B., and Sokol, H. (2016). Fecal microbiota transplantation in inflammatory bowel disease: the quest for the holy grail. *Mucosal Immunol.* 9, 1360–1365. doi: 10.1038/mi.2016.67

Pinto-Sanchez, M. I., Hall, G. B., Ghajar, K., Nardelli, A., Bolino, C., Lau, J. T., et al. (2017). Probiotic *Bifidobacterium longum* NCC3001 reduces depression scores and alters brain activity: a pilot study in patients with irritable bowel syndrome. *Gastroenterology* 153, 448.e8–459.e8. doi: 10.1053/j.gastro.2017.05.003

Plaza-Diaz, J. (2014). Modulation of immunity and inflammatory gene expression in the gut, in inflammatory diseases of the gut and in the liver by probiotics. *World J. Gastroenterol.* 20:15632. doi: 10.3748/wjg.v20.i42.15632

Plaza-Diaz, J., Gomez-Llorente, C., Abadia-Molina, F., Saez-Lara, M. J., Campaña-Martin, L., Muñoz-Quezada, S., et al. (2014). Effects of *Lactobacillus paracasei* CNCM I-4034, *Bifidobacterium breve* CNCM I-4035 and *Lactobacillus rhamnosus* CNCM I-4036 on hepatic steatosis in zucker rats. *PLOS ONE* 9:e98401. doi: 10.1371/journal.pone.0098401

Quévrain, E., Maubert, M. A., Michon, C., Chain, F., Marquant, R., Tailhades, J., et al. (2016). Identification of an anti-inflammatory protein from *Faecalibacterium prausnitzii*, a commensal bacterium deficient in Crohn's disease. *Gut* 65, 415–425. doi: 10.1136/gutjnl-2014-307649

Ramesh, M., Khanna, S., Messer, J., and Adams, M. (2016). *Prevention of Recurrent C. difficile Infection with RBX2660 | PUNCH CD 2 Results.* Roseville, MN: Rebiotix.

Rao, K., and Safdar, N. (2015). Fecal microbiota transplantation for the treatment of *Clostridium difficile* infection. *J. Hosp. Med.* 11, 56–61. doi: 10.1002/jhm.2449

Rao, K., and Young, V. B. (2017). Probiotics for prevention of *Clostridium difficile* infection in hospitalized patients: is the jury still out? *Gastroenterology* 152, 1817–1819. doi: 10.1053/j.gastro.2017.04.027

Ratner, M. (2015). Microbial cocktails join fecal transplants in IBD treatment trials. *Nat. Biotechnol.* 33, 787–788. doi: 10.1038/nbt0815-787

Reardon, S. (2014). Microbiome therapy gains market traction. *Nature* 509, 269–270. doi: 10.1038/509269a

Rebiotix Media (2015). *Rebiotix Receives Breakthrough Therapy Designation for RBX2660 – A Microbiota Restoration Therapy (MRT) for the Treatment of Recurrent Clostridium difficile Infection.* Available at: http://www.rebiotix.com/wp-content/uploads/rebiotix_receives_breakthrough_therapy_designation_recurrent_clostridium_difficile.pdf

Reichold, A., Brenner, S. A., Spruss, A., Förster-Fromme, K., Bergheim, I., and Bischoff, S. C. (2014). *Bifidobacterium adolescentis* protects from the development of nonalcoholic steatohepatitis in a mouse model. *J. Nutr. Biochem.* 25, 118–125. doi: 10.1016/j.jnutbio.2013.09.011

Reijnders, D., Goossens, G. H., Hermes, G. D., Neis, E. P., van der Beek, C. M., Most, J., et al. (2016). Effects of gut microbiota manipulation by antibiotics on host metabolism in obese humans: a randomized double-blind placebo-controlled trial. *Cell Metab.* 24, 63–74. doi: 10.1016/j.cmet.2016.07.008

Ricci, A., Allende, A., Bolton, D., Chemaly, M., Davies, R., Girones, R., et al. (2017). Update of the list of QPS-recommended biological agents intentionally added to food or feed as notified to EFSA 5: suitability of taxonomic units notified to EFSA until September 2016. *EFSA J.* 15:4663. doi: 10.2903/j.efsa.2017.4663

Rivière, A., Selak, M., Lantin, D., Leroy, F., and De Vuyst, L. (2016). Bifidobacteria and butyrate-producing colon bacteria: importance and strategies for their stimulation in the human gut. *Front. Microbiol.* 7:979. doi: 10.3389/fmicb.2016.00979

Round, J. L., Lee, S. M., Li, J., Tran, G., Jabri, B., Chatila, T. A., et al. (2011). The toll-like receptor 2 pathway establishes colonization by a commensal of the human microbiota. *Science* 332, 974–977. doi: 10.1126/science.1206095

Round, J. L., and Mazmanian, S. K. (2009). The gut microbiota shapes intestinal immune responses during health and disease. *Nat. Rev. Immunol.* 9, 600–600. doi: 10.1038/nri2614

Sanders, M. E. (2008). Probiotics: definition, sources, selection, and uses. *Clin. Infect. Dis.* 46, S58–S61. doi: 10.1086/523341

Sang, L.-X. (2010). Remission induction and maintenance effect of probiotics on ulcerative colitis: a meta-analysis. *World J. Gastroenterol.* 16:1908. doi: 10.3748/wjg.v16.i15.1908

Saulnier, D. M., Ringel, Y., Heyman, M. B., Foster, J. A., Bercik, P., Shulman, R. J., et al. (2013). The intestinal microbiome, probiotics and prebiotics in neurogastroenterology. *Gut Microbes* 4, 17–27. doi: 10.4161/gmic.22973

Savcheniuk, O., Kobyliak, N., Kondro, M., Virchenko, O., Falalyeyeva, T., and Beregova, T. (2014). Short-term periodic consumption of multiprobiotic from childhood improves insulin sensitivity, prevents development of non-alcoholic fatty liver disease and adiposity in adult rats with glutamate-induced obesity. *BMC Complement. Altern. Med.* 14:247. doi: 10.1186/1472-6882-14-247

Sbahi, H., and Di Palma, J. A. (2016). Faecal microbiota transplantation: applications and limitations in treating gastrointestinal disorders. *BMJ Open Gastroenterol.* 3:e000087. doi: 10.1136/bmjgast-2016-000087

Schneeberger, M., Everard, A., Gómez-Valadés, A. G., Matamoros, S., Ramírez, S., Delzenne, N. M., et al. (2015). *Akkermansia muciniphila* inversely correlates with the onset of inflammation, altered adipose tissue metabolism and metabolic disorders during obesity in mice. *Sci. Rep.* 5:16643. doi: 10.1038/srep16643

Scott, K. P., Antoine, J. M., Midtvedt, T., and van Hemert, S. (2015). Manipulating the gut microbiota to maintain health and treat disease. *Microb. Ecol. Health Dis.* 26:25877. doi: 10.3402/mehd.v26.25877

Seres Therapeutics (2015). *Seres Therapeutics, Inc. Announces FDA Orphan Drug Designation for SER-109 for the Prevention of Recurrent Clostridium difficile Infection in Adults.* Available at: http://ir.serestherapeutics.com/phoenix.zhtml?c=254006&p=irol-newsArticle&ID=2081167

Seres Therapeutics (2017). *Inflammatory Bowel Disease. Serestherapeutics.Com.* Available at: http://www.serestherapeutics.com/pipeline/products/inflammatory-bowel-disease

Shah, N. P., Ding, W. K., Fallourd, M. J., and Leyer, G. (2010). Improving the stability of probiotic bacteria in model fruit juices using vitamins and antioxidants. *J. Food Sci.* 75, M278–M282. doi: 10.1111/j.1750-3841.2010.01628.x

Shi, Y., Dong, Y., Huang, W., Zhu, D., Mao, H., and Su, P. (2016). Fecal microbiota transplantation for ulcerative colitis: a systematic review and meta-analysis. *PLOS ONE* 11:e0157259. doi: 10.1371/journal.pone.0157259

Sokol, H., Galperine, T., Kapel, N., Bourlioux, P., Seksik, P., Barbut, F., et al. (2016). Faecal microbiota transplantation in recurrent *Clostridium difficile* infection:

recommendations from the French group of faecal microbiota transplantation. *Dig. Liver Dis.* 48, 242–247. doi: 10.1016/j.dld.2015.08.017

Sokol, H., Pigneur, B., Watterlot, L., Lakhdari, O., Bermudez-Humaran, L. G., Gratadoux, J.-J., et al. (2008). *Faecalibacterium prausnitzii* is an anti-inflammatory commensal bacterium identified by gut microbiota analysis of Crohn disease patients. *Proc. Natl. Acad. Sci. U.S.A.* 105, 16731–16736. doi: 10.1073/pnas.0804812105

Steenbergen, L., Sellaro, R., van Hemert, S., Bosch, J. A., and Colzato, L. S. (2015). A randomized controlled trial to test the effect of multispecies probiotics on cognitive reactivity to sad mood. *Brain Behav. Immun.* 48, 258–264. doi: 10.1016/j.bbi.2015.04.003

Surawicz, C. M., Brandt, L. J., Binion, D. G., Ananthakrishnan, A. N., Curry, S. R., Gilligan, P. H., et al. (2013). Guidelines for diagnosis, treatment, and prevention of *Clostridium difficile* infections. *Am. J. Gastroenterol.* 108, 478–498. doi: 10.1038/ajg.2013.4

Timmerman, H. M., Koning, C. J. M., Mulder, L., Rombouts, F. M., and Beynen, A. C. (2004). Monostrain, multistrain and multispecies probiotics—a comparison of functionality and efficacy. *Int. J. Food Microbiol.* 96, 219–233. doi: 10.1016/j.ijfoodmicro.2004.05.012

Timmerman, H. M., Niers, L. E. M., Ridwan, B. U., Koning, C. J. M., Mulder, L., Akkermans, L. M. A., et al. (2007). Design of a multispecies probiotic mixture to prevent infectious complications in critically ill patients. *Clin. Nutr.* 26, 450–459. doi: 10.1016/j.clnu.2007.04.008

Troy, E. B., and Kasper, D. L. (2010). Beneficial effects of *Bacteroides fragilis* polysaccharides on the immune system. *Front. Biosci.* 15, 25–34. doi: 10.2741/3603

Udayappan, S., Manneras-Holm, L., Chaplin-Scott, A., Belzer, C., Herrema, H., Dallinga-Thie, G.-M., et al. (2016). Oral treatment with *Eubacterium hallii* improves insulin sensitivity in db/db mice. *NPJ Biofilms Microbiomes* 2:16009. doi: 10.1038/npjbiofilms.2016.9

van der Lelie, D., Taghavi, S., Henry, C., and Gilbert, J. A. (2017). The microbiome as a source of new enterprises and job creation: considering clinical faecal and synthetic microbiome transplants and therapeutic regulation. *Microb. Biotechnol.* 10, 4–5. doi: 10.1111/1751-7915.12597

van Minnen, L. P., Timmerman, H. M., Lutgendorff, F., Verheem, A., Harmsen, W., Konstantinov, S. R., et al. (2007). Modification of intestinal flora with multispecies probiotics reduces bacterial translocation and improves clinical course in a rat model of acute pancreatitis. *Surgery* 141, 470–480. doi: 10.1016/j.surg.2006.10.007

van Nood, E., Speelman, P., Nieuwdorp, M., and Keller, J. (2014). *Fecal Microbiota Transplantation.* New York, NY: Medscape.

Venturi, A., Gionchetti, P., Rizzello, F., Johansson, R., Zucconi, E., Brigidi, P., et al. (1999). Impact on the composition of the faecal flora by a new probiotic preparation: preliminary data on maintenance treatment of patients with ulcerative colitis. *Aliment. Pharmacol. Ther.* 13, 1103–1108. doi: 10.1046/j.1365-2036.1999.00560.x

Vermeire, S., Joossens, M., Verbeke, K., Wang, J., Machiels, K., Sabino, J., et al. (2015). Donor species richness determines faecal microbiota transplantation success in inflammatory bowel disease. *J. Crohns Colitis* 10, 387–394. doi: 10.1093/ecco-jcc/jjv203

Wallace, C. J. K., and Milev, R. (2017). The effects of probiotics on depressive symptoms in humans: a systematic review. *Ann. Gen. Psychiatry* 16, 14. doi: 10.1186/s12991-017-0141-7

Wang, J., Tang, H., Zhang, C., Zhao, Y., Derrien, M., Rocher, E., et al. (2014). Modulation of gut microbiota during probiotic-mediated attenuation of metabolic syndrome in high fat diet-fed mice. *ISME J.* 9, 1–15. doi: 10.1038/ismej.2014.99

Wexler, H. M. (2007). *Bacteroides*: the good, the bad, and the nitty-gritty. *Clin. Microbiol. Rev.* 20, 593–621. doi: 10.1128/cmr.00008-07

WHO/FAO (2006). *Probiotics in Food Health and Nutritional Properties and Guidelines for Evaluation.* Rome: Food and Agriculture Organization of the United Nations.

Yan, F., and Polk, D. B. (2011). Probiotics and immune health. *Curr. Opin. Gastroenterol.* 27, 496–501. doi: 10.1097/mog.0b013e32834baa4d

Yang, J.-Y., Lee, Y.-S., Kim, Y., Lee, S.-H., Ryu, S., Fukuda, S., et al. (2016). Gut Commensal *Bacteroides acidifaciens* prevents obesity and improves insulin sensitivity in mice. *Mucosal Immunol.* 10, 104–116. doi: 10.1038/mi.2016.42

Yin, Y.-N. (2010). Effects of four *Bifidobacteria* on obesity in high-fat diet induced rats. *World J. Gastroenterol.* 16:3394. doi: 10.3748/wjg.v16.i27.3394

Yoon, J. S., Sohn, W., Lee, O. Y., Lee, S. P., Lee, K. N., Jun, D. W., et al. (2013). Effect of multispecies probiotics on irritable bowel syndrome: a randomized, double-blind, placebo-controlled trial. *J. Gastroenterol. Hepatol.* 29, 52–59. doi: 10.1111/jgh.12322

Youngster, I., Russell, G., Pindar, C., Sauk, J., and Hohmann, E. (2014). 1798Oral, frozen fecal microbiota capsules for relapsing *Clostridium difficile* infection. *Open Forum Infect. Dis.* 1(Suppl. 1), S62–S62. doi: 10.1093/ofid/ofu051.170

Zhou, D. (2016). Impact of sanitary living environment on gut microbiota. *Precis. Med.* 2:e1161. doi: 10.14800/pm.1161

Zipursky, J. S., Sidorsky, T. I., Freedman, C. A., Sidorsky, M. N., and Kirkland, K. B. (2014). Patient attitudes toward the use of fecal microbiota transplantation in the treatment of recurrent *Clostridium difficile* infection. *Clin. Infect. Dis.* 55, 1652–1658. doi: 10.1093/cid/cis809

7

Lactobacillus paraplantarum 11-1 Isolated from Rice Bran Pickles Activated Innate Immunity and Improved Survival in a Silkworm Bacterial Infection Model

*Satoshi Nishida[1,2,3], Masaki Ishii[1], Yayoi Nishiyama[4], Shigeru Abe[4], Yasuo Ono[3] and Kazuhisa Sekimizu[1,2,4]**

[1] Genome Pharmaceuticals Institute Co. Ltd., Tokyo, Japan, [2] Laboratory of Microbiology, Graduate School of Pharmaceutical Sciences, The University of Tokyo, Tokyo, Japan, [3] Department of Microbiology and Immunology, Teikyo University School of Medicine, Tokyo, Japan, [4] Teikyo University Institute of Medical Mycology, Tokyo, Japan

***Correspondence:**
Kazuhisa Sekimizu
sekimizu@main.teikyo-u.ac.jp

Lactic acid bacteria (LAB) have high immune system-stimulating activity and are considered beneficial for human health as probiotics in the gut. The innate immune system is highly conserved between mammals and insects. Microbe-associated molecular patterns (e.g., peptidoglycan and β-glucan) induce cytokine maturation, which, in silkworm larvae, leads to muscle contraction. The purpose of this study is to find a novel probiotic by using silkworm muscle contraction assay. In the present study, we isolated LAB derived from rice bran pickles. We selected highly active LAB to activate the innate immune system of the silkworm, which was assayed based on silkworm muscle contraction. Of various LAB, *L. paraplantarum* 11-1 strongly stimulated innate immunity in the silkworm, leading to stronger silkworm contraction than a dairy-based LAB. Silkworms fed a diet containing *L. paraplantarum* 11-1 exhibited tolerance against the pathogenicity of *Pseudomonas aeruginosa*. These findings suggest that *L. paraplantarum* 11-1 could be a useful probiotic for activating innate immunity.

Keywords: Lactic acid bacteria, *Lactobacillus* sp., silkworm, innate immunity, infection, *Pseudomonas aeruginosa*

INTRODUCTION

Innate immunity is highly conserved between invertebrates and vertebrates. In mammals, dendritic cells and macrophages produce cytokines in response to microbial pathogens (Janeway and Medzhitov, 2002), whereas in insects, hemocytes and fat bodies recognize microbial pathogens and induce an anti-microbial response (Brennan and Anderson, 2004). Especially in silkworms, immune cells produce reactive oxygen species to activate proteases, resulting in cytokine release. Our group discovered an active cytokine, paralytic peptide, that induces muscle contraction in silkworms (Ishii et al., 2008). We used silkworm muscle specimens to screen for innate immunity-activating substances and found that lactic acid bacteria (LAB) strongly induce silkworm muscle contraction (Dhital et al., 2011; Fujiyuki et al., 2012; Nishida et al., 2016). This screening method has several advantages compared with conventional screening using mammalian innate immune cells such as macrophages. First, the silkworm does not respond to lipopolysaccharides, which often produces a false-positive response in mammalian macrophages. Second, insect whole body assays reflect the absorption, distribution, metabolism, excretion, and toxicity factors that govern the therapeutic effects of medicines. Therefore, substances with less effective pharmacokinetics/pharmacodynamics and/or are toxic in the silkworm muscle contraction assay would be excluded by these tests.

LAB are traditionally used for fermenting foods, dairy products, and probiotics. LAB are Gram-positive, catalase-negative, form no spores, and are immotile. Foods fermented with LAB could be beneficial for human health by activating innate immunity (Ichikawa et al., 2012; Kawashima et al., 2013). In our previous report, we isolated a dairy-based LAB to activate the innate immune system in the silkworm (Nishida et al., 2016). LAB isolated from dairy products have been characterized well, whereas LAB from fermented pickles have not. The purpose of this study is to find a novel probiotic to activate the innate immune system in the silkworm by screening LAB from non-dairy products, such as fermented pickles.

In this work, we isolated LAB from rice bran pickles and Korean pickles (kimchi). We evaluated the innate-immunity stimulating activity of LAB in silkworms. We selected a highly active LAB based on the results of the silkworm muscle contraction assay. Isolated *L. paraplantarum* 11-1 exhibited high activity in the silkworm contraction assay. Silkworms that ingested an artificial diet containing *L. paraplantarum* 11-1 exhibited tolerance against the pathogenicity of *Pseudomonas aeruginosa*. To the best of our knowledge, this is the first report of a probiotic effect of *L. paraplantarum* against *P. aeruginosa* infection. This LAB might be valuable as a probiotic for activating innate immunity. The infection model used in this study has the potential to be used to study a novel probiotic against *P. aeruginosae*.

MATERIALS AND METHODS

Materials

Gifu Anaerobic Medium (GAM) broth and GAM agar were purchased from Nissui (Tokyo, Japan). MRS broth and MRS agar were purchased from Becton Dickinson (Franklin Lakes, NJ, USA). $CaCO_3$-MRS agar was prepared by adding $CaCO_3$ (final concentration: 1%, Wako, Osaka, Japan) to the MRS agar after autoclaving. An AnaeroPak (Mitsubishi Gas Chemicals, Tokyo, Japan) was used for anaerobic culturing on agar plates. Saline was prepared as 0.9% NaCl (Wako, Osaka, Japan). Lysogeny broth (LB) medium was prepared with 1% bacto tryptone (Becton Dickinson, Franklin Lakes, NJ, USA), 0.5% bacto yeast extract (Becton Dickinson, Franklin Lakes, NJ, USA), and 1% NaCl (Wako, Osaka, Japan). An LB agar plate was prepared with LB medium containing 1.5% (w/v) agar (Nacalai Tesque, Kyoto, Japan).

DNA Sequencing

Fragments containing 16S rDNA were amplified with polymerase chain reaction using KOD FX Neo (Toyobo, Tokyo, Japan) with primers 9F and 1541R (Hashimoto et al., 2007). The DNA sequences were determined with direct sequencing, BigDye Terminator v3.1 Cycle Sequencing Kit and ABI PRISM 3100 Genetic Analyzer (ThermoFisher Applied Biosystems, Foster City, CA, USA). Sequences were analyzed with the NCBI BLASTN 2.2.27+ (Zhang et al., 2000), 16S ribosomal RNA sequences database (Bacteria and Archaea 7545 sequences). DNA sequences are currently in preparation for submission to the GenBank.

Characterization of LAB

Fluid from the pickles was spread on MRS agar. After incubation at 30°C for 2 days, white colonies appeared on each plate. Isolated bacteria were Gram-stained with Gram-color (Merck, Kenilworth, NJ, USA). For scanning electron microscopy (SEM), bacterial cells were pre-fixed with 2.5% glutaraldehyde in 0.1 M cacodylate buffer (pH 7.2), post-fixed with 1% osmium tetroxide in the same buffer, and freeze-dried in *t*-butyl alcohol. The sample was examined with a field-emission SEM (JSM- 7500F, JEOL, Japan). The bacterial colony was suspended in 3% H_2O_2 for a catalase test. *Staphylococcus aureus* RN4220 and *Escherichia coli* JM109 were used as controls. Other identification kits, Api Zym and Api 50 CHL, were purchased from bioMérieux (Marcy l'Etoile, France), and the data were analyzed using the Api web v5.1 database (bioMérieux, Marcy l'Etoile, France).

Silkworm Muscle Contraction Assay

Silkworm muscle contraction was measured as previously reported (Ishii et al., 2008). Briefly, autoclaved bacterial suspension (50 μl) was injected into a silkworm muscle specimen. The contraction value was determined as (prelength-postlength)/prelength. The sample amount (mg) that induced a contraction value of 0.15 was defined as 1 unit.

Silkworm Infection Model

The silkworm infection model was described previously (Hamamoto et al., 2004). Pathogens used in the infection model were *P. aeruginosa* PAO1 (Stover et al., 2000) and methicillin-sensitive *S. aureus* 1 (MSSA1) (Akimitsu et al., 1999) from our laboratory stock. Pathogenic bacteria grown in LB medium overnight were diluted with saline (0.9% NaCl) and injected into fifth instar larva ($n = 7$) fed overnight. Survival of silkworm larva was counted for 5 days.

Statistical Analysis

Statistical analysis was performed with Microsoft Excel 2007 for Windows (Redmond, WA, USA) and Excel Statistics 2008 (Social Survey Research Information, Tokyo, Japan). Survival plots were generated by the Kaplan-Meier method and analyzed by the log-rank test. Activity was compared with the Mann-Whitney *U*-test. Differences having a $P < 0.05$ were considered to be statistically significant. Survival curve was plotted using Kaleidagraph 4.1.4 (Synergy Software, Reading, PA, USA) and LD_{50} values were determined from fitting curve of the logistic equation, $y = a + (b - a)/(1 + (x/c)^\wedge d)$, y is the fraction of larva killed, x is the number of viable cells injected, c is LD_{50}, a, b and d is the constant of fitting curve. Curve fitting was applied with Levenberg-Marquardt algolism.

RESULTS

Isolation and Characterization of LAB

We selected Gram-positive bacteria on MRS agar, as LAB generally recognized as safe are Gram-positive bacteria. Colonies were re-streaked on $CaCO_3$-MRS medium to confirm lactic-acid fermentation. Lactate-fermenting and Gram-positive bacteria were subjected to the silkworm contraction assay. LAB tested for the contraction assay was sequenced for 16S rDNA (**Table 1**).

In order to investigate morphological and ultrastructural appearance of isolated bacteria, we performed Gram staining and SEM. Gram stains of LAB displayed a Gram-positive bacillus with homogeneous morphology (**Figure 1**). SEM revealed that LAB was characterized as a rod shaped bacterium (**Figure 2**).

The silkworm muscle contraction activity of LAB is shown in **Table 1**. LAB isolated from pickles showed diverse activity. *L. paraplantarum* 11-1 exhibited the highest activity, 165 U/mg, which was higher than that of the LAB in a previous report from our laboratory (Nishida et al., 2016). The activity of the other isolated LABs was as follows: *Lactobacillus sakei* 4, 6.7 U/mg; *Pediococcus ethanolidurans* 11-2, 2.7 U/mg; and *Leuconostoc citreum* A, 43 U/mg.

BLAST analysis of the 16S rDNA sequence of the 11-1 strain revealed that the 11-1 strain had 98% homology with *L. paraplantarum* DSM10667 (NR_025447.1) and *L. plantarum* WCFS1 (NR_075041.1). Strain 11-1 was more similar to *L. paraplantarum* DSM10667 than *L. plantarum* WCFS1. Therefore, we identified the 11-1 strain as *L. paraplantarum*. We then determined the growth characteristics of *L. paraplantarum* 11-1. *L. paraplantarum* 11-1 had strict temperature sensitivity as it grew in MRS medium at 30°C, but not at 16° or 37°C (**Table 2**). Growth of *L. paraplantarum* 11-1 in MRS medium was sensitive to salt higher than 5% NaCl in the medium and resistant to acidic conditions (pH 4.0). In contrast, *L. plantarum* JCM1057 grew at a wide-range of temperatures (16°, 30°, and 37°C) and its growth was resistant to salt (5, 8, and 10% NaCl).

We next examined the ability of *L. paraplantarum* 11-1 to ferment carbohydrates using Api 50 CHL (**Table 3**). *L. paraplantarum* 11-1 exhibited different characteristics from *L. paraplantarum* DSM10667 (CNRZ 1885^T) in 5 of 49 sugars and derivatives utilized. Amygdalin, lactose, melibiose, melezitose, and gluconate were not utilized by *L. paraplantarum* 11-1, whereas α-methyl-D-glucoside was utilized. On the other hand, *L. plantarum* JCM1057 utilized three different sugars than plant-derived *L. plantarum* ATCC14917^T (Bringel et al., 1996; Curk et al., 1996). The carbohydrate fermentation scores of *L. paraplantarum* 11-1 matched 90.5% of those of *Carnobacterium maltaromaticum* in the Api web v5.1 database, whereas those of *L. plantarum* JCM1057 matched 99.2% of those of *L. plantarum* 1. The possibility that strain 11-1 was *C. maltaromaticum* was excluded due to the low similarity of the 16S rDNA sequences. The 16S rDNA sequence of strain 11-1 exhibited 98% similarity with *L. paraplantarum* DSM10667 (NR_025447.1) and 91% similarity with *C. maltaromaticum* DSM 20342 (NR_044710.2).

We also examined enzymatic characteristics of strain 11-1 using the Api Zym test and compared them with those of other related strains (Curk et al., 1996; Oberg et al., 2016) (**Table 4**). The enzymatic characteristics data of *L. paraplantarum* are unavailable, and therefore we compared the data of strain 11-1 and control strain *L. plantarum* JCM 1057, and previously reported data of *L. plantarum* and *L. curvatus*. *L. paraplantarum* 11-1 exhibited different activities (acid phosphatase) of 19 enzymes compared with *L. curvatus* WSU01. In contrast, *L. paraplantarum* 11-1 exhibited 5 different activities (esterase (C4), β-galactosidase, α-glucosidase, β-glucosidase, β-glucosaminidase) of 19 enzymes compared with *L. plantarum* JCM 1057. The enzymatic characteristics of *L. paraplantarum* 11-1 were more similar to those of *L. curvatus* WSU01 than *L. plantarum* JCM 1057.

Probiotic Effect of *L. paraplantarum* 11-1

To evaluate the probiotic effect of *L. paraplantarum* 11-1, we used the silkworm infection model (**Figure 3**). Injection of *P. aeruginosa* into silkworm larvae had time-dependent and dose-dependent silkworm killing effects. Silkworms were fed a diet containing *L. paraplantarum* 11-1 viable cells without apparent problems. Feeding silkworms a diet containing *L. paraplantarum* 11-1 viable cells increased the number of animals that survived after injection of *P. aeruginosa*, resulting in a ~100-fold higher LD_{50}. We then tested the infection model with the Gram-positive bacteria *S. aureus* (**Figure 4**). Feeding the silkworm a diet containing *L. paraplantarum* 11-1 viable cells increased the number of animals that survived after injection of MSSA, resulting in a ~2-fold higher LD_{50}.

TABLE 1 | Identification of bacteria and its activity of silkworm muscle contraction assay.

Strain	Origin	Gram stain	Identification (References)	GenBank Accession no.	ID %	Activity (U/mg)
4	Rice bran pickles	Gram-positive Bacilli	*Lactobacillus sakei* 23K (Chaillou et al., 2005)	NR_075042.1	99	6.7
11-1	Rice bran pickles	Gram-positive Bacilli	*Lactobacillus paraplantarum* DSM10667 (Bringel et al., 1996; Curk et al., 1996)	NR_025447.1	98	165 ± 35[a]
11-2	Rice bran pickles	Gram-positive Cocci	*Pediococcus ethanolidurans* Z-9 (Liu et al., 2006)	NR_043291.1	98	2.7
A	Kimchi	Gram-positive Cocci	*Leuconostoc citreum* KM20 (Kim et al., 2008)	NR_074694.1	100	43

[a]*Mean ± SE (n = 2).*

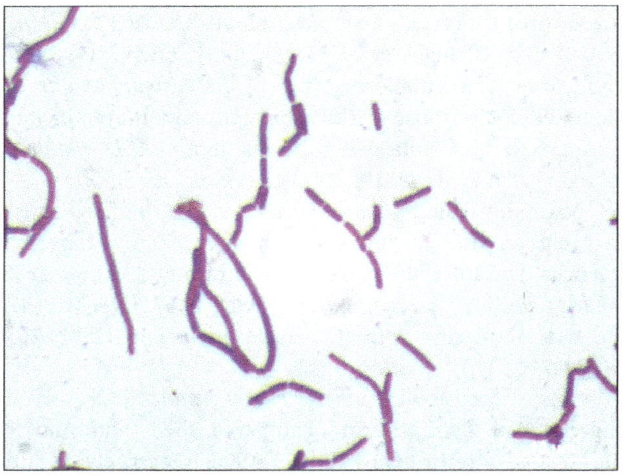

FIGURE 1 | Gram staining of *L. paraplantarum* 11-1. An *L. paraplantarum* 11-1 colony on $CaCO_3$-MRS agar was Gram-stained (Merck). The image was captured with a charge-coupled device camera (Hamamatsu Photonics) using an Olympus phase-contrast microscope at 1,000× magnification.

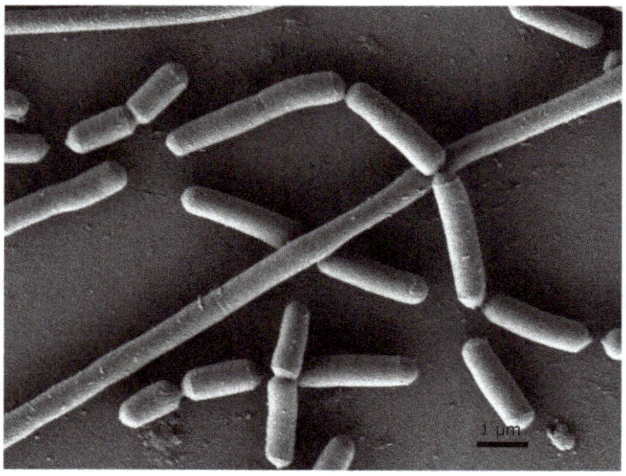

FIGURE 2 | Scanning electron micrograph (SEM) of *L. paraplantarum* 11-1. The sample was examined with a field-emission SEM (JSM- 7500F, JEOL, Japan). The sample was depicted at 10,000× magnification.

DISCUSSION

Isolation of LAB with High Innate Immunity-Stimulating Activity

In general, LAB are thought to be beneficial for human health as probiotics in the gut. LAB were recently reported to have high immunity stimulating activity (Ichikawa et al., 2012; Kawashima et al., 2013). Pickles are a food that is fermented with LAB (Hammes, 2009). Fermented-vegetable foods such as pickles are potential sources of non-dairy LAB. In this study, we isolated LAB from pickles by streaking samples of pickle fluid on MRS agar, a selection plate for LAB (de Man et al., 1960). We confirmed the Gram-positive feature of the isolated bacteria

TABLE 2 | Growth of LAB in MRS under different conditions.

Growth in MRS	*L. paraplantarum* 11-1	*L. plantarum* JCM 1057
16°C	−	+
30°C	+	+
37°C	−	+
43°C	−	−
pH 4, 30°C	+	+
pH 6, 30°C	+	+
pH 7, 30°C	+	+
5% NaCl	−	+
8% NaCl	−	+
10% NaCl	−	+

and its lactic acid production on $CaCO_3$-MRS agar, in which lactic acid solubilizes $CaCO_3$ to form a transparent zone around the colony. Gram staining and SEM characterized LAB as a Gram-positive bacillus and a rod shaped bacterium respectively. (**Figures 1**, **2**). Pleomorphism, defined as variation in size or shape of a bacterial cell, is described for different Lactobacillicae in response to the absence of deoxyribosides, vitamin B_{12}, or divalent cation. Culture broth composition is correlated with the morphology of *L. acidophilus* NCFM (Senz et al., 2015). Different sizes in microscopy morphology might depend on nutrient composition in culture medium. Next, we determined the 16S rDNA sequences of each isolate. The identity of strain 11-1 as *L. paraplantarum* was based on 98% similarity between strain 11-1 and *L. paraplantarum* DSM10667 (NR_025447.1).

L. plantarum and *L. paraplantarum* are closely related and heterofermentive. *L. paraplantarum* is isolated from beer and human feces. *L. plantarum* is a nonpathogenic LAB colonizing in fermented foods and in the human mouth and gut. Therefore, *L. plantarum* is normal human gut microbiota (Bernardeau et al., 2008; Hammes, 2009). The *L. plantarum* WCFS1 genome was sequenced and a recombinant DNA technique was established to construct a strain expressing a specific antigen (Grangette et al., 2001; Seegers, 2002; Kleerebezem et al., 2003; Wells and Mercenier, 2008; Siezen et al., 2012).

Innate-Immunity Activation in Silkworms

Multiple studies demonstrate the validity of silkworm contraction assay for innate immune activation (Ishii et al., 2008; Dhital et al., 2011; Fujiyuki et al., 2012). We determined the activity of LAB to stimulate innate immunity in silkworms using a muscle contraction assay (Ishii et al., 2008). When *L. paraplantarum* 11-1 was injected into the silkworm body fluid, the insect cytokine paralytic peptide was activated upon innate immune stimulation, resulting in silkworm muscle contraction. Compared with a conventional method using macrophages, the muscle contraction assay does not require cell culture and is insensitive to lipopolysaccharides, which often cause a false-positive response in test samples. We isolated several LABs that exhibited a variety of muscle contraction activities (Nishida et al., 2016). Among them, *L. paraplantarum* 11-1 exhibited the highest activity (Supplemental Figure 1).

TABLE 3 | Growth characteristics of LAB.

Carbohydrate	11-1 (This study)	*L. plantarum* JCM 1057 (This study)	*L. paraplantarum* DSM 10667[T] (CNRZ 1885[T])[a]	*L. plantarum* subsp. *plantarum* ATCC 14917[T][a]
Glycerol	–	–	–	–
Erythritol	–	–	–	–
D-Arabinose	–	–	–	–
L-Arabinose	–	+	–	+
Ribose	±	+	±	+
D-Xylose	–	–	–	–
L-Xylose	–	–	–	–
Adonitol	–	–	–	–
β-Methyl-D-xyloside	–	–	–	–
Galactose	+	+	+	+
D-Glucose	+	+	+	+
D-Fructose	+	+	+	+
D-Mannose	+	+	+	+
L-Sorbose	–	–	–	–
Rhamnose	–	±	–	–
Dulcitol	–	–	–	–
Inositol	–	–	–	–
Mannitol	+	+	+	+
Sorbitol	–	+	–	+
α-Methyl-D-mannoside	–	+	–	+
α-Methyl-D-glucoside	+	+	–	–
N-Acetyl glucosamine	+	+	+	+
Amygdalin	–	+	+	+
Arbutin	+	+	+	+
Esculin	+	+	+	+
Salicin	+	+	+	+
Cellobiose	+	+	+	+
Maltose	+	+	+	+
Lactose	–	+	+	+
Melibiose	–	+	+	+
Saccharose	+	+	+	+
Trehalose	+	+	+	+
Inulin	–	–	–	–
Melezitose	–	+	+	+
D-Raffinose	–	±	+	+
Starch	–	–	–	–
Glycogen	–	–	–	–
Xylitol	–	–	–	–
β-Gentiobiose	+	+	+	+
D-Turanose	–	+	–	+
D-Lyxose	–	–	–	–
D-Tagatose	–	–	–	–
D-Fucose	–	–	–	–
L-Fucose	–	–	–	–
D-Arabitol	–	±	–	±
L-Arabitol	–	–	–	–
Gluconate	–	+	+	+
2-Keto-gluconate	–	–	–	–
5-Keto-gluconate	–	–	–	–

[a]*Data from Curk et al. (1996).*

TABLE 4 | Enzymatic characteristics of LAB.

Enzyme	11-1 (This study)	*L. plantarum* JCM 1057 (This study)	*L. curvatus* WSU01[a]	*L. planturum* ($n = 7$)[b]	*L. curvatus* ($n = 24$)[b]
Alkaline phosphatase	–	–	–	–	–
Esterase (C4)	–	+	–	–	–
Esterase lipase (C8)	–	–	–	–	–
Lipase (C14)	–	–	–	ND	ND
Leucine aminopeptidase	+	+	+	+	+
Valine aminopeptidase	+	+	+	+	+
Cystine aminopeptidase	–	–	–	–	±
Trypsin	–	–	–	ND	ND
Chymotrypsin	–	–	–	ND	ND
Acid phosphatase	+	+	–	+	±
Phosphohydrolase	+	+	+	±	±
α-Galactosidase	–	–	–	±	–
β-Galactosidase	–	+	–	+	+
β-Glucuronidase	–	–	–	–	–
α-Glucosidase	–	+	–	+	–
β-Glucosidase	–	+	–	+	±
β-Glucosaminidase	–	+	–	+	±
α-Mannosidase	–	–	–	–	–
α-Fucosidase	–	–	–	ND	ND

[a,b]*Data from Oberg et al. (2016) and Papamanoli et al. (2003) respectively.*

Silkworm Acquired Tolerance to Bacterial Infection by Ingesting *L. paraplantarum* 11-1

Use of silkworms as a surrogate animal for animal tests poses the fewer ethical, financial, and logistical problem than mammalian tests. In addition, silkworms are large enough to inject a precise amount of samples compared to other insect (Sekimizu et al., 2012). The infection model described here also has the potential to be used to study novel probiotics for *in vivo* activity against *P. aeruginosae*.

We have used the silkworm as a surrogate animal to test the probiotic effect of LAB (Nishida et al., 2016). Silkworms were fed a diet containing LAB. Silkworms fed LAB exhibited tolerance to the lethality of *P. aeruginosa* and *S. aureus* infections. Our previous results demonstrated that silkworms acquire tolerance to *P. aeruginosa* infection by ingesting a diet containing *Lactococcus lactis* or peptidoglycans of *Lactobacillus plantarum* (Miyashita et al., 2015; Nishida et al., 2016). In this study, we demonstrated that ingesting *L. paraplantarum* 11-1 extended the survival of silkworm after infection with *P. aeruginosa*. These findings suggest that activation of the innate immune system induced tolerance against microbial infection.

LAB in dairy and fermented products are expected to benefit human health. Reports on the probiotic effects of LAB in animal infection models, however, are limited. Oral administration of heat-killed *L. casei* protects against

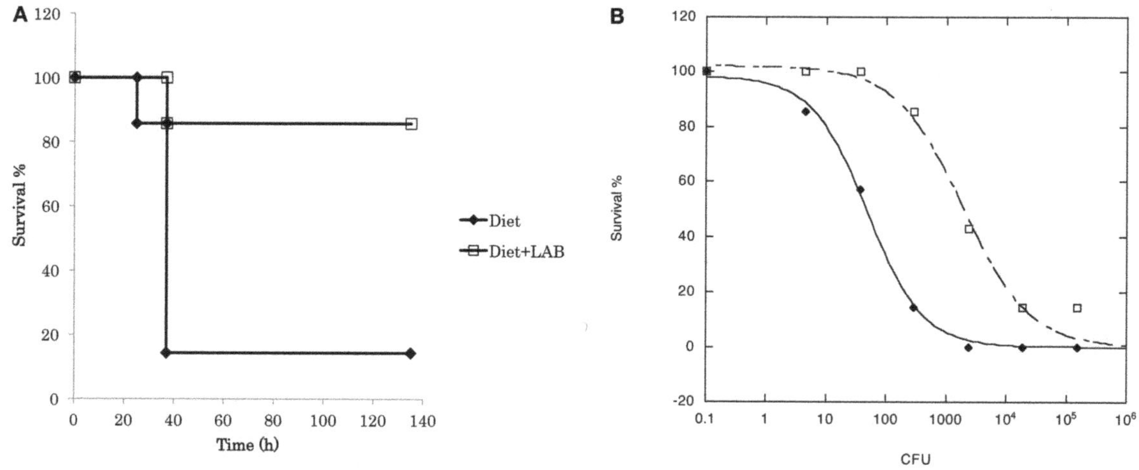

FIGURE 3 | Probiotic effect of *L. paraplantarum* 11-1 on *P. aeruginosa* infection. (A) Time course of survival of silkworms fed a diet with or without *L. paraplantarum* 11-1 viable cells (1 × 10^7 cfu/larva) after *P. aeruginosa* PAO1 infection. Survival of silkworms fed a diet with *L. paraplantarum* 11-1 was significantly higher than that of silkworms fed a normal diet ($p = 0.038$). **(B)** Dose response of *P. aeruginosa* PAO1 on silkworm survival after 2 days. *P. aeruginosa* PAO1 was injected into 5th instar larva fed a diet with or without *L. paraplantarum* 11-1 viable cells.

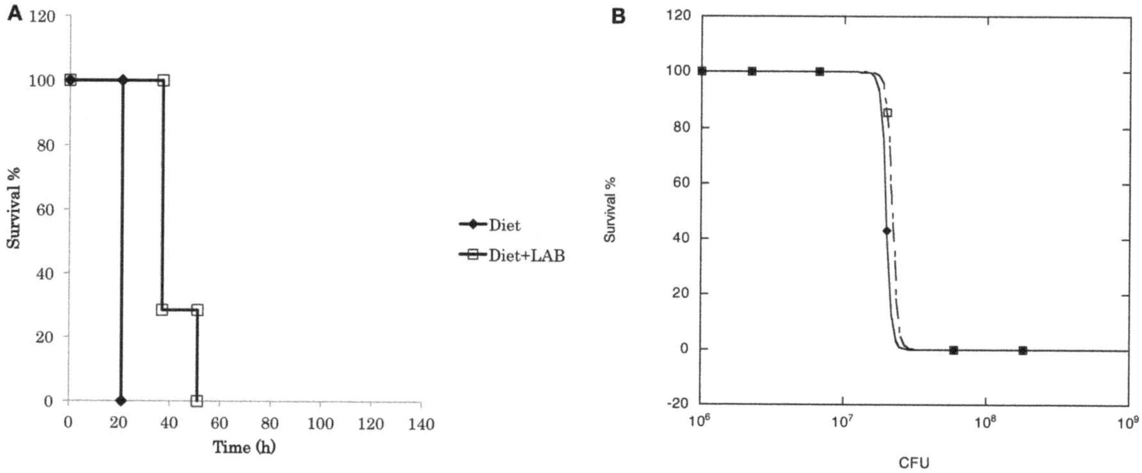

FIGURE 4 | Probiotic effect of *L. paraplantarum* 11-1 on *S. aureus* infection. (A) Time course of survival of silkworms fed a diet with or without *L. paraplantarum* 11-1 viable cells (1 × 10^7 cfu/larva) after *S. aureus* MSSA1 infection. Survival of silkworms fed a diet with *L. paraplantarum* 11-1 was significantly higher than that of silkworms fed a normal diet ($p = 0.030$). **(B)** Dose response of *S. aureus* MSSA1 on silkworm survival after 2 days. *S. aureus* MSSA1 was injected into 5th instar larva fed a diet with or without *L. paraplantarum* 11-1 viable cells.

P. aeruginosa infection in mice (Miake et al., 1985; Setoyama et al., 1985). *Bifidobacterium longum* prevents *P. aeruginosa* gut-derived sepsis in a mouse model (Matsumoto et al., 2008). *Bifidobacterium* protects germ-free mice from *E. coli* O157 infection (Fukuda et al., 2011). Our data indicate that the silkworm is a useful model animal for evaluating the probiotic effects of LAB. *P. aeruginosa* is the most commonly isolated antibiotic-resistant Gram-negative bacteria in ventilator-assisted pneumonia. Oral administration of a probiotic delays respiratory tract colonization and infection by *P. aeruginosa* in human (Forestier et al., 2008). Searching novel probiotics would be matching potential medical needs. Further study on the prevention of *P. aeruginosa* in silkworm infection model would be required for the translation of probiotics to benefit human health.

ETHICS STATEMENT

This study was exempted by The University of Tokyo Life Science Research Ethics and Safety Committee, and Teikyo University Animal Ethics Committee.

AUTHOR CONTRIBUTIONS

SN designed and conducted the experiments, and performed data analysis. MI and YN conducted the experiment of Gram stain and SEM. SN and KS wrote the manuscript. MI, YN, SA, and YO reviewed and edited the manuscript. SN, YO, and KS revised the manuscript.

ACKNOWLEDGMENTS

This work was supported by a grant from Genome Pharmaceuticals Institute Co. Ltd. We thank other members of the Laboratory of Microbiology at the University of Tokyo for helpful discussions. We especially thank Dr. Kataoka, Mr. Yamashita, and Ms. Hashimoto at Genome Pharmaceuticals Institute Co. Ltd. for experimental help.

REFERENCES

Akimitsu, N., Hamamoto, H., Inoue, R., Shoji, M., Akamine, A., Takemori, K., et al. (1999). Increase in resistance of methicillin-resistant *Staphylococcus aureus* to beta-lactams caused by mutations conferring resistance to benzalkonium chloride, a disinfectant widely used in hospitals. *Antimicrob. Agents. Chemother.* 43, 3042–3043.

Bernardeau, M., Vernoux, J. P., Henri-Dubernet, S., and Guéguen, M. (2008). Safety assessment of dairy microorganisms: the *Lactobacillus* genus. *Int. J. Food Microbiol.* 126, 278–285. doi: 10.1016/j.ijfoodmicro.2007.08.015

Brennan, C. A., and Anderson, K. V. (2004). *Drosophila*: The genetics of innate immune recognition and response. *Annu. Rev. Immunol.* 22, 457–483. doi: 10.1146/annurev.immunol.22.012703.104626

Bringel, F., Curk, M. C., and Hubert, J. C. (1996). Characterization of lactobacilli by southern-type hybridization with a *Lactobacillus plantarum pyrDFE* probe. *Int. J. Syst. Bacteriol.* 46, 588–594. doi: 10.1099/00207713-46-2-588

Chaillou, S., Champomier-Vergès, M. C., Cornet, M., Crutz-Le Coq, A. M., Dudez, A. M., Martin, V., et al. (2005). The complete genome sequence of the meat-borne lactic acid bacterium *Lactobacillus sakei* 23K. *Nat. Biotechnol.* 23, 1527–1533. doi: 10.1038/nbt1160

Curk, M. C., Hubert, J. C., and Bringel, F. (1996). *Lactobacillus paraplantarum* sp. nov., a new species related to *Lactobacillus plantarum. Int. J. Syst. Bacteriol.* 46, 595–598. doi: 10.1099/00207713-46-2-595

de Man, J. D., Rogosa, M., and Sharpe, M. E. (1960). A medium for the cultivation of *Lactobacilli. J. Appl. Bacteriol.* 23, 130–135. doi: 10.1111/j.1365-2672.1960.tb00188.x

Dhital, S., Hamamoto, H., Urai, M., Ishii, K., and Sekimizu, K. (2011). Purification of innate immunostimulant from green tea using a silkworm muscle contraction assay. *Drug Discov. Ther.* 5, 18–25. doi: 10.5582/ddt.v5.1.18

Forestier, C., Guelon, D., Cluytens, V., Gillart, T., Sirot, J., and De Champs, C. (2008). Oral probiotic and prevention of *Pseudomonas aeruginosa* infections: a randomized, double-blind, placebo-controlled pilot study in intensive care unit patients. *Crit. Care.* 12, R69. doi: 10.1186/cc6907

Fujiyuki, T., Hamamoto, H., Ishii, K., Urai, M., Kataoka, K., Takeda, T., et al. (2012). Evaluation of innate immune stimulating activity of polysaccharides using a silkworm (*Bombyx mori*) muscle contraction assay. *Drug Discov. Ther.* 6, 88–93. doi: 10.5582/ddt.2012.v6.2.88

Fukuda, S., Toh, H., Hase, K., Oshima, K., Nakanishi, Y., Yoshimura, K., et al. (2011). Bifidobacteria can protect from enteropathogenic infection through production of acetate. *Nature.* 469, 543–547. doi: 10.1038/nature09646

Grangette, C., Müller-Alouf, H., Goudercourt, D., Geoffroy, M. C., Turneer, M., and Mercenier, A. (2001). Mucosal immune responses and protection against tetanus toxin after intranasal immunization with recombinant *Lactobacillus plantarum. Infect. Immun.* 69, 1547–1553. doi: 10.1128/IAI.69.3.1547-1553.2001

Hamamoto, H., Kurokawa, K., Kaito, C., Kamura, K., Manitra Razanajatovo, I., Kusuhara, H., et al. (2004). Quantitative evaluation of the therapeutic effects of antibiotics using silkworms infected with human pathogenic microorganisms. *Antimicrob. Agents Chemother.* 48, 774–779. doi: 10.1128/AAC.48.3.774-779.2004

Hammes, W. P. (2009). "*Lactobacillus*," in *Bergey's Manual of Systematics of Archaea and Bacteria*, eds W. B. Whitman, P. DeVos, J. Chun, S. Dedysh, B. Hedlund, P. Kämpfer, F. Rainey, and M.Trujillo (Hoboken, NJ: John Wiley and Sons, Inc.), 1–21. doi: 10.1002/9781118960608.gbm00604

Hashimoto, M., Taguchi, T., Nishida, S., Ueno, K., Koizumi, K., Aburada, M., et al. (2007). Isolation of 8′-phosphate ester derivatives of amicoumacins: structure-activity relationship of hydroxy amino acid moiety. *J. Antibiot.* 60, 752–756. doi: 10.1038/ja.2007.99

Ichikawa, S., Miyake, M., Fujii, R., and Konishi, Y. (2012). MyD88 associated ROS generation is crucial for *Lactobacillus* induced IL-12 production in macrophage. *PLoS ONE* 7:e35880. doi: 10.1371/journal.pone.0035880

Ishii, K., Hamamoto, H., Kamimura, M., and Sekimizu, K. (2008). Activation of the silkworm cytokine by bacterial and fungal cell wall components via a reactive oxygen species-triggered mechanism. *J. Biol. Chem.* 283, 2185–2191. doi: 10.1074/jbc.M705480200

Janeway, C. A. Jr., and Medzhitov, R. (2002). Innate immune recognition. *Annu. Rev. Immunol.* 20, 197–216. doi: 10.1146/annurev.immunol.20.083001.084359

Kawashima, T., Kosaka, A., Yan, H., Guo, Z., Uchiyama, R., Fukui, R., et al. (2013). Double-Stranded RNA of intestinal commensal but not pathogenic bacteria triggers production of protective interferon-β. *Immunity.* 38, 1187–1197. doi: 10.1016/j.immuni.2013.02.024

Kim, J. F., Jeong, H., Lee, J. S., Choi, S. H., Ha, M., Hur, C. G., et al. (2008). Complete genome sequence of *Leuconostoc citreum* KM20. *J. Bacteriol.* 190, 3093–3094. doi: 10.1128/JB.01862-07

Kleerebezem, M., Boekhorst, J., van Kranenburg, R., Molenaar, D., Kuipers, O. P., Leer, R., et al. (2003). Complete genome sequence of *Lactobacillus plantarum* WCFS1. *Proc. Natl. Acad. Sci. U.S.A.* 100, 1990–1995. doi: 10.1073/pnas.0337704100

Liu, L., Zhang, B., Tong, H., and Dong, X. (2006). *Pediococcus ethanolidurans* sp. nov., isolated from the walls of a distilled-spirit-fermenting cellar. *Int. J. Syst. Evol. Microbiol.* 56, 2405–2408. doi: 10.1099/ijs.0.64407-0

Matsumoto, T., Ishikawa, H., Tateda, K., Yaeshima, T., Ishibashi, N., and Yamaguchi, K. (2008). Oral administration of *Bifidobacterium longum* prevents gut-derived *Pseudomonas aeruginosa* sepsis in mice. *J. Appl. Microbiol.* 104, 672–680. doi: 10.1111/j.1365-2672.2007.03593.x

Miake, S., Nomoto, K., Yokokura, T., Yoshikai, Y., Mutai, M., and Nomoto, K. (1985). Protective effect of *Lactobacillus casei* on *Pseudomonas aeruginosa* infection in mice. Infect. *Immun.* 48, 480–485.

Miyashita, A., Takahashi, S., Ishii, K., Sekimizu, K., and Kaito, C. (2015). Primed immune responses triggered by ingested bacteria lead to systemic infection tolerance in silkworms *PLoS ONE* 10:e0130486. doi: 10.1371/journal.pone.0130486

Nishida, S., Ono, Y., and Sekimizu, K. (2016). Lactic acid bacteria activating innate immunity improve survival in bacterial infection model of silkworm. *Drug Discov. Ther.* 10, 49–56. doi: 10.5582/ddt.2016.01022

Oberg, C. J., Oberg, T. S., Culumber, M. D., Ortakci, F., Broadbent, J. R., and McMahon, D. J. (2016). *Lactobacillus wasatchensis* sp. nov., a non-starter lactic acid bacteria isolated from aged Cheddar cheese. *Int. J. Syst. Evol. Microbiol.* 66, 158–164. doi: 10.1099/ijsem.0.000689

Papamanoli, E., Tzanetakis, N., Litopoulou-Tzanetaki, E., and Kotzekidou, P. (2003). Characterization of lactic acid bacteria isolated from a Greek dry-fermented sausage in respect of their technological and probiotic properties. *Meat Sci.* 65, 859–867. doi: 10.1016/S0309-1740(02)00292-9

Seegers, J. F. (2002). Lactobacilli as live vaccine delivery vectors: progress and prospects. *Trends Biotechnol.* 20, 508–515. doi: 10.1016/S0167-7799(02)02075-9

Sekimizu, N., Paudel, A., and Hamamoto, H. (2012). Animal welfare and use of silkworm as a model animal. *Drug Discov. Ther.* 6, 226–229. doi: 10.5582/ddt.2012.v6.4.226

Senz, M., van Lengerich, B., Bader, J., and Stahl, U. (2015). Control of cell morphology of probiotic *Lactobacillus acidophilus* for enhanced cell stability during industrial processing. *Int. J. Food Microbiol.* 192, 34–42. doi: 10.1016/j.ijfoodmicro.2014.09.015

Setoyama, T., Nomoto, K., Yokokura, T., and Mutai, M. (1985). Protective effect of lipoteichoic acid from *Lactobacillus casei* and *Lactobacillus fermentum* against *Pseudomonas aeruginosa* in mice. *J. Gen. Microbiol.* 131, 2501–2503. doi: 10.1099/00221287-131-9-2501

Siezen, R. J., Francke, C., Renckens, B., Boekhorst, J., Wels, M., Kleerebezem, M., et al. (2012). Complete resequencing and reannotation of the *Lactobacillus plantarum* WCFS1 genome. *J. Bacteriol.* 194, 195–196. doi: 10.1128/JB.06275-11

Stover, C. K., Pham, X. Q., Erwin, A. L., Mizoguchi, S. D., Warrener, P., Hickey, M. J., et al. (2000). Complete genome sequence of *Pseudomonas aeruginosa* PAO1, an opportunistic pathogen. *Nature.* 406, 959–964. doi: 10.1038/35023079

Wells, J. M., and Mercenier, A. (2008). Mucosal delivery of therapeutic and prophylactic molecules using lactic acid bacteria. *Nat. Rev. Microbiol.* 6, 349–362. doi: 10.1038/nrmicro1840

Zhang, Z., Schwartz, S., Wagner, L., and Miller, W. (2000). A greedy algorithm for aligning DNA sequences. *J. Comput. Biol.* 7, 203–214. doi: 10.1089/10665270050081478

8

Probiotic *Lactobacillus sakei* proBio-65 Extract Ameliorates the Severity of Imiquimod Induced Psoriasis-Like Skin Inflammation in a Mouse Model

Irfan A. Rather[1†], Vivek K. Bajpai[2†], Yun Suk Huh[3], Young-Kyu Han[2], Eijaz A. Bhat[4], Jeongheui Lim[5*], Woon K. Paek[5] and Yong-Ha Park[1*]*

[1] Department of Applied Microbiology and Biotechnology, School of Biotechnology, Yeungnam University, Gyeongsan, South Korea, [2] Department of Energy and Materials Engineering, Dongguk University, Seoul, South Korea, [3] Department of Biological Engineering, Inha University, Incheon, South Korea, [4] Department of Biochemistry, Yeungnam University, Gyeongsan, South Korea, [5] National Science Museum, Ministry of Science, ICT and Future Planning, Daejeon, South Korea

***Correspondence:**
Young-Kyu Han
ykenergy@dongguk.edu
Jeongheui Lim
jhlim1226@naver.com;
jeongheuilim@gmail.com
Yong-Ha Park
peter@ynu.ac.kr

†These authors have contributed equally to this work.

This study was designed to evaluate the protective effect of ethanol extract (SEL001) isolated from a potent probiotic strain *Lactobacillus sakei* proBio-65 on imiquimod (IMQ)-induced psoriasis-like skin inflammation in a mouse model. Histopathological and histomorphometrical changes in the ear and dorsal skin tissues were observed under hematoxylin and eosin stain for general histopathological architectures or Masson's trichrome stain for collagen fibers. The expression profile of psoriasis-associated specific genes was determined using Real-Time PCR analysis. As a result, topical application of IMQ resulted in a significant increase of mean total and epithelial (epidermis) thicknesses, the number of inflammatory cells infiltrated in the dermis, and the decrease of dermis collagen fiber occupied regions in the ear tissues of IMQ and IMQ plus vaseline treated groups when compared to the intact control group. A significant increase of epithelial thickness and number of inflammatory cells infiltrated in the dermis of dorsal skin tissues were also noticed in IMQ and IMQ plus vaseline treated groups as compared to the intact control group, suggesting classic IMQ-induced hypersensitive psoriasis. IMQ-induced hypersensitive psoriasis related histopathological changes to the ear and dorsal skin tissues were significantly inhibited by the treatment of a standard drug clobetasol and SEL001. Further, mRNA expression analysis indicated a significant increase in gene expression levels of pro-inflammatory cytokines, including IL-19, IL-17A, and IL-23 in IMQ and IMQ plus vaseline treated groups than that of the control. Clobetasol and SEL001 treated groups resulted in a lower gene expression level of IL-19, IL-17A, and IL-23 as compared to IMQ and IMQ plus vaseline treated groups. These results enforce that SEL001 could be a novel treatment for psoriasis and an alternative to other drugs that pose a number of side effects on the skin.

Keywords: psoriasis, skin inflammation, *Lactobacillus sakei*, lactic acid bacteria, imiquimod

INTRODUCTION

The skin is one of the vital organs of the body that serves as a barrier from the outside environment. Psoriasis is a chronic skin disorder with unknown trigger, which is characterized by inflammation, thickening, and abnormal epidermal proliferation with up to 4% of prevalence in the general population (Griffiths and Barker, 2007). The pathogenesis of psoriasis is multifactorial and, as a perpetual incendiary skin issue, irregularity amongst pro- and anti-inflammatory mediators may play a vital part in the development and progression of this skin disorder (Li et al., 2016). Due to its incomplete etiology, there is still no permanent cure; however, genetic predisposition and environments stimuli might have a disease causing role. While the pathogenesis of psoriasis is not fully elucidated, it is extensively putative that pro-inflammatory cytokines have a key role in both development and maintenance of psoriatic lesions. A number of studies have reported the presence of immune-derived cytokines in psoriatic skin lesions and serum, suggesting their role in the pathogenesis of psoriasis (Kagami et al., 2010; Res et al., 2010; Zhang et al., 2010; Mudigonda et al., 2012; Tokura, 2012; Yoo et al., 2012; El Malki et al., 2013; Wang et al., 2013). Specifically, tissue alterations seen in psoriasis are driven by the exaggerated production of pro-inflammatory cytokines and the lesion development is critically dependent on IL-23 and IL-17 (Lee et al., 2004; Piskin et al., 2006; van der Fits et al., 2009). One of the pro-inflammatory cytokines, IL-19 has a key role in psoriatic pathogenesis and upregulates in psoriatic lesions during disease progression (Li et al., 2005), thus, controlling the level of these pro-inflammatory cytokines is necessary to treat this chronic disease.

The effect of the concurrent presence of IL-17 and IL-19 in psoriasis lesions might have impact on various levels of the pathogenic progression. The two cytokines upregulate the expression of β-defensins and S100A proteins thereby increases the antibacterial competence of keratinocytes. Moreover, their role in impeding infections may uphold the process to infiltrate immune cells to skin and increase the inflammation (Wolf et al., 2008). The process could be further regulated by tight coordination of IL-19 and IL-17 which in turn could attract particular T-helper type 1-cells, dendritic cells and neutrophilic granulocytes thereby directly increasing the secretion of chemokines. In addition, IL-19 and IL-17 promote the maintenance and effector function of T helper type 17-cells synergistically through the production of several mediators. Of note, T helper type 17-cells are critical for pathogenicity, IL-23 drives their proliferation, survival, and cytokine production (Ouyang et al., 2008). In addition, IL-19 and IL-17 are known to induce other interleukins which contributes to the psoriasis typical epidermal alterations. Topical application of IMQ, a TLR7/8 ligand and potent immune activator, can induce and exacerbate psoriasis, a chronic inflammatory skin disorder (van der Fits et al., 2009), and has been used as activator for valuable psoriasis animal model (Qin et al., 2014; Bai et al., 2016). Additionally, psoriasis may be linked with genuine comorbidities, for example, metabolic disorder and cardiovascular sickness, likely mirroring a systemic provocative part of the infection (Perera et al., 2012). At present, there are a number of temporary treatments for psoriasis ranging from tropical medicine, heliotherapy, and systematic to biological treatments (Gustafson et al., 2013). Nevertheless, the outcome of these treatments may result in severe side effects, thus, demands a much safer treatment to render this disease.

Probiotics are known as beneficial microorganisms that, when administered in adequate amounts, confer health benefits to the host (Joint FAO/WHO, 2001). The effect of probiotics on the skin could be mediated by the modulation of both the innate and the adaptive immune responses in the host. Modulation of an immune system is one of the beneficial effects of probiotics in human health. Recently, we reported that oral administration of heat-killed *Lactobacillus sakei* proBio65 inhibited immunoglobulin E-mediated histamine and β-hexosaminidase in NC/Nga mice, suggesting that *L. sakei* has an inhibitory effect on atopic dermatitis-like skin lesion (Park et al., 2008; Kim et al., 2013). Oral administration of *L. casei* has been seen to reduce antigen-specific skin inflammation by controlling the size of the CD8+ effector pool (Chapat et al., 2004). In addition, *L. casei* DN-114001 alleviates T-cell mediated skin inflammation (Hacini-Rachinel et al., 2009). Recently, *L. pentosus* GML-77 has been seen to inhibit skin lesions in IMQ-induced psoriasis in mice (Wu et al., 2017).

Use of probiotics and their cellular components in preventive medicine to maintain a healthy function is well documented (Matsumoto et al., 2005; Tojo et al., 2014). Probiotics have been proposed as therapeutic agents in various pathological conditions, including intestinal chronic inflammation, atopic dermatitis and gut homeostasis (Park et al., 2014; Tojo et al., 2014; Plaza-Díaz et al., 2017). Previously, we confirmed the therapeutic potential of SEL001 like products of plant and microbial origin *in vitro* and *in vivo* using a diabetic animal model (Shukla et al., 2011; Bajpai et al., 2016). Various studies have also shown that probiotics, such as *L. sakei* probio65 exhibit a wide range of pharmacological effects such as anti-atopic dermatitis in animals and humans (Park et al., 2008, 2014; Kim and Pyo, 2012; Kim et al., 2013, 2015c).

Although a number of studies have emphasized the therapeutic role of probiotics in various inflammatory conditions, there is no report available on the anti-inflammatory effects of SEL001 of probiotic origin in a psoriasis model of inflammation. Since the IMQ-induced psoriasis model highly resembles human psoriasis lesions (van der Fits et al., 2009), in this study, we investigated the effect of topical application of SEL001, a probiotic product isolated from *L. sakei* proBio65 in an IMQ-induced psoriasis mouse model.

MATERIALS AND METHODS

Preparation of SEL001

To prepare the ethanolic extract of *Lactobacillus sakei* Probio65 hereby called SEL001, 48 h grown culture of strain *L. sakei* probio65 was mixed with ethanol (1:2 ratio) and the flask containing mixture of bacterial culture and ethanol

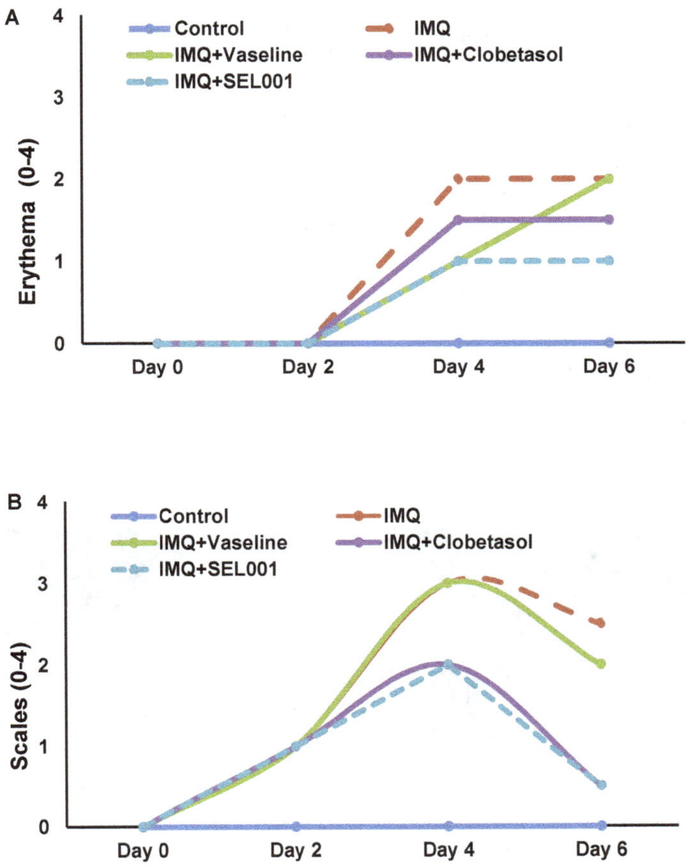

FIGURE 1 | Erythema and scales score of the dorsal skin of the mice. The scoring was performed on 0 day, 2 day, 4 day, and 6 day using the Psoriasis Area Severity Index (PASI). **(A)** Erythema score and **(B)** scales score.

was incubated at 150 rpm for 6 h at room temperature. Following the incubation, the mixture was centrifuged (8,000 *g* for 10 min) and the cell pellet was discarded. Resulting supernatant was filter sterilized and subjected to freeze drying until get a dry-powdered material, which was served as SEL001.

Chemical Composition Analysis of SEL001

Gas chromatography–mass spectrometry (GC–MS) was explored to identify the chemical composition of SEL001. Briefly, dried SEL001 derived from the probiotic strain *L. sakei* probio65 was dissolved in 95% v/v methanol and two microliter of this solution was injected for GC-MS analysis. The protocol was followed as reported by Ravi et al. (2013).

Animals

Thirty ICR mice of 6 weeks age were occupied from Samtaco Bio Co. (Korea), and were kept in cages at constant levels of temperature and humidity on 12 h light/dark cycles. The animals were acclimatized for 1 week and their backs were shaved using pet electric shaver (GSAK CO., LTD., Korea). The animals had free access to water and feed throughout the trial. Animal management and institutional approval for research protocols were supported and approved by the Animal Ethical Committee of the Yeungnam University (YNU-ANETCOMM-2016-00123), Gyeongsan, Korea.

IMQ-Induced Psoriasis Model and Treatment

The mice were divided into five groups; a control group, an IMQ group, an IMQ+vaseline group, an IMQ-clobetasol group, and an IMQ+SEL001. Each group contains 6 mice and were housed as 2 mice per cage.

In this study a total of four topical treatments were used such as, IMQ, vaseline, clobetasol, and SEL001. IMQ was used to induce psoriasis like skin inflammation in mouse mode. Further, the treatment groups received vaseline, clobetasol and SEL001 topically 1 h before topical application of IMQ. Clobetasol propionate, a corticosteroid drug is used to treat various skin diseases, including psoriasis, therefore, it was used a gold standard, and SEL001 was used as a test sample against IMQ-induced psoriasis. Except for the control group, all other groups received a daily dose of 62.5 mg of 5% IMQ cream/cm^2 (Aldara; MEDA AS) applied their backs and 20 mg on the right ear once a day for six consecutive days as previously described (van

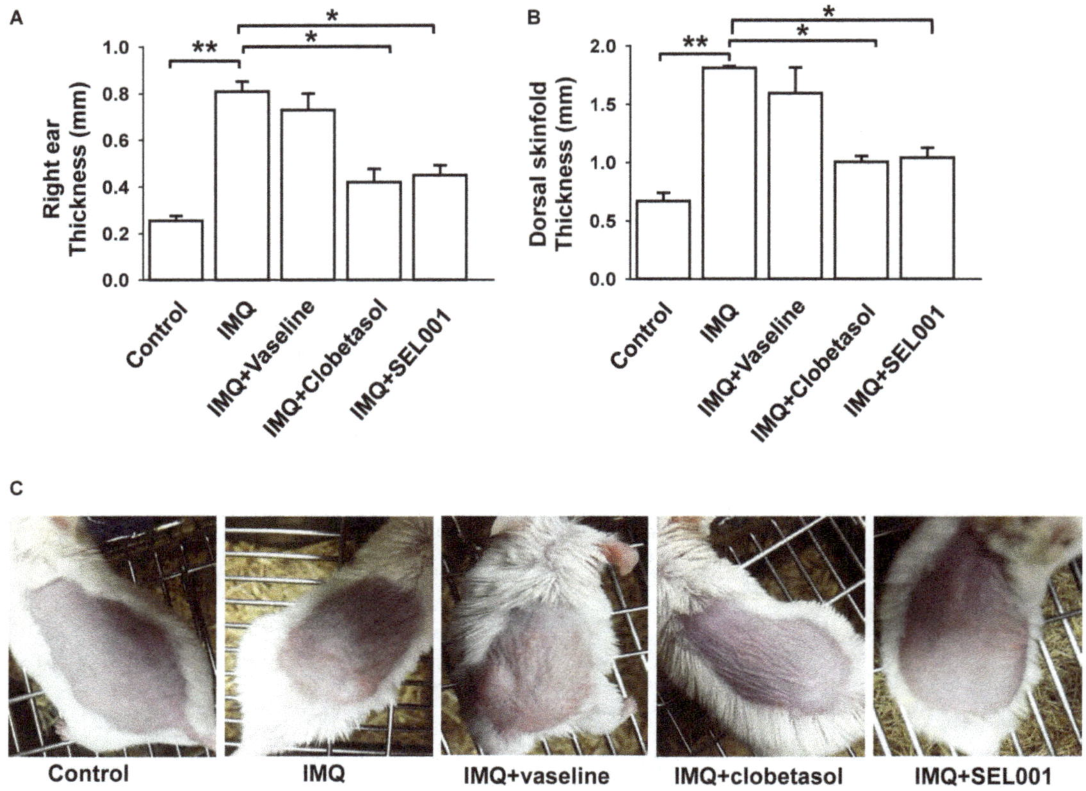

FIGURE 2 | Caliper measurement and visual appearance of skin. **(A)** Skin fold thickness on the backs of the mice, **(B)** right ear thickness, and **(C)** visual appearance on day 6. Columns represent means ± standard deviation of skin/ear measurements day 6. $^{**}p < 0.001$ or $^{*}p < 0.05$ is significant, analyzed by one-way ANOVA test.

der Fits et al., 2009; Nadeem et al., 2015; Rather et al., 2016). Further, IMQ+vaseline group received a daily dose of 62.5 mg of 5% IMQ cream plus vaseline cream (80 mg/cm^2 on back and 20 mg on the right ear); IMQ plus clobetasol group received a daily dose of 62.5 mg of 5% IMQ cream plus clobetasol (80 mg/cm^2 on back and 20 mg on the right ear), and IMQ plus SEL001 group received a daily dose of 62.5 mg of 5% IMQ cream plus SEL001 (50 mg/cm^2 on back and 10 mg on the right ear).

Scoring of Skin Inflammation Severity

On days 0, 2, 4, and 6, all animas were assessed using 2 elements of the Psoriasis Area Severity Index (PASI), to consign a score of 0–4 (0, none; 1, moderate; 3, severe; 4, very severe) for both erythema and scaling parameters. Further, back skin and ear thickness were measured by using electronic caliper (Shenzhen Liweihui Technology Co., Ltd., China). After day 6, animals were euthanized and the shaved skin area of the back and ear was excised. Two lesions of the skin of each mouse were taken for histological and mRNA expression analysis.

Histological Process

Approximated regions of an individual ear and dorsal skin tissues were sampled and they were crossly trimmed. All trimmed ear and dorsal skin tissues were re-fixed in 10% neutral buffered formalin (NBF), again for 24 h. After paraffin embedding, 3–4 μm sections were prepared. Representative sections were stained with hematoxylin and eosin (HE) for general histological architectures or Masson's trichrome (MT) for collagen fibers in the dermis of the ear and dorsal back skin tissues (Kim et al., 2015a; Bai et al., 2016). The histological profiles of individual cross trimmed ear and dorsal skin tissues were observed under a light microscope (Model Eclipse 80*i*, Nikon, Tokyo, Japan). Histological evaluation was performed on the two fields in each part of the ear and dorsal skin tissues; consequently, six histological fields of an ear and dorsal back skin tissues in each group were considered for further histomorphometric analysis. The histopathological analysis was done by the histopathologist who was unaware of group distribution. To observe more detailed changes, mean total and epithelial thicknesses of ear and dorsal skin tissues (μm), mean numbers of inflammatory cells infiltrated in dermis of ear and dorsal skin tissues (cells/mm^2 of dermis) and mean collagen fiber occupied regions in dermis of ear and dorsal skin tissues (%/mm^2 of dermis) were calculated using a computer-based automated image analyzer (*i*Solution FL ver 9.1, IMT *i*-solution Inc., Vancouver, QC, Canada) according to our previously established methods (Qin et al., 2014; Kim et al., 2015b; Bai et al., 2016). At least five

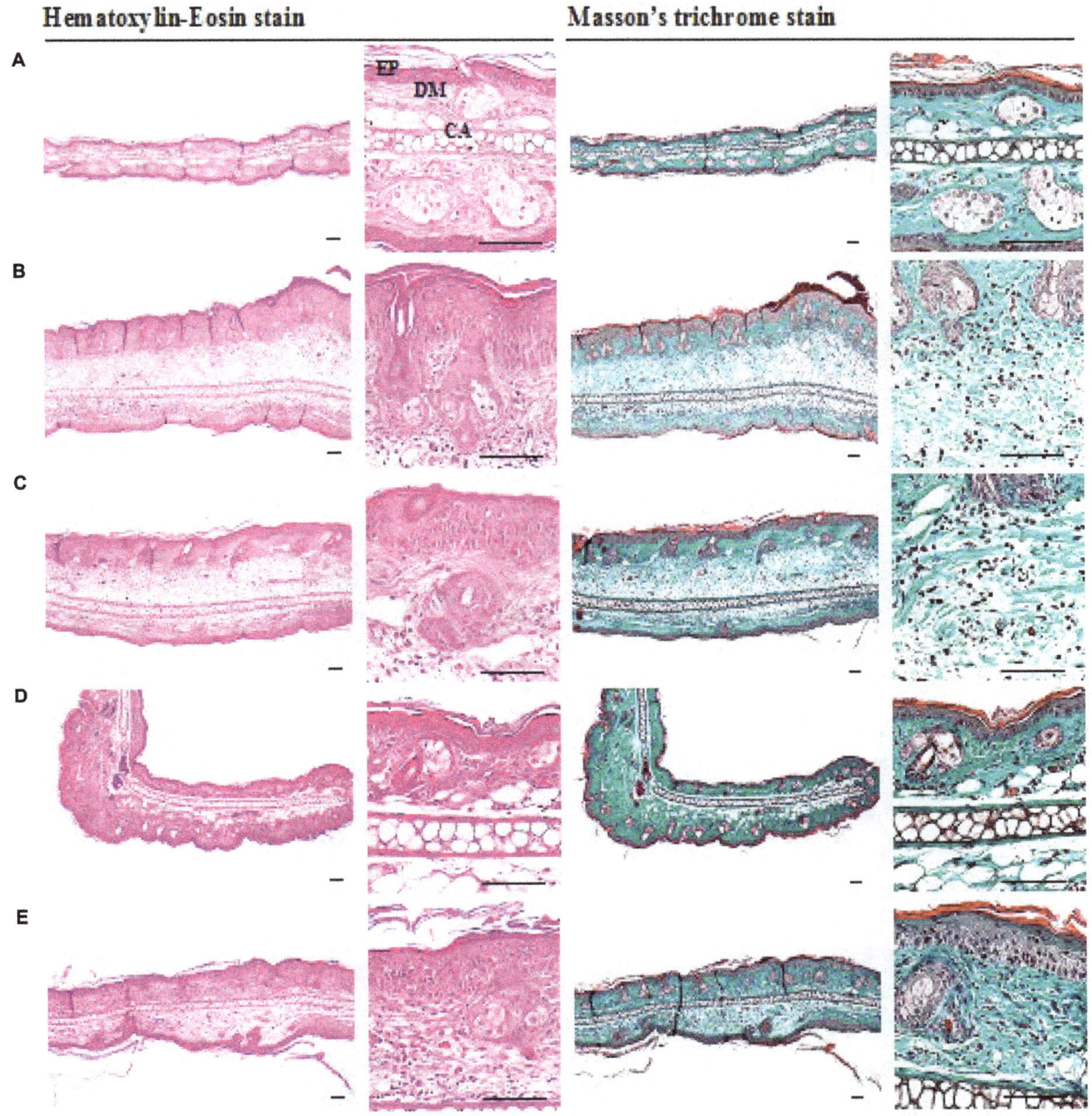

FIGURE 3 | Histopathological images of ear tissues of IMQ-induced psoriasis mice. **(A)** Control, **(B)** IMQ, **(C)** IMQ+vaseline, **(D)** IMQ+clobetasol, and **(E)** IMQ+SEL001. A noticeable increase of total and epithelial (epidermis) thicknesses, inflammatory cell infiltrations in the dermis, and decreases of dermis collagen fibers were observed in ear tissues of IMQ and IMQ+vaseline as compared with intact control, respectively. However, these IMQ-induced hypersensitive psoriasis related histopathological changes on the ear tissues were significantly inhibited by treatment of test material SEL001 and reference drug clobetasol in the current histopathological inspection. No meaningful histopathological changes in the ear tissues were demonstrated in IMQ+vaseline as compared with those of IMQ control [IMQ = Imiquimod; EP = Epithelium/Epidermis; DM = Dermis; CA = Ear cartilage].

repeated measurements were considered to calculate each mean histomorphometric value, whenever possible, in this histopathological evaluation.

Statistical Analysis

The data obtained were analyzed by one-way ANOVA test followed by least significant differences (LSD) multi-comparison test to determine which pairs of group comparison were significantly different. Differences were considered significant at $p < 0.05$.

Quantitative Real-Time (RT) Reverse Transcriptase Polymerase Chain Reaction (PCR)

The extraction of RNA was done using Trizol™ reagent (Invitrogen, United States) following manufacturer's instructions.

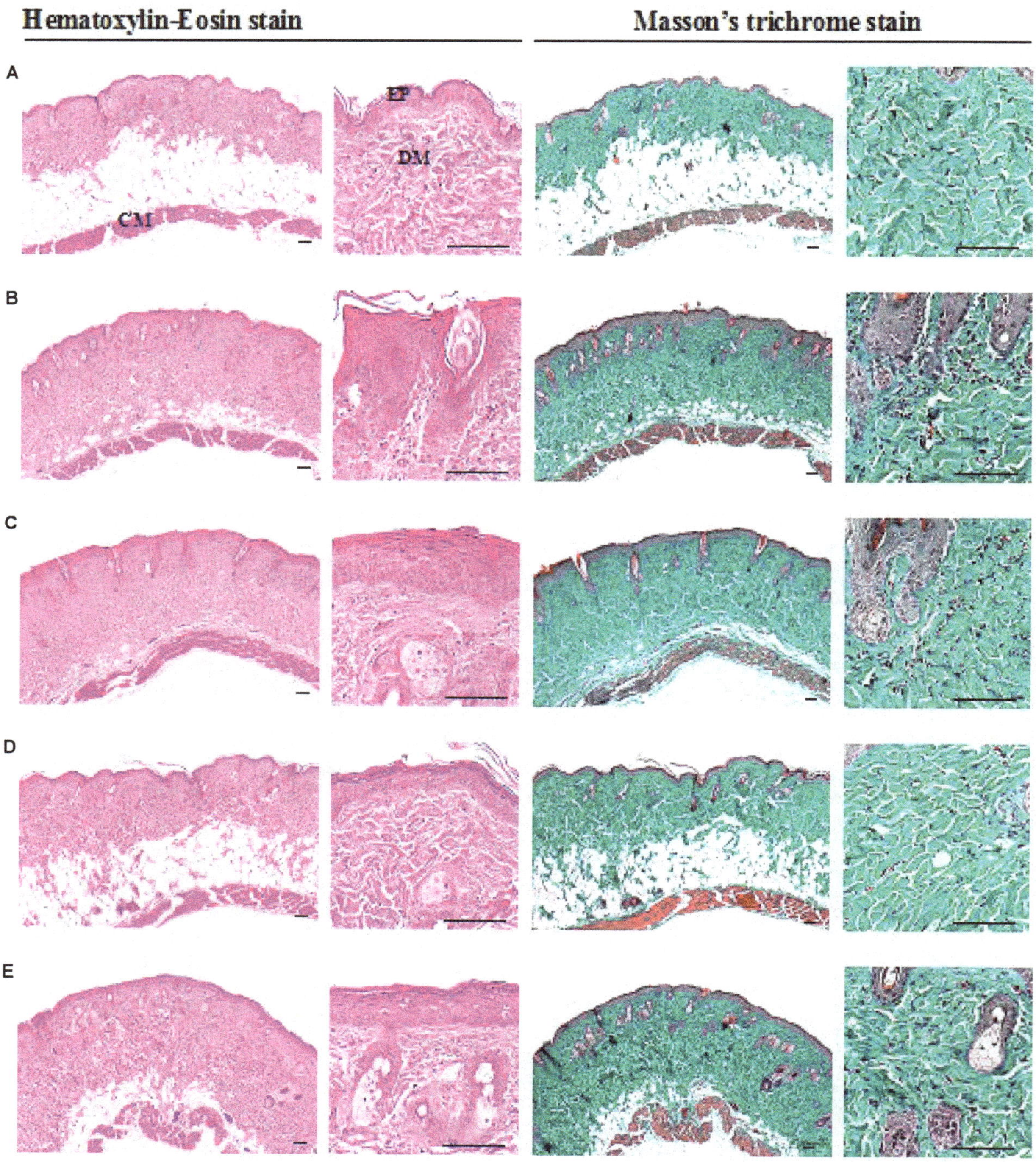

FIGURE 4 | Histopathological images of dorsal skin tissues of IMQ-induced psoriasis mice. **(A)** Control, **(B)** IMQ, **(C)** IMQ+vaseline, **(D)** IMQ+clobetasol, and **(E)** IMQ+SEL001. Increase of dorsal skin epithelial thickness and inflammatory cell infiltrations in dermis of dorsal skin were noticed in IMQ control and IMQ+vaseline as compared with intact control, respectively. But no significant changes on the dorsal back skin total thicknesses and collagen fiber occupied regions in the dermis were demonstrated in IMQ control and IMQ+vaseline as compared with intact control and no significant histopathological changes in the dorsal skin tissues were demonstrated in IMQ+vaseline as compared with those of IMQ control. These IMQ-induced hypersensitive psoriasis related histopathological changes on the dorsal skin tissues were significantly inhibited by treatment of SEL001 and clobetasol.

The extracted RNA was diluted in RNase-free water and quantified using Nano Drop by measuring the absorbance at 260 and 280 nm. Further, 1 μg of RNA was converted to cDNA using Maxime RT premix (iNtRON Biotechnology). Transcription levels of genes were quantitatively determined using RT-PCR (Stratagene 246 mix 3000p QPCR System, Agilent Technologies, Santa Clara, CA, United States) by employing power SYBR green (Roche Diagnostics Gmbh, Mannheim, Germany). The

PCR reactions for each sample were run in duplicate, and for every gene, the transcription levels were normalized with β-actin. The primers used in this study were purchased from Microgen (Korea).

RESULTS

Chemical Composition of SEL001

The GC–MS analysis of ethanolic extract of a probiotic strain *L. sakei* probio65 (SEL001) resulted in the identification of various compounds which included organic acids, amino acids, phenols, imidazole derivatives, and sugar alcohols along with some other organic compounds. The major composition of the SEL001 contained D-lactic acid (33.86%), propanoic acid (16.65%), glycerol (16.6%), L-lactic acid (6.03%), *myo*-inositol (1.86%), 1,3-butandiol (1.35%), 4-(methylsulfanylphenyl) carbamic acid (1.32%), 3,6-dioxa-2,7-disilaoctane (1.31%), pyrrolo[1,2-1] pyrazine-1,4-dione (1.26%), and valine (1.12%).

Erythema and Scaling

The severity of psoriasis during the 6-day trial was scored on 0, 2nd, 4th and 6th day following Psoriasis Area Severity Index (PASI). By applying IMQ on dorsal skin, psoriasis-like skin became apparent on second day onward. No significant changes in skin condition were seen on the second day in groups applied with vaseline, clobetasol or SEL001. However, from day three onward, erythema and scales were more visible. The erythema and scaling on mice back showed a dramatic increase in all groups as seen on day 4. However, a significant increase in erythema and scaling scores was seen in IMQ group when compared to control. In case of IMQ+vaseline group, a steady rate in erythema and slight decrease in scaling was observed from day 4 to day 6. In case of IMQ+clobetasol and IMQ+SEL001 the erythema scores were significantly less when compared to IMQ group ($p < 0.01$), and the scaling scores significantly decreased from day 4 to day 6+. Nevertheless, the erythema score in IMQ+clobetasol and IMQ+SEL001 was not completely normalized when compared to control group. The total mean scores for erythema and scales are shown in **Figures 1A,B**, from 0 day to day 6.

Skin and Ear Thickness

The ear thickness of right ear significantly increased in IMQ and IMQ+vaseline groups. In case of IMQ+clobetasol and IMQ+SEL001, the ear thickness was significantly reduced (**Figure 2A**). In addition, similar results were seen in dorsal skin thickness. The dorsal skinfold thickness of the mice in IMQ group and IMQ+vaseline showed a significant increase by topical application of IMQ treatment as compared with the intact control group ($p < 0.01$). The skinfold thickness in IMQ+clobetasol and IMQ+SEL001 group was significantly reduced compared to the IMQ group ($p < 0.01$) (**Figure 2B**). **Figure 2C** shows the visual appearance of IMQ-induced skin after 6 days of treatment. The skinfold thickness and ear thickening in IMQ+clobetasol and IMQ+SEL001 were not completely normalized when compared to control group. Nevertheless, the effect of clobetasol and SEL001 was promising.

Histological Analysis

A significant increase in epithelial thickness and number of inflammatory cells infiltrated in the dermis of ear tissues were observed in IMQ and IMQ+vaseline group compared

TABLE 1 | Histomorphometrical analysis of ear tissues from control or IMQ-induced psoriasis mice.

Groups	Total thickness (μm)	Epithelial thickness (μm)	Inflammatory cell numbers (cells/mm^2 of dermis)	Collagen occupied regions (%/mm^2 of dermis)
Control	228.70 ± 23.62	20.14 ± 2.67	21.83 ± 3.54	66.92 ± 5.43
IMQ	651.42 ± 133.75^a	84.97 ± 13.00^a	566.50 ± 125.43^a	42.56 ± 4.54^a
IMQ+vaseline	653.42 ± 104.38^a	83.30 ± 13.78^a	550.17 ± 135.19^a	41.65 ± 6.66^a
IMQ+clobetasol	343.09 ± 86.69^{bcd}	34.43 ± 10.71^{bcd}	156.83 ± 38.59^{bcd}	60.88 ± 1.07^{cd}
IMQ+SEL001	426.78 ± 90.28^{acd}	46.16 ± 13.00^{acd}	286.00 ± 71.55^{acd}	53.56 ± 6.61^{acd}

Values are expressed as mean ± SD of six ear histological fields. IMQ = Imiquimod, SEL001 = Test material; LSD = Least-significant differences multi-comparison. $^a p < 0.01$ and $^b p < 0.05$ as compared with control by LSD test; $^c p < 0.01$ as compared with IMQ by LSD test; $^d p < 0.01$ as compared with IMQ+vaseline by LSD test.

TABLE 2 | Histomorphometrical analysis of dorsal skin tissues taken from control or IMQ-induced psoriasis mice.

Groups	Total thickness (μm)	Epithelial thickness (μm)	Inflammatory cell numbers (cells/mm^2 of dermis)	Collagen occupied regions (%/mm^2 of dermis)
Control	807.56 ± 104.99	24.30 ± 6.19	43.33 ± 10.44	68.91 ± 10.00
IMQ	797.82 ± 105.24	65.11 ± 5.47^a	319.83 ± 139.20^d	67.82 ± 11.00
IMQ+vaseline	814.14 ± 76.68	66.41 ± 10.91^a	320.17 ± 116.10^d	67.51 ± 11.54
IMQ+clobetasol	792.12 ± 91.95	34.44 ± 10.47^{bc}	37.00 ± 8.44^{ef}	69.07 ± 10.28
IMQ+SEL001	803.39 ± 78.65	44.54 ± 11.40^{abc}	79.67 ± 17.01^{def}	70.84 ± 10.42

Values are expressed as mean ± SD of six ear histological fields. IMQ = Imiquimod, SEL001 = Test material; LSD = Least-significant differences multi-comparison. $^a p < 0.01$ as compared with control by LSD test; $^b p < 0.01$ as compared with IMQ by LSD test; $^c p < 0.01$ as compared with IMQ+vaseline by LSD test; $^d p < 0.01$ as compared with control by MW test; $^e p < 0.01$ as compared with IMQ by MW test; $^f p < 0.01$ as compared with IMQ+vaseline by MW test.

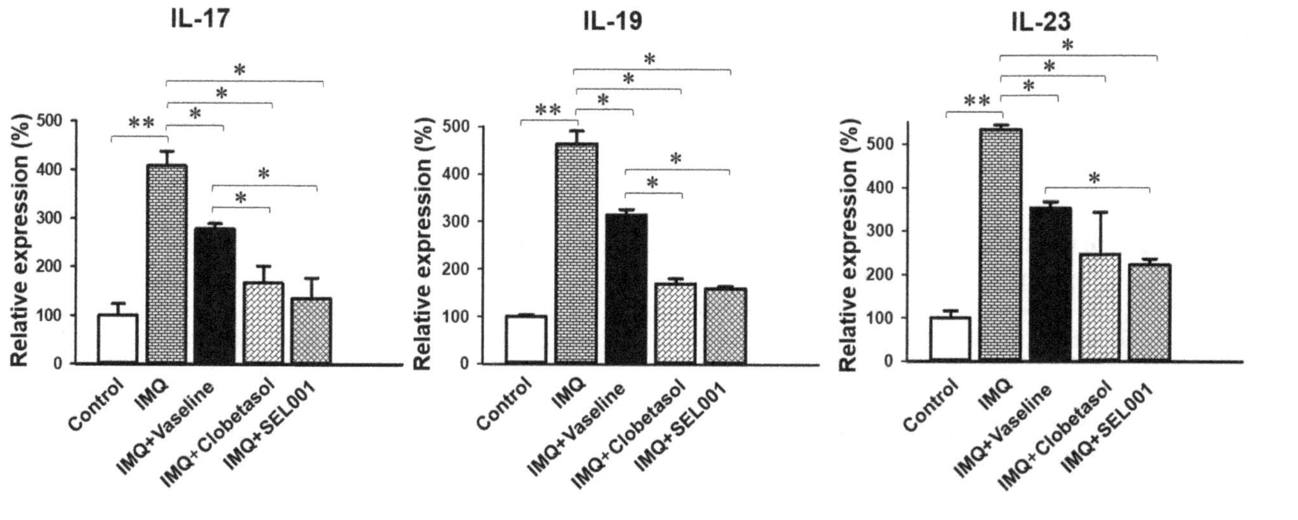

FIGURE 5 | mRNA expression profile. The data is expressed as mean ± standard deviation, $^{**}p < 0.001$ or $^{*}p < 0.05$ is significant, analyzed by one-way ANOVA test.

to control group ($p < 0.01$), as shown in **Figure 3**. In addition, a significant increase in dorsal skin epithelial thickness and the number of inflammatory cells infiltrated in dermis of dorsal skin were also noticed in IMQ group and IMQ+vaseline group as compared with control group ($p < 0.01$), as shown in **Figure 4**. Moreover, no significant changes in total dorsal skin thickness and collagen fiber occupied regions in the dermis were observed in the IMQ group and IMQ+vaseline group as compared with the control group, and no significant histopathological changes in the ear and dorsal skin tissues were observed in the IMQ+vaseline group as compared with those of IMQ group. These IMQ-induced hypertensive psoriasis related histopathological changes in both ear and dorsal skin tissues were significantly inhibited in IMQ+clobetasol and IMQ+SEL001 groups ($p < 0.01$) as shown in **Tables 1, 2**.

Gene Expression Analysis

Topical treatment of IMQ on the dorsal skin of mice showed an intense change in the gene expression level compared to the intact control, and/or mice treated with IMQ+clobetasol and IMQ+SEL001. The RNA expression analysis indicated an increase in gene expression of IL-19, IL-17A, and IL-23 in the IMQ group when compared with control group a pronounced drop of IL-19 was induced by clobetasol and SEL001 as seen in IMQ+clobetasol and IMQ+SEL001 groups. Similarly, a downregulation of gene expression level of IL-19, IL-17A, and IL-23 was seen in IMQ+clobetasol and IMQ+SEL001 groups compared to IMQ group and IMQ+vaseline group (**Figure 5**).

DISCUSSION

We have previously shown that *L. sakei* pro65 has a potent effect against atopic dermatitis both in the mouse model as well as in human clinical trial (Park et al., 2008; Woo et al., 2010). *Lactobacillus sakei* pro65 significantly reduced the IgE expression level in DNCB induced AD animal model (Kim et al., 2013). Furthermore, in our previous study, we showed *L. sakei* pro65 extract has antioxidant, anti-diabetic and tyrosinase inhibitory effects (Bajpai et al., 2016). Therefore, this study was designed to evaluate the effect of SEL001 on IMQ-induced psoriasis-like skin inflammation in a mouse model. Interestingly, chemical composition analysis of SEL001 confirmed the presence of various bioactive substances in SEL001, including organic acids, amino acids, phenols, imidazole derivatives, and sugar alcohols. As reported previously, these compounds or SEL001 like products of different origins containing phenolics and organic acids have been found to exhibit significant anti-inflammatory effects in various *in vitro* and *in vivo* models (Lee et al., 2006; Beh et al., 2017; Hearps et al., 2017). However, no effective agent has been developed against chronic psoriasis using the probiotic approach, which are known to be Generally Recognized As Safe (GRAS) in nature with no or less adversary effect for human application. Moreover, the SEL001 was found to contain important sugar alcohols, including *myo*-inositol. It has been reported that *myo*-inositol has been implicated with curing inflammatory disorders in animal mouse model (Claxson et al., 1990), suggesting that anti-inflammatory effect observed in this study might be mediated through *myo*-inositol. However, synergistic effects of other active components present in the SEL001 cannot be ruled out. As expected, the application of IMQ resulted in an increase in skin thickness and PASI score for both erythema and scaling. IMQ induced psoriasis model is considered as similar to human psoriasis (Leslie van der et al., 2009; Rather et al., 2016). Nevertheless, it was shown that IMQ induced skin lesions in humans differ to some extent from native psoriasis plaques (Vinter et al., 2015).

In the current histopathological inspection, skin protective effects of SEL001 were observed on the IMQ-induced hypersensitive psoriasis in a mouse model through well-documented histopathology-histomorphometric methods (Qin et al., 2014; Kim et al., 2015a,b; Bai et al., 2016). The results of representative histological profiles and histomorphometric analysis of the ear and dorsal back skin tissues are shown in **Figures 3** and **4**, respectively.

As reported previously, histopathologically, IMQ-induced hypersensitive psoriasis-like inflammation increased the epidermis hyperplasia and hypertrophy, and dermis inflammatory cell infiltrations in the ear and dorsal skin (van der Fits et al., 2009; Kim et al., 2015a; Bai et al., 2016), and similar results were observed in IMQ and IMQ+vaseline groups in this study. Significant increase of mean total and epidermal thicknesses, numbers of inflammatory cells infiltrated in the dermis, and decrease of dermis collagen fiber occupied regions were observed in the ear tissues of IMQ and IMQ+vaseline groups when compared with the control group. In addition, a significant increase of dorsal skin epithelial thicknesses and number of inflammatory cells infiltrated in the dermis of dorsal back skin were also noticed in IMQ and IMQ+vaseline groups as compared with control group, suggesting classic IMQ-induced hypersensitive psoriasis.

Moreover, no significant changes in the dorsal skin total thicknesses and collagen fiber occupied regions in dermis were demonstrated in IMQ group and IMQ+vaseline group as compared with control group. Also, in the present histopathological measurement, no significant histopathological changes in the tissue of both ear and dorsal skin were observed in IMQ+vaseline group as compared with those of IMQ group, suggesting that vaseline treatment did not show any effect on IMQ-induced hypersensitive psoriasis related histopathology in the ear and dorsal skin tissues. On the other hand, these IMQ-induced hypersensitive psoriasis related histopathological changes in both ear and dorsal skin tissues were significantly inhibited by the treatment of clobetasol and SEL001. Based on histopathological findings, SEL001 has obvious protective effects on the IMQ-induced hypersensitive psoriasis related histopathology in the ear and dorsal skin tissues. The decrease of collagen fibers in the dermis has been indicated edematous changes related to inflammations, as also considered in previous reports (Kim et al., 2015a,b). Decrease in the gene expression of IL-19, IL-17A, and IL-23 levels further confirms the potent effect of SEL001 on IMQ-induced psoriasis.

CONCLUSION

In summary, in this study, the SEL001 ameliorates the severity of IMQ-induced psoriasis like skin inflammation in mice. Topical application of SEL001 significantly reduced the skin thickening, and improved the erythema and scaling scores. These findings were further supported by improvements in histoclinical symptoms. SEL001 significantly inhibited IMQ-induced skin epithelial thicknesses and dermis inflammatory cell infiltrations. Furthermore, treatment with SEL001 decreased the expression level of psoriasis-associated pro-inflammatory cytokines, such as IL-17A, IL-19, and IL-23, proposing that altogether these changes might be mediators of the positive effects of SEL001 observed in the psoriasis-like skin inflammation model used in this study.

AUTHOR CONTRIBUTIONS

IR and VB performed the experiments and analyzed the data. EB and WP helped in the interpretation of the data. JL and Y-HP participated in the design of the study and the interpretation of the data. IR and VB wrote the manuscript. All authors read and approved the manuscript.

FUNDING

This work was supported by National Research Foundation of Korea (2013M3A9A504705 and 2017M3A9A5048999).

REFERENCES

Bai, S., Zhang, Z., Hou, S., and Liu, X. (2016). Influence of different types of contact hypersensitivity on imiquimod-induced psoriasis-like inflammation in mice. *Mol. Med. Rep.* 14, 671–680. doi: 10.3892/mmr.2016.5299

Bajpai, V. K., Rather, I. A., and Park, Y. H. (2016). Partially purified exo-polysaccharide from *Lactobacillus sakei* Probio 65 with antioxidant, α-glucosidase and tyrosinase inhibitory potential. *J. Food Biochem.* 40, 264–274. doi: 10.1111/jfbc.12230

Beh, B. K., Mohamad, N. E., Yeap, S. K., Ky, H., Boo, S. Y., and Chua, J. Y. H. (2017). Anti-obesity and anti-inflammatory effects of synthetic acetic acid vinegar and Nipa vinegar on high-fat diet-induced obese mice. *Sci. Rep.* 7:e6664. doi: 10.1038/s41598-017-06235-7

Chapat, L., Chemin, K., Dubois, B., Bourdet-Sicard, R., and Kaiserlian, D. (2004). *Lactobacillus casei* reduces CD8$^+$ T cell-mediated skin inflammation. *Eur. J. Immunol.* 34, 2520–2528. doi: 10.1002/eji.200425139

Claxson, A., Morris, C., Blake, D., Sirén, M., Halliwell, B., and Gustafsson, T. (1990). The anti-inflammatory effects of D-myo-inositol-1.2.6-trisphosphate (PP56) on animal models of inflammation. *Agents Actions* 29, 68–70. doi: 10.1007/BF01964724

El Malki, K., Karbach, S. H., Huppert, J., Zayoud, M., Reisig, S., Schuler, R., et al. (2013). An alternative pathway of imiquimod-induced psoriasis-like skin inflammation in the absence of interleukin-17 receptor a signaling. *J. Invest. Dermatol.* 133, 441–451. doi: 10.1038/jid.2012.318

Griffiths, C. E., and Barker, J. N. (2007). Pathogenesis and clinical features of psoriasis. *Lancet* 370, 263–271. doi: 10.1016/S0140-6736(07)61128-3

Gustafson, C. J., Watkins, C., Hix, E., and Feldman, S. R. (2013). Combination therapy in psoriasis: an evidence based review. *Am. J. Clin. Dermatol.* 14, 9–25. doi: 10.1007/s40257-012-0003-7

Hacini-Rachinel, F., Nancey, S., Boschetti, G., Sardi, F., Doucet-Ladevèze, R., Pierre-Yves, D., et al. (2009). CD4$^+$ T cells and *Lactobacillus casei* control relapsing colitis mediated by CD8$^+$ T cells. *J. Immunol.* 183, 5477–5486. doi: 10.4049/jimmunol.0804267

Hearps, A. C., Tyssen, D., Srbinovski, D., Bayigga, L., Diaz, D. J., and Aldunate, M. (2017). Vaginal lactic acid elicits an anti-inflammatory response from human cervicovaginal epithelial cells and inhibits production of pro-inflammatory mediators associated with HIV acquisition. *Mucosal Immunol.* 10, 1480–1490. doi: 10.1038/mi.2017.27

Joint FAO/WHO (2001). *Expert Committee on Food Additives and World Health Organization. Food & Agriculture Organization. Safety Evaluation of Certain Mycotoxins in Food. Issue 74. Meeting, 2001.* Geneva: World Health Organization

Kagami, S., Rizzo, H. L., Lee, J. J., Koguchi, Y., and Blauvelt, A. (2010). Circulating Th17, Th22, and Th1 cells are increased in psoriasis. *J. Invest. Dermatol.* 130, 1373–1383. doi: 10.1038/jid.2009.399

Kim, C. G., Kang, M., Lee, Y. H., Min, W. G., Kim, Y. H., Kang, S. J., et al. (2015a). Bathing effects of various seawaters on allergic (atopic) dermatitis-like skin lesions induced by 2,4-dinitrochlorobenzene in hairless mice. *Evid. Based Complement. Alternat. Med.* 2015, 179–185. doi: 10.1155/2015/179185

Kim, K. H., Park, S. J., Lee, Y. J., Lee, J. E., Song, C. H., Choi, S. H., et al. (2015b). Inhibition of UVB-induced skin damage by exopolymers from *Aureobasidium pullulans* SM-2001 in hairless mice. *Basic Clin. Pharmacol. Toxicol.* 116, 73–86. doi: 10.1111/bcpt.12288

Kim, H., Rather, I. A., Kim, H., Kim, S., Kim, T., and Jang, J. (2015c). A double-blind, placebo controlled-trial of a probiotic strain *Lactobacillus sakei* probio-65 for the prevention of canine atopic dermatitis. *J. Microbiol. Biotechnol.* 25, 1966–1969. doi: 10.4014/jmb.1506.06065

Kim, J. Y., Park, B. K., Park, H. J., Park, Y. H., Kim, B. O., and Pyo, S. (2013). Atopic dermatitis-mitigating effects of new *Lactobacillus* strain, *Lactobacillus sakei* probio 65 isolated from Kimchi. *J. Appl. Microbiol.* 115, 517–526. doi: 10.1111/jam.12229

Kim, J. Y., and Pyo, S. (2012). Oral administration of dead *Lactobacillus sakei* inhibits atopic dermatitis-like skin lesion in NC/Nga mice. *FASEB J.* 26:e364. doi: 10.1111/jam.12229

Lee, E., Trepicchio, W. L., Oestreicher, J. L., Pittman, D., Wang, F., Chamian, F., et al. (2004). Increased expression of interleukin 23 p19 and p40 in lesional skin of patients with psoriasis vulgaris. *J. Exp. Med.* 199, 125–130. doi: 10.1084/jem.20030451

Lee, J. Y., Jang, Y. W., Kang, H. S., Moon, H., Sim, S. S., and Kim, C. J. (2006). Anti-inflammatory action of phenolic compounds from *Gastrodia elata* root. *Arch. Pharm. Res.* 29, 849–858. doi: 10.1007/BF02973905

Leslie van der, F., Sabine, M., Jane, S. A. V., Marius, K., Louis, B., Jon, D. L., et al. (2009). Imiquimod-induced psoriasis-like skin inflammation in mice is mediated via the IL-23/IL-17 axis. *J. Immunol.* 182, 5836–5845. doi: 10.4049/jimmunol.0802999

Li, H. H., Lin, Y. C., Chen, P. J., Hsiao, C. H., Lee, J. Y., Chen, W. C., et al. (2005). Interleukin-19 upregulates keratinocyte growth factor and is associated with psoriasis. *Br. J. Dermatol.* 153, 591–595. doi: 10.1111/j.1365-2133.2005.06665.x

Li, R., Wang, J., Wang, X., Zhou, J., Wang, M., Ma, H., et al. (2016). Increased βTrCP are associated with imiquimod-induced psoriasis-like skin inflammation in mice via NF-κB signaling pathway. *Gene* 592, 164–171. doi: 10.1016/j.gene.2016.07.066

Matsumoto, S., Hara, T., Hori, T., Mitsuyama, K., Nagaoka, M., and Tomiyasu, N. (2005). Probiotic *Lactobacillus*-induced improvement in murine chronic inflammatory bowel disease is associated with the down-regulation of pro-inflammatory cytokines in lamina propria mononuclear cells. *Clin. Exp. Immunol.* 140, 417–426. doi: 10.1111/j.1365-2249.2005.02790.x

Mudigonda, P., Mudigonda, T., Feneran, A. N., Alamdari, H. S., Sandoval, L., and Feldman, S. R. (2012). Interleukin-23 and interleukin-17: importance in pathogenesis and therapy of psoriasis. *Dermatol. Online J.* 18:1.

Nadeem, A., Al-Harbi, N. O., Al-Harbi, M. M., El-Sherbeeny, A. M., Ahmad, S. F., and Siddiqui, N. (2015). Imiquimod-induced psoriasis-like skin inflammation is suppressed by BET bromodomain inhibitor in mice through RORC/IL-17A pathway modulation. *Pharmacol. Res.* 99, 248–257. doi: 10.1016/j.phrs.2015.06.001

Ouyang, W., Kolls, J. K., and Zheng, Y. (2008). The biological functions of T helper 17 cell effector cytokines in inflammation. *Immunity* 28, 454–467. doi: 10.1016/j.immuni.2008.03.004

Park, C. W., Young, M., Jung, Y. M., Kim, H., Jeong, Y., Lee, H. K., et al. (2008). New functional probiotic *Lactobacillus sakei* probio 65 alleviates atopic symptoms in the mouse. *J. Med. Food* 11, 405–412. doi: 10.1089/jmf.2007.0144

Park, S. B., Im, M., Lee, Y., Lee, J. H., Lim, J., and Park, Y. H. (2014). Effect of emollients containing vegetable-derived *Lactobacillus* in the treatment of atopic dermatitis symptoms: split-body clinical trial. *Ann. Dermatol.* 26, 150–155. doi: 10.5021/ad.2014.26.2.150

Perera, G. K., Di Meglio, P., and Nestle, F. O. (2012). Psoriasis. *Annu. Rev. Pathol.* 7, 385–422. doi: 10.1146/annurev-pathol-011811-132448

Piskin, G., Sylva-Steenland, R. M. R., Bos, J. D., and Teunissen, M. B. M. (2006). In vitro and in situ expression of IL-23 by keratinocytes in healthy skin and psoriasis lesions: enhanced expression in psoriatic skin. *J. Immunol.* 176, 1908–1915. doi: 10.4049/jimmunol.176.3.1908

Plaza-Díaz, J., Ruiz-Ojeda, F. J., Vilchez-Padial, L. M., and Gil, A. (2017). Evidence of the anti-inflammatory effects of probiotics and synbiotics in intestinal chronic diseases. *Nutrients* 9:e555. doi: 10.3390/nu9060555

Qin, S., Wen, J., Bai, X. C., Chen, T. Y., Zheng, R. C., Zhou, G. B., et al. (2014). Endogenous n-3 polyunsaturated fatty acids protect against imiquimod-induced psoriasis-like inflammation via the IL-17/IL-23 axis. *Mol. Med. Rep.* 9, 2097–2104. doi: 10.3892/mmr.2014.2136

Rather, I. A., Bajpai, V. K., Han, J. H., and Nam, G. J. (2016). Imiquimod-induced psoriasis-like skin inflammation in mouse mode. *Bangladesh J. Pharmacol.* 11, 849–885. doi: 10.1111/exd.13269

Ravi, B., Rentitta, R. E., Pradha, M. L., Issac, R., and Naidu, S. (2013). Evaluation of antidiabetic potential of oyster mushroom (*Pleurotus ostreatus*) in alloxan-induced diabetic mice. *Immunopharmacol. Immunotoxicol.* 35, 101–109. doi: 10.3109/08923973.2012.710635

Res, P. C., Piskin, G., de Boer, O. J., van der Loos, C. M., Teeling, P., Bos, J. D., et al. (2010). Overrepresentation of IL-17A and IL- 22 producing CD8 T cells in lesional skin suggests their involvement in the pathogenesis of psoriasis. *PLoS One* 5:e14108. doi: 10.1371/journal.pone.0014108

Shukla, S., Mehta, A., Mehta, P., and Bajpai, V. K. (2011). Evaluation of comparative antidiabetic effects of ethanol extracts of *Caesalpinia bonducella* and *Stevia rebaudiana* in normal and alloxan-induced experimental rats. *Rom. Biotechnol. Lett.* 16, 6187–6199.

Tojo, R., Suárez, A., Clemente, M. G., De los Reyes-Gavilán, C. G., Margolles, A., and Gueimonde, M. (2014). Intestinal microbiota in health and disease: role of bifidobacteria in gut homeostasis. *World J. Gastroenterol.* 20, 15163–15176. doi: 10.3748/wjg.v20.i41.15163

Tokura, Y. (2012). Th17 cells and skin diseases. *Nihon Rinsho Meneki Gakkai Kaishi* 35, 388–392. doi: 10.2177/jsci.35.388

van der Fits, L., Mourits, S., Voerman, J. S., Kant, M., Boon, L., Laman, J. D., et al. (2009). Imiquimod-induced psoriasis-like skin inflammation in mice is mediated via the IL-23/IL-17 axis. *J. Immunol.* 182, 5836–5845. doi: 10.4049/jimmunol.0802999

Vinter, H., Iversen, L., Steiniche, T., Kragballe, K., and Johansen, C. (2015). Aldara®-induced skin inflammation: studies of patients with psoriasis. *Br. J. Dermatol.* 172, 345–353. doi: 10.1111/bjd.13236

Wang, W. J., Yin, X. Y., Zuo, X. B., Cheng, H., Du, W. D., Zhang, F. Y., et al. (2013). Gene-gene interactions in IL23/Th17 pathway contribute to psoriasis susceptibility in Chinese Han population. *J. Eur. Acad. Dermatol. Venereol.* 27, 1156–1162. doi: 10.1111/j.1468-3083.2012.04683.x

Wolf, R., Howard, O. M., Dong, H. F., Voscopoulos, C., Boeshans, K., and Winston, J. (2008). Chemotactic activity of S100A7 (Psoriasin) is mediated by the receptor for advanced glycation end products and potentiates inflammation with highly homologous but functionally distinct S100A15. *J. Immunol.* 181, 1499–1506. doi: 10.4049/jimmunol.181.2.1499

Woo, S. I., Kim, J. Y., Lee, Y. J., Kim, N. S., and Hahn, Y. S. (2010). Effect of *Lactobacillus sakei* supplementation in children with atopic eczema-dermatitis syndrome. *Ann. Allery Asthama Immunol.* 104, 343–348. doi: 10.1016/j.anai.2010.01.020

Wu, C.-S., Chui, W.-H., Chen, Y.-H., Chao, Y.-H., Lin, C.-C., Li, Y.-R., et al. (2017). *Lactobacillus pentosus* GMNL-77 inhibits skin lesions in imiquimod-induced psoriasis-like mice. *J. Dermatol. Sci.* 86, e17–e18. doi: 10.1016/j.jdermsci.2017.02.050

Yoo, I. S., Lee, J. H., Song, S. T., Kim, J. H., Lee, H. J., and Kang, S. W. (2012). T-helper 17 cells: the driving force of psoriasis and psoriatic arthritis. *Int. J. Rheum. Dis.* 15, 531–537. doi: 10.1111/j.1756-185X.2012.01813.x

Zhang, L., Yang, X. Q., Cheng, J., Hui, R. S., and Gao, T. W. (2010). Increased Th17 cells are accompanied by FoxP3(+) Treg cell accumulation and correlated with psoriasis disease severity. *Clin. Immunol.* 135, 108–117. doi: 10.1016/j.clim.2009.11.008

9

Bile Salt Hydrolase Activities: A Novel Target to Screen Anti-*Giardia* Lactobacilli

Thibault Allain[1,2], Soraya Chaouch[2], Myriam Thomas[3,4], Marie-Agnès Travers[2†], Isabelle Valle[3,4], Philippe Langella[1], Philippe Grellier[2], Bruno Polack[3,4], Isabelle Florent[2*] and Luis G. Bermúdez-Humarán[1*]

[1] INRA, Commensal and Probiotics-Host Interactions Laboratory, Micalis Institute, AgroParisTech, Paris, France, [2] UMR 7245, Muséum National d'Histoire Naturelle, Centre National de la Recherche Scientifique, Sorbonne Universités, Paris, France, [3] INRA, Ecole Nationale Vétérinaire d'Alfort, BIPAR, ENVA, ANSES, UMR, Université Paris-Est, Champs-sur-Marne, France, [4] INRA, Laboratoire de Santé Animale, BIPAR, ENVA, ANSES, UMR, Maisons-Alfort, France

***Correspondence:**
Luis G. Bermúdez-Humarán
luis.bermudez@inra.fr
Isabelle Florent
isabelle.florent@mnhn.fr

†Present address:
Marie-Agnès Travers,
Laboratoire de Génétique et Pathologie des Mollusques Marins, SG2M-LGPMM, Ifremer, La Tremblade, France

Giardia duodenalis is a protozoan parasite responsible for giardiasis, a disease characterized by intestinal malabsorption, diarrhea and abdominal pain in a large number of mammal species. Giardiasis is one of the most common intestinal parasitic diseases in the world and thus a high veterinary, and public health concern. It is well-established that some probiotic bacteria may confer protection against this parasite *in vitro* and *in vivo* and we recently documented the implication of bile-salt hydrolase (BSH)-like activities from strain La1 of *Lactobacillus johnsonii* as mediators of these effects *in vitro*. We showed that these activities were able to generate deconjugated bile salts that were toxic to the parasite. In the present study, a wide collection of lactobacilli strains from different ecological origins was screened to assay their anti-giardial effects. Our results revealed that the anti-parasitic effects of some of the strains tested were well-correlated with the expression of BSH-like activities. The two most active strains *in vitro*, La1 and *Lactobacillus gasseri* CNCM I-4884, were then tested for their capacity to influence *G. duodenalis* infection in a suckling mice model. Strikingly, only *L. gasseri* CNCM I-4884 strain was able to significantly antagonize parasite growth with a dramatic reduction of the trophozoites load in the small intestine. Moreover, this strain also significantly reduced the fecal excretion of *Giardia* cysts after 5 days of treatment, which could contribute to blocking the transmission of the parasite, in contrast of La1 where no effect was observed. This study represents a step toward the development of new prophylactic strategies to combat *G. duodenalis* infection in both humans and animals.

Keywords: *Giardia duodenalis*, lactobacilli, *Lactobacillus johnsonii*, *Lactobacillus gasseri*, probiotics, bile salt hydrolases

INTRODUCTION

Giardia duodenalis (also known as *G. lamblia* or *G. intestinalis*) is the etiologic agent of the zoonotic disease giardiasis, one of the most common waterborne parasitic infections globally. *G. duodenalis* is a flagellate protozoan (Excavata, Diplomonad) that infects a broad diversity of animals such as humans, mammals, reptiles and birds (Thompson and Monis, 2004, 2012). Transmission can occur by ingestion of viable cysts from contaminated water and soil, or directly by contact with an infected animal's feces (Gardner and Hill, 2001). After ingestion, exposure to gastric acid and proteases in the stomach leads to excystation and liberation of replicative trophozoite stages that adhere transiently to the proximal small intestine and persist for several days (for up to several months in some cases) (Reiner et al., 2003). After this replicative and pathogenic stage, trophozoites are carried into the colon and progressively encyst. Cysts, released through host feces, may then survive in the environment for several months and remain infectious at low doses (Thompson et al., 1993).

The main clinical symptoms of giardiasis are acute or chronic diarrhea, abdominal pain, intestinal malabsorption, steatorrhea, and weight loss (Farthing, 1996; Buret, 2007). Considered as a public health threat and a veterinary concern worldwide, giardiasis is responsible for many waterborne diarrhea outbreaks in developed countries (Roxstrom-Lindquist et al., 2006; Buret, 2007). In humans, it affects mainly children, and undernourished or immunosuppressed individuals. Even though giardiasis can be self-limited, standard antibiotic therapies including 5-nitroimidazole and benzimidazole drugs are needed to treat long-term infections (Savioli et al., 2006). In mammals, *G. duodenalis* infections are common in companion animals, small ruminants and cattle, for which alternative treatments are very limited (Harris et al., 2001).

The increasing number of clinical trial failures and the emergence of resistant *Giardia* strains in both medical and veterinary applications have encouraged the development of new therapeutic strategies (Harris et al., 2001; Upcroft and Upcroft, 2001). In this context, it has been established that gut microbiota plays a pivotal role in the protection against enteropathogens through the production of antimicrobial compounds and by competition for nutrients and attachment to the mucosal surface (Travers et al., 2011; Bengmark, 2013). In particular, probiotic bacteria such as some strains of lactobacilli have been shown to confer host health benefits by enhancing innate and adaptive immune responses (Sanders, 2008; Martin et al., 2013; Sokol, 2014). Moreover, pre-clinical studies suggest that colonization of the small intestine by *G. duodenalis* trophozoites depends on the composition of host gut microbiota (Singer and Nash, 2000; Barash et al., 2017; Bartelt et al., 2017). In recent years, probiotic-based therapies have been explored to treat giardiasis (Allain et al., 2017). For instance, some lactobacilli strains such *Lactobacillus johnsonii* La1 (also known as NCC533 but hereafter named La1), *Lactobacillus casei* MTCC1423 and *Lactobacillus rhamnosus* GG (LGG), have been shown to display anti-giardial properties by (i) antagonizing the proliferation of trophozoites and, (ii) reducing the severity of infection in several murine models (Humen et al., 2005; Shukla et al., 2008; Goyal et al., 2011; Travers et al., 2011). While the molecular mechanisms remain poorly understood, we have recently discovered the involvement of deconjugated bile salts, generated by the hydrolysis of conjugated bile salts from bile by La1 strain, as one of the mechanisms contributing to the inhibition of *Giardia* trophozoite growth *in vitro* (Perez et al., 2001; Travers et al., 2016). Our hypothesis was that these deconjugated bile salts were produced by bile salt hydrolase (BSH)-like enzymes released or secreted by this strain (Travers et al., 2016).

In the current study, we screened a wide collection of lactobacilli strains from various environmental origins in order to determine their ability to display an anti-giardial effect. *In vitro* analysis from supernatant-lactobacilli samples led to the identification of several strains having a strong inhibitory activity against *G. duodenalis* growth (up to the level previously reported for La1). In parallel, we showed that the *in vitro* anti-*Giardia* activity displayed by some of these lactobacilli strains is clearly correlated with their BSH-like activities *in vitro*. The two strains displaying the strongest inhibitory effects: La1 and *Lactobacillus gasseri* CNCM I-4884, were then evaluated *in vivo* in a suckling mice model challenged with the WB6 strain of *G. duodenalis*. Our results showed that *L. gasseri* CNCM I-4884 displayed a higher anti-giardial effect *in vivo* than La1, with an almost complete clearance of *Giardia* infection in suckling mice. These findings show that a screening based on the detection of BSH activities is a promising tool to identify new anti-*Giardia* lactobacilli strains. Overall, our study opens new therapeutic strategies for both preventing and treating giardiasis in humans.

MATERIALS AND METHODS

Giardia duodenalis Culture Conditions

Giardia duodenalis was grown *in vitro* as recently described (Travers et al., 2016). Trophozoites of *G. duodenalis* strain WB clone 6 (WB6) assemblage A1 (ATCC 50803) were grown in Keiser's modified TYI-S-33 medium (KM) (Morrison et al., 2007). KM medium was supplemented with 10% heat-inactivated fetal calf serum (FCS, reference A15-101, PAA Laboratories, GE healthcare), adjusted to pH 6.0, and sterilized with a 0.22 μm filter. *G. duodenalis* WB6 trophozoites were subcultured in anaerobic conditions at 5×10^4 cells per ml after chilling on ice for 10 min and centrifuged at $700 \times g$, 5 min. Aliquots were frozen in liquid nitrogen and stored at −80°C until further use. For *in vitro* and *in vivo* experiments, 48 h old cultures of confluent trophozoites were pelleted at $700 \times g$, 5 min after chilling on ice for 10 min, and resuspended at the needed concentrations.

Bacterial Strains and Culture Conditions

The bacteria collection used in this study comprises 29 lactobacilli isolated from different biotopes (**Table 1**). The strains were grown in Man Rogosa Sharpe (MRS, Difco) medium on agar plates over night at 37°C in anaerobic conditions (GasPack Plus, BBL). Bacteria were then subcultured for 16 h at 37°C in MRS broth and were subsequently grown in Keiser's modified TYI-S-33 medium supplemented with 10% heat-inactivated FCS (see above) to stationary phase. An intermediary subculture in modified TYI-S-33 medium was used for some strains as previously described (Perez et al., 2001). Bacterial supernatants were then collected after centrifugation at $10{,}000 \times g$ for 10 min, sterilized with a 0.22 μm filter and the pH was adjusted to 6.2 with 5N NaOH.

Bile Salt Hydrolase Assays

The bacterial strains were tested for Tauro-deoxycholic acid (TDCA) and Glyco-deoxycholic acid (GDCA) hydrolase activities on MRS-agar plates supplemented with either 0.5%

TABLE 1 | List of tested lactobacilli strains with their characteristics and bile salt hydrolase activity specificities.

Lactobacillus species	Strain[1]	Origin	TDCA (0.5%) hydrolase activity	TDCA hydrolase activity score[2]	GDCA (0.5%) hydrolase activity	GDCA hydrolase activity score[2]
L. acidophilus	ATCC4356	Feces, human	P	+	N	–
L. brevis	CNRZ1845	Malt (beer)	P	+	P	+
L. casei	ATCC393	Cheese	N	–	N	–
L. crispatus	CIP103606	Unknown	N	–	P	++
L. curvatus	CNRZ1335	Fermented sausage/mea	N	–	N	–
L. gasseri	ATCC33323	Vaginal tract, human	N	–	N	–
L. gasseri	CNCM I-4884 ATCC29601	Cariouth tooth, human	P	+++	P	++
L. helveticus	CNRZ1109	Lactic starter	N	–	N	–
L. helveticus	ATCC11977	Lactic starter (cheese)	N	–	P	++
L. johnsonii	CNRZ217	Feces, rat	N	–	P	+
L. johnsonii	CNRZ218	Feces, rat	P	+	P	++
L. johnsonii	CNRZ1897	Fermented milk	P	+++	ND	ND
L. johnsonii	CIP103614	Vaginal tract, human	P	++	N	–
L. johnsonii	CIP103786	Cheese	P	+	P	++
L. johnsonii	CIP103652	Unknown	P	++	N	–
L. johnsonii	CIP103653	Unknown	P	++	N	–
L. johnsonii	CIP103654	Pharmaceutical preparation	P	+	P	+
L. johnsonii	CIP103781	Unknown	P	+++	P	++
L. johnsonii	CIP103782	Urethran, human	P	+	N	–
L. johnsonii	ATCC33200	Blood, human	P	++	P	++
L. johnsonii	La1 (NCC533)	Feces, human	P	+++	P	++
L. paracasei	CNRZ315	Unknown	N	–	N	–
L. pentosus	CNRZ1218	Cheese	N	–	N	–
L. plantarum	CNRZ738	Silage	N	–	P	+
L. rhamnosus	CNRZ317	Unknown	N	–	N	–
L. rhamnosus	CNRZ2084	Fermented milk	N	–	N	–
L. reuteri	CNRZ431	Sourdough	N	–	N	–
L. sakei	CNRZ1332	Moto, starter of sake	N	–	N	–
L. zeae	CNRZ2269	Corn steep liquor	N	–	N	–

P, positive; N, negative; ND, non-determined. [1]Strains were obtained from different collections: CIP, Collection de l'Institut Pasteur, France; CNRZ/CIRM, Centre International de Ressources Microbiennes; CNCM, Collection Nationale de Cultures de Microorganismes, Institut Pasteur, France; ATCC, American Type Culture Collection, United States. [2]TDCA/GDCA hydrolase activity score were determined on the size of the halo zone (diameter): (–): no detected halo; (+): <8 mm; (++): 9 mm to 12 mm; (+++): >13 mm.

TDCA (Sigma–Aldrich) or 0.5% GDCA (Merck) following the protocol described by Moser and Savage (2001). MRS plates with 0.5% TDCA were first incubated at 37°C in anaerobic conditions for 24 h prior to inoculation. Strains were grown anaerobically for 16 h at 37°C in MRS broth, then streaked on MRS-agar plates, supplemented or not, with 0.5% TDCA or 0.5% GDCA and incubated at 37°C in anaerobic conditions for 48–72 h. BSH activity can be easily detected when unconjugated deoxycholic acid precipitates in the MRS-agar plate, forming an iridescent halo below and around active colonies. These assays were performed in duplicates, and included two biological replicates. BSH activity score was determined as indicated in **Table 1**.

In Vitro Anti-giardial Assays

Filtered bacterial supernatants (500 μl) were co-incubated with fresh cultures of *Giardia* trophozoites (1.33×10^5 parasites/ml in KM medium, pH 6.0, supplemented with 10% heat-inactivated FCS) at a volumetric ratio of 1–3, in the presence or absence of bovine bile (0.6 g/L) at 37°C in anaerobic conditions for 22 h. BSH from *Clostridium perfringens* (1 U) (reference C4018, Sigma–Aldrich) was used as a positive control for *Giardia* growth inhibition as previously described (Travers et al., 2016). Samples were then ice-chilled for 10 min and trophozoite load was determined using hemocytometer (flagella mobility was used to screen parasite viability). The inhibition rates were determined by counting the number of living trophozoites and establishing ratios compared to the controls (in percentage). Experiments were conducted in duplicates and included three biological replicates.

Assessment of Anti-giardial Activity *in Vivo*

Cultures of *G. duodenalis* trophozoites WB6 were grown in Keister's modified TYI-S-33 medium with 10% heat-inactivated FCS. Lactobacilli strains (La1, *L. gasseri* CNCM I-4884 and *L. curvatus* CNRZ1335) were cultured in MRS broth for 16 h at 37°C in anaerobic conditions from precultures. Bacteria were then harvested by centrifugation at 7000 × *g* for 15 min, washed two times and resuspended in a corresponding volume of sterile PBS/Glycerol 15% to obtain a final concentration of 2.5×10^{10} CFU/ml for intragastric administrations (5×10^8 CFU per neonatal mouse). Mice used for reproduction were non-inbred mice of the OF1 strain (Charles River, Saint-Germain-Nuelles, France). All experiments were conducted in a filtered air chamber and manipulations were performed under a laminar flow hood to prevent contamination of the environment by cysts of *G. duodenalis* and other pathogens.

Lactobacilli strains were administered daily by intragastric gavage in a volume of 20 μl (5×10^8 CFU) to 5 days old neonatal mice from day 5 to day 15 (n = 9–12 per group) (**Figure 2**). Control animals (n = 8) received PBS with glycerol 15% instead of bacterial suspensions. Neonatal mice were then challenged with trophozoites at day 10 by intragastric gavage in a volume of 100 μl (10^5 trophozoites). Mice were sacrificed by cervical dislocation at day 16. The small intestine and colon contents were examined for the presence of trophozoites and cysts, by counting the parasite burden, using a hemocytometer. The counting of trophozoites was performed from the small intestine (resuspended in 5 ml of ice-chilled sterile PBS), while cysts were enumerated in the colon and caecum (resuspended in 5 ml of ice-chilled 2.5% Potassium dichromate). The minimum threshold of counting values for statistical analysis was set at 10^3 trophozoites.

Statistical Analysis

Results were expressed as means ± standard error of the mean (SEM). Comparison between groups was assessed by one or two-way analysis of variance (ANOVA), *t*-test, Mann–Whitney and Kruskal–Wallis. Correlation tests were performed using Spearman's Rank Correlation Test. Statistical significance was calculated at *p*-values under 0.05 at 95% confidence interval.

Ethics Statement

All protocols were carried out in accordance with the institutional ethical guidelines of the ethics committee ANSES's Animal Health Laboratory at Maisons-Alfort on the campus of the French National Veterinary School of Alfort (ENVA), which approved this study.

RESULTS

BSH Activities of Lactobacilli Strains

The 29 strains tested in this study were able to grow in MRS-agar supplemented with 0.5% TDCA whereas only 25 grew in MRS-agar supplemented with 0.5% GDCA, supporting that GDCA has a higher bactericidal activity than TDCA *in vivo* (Begley et al., 2006). TDCA/GDCA hydrolase activity is a well-recognized indicator of BSH activity in bacteria (Bustos et al., 2012). A semi-quantitative method was used to monitor the BSH activity by measuring the halo zone of positive strains after 48–72 h of incubation. Among the 29 strains, 6 exhibited TDCA hydrolase activity, 4 exhibited GDCA hydrolase activity and 8 displayed both TDCA and GDCA hydrolase activities (**Table 1**). No halo was detected for 11 strains. Interestingly, all *L. johnsonii* strains tested displayed at least one type of BSH activity. Among the strains harboring both tauro and glyco-specific BSH activities, La1, *L. gasseri* CNCM I-4884 and *L. johnsonii* CIP103782 exhibited the highest BSH scores (**Table 1** and **Figure 1A**).

Characterization of Anti-giardial Lactobacilli Strains

We screened the 29 lactobacilli strains for their inhibitory abilities against *G. duodenalis*. For this, bacterial supernatants were co-incubated for 22 h at 37°C with *Giardia* trophozoite cultures in KM growth medium supplemented, or not, with bovine bile (0.6 g/L). Living trophozoites were enumerated using hemocytometer. Parasite cultures that were grown without bile did not display major differences when compared to trophozoites grown in KM supplemented with bile, showing that cholesterol and lipids from fetal bovine serum are sufficient to fulfill the lipid uptake requirements of *Giardia* and that bile components are not toxic for *Giardia* (Travers et al., 2016).

When co-incubated with *Giardia* in KM supplemented with bovine bile, 19 bacterial supernatants exhibited significant antagonistic effects on *Giardia* growth, with a wide range of inhibition levels (**Figure 1A**). Six strains showed growth inhibition levels from 15 to 30%, 10 exhibited growth inhibition levels from 30 to 70%, and 12 strains displayed a strong reduction of trophozoites by 70–100% ($p < 0.001$). Only supernatant of *L. gasseri* CNCM I-4884 were as efficient as that of La1 to antagonize *Giardia* growth *in vitro* (100%). Using Spearman's Rank Correlation Test, we observed a positive correlation between inhibition levels and BSH activity score ($r = 0.86$; $p < 0.0001$) of bacterial strains (**Figure 1B**). Inhibition assays were then divided into two groups: (i) BSH negative (strains with no detected BSH activity) and (ii) BSH positive (strains displaying either TDCA, GDCA, or both BSH activities). We observed that *Giardia* growth inhibitory activity of BSH positive strains were twofold higher relative to BSH negative strains (Student's *t*-test; $p < 0.0001$) (**Figure 1C**). Moreover, the cytotoxic effect on *Giardia* was lost when trophozoites were co-incubated with bacterial supernatant in the absence of bile (**Figure 1D**). However, a very weak inhibition was still observed for a majority of the strains (range between 5 and 15%), which can be explained by the presence of other extracellular compounds released by lactobacilli (e.g., bacteriocins) that are also potentially deleterious to *Giardia* growth. Taken together, these *in vitro* results strongly suggest that the anti-giardial effect displayed by lactobacilli strains tested in this study is mostly bile-dependent.

In Vivo Effect of Orally Administered Lactobacilli against *G. duodenalis*

In vivo experiments were performed in order to assess the potential of newly identified anti-giardial lactobacilli strains to antagonize *G. duodenalis in vivo*. Bacterial suspensions, or PBS/glycerol were daily administered by intragastric gavage (5×10^8 CFU) to neonatal mice from day 5 to day 15 (**Figure 2**). The persistence of lactobacilli in suckling mice and administration route were determined in previous

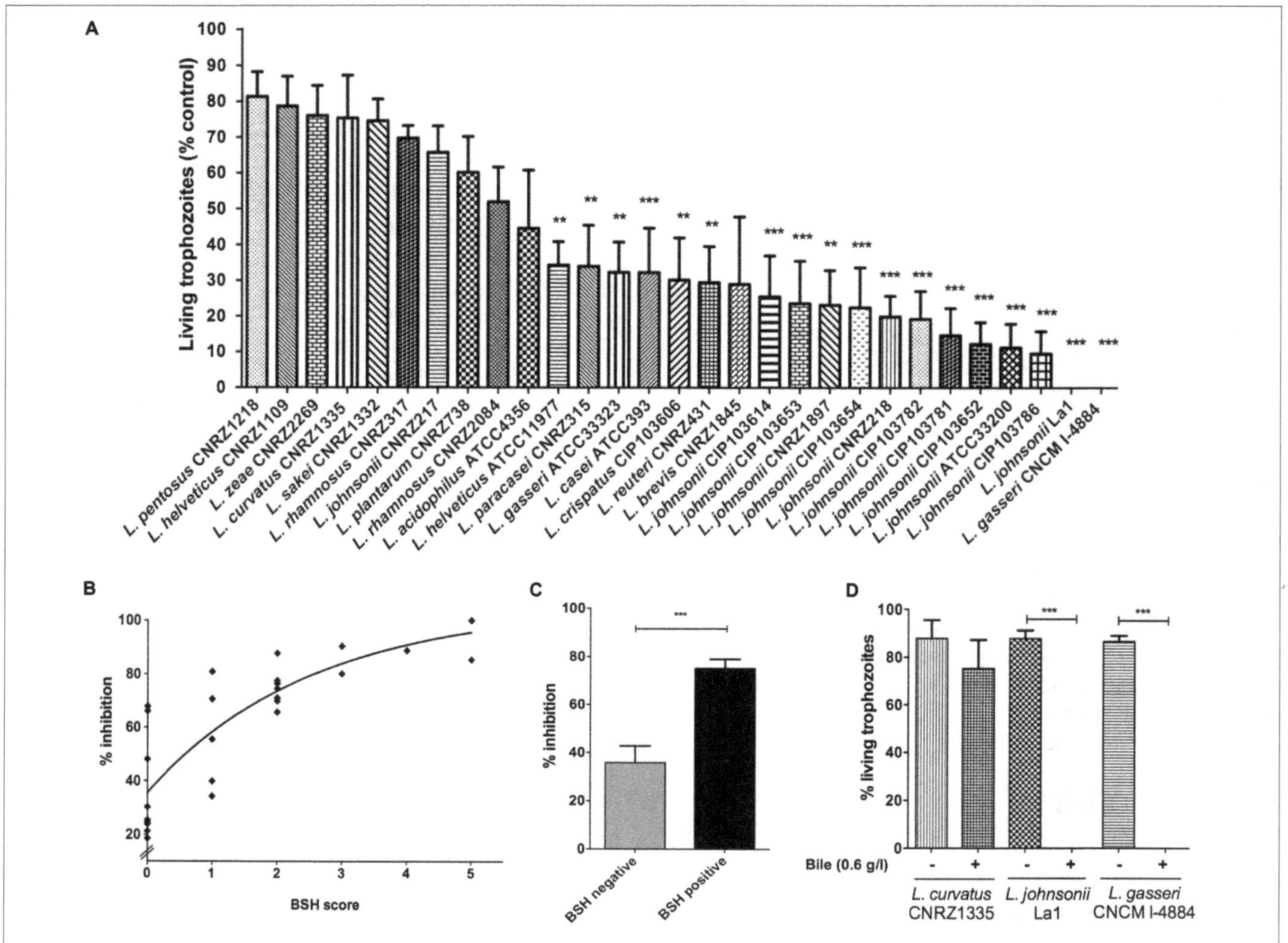

FIGURE 1 | Bile-salt hydrolase (BSH) and anti-*Giardia in vitro* activities of different lactobacilli strains. **(A)** Percentage of living *Giardia duodenalis* trophozoites when cultivated 22 h with lactobacilli supernatants. *G. duodenalis* trophozoites were enumerated after 22 h of co-incubation at 37°C in anaerobic conditions (values are represented with bile supplementation). Values are mean ± SEM. **(B)** Spearman's rank correlation test between percentage of inhibition of lactobacilli strains and their BSH activity score. BSH score was determined depending on the size of the halo zone (+ = 1; ++ = 2; +++ = 3, **Table 1**) and the ability to deconjugate either tauro-conjugated bile salts or glyco-conjugated bile salts or both (addition of BSH score for each substrate specificity). A positive correlation is observed ($r = 0.86$; $p < 0.0001$). **(C)** Inhibition assays according to Bile Salt Hydrolase activities. Lactobacilli strains were divided into two groups: (i) BSH negative (strains with no detected BSH activity), (ii) BSH positive (strains exhibiting either TDCA, GDCA, or both BSH activities). *G. duodenalis* trophozoites were enumerated after 22 h of co-incubation at 37°C in anaerobic conditions (values are represented with bile supplementation). Values are in mean ± SEM. **(D)** Percentage of living *G. duodenalis* trophozoites when co-cultivated 22 h with lactobacilli strains supernatants, with or without bile supplementation (bovine bile 0.6 g/L). *G. duodenalis* trophozoites were enumerated after 22 h of co-incubation at 37°C in anaerobic conditions. Values are mean ± SEM. $^{**}p \leq 0.01$; $^{***}p \leq 0.001$.

experiments (**Supplementary Figure S1**). Mice were challenged with *G. duodenalis* WB6 trophozoites at day 10 by intragastric gavage (1×10^5 trophozoites) and sacrificed at day 16 (**Figure 2**). In preliminary experiments, we showed that this parasite strain was able to persist and colonize in OF1 suckling mice model, the peak of trophozoite load being reached at day 16 (i.e., 6 days post-inoculation) (**Supplementary Figure S2**). On the other hand, we demonstrated that lactobacilli strains can persist in the gut up to 3–4 days after intragastric gavage.

Mice were divided into four groups with a minimum of eight animals per group. The parasite burden in mice treated with PBS/glycerol was 20-fold higher than the initial dose showing that trophozoites were able to colonize, multiply, and persist in the small intestine. As shown in **Figure 3A**, mice treated with *L. curvatus* CNRZ1335 were not protected against *G. duodenalis* challenge as they present a similar profile in trophozoite colonization and proliferation. In contrast, mice treated with *L. gasseri* CNCM I-4884 exhibited an 18-fold reduction in the trophozoites load in the small intestine (~93%) ($p < 0.001$) compared to the PBS/glycerol group (**Figure 3A**). Mice fed with the probiotic strain La1 exhibited a twofold reduction in the trophozoites load compared to controls (~43%). Interestingly, *L. gasseri* CNCM I-4884 was more efficient than La1 in preventing *G. duodenalis* proliferation *in vivo*.

Cysts enumerations were performed in both colon and caecum. We observed a significant reduction (−81%) ($p < 0.01$) in cyst formation in groups treated with *L. gasseri* CNCM I-4884 compared to both PBS/glycerol and *L. curvatus*-treated groups.

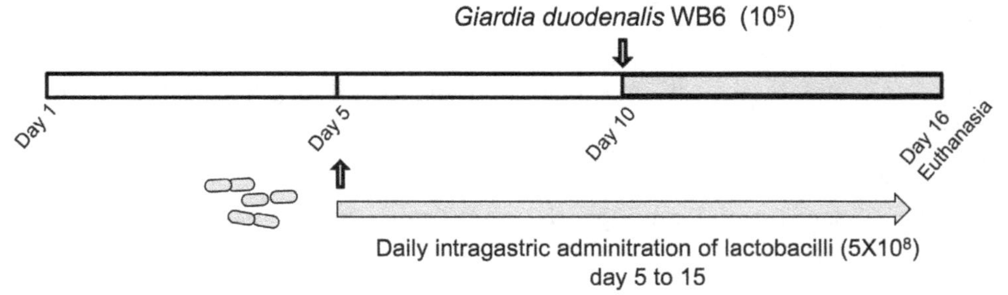

FIGURE 2 | Experimental design of *G. duodenalis* infection in OF1 suckling mice model. Lactobacilli strains were administered daily by intragastric gavage (5×10^8 CFU) to 5 days old OF1 suckling mice from day 5 to day 15. Control animals received PBS/glycerol 15%. Mice were challenged with *G. duodenalis* WB6 trophozoites (10^5) at day 10 by intragastric gavage. Mice were sacrificed by cervical dislocation at day 16.

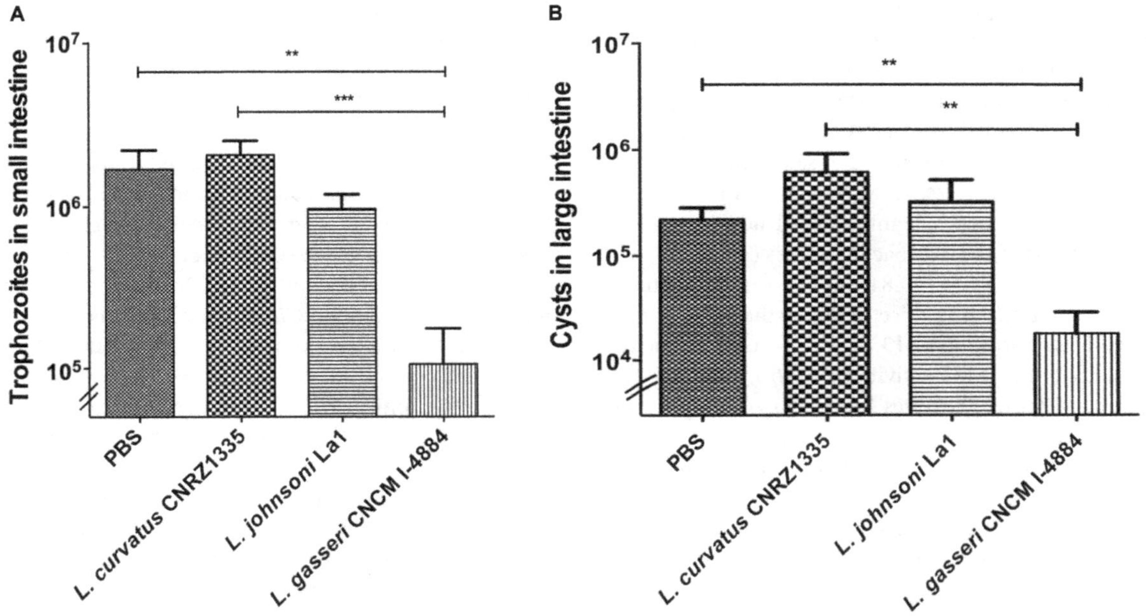

FIGURE 3 | *In vivo* activities of *Lactobacillus gasseri* CNCM I-4884 and La1 lactobacilli strains against *G. duodenalis.* **(A)** *G. duodenalis* trophozoites enumeration after administration to animals. Suckling mice received either PBS ($n = 8$), La1 ($n = 12$), *L. gasseri* CNCM I-4884 ($n = 10$) or *L. curvatus* CNRZ1335 ($n = 9$) by intragastric gavage (5×10^8 CFU/mice) daily from day 5, before inoculation with *G. duodenalis* WB6 trophozoites (10^5 trophozoites per animal) at day 10. Gavages were performed until day 15. Small intestines were resuspended in PBS and trophozoites were counted using a hemocytometer. Values are mean ± SEM; $p < 0.05$. **(B)** *G. duodenalis* cysts counting in colon and caecum. Suckling mice received either PBS/glycerol 15%, La1, *L. gasseri* CNCM I-4884 or *L. curvatus* CNRZ1335 by intragastric gavage (5×10^8 CFU/mice) daily from day 5 before inoculation with *G. duodenalis* WB6 trophozoites (10^5 trophozoites per animal) at day 10. Gavages were performed until day 15 (n = 8–12/group). Colons and caeca were resuspended in 5 ml of ice-chilled 2.5% potassium dichromate and cysts were counted using a hemocytometer. Values are mean ± SEM. $^{**}p \leq 0.01$; $^{***}p \leq 0.001$.

No significant reduction was observed in the group treated with either La1 or *L. curvatus* CNRZ1335 compared to control groups treated with PBS/glycerol (**Figure 3B**).

DISCUSSION

Several studies have demonstrated that probiotics might play key roles against enteropathogens including intestinal protototozan parasites (see Travers et al., 2011, for a review). In the last 10 years, several lactobacilli strains have been studied for their ability to prevent the establishment of *G. duodenalis in vivo* and to reduce the severity of giardial infections (Humen et al., 2005; Shukla et al., 2008; Goyal et al., 2011; Goyal and Shukla, 2013). In some instances, *in vitro* assays were designed to decipher the molecular mechanisms involved in these protective effects. For the probiotic strain La1 of *L. johnsonii,* previously known to antagonize *Giardia* growth *in vitro* and *in vivo,* Perez and collaborators established the presence of an active principle in the supernatant of this probiotic strain (Perez et al., 2001; Humen et al., 2005). More recently, we undertook the molecular characterization of this active principal from La1 and discovered at least one possible mechanism of action: the involvement of bacterial BSH-like activities, that would mediate anti-giardial effect by generating deconjugated bile salts (toxic for the parasite) from non-toxic conjugated bile salts (Travers et al., 2016). BSH are common in *Lactobacillus* and *Bifidobacterium*, playing an important role for colonization and persistence in the gut (Tanaka et al., 1999; Begley et al., 2006; Denou et al., 2008). Therefore, we looked for other probiotic strains (closely related or not to La1) exhibiting anti-giardial activities. We thus selected 29 lactobacilli strains from diverse origins and screened their supernatants for their putative anti-giardial activities *in vitro* while, in parallel, we analyzed their BSH activities and properties. Among the supernatants issued from the 29 analyzed strains, 19 were found to display anti-parasitic activities on fresh trophozoites *Giardia* cultures. Interestingly, these 19 strains also displayed the highest BSH scores, indicating a correlation between these two properties. These results thereby suggest that a screening method based on BSH activities may predict potential anti-giardial activity in lactobacilli. Interestingly, *L. gasseri* CNCM I-4884 and La1 strains (which killed 100% of trophozoites *in vitro*) displayed both TDCA and GDCA specific BSH activities. We therefore propose that this dual or combined BSH activity would contribute to reinforce the release of deconjugated bile salt toxic for *Giardia*, from a larger panel of substrates. However, no clear relationships appeared between the observed anti-giardial activity and the environmental origins of the lactobacilli isolates (**Table 1**).

Lactobacillus gasseri CNCM I-4884 and La1 were subsequently administrated to OF1 suckling mice to assess their antagonistic effects *in vivo*. *L. curvatus* CNRZ1335, which displayed neither anti-giardial activity nor BSH activities *in vitro*, was used as a negative control. High trophozoites burden in controls showed efficient colonization and proliferation of the *G. duodenalis* WB6 in the OF1 mice (Shukla et al., 2008). Mice treated with *L. gasseri* CNCM I-4884 exhibited a dramatic reduction of viable trophozoites in their small intestines, 6 days post-challenge. La1 strain supplementation also lead to a reduction of trophozoites in mice intestines, but to a much lesser extent than *L. gasseri* CNCM I-4884. Previous studies have reported anti-giardial properties of lactobacilli strains. For instance, *L. casei* MTCC1423 and LGG strains reduced the duration and the severity of *G. duodenalis* infection (Portland strain) in C57BL/6 mice in 7–14 days (Shukla et al., 2008; Goyal et al., 2011) and La1 antagonized *Giardia* (WB6) in Mongolian gerbils in 7–21 days (Humen et al., 2005). However, no correlation between the anti-giardial effects and a BSH-like activity was established in these studies. Strikingly, in the current study, administration of *L. gasseri* CNCM I-4884 led to a stronger reduction of trophozoites load in a short period of time. Cyst formation is another important indication of the control of infectious parasite development (Lujan et al., 1997). A treatment capable of preventing trophozoite differentiation into cysts is indeed essential to minimize their spreading in the environment via animals' feces. We observed that mice fed with *L. gasseri* CNCM I-4884 exhibited a dramatic reduction of cyst excretion 6 days post-challenge compared to untreated infected mice. This is in concordance with previous results showing that other lactobacilli such as *L. casei* MTCC 1423 and LGG were effective in eliminating cysts after 7 days of treatment. In contrast, no cyst reduction was observed in mice treated with La1 although its ability to eliminate cysts has been previously reported in mongolian gerbils (Humen et al., 2005). The differences in terms of *in vivo* efficiency between *L. gasseri* CNCM I-4884 and La1, both BSH-positive strains, can be explained by either a better hydrolysis of conjugated bile salts *in vivo*, a higher ability for competing for biological niches in the small intestine, and a better persistence in the gut.

To date, the underlying mechanisms involved in the antagonistic effect of lactobacilli against *Giardia* is an emerging field. Besides the role of BSH-like activities that we have previously reported for La1 (Travers et al., 2016), and now for other *Lactobacillus* strains, other mechanisms have been identified. Among them, the role of anti-microbial peptides in the anti-giardial activity of lactobacilli has been explored. Indeed, when administered orally, P106, a derived bacteriocin isolated from *L. acidophilus*, was shown to reduce the trophozoite burden in mice at high concentrations (Amer et al., 2014). However, the ability to produce anti-microbial peptides is strain dependent and highly variable and this cannot be extrapolated to all anti-giardial strains. Also, probiotic lactobacilli are known to enhance the mucosal immune system, which participate in clearing enteropathogens from the gut (Howarth and Wang, 2013). The immunomodulatory properties of lactobacilli have also been proposed to explain their anti-giardial properties (Goyal and Shukla, 2013; Allain et al., 2017; Barash et al., 2017; Bartelt et al., 2017; Fink and Singer, 2017). In our study, the local and systemic response to *Giardia* infection has not been assessed due to the fact that suckling mice have an immature immune system (Basha et al., 2014).

While the anti-giardial properties of lactobacilli appear to be multifactorial, there is a clear contribution of BSH-activities. However, further experiments are necessary to investigate the potential of BSH in treating giardiasis, including the direct effect of BSHs *in vitro* and *in vivo*. Knockout mutant strains for all BSH genes (several BSH genes are commonly found in lactobacilli) are still needed to evaluate the relative contribution of each one of these enzymes. To summarize, this study shows BSH activity as a key screening parameter to identify anti-*Giardia* lactobacilli strains. In addition, *L. gasseri* CNCM I-4884, which displayed both high anti-giardial and BSH activities *in vitro*, antagonizes *Giardia* survival in OF1 mice. This study represents a significant step toward the development of new prophylactic strategies, with both human and veterinary applications.

AUTHOR CONTRIBUTIONS

IF, BP, PG, TA, and LB-H conceived and designed the study. TA, BP, SC, and MT performed all the experiments. M-AT, IV, and PL discussed the experiments and results. TA, IF, and LB-H wrote the manuscript.

FUNDING

This work was partially funded by Région Île-de-France-DIM (Maladies Infectieuses, Parasitaires et Nosocomiales Émergentes, program no. 120092).

ACKNOWLEDGMENTS

The authors thank Dr. Cissé Sow (MHNH) and Yasmine Kirati (Mett) for their technical help in preliminary experiments. They also thank Dr. Saulius Kulakauskas (INRA, Jouy-en-Josas) who provided some strains of lactic acid bacteria.

SUPPLEMENTARY MATERIAL

FIGURE S1 | Persistence of *L. johnsonii* La1 strain (Ery^r) in OF1 suckling mice. Each mouse received a single administration of 5 × 10^8 CFU of *L. johnsonii* La1 Ery^r either by oral gavage (days 1, 2, and 3; $n = 4$) or intragastric gavage (days 1, 2, 3, and 4; $n = 4$). *L. johnsonii* La1 was transformed with a plasmid harboring an erythromycin (Ery)-resistance gene as described previously (Allain et al., 2016). Values are in mean ± SEM.

FIGURE S2 | Kinetics of infection of *G. duodenalis* strain WB6 in OF1 suckling mice. **(A)** *G. duodenalis* trophozoites enumeration in small intestine after single gavage (day 0). Trophozoite burden was measured at days 3, 6, 8, 10, 12, 15, and 18 ($n = 10$). Small intestines were resuspended in PBS and trophozoites were counted using a hemocytometer **(B)** *G. duodenalis* cysts enumeration in large intestine after single gavage (day 0). Cysts were measured at days 3, 6, 8, 10, 12, 15, and 18 ($n = 10$). Large intestines were resuspended in 2.5% Potassium dichromate and cysts were counted using a hemocytometer. Values are in mean ± SEM.

REFERENCES

Allain, T., Amat, C. B., Motta, J. P., Manko, A., and Buret, A. G. (2017). Interactions of *Giardia sp.* with the intestinal barrier: epithelium, mucus, and microbiota. *Tissue Barriers* 5:e1274354. doi: 10.1080/21688370.2016.1274354

Allain, T., Mansour, N. M., Bahr, M. M., Martin, R., Florent, I., Langella, P., et al. (2016). A new lactobacilli *in vivo* expression system for the production and delivery of heterologous proteins at mucosal surfaces. *FEMS Microbiol. Lett.* 363:fnw117. doi: 10.1093/femsle/fnw117

Amer, E. I., Mossallam, S. F., and Mahrous, H. (2014). Therapeutic enhancement of newly derived bacteriocins against *Giardia lamblia*. *Exp. Parasitol.* 146, 52–63. doi: 10.1016/j.exppara.2014.09.005

Barash, N. R., Maloney, J. G., Singer, S. M., and Dawson, S. C. (2017). *Giardia* alters commensal microbial diversity throughout the murine gut. *Infect. Immun.* 85, e00948-e16. doi: 10.1128/IAI.00948-16

Bartelt, L. A., Bolick, D. T., Mayneris-Perxachs, J., Kolling, G. L., Medlock, G. L., Zaenker, E. I., et al. (2017). Cross-modulation of pathogen-specific pathways enhances malnutrition during enteric co-infection with *Giardia lamblia* and enteroaggregative *Escherichia coli*. *PLOS Pathog.* 13:e1006471. doi: 10.1371/journal.ppat.1006471

Basha, S., Surendran, N., and Pichichero, M. (2014). Immune responses in neonates. *Expert Rev. Clin. Immunol.* 10, 1171–1184. doi: 10.1586/1744666X.2014.942288

Begley, M., Hill, C., and Gahan, C. G. (2006). Bile salt hydrolase activity in probiotics. *Appl. Environ. Microbiol.* 72, 1729–1738. doi: 10.1128/AEM.72.3.1729-1738.2006

Bengmark, S. (2013). Gut microbiota, immune development and function. *Pharmacol. Res.* 69, 87–113. doi: 10.1016/j.phrs.2012.09.002

Buret, A. G. (2007). Mechanisms of epithelial dysfunction in giardiasis. *Gut* 56, 316–317. doi: 10.1136/gut.2006.107771

Bustos, A. Y., Saavedra, L., De Valdez, G. F., Raya, R. R., and Taranto, M. P. (2012). Relationship between bile salt hydrolase activity, changes in the internal pH and tolerance to bile acids in lactic acid bacteria. *Biotechnol. Lett.* 34, 1511–1518. doi: 10.1007/s10529-012-0932-5

Denou, E., Pridmore, R. D., Berger, B., Panoff, J. M., Arigoni, F., and Brussow, H. (2008). Identification of genes associated with the long-gut-persistence phenotype of the probiotic *Lactobacillus johnsonii* strain NCC533 using a combination of genomics and transcriptome analysis. *J. Bacteriol.* 190, 3161–3168. doi: 10.1128/JB.01637-07

Farthing, M. J. (1996). Giardiasis. *Gastroenterol. Clin. North Am.* 25, 493–515. doi: 10.1016/S0889-8553(05)70260-0

Fink, M. Y., and Singer, S. M. (2017). The intersection of immune responses, microbiota, and pathogenesis in giardiasis. *Trends Parasitol.* 33, 901–913. doi: 10.1016/j.pt.2017.08.001

Gardner, T. B., and Hill, D. R. (2001). Treatment of giardiasis. *Clin. Microbiol. Rev.* 14, 114–128. doi: 10.1128/CMR.14.1.114-128.2001

Goyal, N., and Shukla, G. (2013). Probiotic *Lactobacillus rhamnosus* GG modulates the mucosal immune response in *Giardia intestinalis*-infected BALB/c mice. *Dig. Dis. Sci.* 58, 1218–1225. doi: 10.1007/s10620-012-2503-y

Goyal, N., Tiwari, R. P., and Shukla, G. (2011). *Lactobacillus rhamnosus* GG as an effective probiotic for murine giardiasis. *Interdiscip. Perspect. Infect. Dis.* 2011:795219. doi: 10.1155/2011/795219

Harris, J. C., Plummer, S., and Lloyd, D. (2001). Antigiardial drugs. *Appl. Microbiol. Biotechnol.* 57, 614–619. doi: 10.1007/s002530100720

Howarth, G. S., and Wang, H. (2013). Role of endogenous microbiota, probiotics and their biological products in human health. *Nutrients* 5, 58–81. doi: 10.3390/nu5010058

Humen, M. A., De Antoni, G. L., Benyacoub, J., Costas, M. E., Cardozo, M. I., Kozubsky, L., et al. (2005). *Lactobacillus johnsonii* La1 antagonizes *Giardia intestinalis* In Vivo. *Infect. Immun.* 73, 1265–1269. doi: 10.1128/IAI.73.2.1265-1269.2005

Lujan, H. D., Mowatt, M. R., and Nash, T. E. (1997). Mechanisms of *Giardia lamblia* differentiation into cysts. *Microbiol. Mol. Biol. Rev.* 61, 294–304.

Martin, R., Miquel, S., Ulmer, J., Kechaou, N., Langella, P., and Bermudez-Humaran, L. G. (2013). Role of commensal and probiotic bacteria in human health: a focus on inflammatory bowel disease. *Microb. Cell Fact.* 12:71. doi: 10.1186/1475-2859-12-71

Morrison, H. G., Mcarthur, A. G., Gillin, F. D., Aley, S. B., Adam, R. D., Olsen, G. J., et al. (2007). Genomic minimalism in the early diverging intestinal parasite *Giardia lamblia*. *Science* 317, 1921–1926. doi: 10.1126/science.1143837

Moser, S. A., and Savage, D. C. (2001). Bile salt hydrolase activity and resistance to toxicity of conjugated bile salts are unrelated properties in lactobacilli. *Appl. Environ. Microbiol.* 67, 3476–3480. doi: 10.1128/AEM.67.8.3476-3480.2001

Perez, P. F., Minnaard, J., Rouvet, M., Knabenhans, C., Brassart, D., De Antoni, G. L., et al. (2001). Inhibition of *Giardia intestinalis* by extracellular factors from Lactobacilli: an In Vitro study. *Appl. Environ. Microbiol.* 67, 5037–5042. doi: 10.1128/AEM.67.11.5037-5042.2001

Reiner, D. S., Hetsko, M. L., Meszaros, J. G., Sun, C. H., Morrison, H. G., Brunton, L. L., et al. (2003). Calcium signaling in excystation of the early diverging eukaryote, *Giardia lamblia*. *J. Biol. Chem.* 278, 2533–2540. doi: 10.1074/jbc.M208033200

Roxstrom-Lindquist, K., Palm, D., Reiner, D., Ringqvist, E., and Svard, S. G. (2006). Giardia immunity-an update. *Trends Parasitol.* 22, 26–31. doi: 10.1016/j.pt.2005.11.005

Sanders, M. E. (2008). Probiotics: definition, sources, selection, and uses. *Clin. Infect. Dis.* 46(Suppl. 2), S58–S61. doi: 10.1086/523341

Savioli, L., Smith, H., and Thompson, A. (2006). Giardia and Cryptosporidium join the 'Neglected Diseases Initiative'. *Trends Parasitol.* 22, 203–208. doi: 10.1016/j.pt.2006.02.015

Shukla, G., Devi, P., and Sehgal, R. (2008). Effect of *Lactobacillus casei* as a probiotic on modulation of giardiasis. *Dig. Dis. Sci.* 53, 2671–2679. doi: 10.1007/s10620-007-0197-3

Singer, S. M., and Nash, T. E. (2000). The role of normal flora in *Giardia lamblia* infections in mice. *J. Infect. Dis.* 181, 1510–1512. doi: 10.1086/315409

Sokol, H. (2014). Probiotics and antibiotics in IBD. *Dig. Dis.* 32(Suppl. 1), 10–17. doi: 10.1159/000367820

Tanaka, H., Doesburg, K., Iwasaki, T., and Mierau, I. (1999). Screening of lactic acid bacteria for bile salt hydrolase activity. *J. Dairy Sci.* 82, 2530–2535. doi: 10.3168/jds.S0022-0302(99)75506-2

Thompson, R. C., and Monis, P. (2012). *Giardia*–from genome to proteome. *Adv. Parasitol.* 78, 57–95. doi: 10.1016/B978-0-12-394303-3.00003-7

Thompson, R. C., and Monis, P. T. (2004). Variation in *Giardia*: implications for taxonomy and epidemiology. *Adv. Parasitol.* 58, 69–137. doi: 10.1016/S0065-308X(04)58002-8

Thompson, R. C., Reynoldson, J. A., and Mendis, A. H. (1993). Giardia and giardiasis. *Adv. Parasitol.* 32, 71–160. doi: 10.1016/S0065-308X(08)60207-9

Travers, M. A., Florent, I., Kohl, L., and Grellier, P. (2011). Probiotics for the control of parasites: an overview. *J. Parasitol. Res.* 2011:610769. doi: 10.1155/2011/610769

Travers, M. A., Sow, C., Zirah, S., Deregnaucourt, C., Chaouch, S., Queiroz, R. M., et al. (2016). Deconjugated bile salts produced by extracellular bile-salt hydrolase-like activities from the probiotic *Lactobacillus johnsonii* La1 Inhibit *Giardia duodenalis In vitro* Growth. *Front. Microbiol.* 7:1453. doi: 10.3389/fmicb.2016.01453

Upcroft, P., and Upcroft, J. A. (2001). Drug targets and mechanisms of resistance in the anaerobic protozoa. *Clin. Microbiol. Rev.* 14, 150–164. doi: 10.1128/CMR.14.1.150-164.2001

10

Gene Replacement and Fluorescent Labeling to Study the Functional Role of Exopolysaccharides in *Bifidobacterium animalis* subsp. *lactis*

Nuria Castro-Bravo[1], Claudio Hidalgo-Cantabrana[1], Miguel A. Rodriguez-Carvajal[2], Patricia Ruas-Madiedo[1]* and Abelardo Margolles[1]

[1] Department of Microbiology and Biochemistry of Dairy Products, Instituto de Productos Lácteos de Asturias – Consejo Superior de Investigaciones Científicas, Villaviciosa, Spain, [2] Department of Organic Chemistry, Universidad de Sevilla, Sevilla, Spain

***Correspondence:**
Patricia Ruas-Madiedo
ruas-madiedo@ipla.csic.es

An extracellular layer of exopolysaccharides (EPS) covers the surface of some *Bifidobacterium animalis* subsp. *lactis* strains, which could be of relevance for its probiotic performance. In order to understand the functional characteristics of *B. animalis* subsp. *lactis*, two isogenic strains that differ in their EPS-producing phenotype, due to a single mutation in the gene Balat_1410, were studied. By means of a double crossover recombination strategy, successfully used for the first time in bifidobacteria, Balat_1410 in the type strain *B. animalis* subsp. *lactis* DSM10140 was replaced by a mutated gene containing a non-synonymous mutation previously associated with the appearance of a mucoid-ropy phenotype. Nuclear magnetic resonance and SEC-MALS analyses showed that the novel strain harboring the mutation acquired a ropy phenotype, due to the production of a high molecular weight (HMW)-EPS that is not produced in the wild-type strain. Fluorescence labeling of both strains with two fluorescent proteins, m-Cherry and Green Fluorescent Protein, was achieved by expressing the corresponding genes under the control of a native selected promoter (the elongation factor Tu promoter). Remarkably, qualitative and quantitative fluorescence analyses demonstrated that the ropy strain displays a lower capability to adhere to human intestinal epithelial cells. In addition, the presence of the HMW-EPS reduced the capability of the producing strain to form biofilms upon three different abiotic surfaces. This work also highlights the fact that different EPS confer variable functional characteristics to the bifidobacterial surface, which may be relevant for the performance of *B. animalis* subsp. *lactis* as a probiotic. The construction of molecular tools allowing the functional characterization of surface structures in next generation probiotics is still a challenging issue that deserves further attention, given the relevant role that such molecules must play in the interaction with the host.

Keywords: *Bifidobacterium*, exopolysaccharide, gene replacement, fluorescent proteins, NMR, SEC-MALS, biofilms

INTRODUCTION

The definition of a probiotic, proposed in 2001 by FAO/WHO, states that is "live microorganisms which when administered in adequate amounts confer a health benefit on the host." The most commonly commercialized probiotics are some species from *Bifidobacterium* and *Lactobacillus* genera that have been accepted as safe due to their long history of use and they are often delivered into food formulations (Hill et al., 2014). Nowadays, it is becoming more evident that certain intestinal commensal microorganisms could be beneficial to correct microbial dysbioses that have been related with some health disorders; however, they have not been used to promote health yet and, in case they will be applied in this context, they would be treated as novel drugs more than food supplements. These microorganisms can be considered as "next generation probiotics" (NGP) and they are termed as "live biotherapeutic products" (LBP) in the new regulatory framework of the Food and Drug Administration (FDA) of United States of America (O'Toole et al., 2017). Some of the proposed NGP belong to genera *Akkermansia, Bacteroides,* and *Faecalibacterium.*

Orally delivered probiotics establish the main contact point with the host at the intestinal mucosa level; in this location, the probiotic-microbiota-cell interplay will drive positive physiological benefits. Despite vast research efforts made into the mechanisms behind the beneficial effects, the manner of probiotic action still remains unclear (Gareau et al., 2010; Wan et al., 2015). The (transitory) contact between bacteria and intestinal epithelial cells might be relevant to initiate this intercellular dialog; the surface microbial associated molecular patterns (MAMPs) interacting with the host pattern recognition receptors (PRR) are involved in triggering the cellular response (Lebeer et al., 2010b; Westermann et al., 2016). One of the most external layers covering the bacterial surface is constituted by exopolysaccharides (EPS), which are carbohydrate polymers whose genetic determinants are present in intestinal bacteria, including most species of the genus *Bifidobacterium* (Ferrario et al., 2016). In fact, some of the beneficial properties attributable to the producing bifidobacteria have been associated with their EPS and their physical-chemical characteristics (Hidalgo-Cantabrana et al., 2014, 2016; Schiavi et al., 2016). Additionally, it has been proven that EPS produced by some NGP, such as *Faecalibacterium prausnitzii*, also has anti-inflammatory properties *in vivo*, thus this bacterium is being proposed as therapeutic agent to treat intestinal inflammatory processes (Rossi et al., 2015).

The development of tools allowing the study of the mechanisms of action, either for well recognized probiotics or NGP, is essential in order to choose those strains which are more valuable for each target population and health benefit. One of the approaches is the use of vectors containing different labeling systems; those applied to lactic acid bacteria and bifidobacteria have recently been reviewed (Landete et al., 2016). A luciferase-based reporter system was developed to monitor the performance of *Bifidobacterium breve* UCC2003 under *in vivo* conditions (Cronin et al., 2008). Different fluorescent proteins have been successfully used as well to label bifidobacteria. In this way, *B. breve, B. longum* subsp. *Longum,* and *B. bifidum* were labeled with cyan fluorescent protein (CFP), green fluorescent protein (GFP), yellow fluorescent protein (YFP) or mCherry under the promoter of the *gap* gene (P_{gap}) of *B. bifidum* (Grimm et al., 2014). Additionally, a GFP fluorescent protein containing a flavin-mono-nucleotide-based cofactor (evoglow-Pp1), which emits fluorescence in the presence/absence of oxygen, was included in a vector under control of the elongation factor Tu (P_{tuf} from *B. longum*) that replicates in *B. longum* and *B. breve* (Landete et al., 2014). This system, which supposes an advantage to study bifidobacteria in strict anaerobic conditions, was latterly validated under the control of other promoters (Montenegro-Rodríguez et al., 2015).

Bifidobacterium animalis subsp. *lactis* is one of the most widely used probiotics and there are several human intervention studies supporting its beneficial effects (Tojo et al., 2014). From an industrial point of view, it is one of the most robust bifidobacterial species which facilitates its inclusion in foods or food supplements (Bogsan et al., 2014). The aims pursued in the current work were: (i) to obtain an EPS-producing variant by means of a double crossover marker-less strategy, which produces a chromosomally stable new variant, (ii) the construction of EPS-producing *B. animalis* subsp. *lactis* strains harboring fluorescent proteins, which have not been reported in literature to date, and (iii) the demonstration that different EPS have an influence on the interaction of the producing strain with biotic and abiotic surfaces. To achieve these goals, a model of *B. animalis* subsp. *lactis* strains, which produced EPS with different physical-chemical characteristics, was initially used. This model was previously developed to demonstrate that a single mutation in the gene Balat_1410, coding for a protein involved in the elongation of the polymer chain, was directly related to a higher abundance of the high molecular weight (HMW)-EPS fraction (about 10^6 Da) that conferred a ropy-mucoid phenotype to the producing strain (Hidalgo-Cantabrana et al., 2015). Indeed, strains producing HMW-EPS are able to attenuate the immune response (López et al., 2012) and they have been proposed for their application in reducing intestinal inflammatory states (Hidalgo-Cantabrana et al., 2016).

MATERIALS AND METHODS

Bifidobacteria Strains, Plasmids and Culture Conditions

The *B. animalis* subsp. *lactis* and *Escherichia coli* strains, as well as the plasmids and oligonucleotides used in this study, are listed in **Table 1**. *E. coli* DH11S (Invitrogen^{TM}, Thermo-Fisher Scientific Inc., Waltham, MA, United States) was grown in Luria-Bertani (LB) broth at 37°C under shaking conditions (200 rpm). Bifidobacterial strains were cultivated in MRSc [MRS (Biokar Diagnostics, Beauvais, Francia) supplemented with 0.25% L-cysteine-HCl (Sigma-Chemical Co., St. Louis, MO, United States)] at 37°C under anaerobic conditions (80% N_2, 10% CO_2, 10% H_2) in a MG500 chamber (Don Whitley Scientific, West Yorkshire, United Kingdom). Bacterial cultures and competent cells were prepared under standardized conditions

TABLE 1 | Bacterial strains, plasmids, and oligonucleotide primers used in this study.

Strains	Description	Reference
E. coli DH11S	*mcrA* Δ(*mrr-hsdRMS-mcrBC*) Δ(*lac-proAB*) Δ(*rec1398*) *deoR rpsL srl-thi*-F' *proAB*$^+$ *lacI*^{q}ZΔM15	Invitrogen
B. animalis subsp. *lactis*		
DSM10140^T	Type strain, Plasmid free, EPS$^+$, no ropy phenotype	DSMZ collection (yogurt isolated)
IPLA-R1	Plasmid free, EPS$^+$, ropy-mucoid phenotype	IPLA collection (bile-salt adapted)
DSM10140-ΔBalat_1410	DSM10140 lacking the gene Balat_1410, no ropy phenotype	Hidalgo-Cantabrana et al., 2015
DSM10140-Balat_1410^{S89L} (=S89L)	DSM10140 mutant obtained after gene integration of Balat_1410^{S89L}, EPS$^+$, ropy-mucoid phenotype	This work
DSM10140-mCherry	DSM10140 harboring pCAS-mCherry	This work
DSM10140-GFP	DSM10140 harboring pCAS- GFP	This work
S89L-mCherry	DSM10140-Balat_1410^{S89L} harboring pCAS-mCherry	This work
S89L-GFP	DSM10140-Balat_1410^{S89L} harboring pCAS- GFP	This work
Plasmids	**Description**	**Reference**
pJL74[a]	*E. coli-Bifidobacterium* cloning vector; Amp^r Sp^r; integrative, non-replicative in *Bifidobacterium*	Hidalgo-Cantabrana et al., 2015
pJL-upst/Balat_1410^{S89L} /dst/ (=pCHC3)	pJL74 containing Balat_1410^{S89L} together with the upstream (3 kb) and downstream (2.7 kb) regions	This work
pAM1[a]	*E. coli-Bifidobacterium* cloning vector; Amp^r Em^r	Alvarez-Martín et al., 2008
pCAS-mCherry	mCherry fluorescent protein gene fused to the elongation factor Tu promoter (P_{tuf}) of *B. animalis* subsp. *lactis* in pAM1	This work
pCAS- GFP	GFP fluorescent protein gene fused to the elongation factor Tu promoter (P_{tuf}) of *B. animalis* subsp. *lactis* in pAM1	This work
Oligonucleotides	**Sequence (5′–3′)**	**Reference**
Balat_1410 -GR-F[b]	TATATA<u>GGGCCC</u>GTCACCTCGTCACCATGAGC[b]	Hidalgo-Cantabrana et al., 2015
Balat_1410 -GR-R[b]	TATATA<u>AGATCT</u>CCACGAGAGCACACGAAGAC	Hidalgo-Cantabrana et al., 2015
In-Balat_1410 -F	GGTATGATGTGCAGATTCGGCTTC	This work
In-Balat_1410 -R	TACATGGCCGAGAACGAGGTAAACC	This work
Spec-F	GGAGAAGATTCAGCCACTGC	Hidalgo-Cantabrana et al., 2015
Spec-R	TTAGTCGTCGTATCTGAACC	Hidalgo-Cantabrana et al., 2015
P_{Tu}_F[b]	TATATA<u>AAGCTT</u>ACATCCGTTACGAATCACGC	This work
mCh_R[b]	TATATA<u>TCTAGA</u>TTATTACTTGTACAGCTCGTCC	This work
GFP_R[b]	TATATA<u>TCTAGA</u>TTATTATTTGTATAGTTCATCC	This work
P_{Tu}_mCh_F[c]	GTCCAGGAGGACAAAAACAT**ATGGTGAGCAAGGGCGAGG**	This work
mCh_P_{Tu}_R[c]	**CCTCGCCCTTGCTCACCAT**ATGTTTTTGTCCTCCTGGAC	This work
P_{Tu}_GFP_F[c]	GTCCAGGAGGACAAAAACAT**ATGCGTAAAGGAGAAGAAC**	This work
GFP_P_{Tu}_R[c]	**GTTCTTCTCCTTTACGCAT**ATGTTTTTGTCCTCCTGGAC	This work

[a]*Amp^r, Em^r, and Sp^r, resistance to ampicillin, erythromycin, and spectinomycin, respectively.* [b]*Restriction enzyme sites are underlined.* [c]*Complementary sequences for splicing overlap extension PCR are bold marked.*

(Hidalgo-Cantabrana et al., 2015) and ampicillin (100 μg/ml), spectinomycin (100 μg/ml) or erythromycin (2.5 μg/ml) were added when required (**Table 1**).

Molecular Techniques

Isolation of Chromosomal and Plasmid DNA, and Plasmid Manipulation

Chromosomal DNA from *B. animalis* subsp. *lactis* was isolated using the GeneElute™ Bacterial Genomic DNA kit (Sigma–Aldrich, Dorset, United Kingdom). Plasmid DNA was isolated from *E. coli* using the Qiagen Plasmid Midi kit (Qiagen, Hilden, Germany), whereas the plasmid isolation from recombinant bifidobacteria was performed by means of the GeneElute™ Plasmid Miniprep kit (Sigma–Aldrich). Manufacturer's recommendations were followed in both cases. For bifidobacterial strains, lysozyme (9 mg/ml, Merck, Darmstadt, Germany) and mutanolysin (5U, Sigma–Aldrich) were added during the lysis step followed by incubation at 37°C for 1 h. DNA concentration was measured in Gene5™ Teck3 Module (BioTek, Vermont, United States).

For plasmid constructions, PCRs were performed using Platinum® Pfx DNA Polymerase (Invitrogen™). Digestions and ligations were made with restriction endonucleases from Takara (Takara Bio Group, Otsu, Japan) and with T4 DNA ligase from Invitrogen™, respectively. All reagents were used according to the manufacturers' instructions. PCR products were checked by electrophoresis in TAE buffer [40 mM TRIS, 20 mM acetic acid, 1 mM EDTA (pH 8)] on 1% agarose gels and then stained with ethidium bromide (0.5 μg/ml). DNA purification from the agarose gels was performed using QIAquick Gel Extraction Kit (QIAgene) and sequenced at Macrogen Inc. (Seoul, South Korea). BLAST algorithm was used for sequence similarity analysis. Finally, Eurx-Taq DNA Polymerase from Roboklon GmbH (Berlin, Germany) was used to check plasmid constructions in *E. coli* and plasmid integration in the bifidobacterial chromosome.

Gene Replacement: Plasmid Construction and Double Crossover Events

The chromosomal DNA from *B. animalis* subsp. *lactis* IPLA-R1 was used as a template for PCR amplification using the specific primers Balat_1410-GR-F/R (**Table 1**) for the construction of the plasmid for gene replacement. These primers amplify 7.1 kb which contain the Balat_1410^{S89L} gene (Hidalgo-Cantabrana et al., 2015) and its flanking regions: upstream (3 kb) and downstream (2.7 kb). The PCR product was digested with *Apa*I and *Bgl*II and cloned into pJL74 previously digested with the same enzymes. Ligation was performed overnight at 16°C and the ligation mixture was purified and transformed into *E. coli* DH11S electrocompetent cells. The resulting plasmid was named pCHC3 (pJL-upst/Balat_1410^{S89L}/dst) and was introduced into *B. animalis* subsp. *lactis* DSM10140-ΔBalat_1410 electrocompetent cells prepared as previously reported (Hidalgo-Cantabrana et al., 2015). After transformation, bifidobacterial cells were immediately recovered in 2 ml of MRSc and incubated at 37°C under anaerobic conditions for 4–6 h before plating onto the same agar-medium containing spectinomycin (100 μg/ml). Plates were then incubated for 48 to 72 h at 37°C in anaerobic conditions. Transformants were checked for plasmid integration into the chromosome (single crossover) by PCR using the specific primers In-Balat_1410-F/R and Spec-F/R (**Table 1**). At this point of the experiment, two of the checked colonies acquired the visually recognizable ropy phenotype (having the integrated plasmid) and they were selected to be grown in 10 ml MRSc without antibiotic. Two subcultures (per day) were made for 5 days to force the loss of the plasmid (second crossover) and, afterward, these bacterial cultures were plated onto agar-MRSc without antibiotics for 48 h. Several colonies were picked up and each of them was grown in agar-MRSc, with and without spectinomycin, to select the non-antibiotic resistant colonies due to the loss of the plasmid. These colonies were checked by PCR using the specific primers In-Balat_1410-F/R and Spec-F/R to analyze the presence of Balat_1410^{S89L} and the absence of spectynomicin-resistance genes into the chromosome; besides, the ropy phenotype, associated with the presence of Balat_1410^{S89L}, was useful for the selection of the right colonies. Thus, one strain with a ropy character, then putatively carrying the Balat_1410^{S89L} gene, and being sensitive to spectynomicin, was selected and named DSM10140-Balat_1410^{S89L}, or S89L in its abbreviated form (**Table 1**). To confirm its genetic background, the chromosomal DNA from S89L was obtained and an inner fragment (1 kb) of Balat_1410^{S89L} gene, containing the mutation (C to T transition) responsible for the ropy trait (Hidalgo-Cantabrana et al., 2015), was amplified using the In-Balat_1410-F/R primers. The genetic background of the *eps* cluster surrounding the insertion and the complete insert was also checked with a set of primers that amplify 1 kb overlapping fragments (data not shown). All these PCR products were sequenced at Macrogen Inc. to confirm the absence of undesirable mutations.

Strain Labeling Using Fluorescence Plasmids

Plasmids harboring fluorescent proteins under the control of the elongation factor Tu promoter from *B. animalis* subsp. *lactis* were constructed using splicing overlap extension PCR strategy to fuse the DNA sequences (Vallejo et al., 1994). The "elongation factor Tu" promoter was amplified from the chromosomal DNA of DSM10140 strain using the specific primers P_{Tu}_F/mCh_P_{Tu}_R (**Table 1**). The gene encoding mCherry fluorescent protein was amplified from the pVG-mCherry plasmid (Grimm et al., 2014) with specific primers P_{Tu}_mCh_F/mCh_R. The PCR products that have complementary tails, between each other, were size-checked in 1% agarose gel. Then, splicing overlap extension PCR was performed to fuse both fragments. The same protocol was followed to fuse the elongation factor Tu promoter to GFP gene: the Tu promoter was amplified using specific primers P_{Tu}_F/GFP_P_{Tu}_R, and GFP gene was obtained from the pVG-GFP plasmid (Grimm et al., 2014) using specific primers P_{Tu}_GFP_F/GFP_R. Fused DNA fragments were checked by electrophoresis and purified from agarose gels. The fused DNA fragments were digested with *Hind*III and *Xba*I at 37°C for 3 h, as well as the plasmid pAM1 (Alvarez-Martín et al., 2008) which was also dephosphorylated. Digestions were also purified from agarose gels and used to perform overnight ligations at 4°C. Electrocompetent *E. coli* DH11S cells were transformed with the ligation mixtures and selection of clones was performed by adding ampicillin (100 μg/ml) to the culture medium. The resulting plasmids were named pCAS-mCherry and pCAS-GFP (**Table 1**). The strains *B. animalis* subsp. *lactis* DSM10140 and S89L were transformed with these plasmids and four fluorescent clones were selected by adding erythromycin (2.5 μg/ml) to the culture medium; the recombinant strains were named as DSM10140-mCherry, DSM10140-GFP, S89L-mCherry and S89L-GFP (**Table 1**).

Qualitative and Quantitative Fluorescence Detection

Fluorescence Scanning

The fluorescent bifidobacterial strains were grown onto the surface of agar-MRSc containing erythromycin, for 3 days at 37°C under anaerobic conditions. The fluorescence of the colonies was checked in the Typhoon 9400 scanner (GE Healthcare, Biosciences, Uppsala, Sweden). GFP was excited with blue laser (488 nm) and emission was detected with 526 nm band-pass filter. In the case of mCherry, excitation was performed with red laser (633 nm) and emission was acquired with 580 nm band-pass filter. These plates were scanned at a resolution of 100 μm pixel size.

Fluorescence Microscopy and Confocal Scanning Laser Microscopy (CSLM)

To visualize the bifidobacteria expressing the fluorescent proteins, overnight grown cultures (in MRSc + erythromycin) were washed, placed on a slide covered with coverslip No.1 (0.13–0.16 mm thick). These preparations were observed with the Leica DMi8 inverted microscope (Leica Microsystems GmbH, Heidelberg, Germany), using a 100× oil immersion objective. The FITC filter cube (excitation 480/40, emission 527/30) and RHOD filter cube (excitation 546/10, emission 585/40) were used for visualization of the bifidobacteria harboring GFP or mCherry proteins, respectively.

Fluorescent (mCherry) bifidobacteria adhered on the top of the intestinal cell line HT29 or into glass slides (as will be described next) were visualized with the Leica TCS AOBS SP8 X confocal inverted microscope [External Service Unit (ESU) of the University of Oviedo, Asturias, Spain]. To visualize DAPI fluorochrom, samples were excited at 405 nm, by a blue-violet laser diode, whereas to detect the mCherry they were excited at 587 nm by a white light laser. Z-stacks of HT29 monolayers or bifidobacterial biofilms upon glass μ-slides were acquired with a 63×/1.4 oil objective. When needed, a 2.50 optical zoom was used to acquire images of detailed regions. Image captures were reordered and processed with the Leica Application Suit X software (version 1.8.1.13759, Leica).

Fluorescence Spectrometry

Fluorescence quantification was performed with overnight cultures of the four fluorescent bifidobacteria, as well as the two parental DSM10140 and S89L strains used as negative controls. Cells were washed with PBS and standardized to an equal $OD_{600\ nm}$; additionally, they were plated in the corresponding (with and without antibiotic) agar-MRSc media. Afterward, the standardized bacterial suspensions were 10-fold concentrated and from them, serial (half) dilutions were prepared in PBS. 96-well Lumitrack™ 600 white polystyrene plates (VWR, Radnor, PA, United States) were filled with 200 μl (per well) of each bifidobacterial dilution. Fluorescence was measured on the Cary Eclipse (Varian Ibérica, S.A. Madrid, Spain) fluorescence spectrometer using the following conditions: 470 nm excitation/525 nm emission, for GFP quantification, and 585 nm excitation/610 nm emission for mCherry quantification. The corresponding fluorescence background, determined from the control samples (parental, non-labeled bifidobacterial suspensions), was subtracted from data obtained for the fluorescent strains. This experiment was performed with three biological replicates. Finally, linear regression equations between the fluorescence emitted and the number of bacteria (Log CFU/ml) were calculated, as well as the corresponding coefficient of determination (R^2) that shows how well the data fits to the linear regression.

Flow Cytometry

Fluorescence of bifidobacterial suspensions, obtained as previously described, were also quantified in the Cytomics FC500 (Beckman Coulter, Barcelona, Spain) located in the ESU from the University of Oviedo. A fix acquisition time of 90 s with "hi" acquisition speed was used. The 488 nm laser was applied for the excitation of both fluorochromes and the selection of the bifidobacterial population was made by means of FSC log/SSC log (size/complexity). This gate was used to plot the FL1 (for GFP detection) vs. FL3 (for mCherry detection) histograms; the filters 525/40 and 620/30 were used for the detectors FL1 and FL3, respectively. The absence of auto-fluorescence was checked in the corresponding non-labeled bacteria (Supplementary Figure S1). In the labeled strains the recorded fluorescence was compensated to avoid the overlapping of both fluorochromes. Finally, serial dilutions of the samples (from 1/2 to 1/100) were measured and the linear regression equations between the "fluorescence emitted" (total number of events multiplied by the mean fluorescence intensity) and the number of bacteria (CFU/ml); the R^2 coefficients were calculated as well (Supplementary Figure S2).

Chemical Analysis of Purified EPS

EPS Purification

The EPS from strains DSM10140, S89L and IPLA-R1 were isolated from the bifidobacterial biomass collected with water from the surface of agar-MRSc plates as previously described (Ruas-Madiedo et al., 2010). Each bacterial suspension was mixed with 1 volume of 2 M NaOH and kept overnight at room temperature under mild shaking. Bacteria were eliminated by centrifugation and the EPS from the supernatant was precipitated with two volumes of chilled absolute ethanol for 48 h at 4°C. Precipitated sediment was collected with ultra-pure water and dialyzed against water, using dialysis tubes of 12–14 kDa molecular mass cut off (Sigma), at 4°C for 3 days with a daily change of water. Finally, each dialyzed sample was freeze-dried in order to obtain the crude-EPS material from each strain. To isolate the HMW EPS-fraction from strains S89L and IPLA-R1, the crude-EPS (25 mg) was dissolved in ultra-pure water (10 ml), dialysed (against water, for 72 h at 4°C) using Spectra/Por Float-A-Lyser 100 kDa MWCO tubes (Sigma), and the content of these dialyzed tubes was freeze-dried (Leivers et al., 2011).

SEC-MALLS Analysis

The molar mass distribution of the crude-EPS and HMW-EPS, as well the quantification of the relative amount of the different size-fractions, were performed by means of size exclusion chromatography (SEC); a chromatographic system (Waters, Milford, MA, United States) coupled in series with a refractive index (RI) detector (Waters) and with a multi-angle laser light scattering detection (MALLS, Dawn Heleos II, Wyatt Europe GmbH, Dembach, Germany) was used as previously described (Nikolic et al., 2012).

NMR Analysis

The HMW-EPS fractions were analyzed by nuclear magnetic resonance (NMR) at the facilities of the University of Seville (Seville, Spain). A sample of 10 mg was deuterium-exchanged several times by freeze-drying from D_2O and then examined in solution (10 mg/750 mL of 99.96% D_2O, Sigma–Aldrich). Spectra were recorded on a Bruker AV500 spectrometer (Bruker BioSciences, Madrid, Spain) operating at 500.13 MHz (^1H). Chemical shifts were given in ppm, using the HDO signal (4.31 ppm at 343 K) as reference (Gottlieb et al., 1997). The 2D heteronuclear one-bond proton-carbon correlation experiment was registered in the ^1H-detection mode via single-quantum coherence (HSQC). A data matrix of 256 × 1K points was used to digitize a spectral width of 5208 in F2 and 22522 Hz in F1. ^{13}C decoupling was achieved by the GARP scheme. Squared-cosine-bell functions were applied in both dimensions, and zero-filling was used to expand the data to 1K × 1K.

Adhesion to HT29

The intestinal epithelial cell line HT29 (ECACC 91072201, European Collection of Cell Cultures, Salisbury, United Kingdom) was used to test the adhesion capability of the fluorescence-labeled and non-labeled bifidobacterial strains; *B. animalis* subsp *lactis* BB-12 was used as reference strain. HT29 was maintained under standard conditions using McCoy's medium (MM, Sigma) supplemented with 10% fetal bovine serum (Sigma) and with a mixture of antibiotics (50 μg/ml penicillin, 50 μg/ml streptomycin, 50 μg/ml gentamicin and 1.25 μg/ml amphotericin B, Sigma). The adhesion experiments were performed upon 11-day old HT29 monolayers grown in microtiter plates. Bifidobacterial suspensions, prepared in MM (without antibiotics), were added to each well at ratio 10:1 (bifidobacteria: HT29) and incubated for 1 h at 37°C/5% CO_2 (Nikolic et al., 2012). For the non-labeled strain the number of bacteria added and bacteria adhered was determined by plating on agar-MRSc and the adhesion percentage was calculated as the ratio between the bacteria adhered with respect to the bacteria added (Nikolic et al., 2012). For the fluorescence-labeled bacteria, the fluorescence was measured by means of flow cytometry, as previously described, and values of absolute fluorescence were used to present the adhesion results. In addition, experiments of competition between the "fluorescence-labeled, ropy" strain and the "non-labeled, non-ropy" strain (or "fluorescence-labeled, non-ropy" vs. "non-labeled, ropy") for adhesion to HT29 were carried out; in this case, both bacteria were added in equal amounts to the cell line (10:1, ratio bacteria: HT29) and the absolute fluorescence was measured.

Bifidobacterial Biofilm Formation upon Abiotic Surfaces

The capability of the ropy and non-ropy EPS-producing bifidobacterial strains to form biofilms was determined using different procedures and abiotic surfaces. A method, based on impedance measurement, recently described by Gutiérrez et al. (2016) to monitor in real time the formation of bacterial biofilms was used. In short, the real time cell analyzer (RTCA) equipment xCelligence RTCA-DP (ACEA Bioscience Inc., San Diego, CA, United States) was introduced in an incubator, at 37°C with 5% CO_2, at least 2 h before the experiments. Bifidobacterial cultures were washed twice with PBS to prepare standardized suspensions in fresh MRSc (~10^9 cfu/ml) which were placed in the wells (100 μl/well) of specific E-plates (ACEA Bioscience Inc.) coated with gold-microelectrodes that are able to transmit the impedance signal. The RTCA software 2.0 (ACEA Bioscience) was used for data collection and the biofilm formation was followed for 46 h, using three biological replicates for each strain; finally, the wells were stained with crystal violet, as will be described next. Biofilms were also formed upon polystyrene plates (96-well microplates Nunc, Thermo-Fisher Scientific Inc.), upon microscope cover glasses (No. 1, 18 mm diameter, Marienfeld GmbH, Lauda-Königshofen, Germany) previously sterilized by autoclaving (121°C, 20 min) which were placed into 6-well microplates (Thermo Fisher Scientific Inc.), and upon the surface of μ-slide-2-well glass bottom (Ibidi GmbH, Martinsried, Germany). After 24-h incubation at 37°C in anaerobic chamber, these biofilms were also stained with crystal violet. Additionally, the fluorescence-labeled bifidobacterial biofilms (incubated in darkness) formed upon cover glasses were visualized under the epifluorescence microscope and those formed upon the surface of μ-slide-2-well glass bottom were detected with the CSLM.

Crystal Violet Staining

The end-point crystal violet method was used to quantify the bifidobacterial biofilm formation upon the three abiotic surfaces used (Gutiérrez et al., 2016). In brief, supernatants from different abiotic-material wells were removed and biofilms washed twice with PBS, dried for 15 min at room temperature and stained with a solution (0.1% w/v) of crystal violet for 15 min. Then, biofilms were gently washed with water, de-stained with a solution (33%) of acetic acid for at least 15 min and, finally, the absorbance of the supernatants was measured at 595 nm in a Microplate Benchmark Plus (Bio-Rad, Hercules, CA, United States) spectrophotometer.

Statistical Analysis

The statistical package IBM SPSS Statistics for Windows Version 22.0 (IBM Corp., Armonk, NY, United States) was used to assess differences among strains by means of one-way ANOVA followed, when needed, by SNK (Student-Newman-Keuls, $p < 0.05$) mean comparison test. The legend of each figure indicates the analysis performed. Finally, the R^2 coefficients, that reflect the adjustment to linear regression equations between different parameters, were calculated.

RESULTS AND DISCUSSION

Generation of a Ropy Strain with a Non-synonymous Mutation in the Gene Balat_1410

In a previous work, an isogenic mutant derived from the type strain *B. animalis* subsp. *lactis* DSM10140 by removing the gene Balat_1410, using a knockout mutation system based on the integrative plasmid pJL74, was constructed (Hidalgo-Cantabrana et al., 2015). Our first aim in the present study was to reintroduce into the genome of *B. animalis* subsp. *lactis* DSM10140-ΔBalat_1410 a mutated Balat_1410 gene containing a non-synonymous, single nucleotide mutation previously associated with the appearance of a mucoid-ropy phenotype in the strain DSM10140-ΔBalat_1410-pAM1-Balat_1410^{S89L} (Hidalgo-Cantabrana et al., 2015). To do that, a double-crossover marker-less strategy previously used for the deletion of the gene, was followed. The strain DSM10140-ΔBalat_1410 was transformed with the plasmid pCHC3 (**Table 1**) containing a fragment of approximately 7 kb amplified from the genome of the strain IPLA-R1 (**Table 1**), that includes the regions immediately located upstream and downstream of the gene Balat_1410 as well as the mutated gene Balat_1410^{S89L} between those regions. Gene integration was achieved as previously described (Hidalgo-Cantabrana et al., 2015), resulting in *B. animalis* subsp. *lactis* DSM10140-Balat_1410^{S89L} (abbreviated as S89L), a strain that has exactly the same genetic background as *B. animalis* subsp. *lactis* DSM10140 which underwent a gene replacement that resulted in a C to T transition in the gene Balat_1410 at position 266, causing a codon change in position 89 (a serine is substituted by a leucine). Although there are several works that have reported gene deletion and interruption systems in bifidobacteria, including *B. breve* (Ruiz et al., 2012), *B. longum* (Fukuda et al., 2011; Hirayama et al., 2012) and *B. animalis* subsp. *lactis* (Arigoni and Delley, 2008; Hidalgo-Cantabrana et al., 2015), to our knowledge this is the first report of a successful gene replacement strategy in bifidobacteria. Due to the lack of genetic tools to introduce specific point mutations in bifidobacterial genomes, our methodology represents a suitable alternative to overcome this limitation.

Analysis of EPS Synthesized by the Recombinant Ropy Strain

In the EPS synthesized by the two ropy strains *B. animalis* subsp. *lactis* IPLA-R1 (parental) and S89L (recombinant) the HMW-EPS fraction (about 1 × 10^6 Da) was present in a higher proportion than in the non-ropy DSM10140 (parental) strain (**Figure 1A**). It should be noticed that the polymer material purified from the three strains, with the procedures used in this study, is the cell-associated EPS but not that liberated into the medium. Previously, the production of the HMW-EPS was correlated with the occurrence of the mucoid-ropy appearance in a recombinant strain harboring the mutated gene in a multi-copy plasmid (Hidalgo-Cantabrana et al., 2015); thus, currently this finding was reinforced with the acquisition of the ropy phenotype in the novel S89L having the single mutation stabilized into the chromosome. After purification of the HMW-EPS fraction from polymers synthesized by IPLA-R1 and S89L strains, one- and two-dimensional NMR analyses revealed an identical

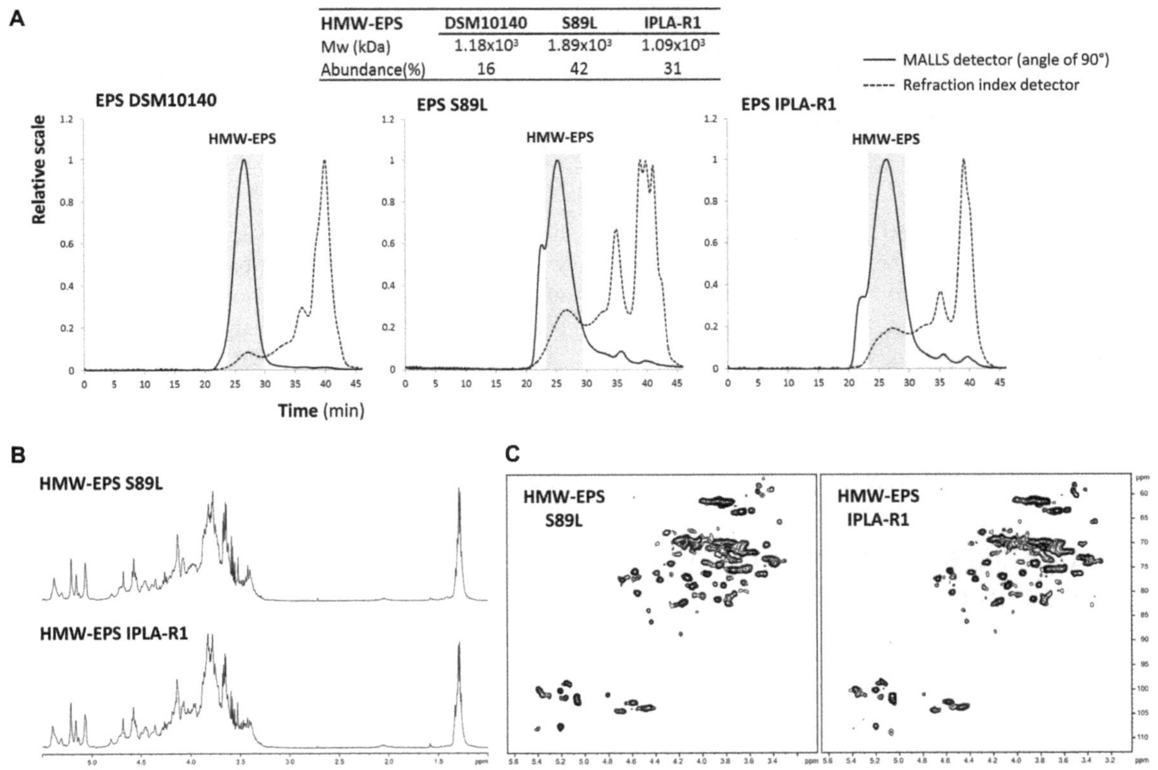

FIGURE 1 | Physical-chemical analysis of EPS isolated from three *B. animalis* subsp. *lactis* strains. SEC-MALLS analysis of the EPS-DSM10140, EPS-S89L and EPS-IPLA-R1 showing the molecular weight (Mw) and relative abundance of the high molecular weight (HMW) fraction in each polymer **(A)**. ^{1}H-NMR (500 MHz, 343 K) spectra **(B)** and 500-MHz ^{1}H-^{13}C- HSQC spectra **(C)** of HMW-EPS purified from EPS-IPLA-R1 and EPS-S89L polymers.

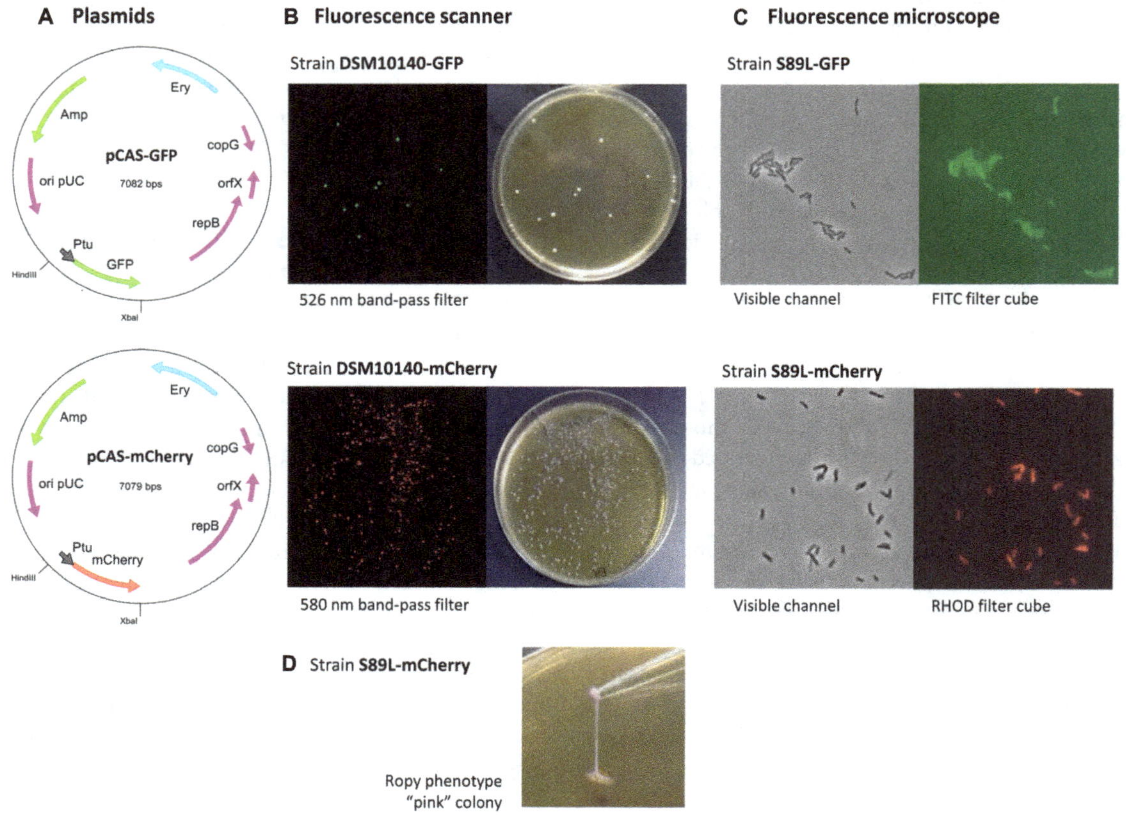

FIGURE 2 | Physical map of pCAS-GFP and pCAS-mCherry, in which the GFP and mCherry genes are located downstream from the elongation factor Tu promoter (P_{tuf}) from *B. animalis* subsp. *lactis* DSM10140 **(A)**. Detection of fluorescence green (top) or red (bottom) colonies of *B. animalis* subsp. *lactis* DSM10140-GFP and DSM10140-mCherry, respectively, using the Typhoon 9400 scanner fluorescence scanner (left hand photographs) and aspect of the colonies visualized with a conventional camera (right hand photographs) **(B)**. Fluorescent *B. animalis* subsp. *lactis* S89L, transformed with pCAS-GFP (top) and pCAS-mCherry (bottom), visualized with the Leica DMi8 inverted microscope using a 100× oil immersion objective **(C)**. Strain *B. animalis* subsp. *lactis* S89L-mCherry showing a colored pink colony with a ropy phenotype denoted for the formation of a long, unbreakable filament **(D)**.

chemical composition (**Figures 1B,C**). These physical-chemical analyses undoubtedly prove that the gene replacement strategy applied to obtain the recombinant S89L strain was successful to introduce the mutation linked to the production of the HMW-EPS. The structural repeating unit of the HMW-EPS was already described for strain IPLA-R1 (Leivers et al., 2011); it is an hexapolysaccharide with 50% rhamnose content, and it is very similar to that reported for strain *B. animalis* subsp. *lactis* LKM512 (Uemura and Matsumoto, 2014).

Expression of Fluorescent Proteins in *B. animalis* subsp. *lactis* and Fluorescence Detection

Bifidobacterium animalis subsp. *lactis* DSM10140 and S89L were transformed with the plasmids pVG-GFP and pVG-mCherry, containing the genes coding for the proteins GFP and mCherry, respectively. It was reported that these plasmids were successfully used for the fluorescent detection of *B. longum*, *B. breve,* and *B. bifidum* strains, grown in similar conditions to those used in our study (Grimm et al., 2014). However, no fluorescence was detected in our *B. animalis* subsp. *lactis* strains using fluorescence spectrometry techniques, suggesting that either the genes are not expressed or the proteins do not emit fluorescence under our experimental conditions. Since gene expression in the plasmids pVG-GFP and pVG-mCherry is under the control of the promoter of the glyceraldehyde-3-phosphate dehydrogenase gene of *B. bifidum* (P_{gap}), a specific promoter of *B. animalis* subsp. *lactis* was investigated which could be suitable to trigger the expression of the GFP and mCherry genes in our strains. Our previous work on bifidobacteria allowed us to depict a detailed protein map of the most abundant cytoplasmic proteins in their soluble proteome (Sánchez et al., 2005, 2007). Indeed, one of the most abundant proteins in the soluble proteome of some bifidobacteria is the elongation factor tu (the product of the *tuf* gene; Sánchez et al., 2005; Wei et al., 2016). Furthermore, previous reports have shown that the P_{tuf} of *B. longum* is a suitable strong and constitutive promoter able to trigger the expression of fluorescent proteins in *B. longum* and *B. breve* (Landete et al., 2014). These previous findings indicate that the *tuf* promoter could be a good candidate for the expression of heterologous genes in *B. animalis* subsp. *lactis*. With this in mind, the promoter of the glyceraldehyde-3-phosphate dehydrogenase, originally present in the plasmids

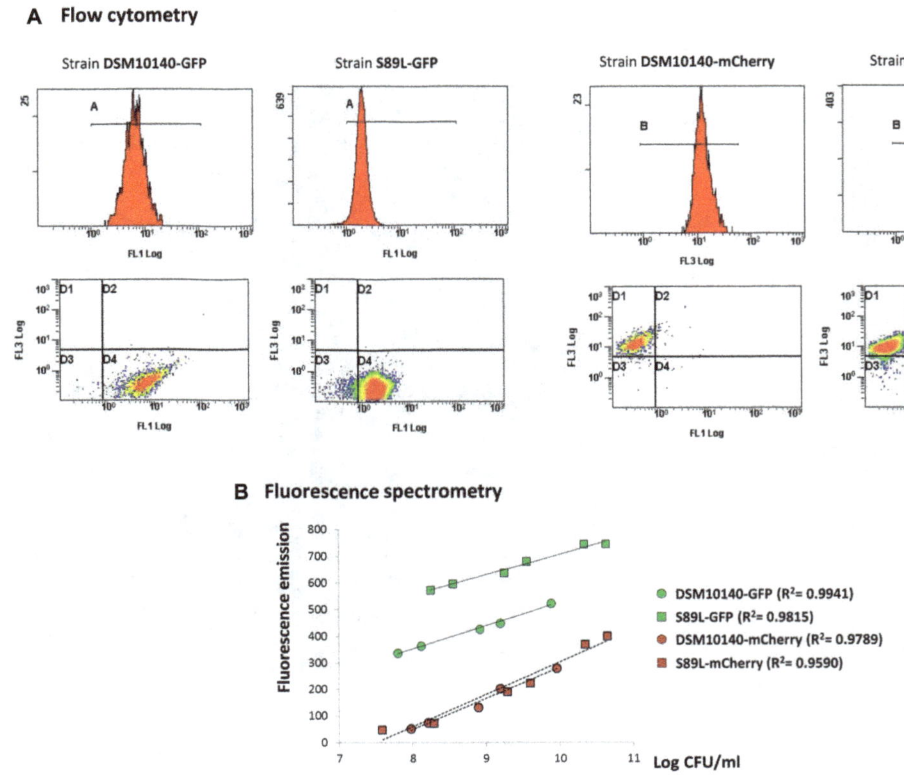

FIGURE 3 | Fluorescence quantification of GFP (the two left panels) and mCherry proteins (the two right panels) of the bifidobacterial strains harboring the corresponding plasmids using the Cytomics FC500 flow cytometer; see Supplementary Figure S2 for correlation with bacterial enumeration in agar-MRSc **(A)**. Linear regression between the fluorescence emitted, recorded by the CaryEclipse fluorescence spectrometer, and the bacterial counts (Log CFU/ml) of seriated dilutions of the fluorescent bifidobacterial suspensions; the coefficients of determination (R^2), showing how well data fit to the regression line equations, are indicated in bold letters **(B)**.

pVG-GFP and pVG-mCherry, was replaced by the upstream region of the *tuf* gene of *B. animalis* subsp. *lactis* DSM10140, containing P_{tuf}, yielding the plasmids pCAS-mCherry and pCAS-GFP (**Table 1** and **Figure 2A**). These plasmids were used to transform *B. animalis* subsp. *lactis* DSM10140 and *B. animalis* subsp. *lactis* S89L; green and red fluorescence in the resulting strains (DSM10140-mCherry, DSM10140-GFP, S89L-mCherry and S89L-GFP) were detected by fluorescence scanning (**Figure 2B**) and fluorescence microscopy (**Figure 2C**). The ropy phenotype, denoted by the formation of a filament, was detected in the strain S89L-mCherrey which also acquired a pink color in the colony (**Figure 2D**). Furthermore, a quantitative analysis of the fluorescently labeled bifidobacteria was performed using flow cytometry (**Figure 3A**), and the fluorescence signal was correlated with bacterial counts by a linear regression analysis (Supplementary Figure S2). Our results showed that the fluorescence quantification of the strains labeled with the two fluorescent proteins correlate with the bacterial counts in agar plates. The coefficients of determination (R^2) obtained in these analysis were in all cases higher than 0.95, indicating the suitability of our approach to quantify fluorescently labeled bifidobacterial populations in a range of 2 log count units (**Figure 3A** and Supplementary Figure S2). Very good fits to the linear regression were also obtained in a range of 3 log count units when the fluorescence quantification was carried out using spectrometric techniques (**Figure 3B**). Previous works have shown that other species, such as *B. longum*, *B. bifidum*, and *B. breve*, can be fluorescently labeled with a variety of proteins, including GFP, m-Cherry, Yellow Fluorescent proteins and Cyan Fluorescent proteins (Grimm et al., 2014; Landete et al., 2014). However, it is worth highlighting that, to the best of our knowledge, this is the first report describing the fluorescent labeling of *B. animalis* subsp. *lactis*, which opens new possibilities to track the functional properties of this *Bifidobacterium* under *in vitro* and *in vivo* conditions.

Regarding the stability of the fluorescence emission of GFP and mCherry, the fluorescence signal of GFP was quite unstable compared with that of m-Cherry. Once the cell growth was stopped, the cells were not able to emit fluorescence for longer than 1 h, independently of the technique used to measure the GFP fluorescence. A quick decrease in the fluorescence in the two *B. animalis* subsp. *lactis* strains analyzed was observed. However, m-Cherry fluorescence was more intense and stable for longer periods of time (a significant decrease of the fluorescent signal after 24 h at RT was not observed) (data not shown). Therefore, the strains labeled with m-Cherry were selected to perform the experiments described in the following sections of this work.

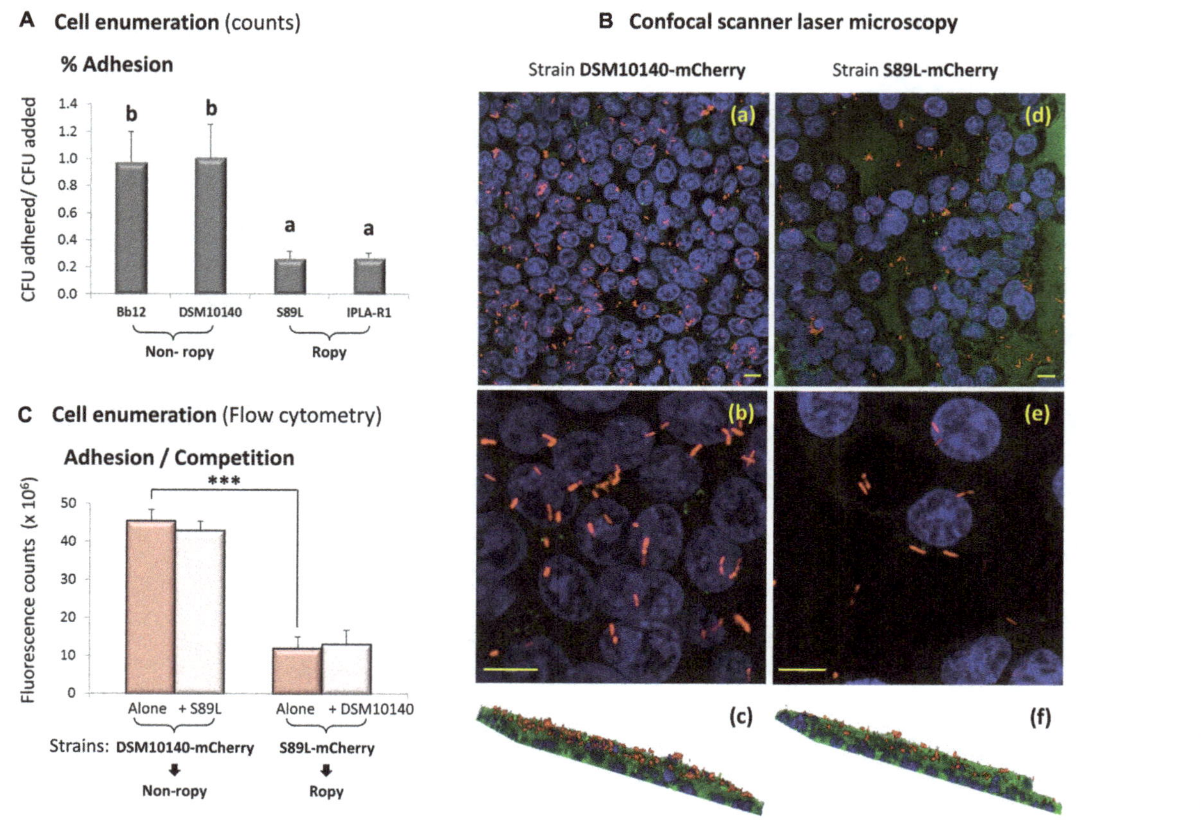

FIGURE 4 | Adhesion to the intestinal cell line HT29 of four *B. animalis* subsp. *lactis* strains: DSM10140 and Bb12 display a non-ropy phenotype and S89L and IPLA-R1 display a ropy phenotype. Bars that do not share a common letter are statistically ($p < 0.05$) different **(A)**. Visualization of DSM10140-mCherry (a, b, and c) and S89L-mCherry (d, e, and f) strains adhered to HT29 using the TCS SPE confocal module of the Leica DMi8 inverted microscope (bars 10 μm). The nucleus was DAPI-stained in blue (excited at 405 nm), the green color corresponds with the auto-fluorescence emitted by cytoplasmic molecules of the cell line, and the fluorescent bifidobacteria were detected in red (excited at 561 nm). The bottom photographs (c and f) represent a rotated 3D-image obtained from the Z- projection (10-XY slides, thickness about 13–15 μm) showing the integrity of the HT29 monolayer covered by a "grass" of fluorescent *B. animalis* subsp. *lactis* strains **(B)**. Adhesion to HT29 of strains DSM10140-mCherry and S89L-mCherry (red bars) quantified by means of flow cytometry; statistical difference between both strains are indicated with asterisks ($p < 0.01$). The pink bars show the adhesion of the fluorescent strains in competition with the non-fluorescent counterpart strains **(C)**.

Application of Fluorescence Labeling to Assess the Role of Ropy EPS in the Adhesion to HT29

In the last consensus statement in the probiotics field revised in 2014, it was considered that the FAO/WHO Guidelines proposed in 2002 (Food, and Agricultural Organization of the United Nations, and World Health Organization [FAO/WHO], 2002) still provide a useful approach to search for and validate probiotic candidates (Hill et al., 2014). Among the *in vitro* tests carried out to study new strains, the capability to adhere to mucus and/or intestinal epithelial cells is extensively analyzed before undertaking *in vivo* studies. In this study, conventional (culturing) techniques have been used to test the adhesion to the human intestinal cell line HT29 of the recombinant *B. animalis* subsp. *lactis* S89L strain in comparison with their isogenic parental strains. The ropy S89L and IPLA-R1 strains, both synthesizing in higher abundance the HMW-EPS, adhered significantly less to HT29 than DSM10140 and Bb12 (a probiotic reference) strains (**Figure 4A**). This result was contrary to that obtained in a previous work with the recombinant (ropy) DSM10140-ΔBalat_1410-pAM1-Balat_1410^{S89L} strain harboring the mutated Balat_1410 gene in the multicopy plasmid pAM1 (Hidalgo-Cantabrana et al., 2015). In fact, the three recombinant strains carrying pAM1 plasmid showed higher adhesion values (above 3%) to HT29 than the values obtained in the current work for the better adherent (around 1%) strains (DSM10140 and Bb12). Thus, in order to clarify this, apparently, contradictory result, the fluorescently labeled strains were used to address their capability to adhere to HT29 by means of different techniques and using the new experimental models in which there is a single copy of Balat_1410 (or Balat_1410^{S89L}) in the chromosome. The CSLM visualization corroborated that the ropy, HMW-EPS producing S89L-mCherry strain adhered to HT29 in lower proportions than the non-ropy DSM10140-mCherry strain (**Figure 4B**). Similarly, the quantitative flow cytometry technique showed about a fivefold reduction ($p < 0.05$) in the adhesion of the first strain with respect to the second (**Figure 4C**). Additionally, the simultaneous addition of a fluorescent strain in combination with its non-labeled counterpart (e.g., strain DSM10140-mCherry and S89L) did not modify the adhesion capability of both fluorescent ropy and non-ropy strains (**Figure 4C**); this indicates that the higher abundance of the HMW-EPS did not represent a disadvantage for *in vitro* competition to adhere to the epithelial cell line. Thus results obtained in the current study support the generalized finding that EPS of high molecular mass make difficult the adhesion of the producing strain to the intestinal epithelium because they could hinder the accessibility of other molecules acting as adhesins (Lebeer et al., 2009; Nikolic et al., 2012; Horn et al., 2014). However, the role of bacterial EPS on the adhesion capability of the producing strain has not been clearly established since it is highly dependent on the producing strain, the intrinsic characteristics of the polymer, as well as on the biological model of study used. As an illustrative example, *in vitro* studies showed that the EPS surrounding *Lactobacillus rhamnosus* GG reduced the adhesion of the strain to the intestinal cell line Caco2 (Lebeer et al., 2009) because the accessibility of the pili acting as strong adhesin to enterocytes was hindered (Lebeer et al., 2012). However, *in vivo* studies showed that this EPS forms a protective shield against host-antimicrobial secreted factors which helps the persistence of strain GG in the gut (Lebeer et al., 2010a). Thus, production of EPS by *L. rhamnosus* GG is relevant to keep an optimal performance, i.e., a balance between protection and adhesion.

Role of Ropy EPS in the Biofilm Formation upon Abiotic Surfaces

Another important role that EPS synthesized by probiotic bacteria could play in the gut ecosystem is the capability of reducing the activity of pathogens in the intestine, including their adhesion to the intestinal epithelium. This has been proved with *in vitro* (Ksonzeková et al., 2016; Zivkovic et al., 2016) as well as *in vivo* studies (Fanning et al., 2012; Chen et al., 2014; Nácher-Vázquez et al., 2015) using different intestinal cell lines and animal models, respectively. It was postulated that the mechanism behind this EPS protection could be the formation of a protective "biofilm-like" layer covering the intestinal epithelium and, therefore, preventing the adhesion of the pathogen or its toxins (Ruas-Madiedo et al., 2010; Fanning et al., 2012). Thus, to test the biofilm-formation ability of our EPS-producing bacteria different methodologies and abiotic surfaces were used as an initial approach before demonstrating this capability in biotic surfaces which, currently, is a challenging issue (**Figure 5**). The recently developed impedance-based method to monitor in real time the bacterial biofilm formation upon gold-microelectrodes of RTCA E-plates (Gutiérrez et al., 2016) showed that the ropy S89L strain presented a lower adhesion ability than the non-ropy DSM10140 parental one during the incubation period (**Figure 5A**). To discard any influence of the abiotic material on the adhesion ability, 24 h-old biofilms were formed upon glass-cover or polystyrene and compared with 46 h-old biofilms made of RTCA E-plates; all biofilms were stained with crystal violet and this method also supported the same tendency between both strains ($p < 0.05$) regardless of the abiotic surface considered

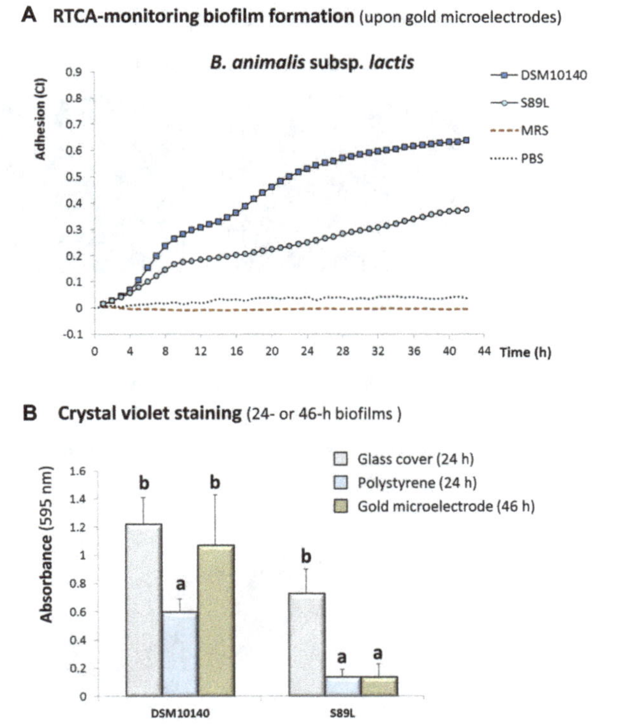

FIGURE 5 | Monitoring in real time the formation of biofilms by strains *B. animalis* subsp. *lactis* DSM10140 and S89L upon (gold-microelectrodes) E-plates in the RTCA (real time cell analyzed) equipment **(A)**. Biofilms formed by the same strains in three abiotic surfaces and stained, at different end-point times, with the crystal violet method; within each strain, bars that do not share a common letter are significantly ($p < 0.05$) different **(B)**.

(**Figure 5B**). However, statistical differences were noted when the behavior of each strain in the three abiotic surfaces was compared; for strain S89L the lowest biofilm formation capability was upon gold and polystyrene, whereas strain DSM10140 showed better adherence to gold (**Figure 5B**). This variability could be related to variations in the hydrophilic/hydrophobic nature of both bacterial surfaces that could suppose variable affinities for materials with different physical properties. In fact, it has been proved that the polar and non-polar characteristics of abiotic surfaces are involved in the differential capability to form biofilms of some pathogens (Meira et al., 2012).

The visualization by epifluorescence microscopy of 24 h-old biofilms formed with the fluorescent-labeled strains showed a higher bacterial density on the glass covered with the non-ropy DSM10140-mCherry strain, in comparison with the ropy S89L-mCherry ones (**Figure 6A**); a quantitative test performed with the same strains confirmed this difference ($p < 0.05$). Similarly, when intact bifidobacterial biofilms formed upon μ-slides were visualized with CSLM a very thin 3-D structure was detected only for strain DSM10140-mCherry whereas only residual bacteria remained attached for strain S89L-mCherry (**Figure 6B**). As far as we could note, this is the first report showing the biofilm formation by *Bifidobacterium* spp. and depending on the type of polymer that is synthesized it could favor or prevent the

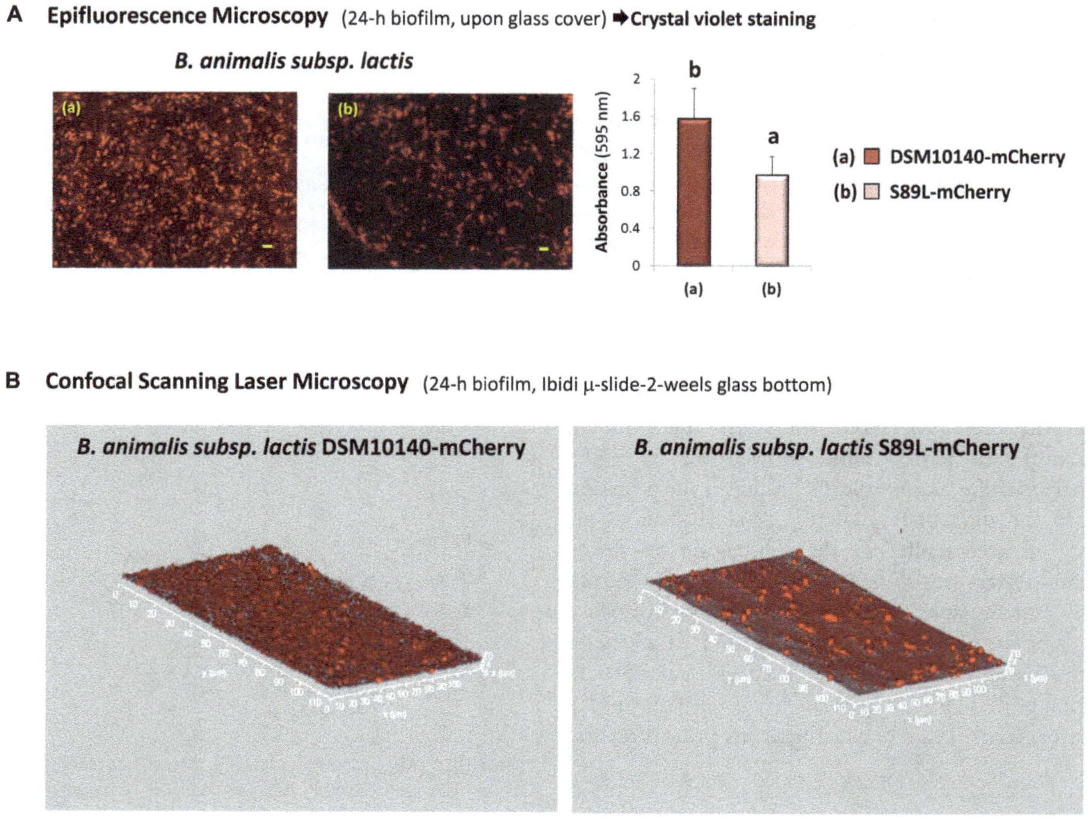

FIGURE 6 | Detection of fluorescence-labeled bifidobacterial DSM10140-mCherry and S89L-mCherry strains upon glass covers using the epifluorescence microscope (bar 5 μm) and crystal violet quantification of the biofilms formed upon the glass covers; bars that do not share a common letter are significantly ($p < 0.05$) different **(A)**. Rotated 3D-images obtained from the Z- projection (thickness about 2–4 μm) showing the biofilm formed by *B. animalis* subsp. *lactis* DSM10140-mCherry upon glass μ-slides and the absence of biofilm by strain S89L-mCherry **(B)**.

adhesion of the bifidobacteria to different abiotic surfaces. As it was indicated above, the presence of a HMW-EPS fraction could reduce the contact of other surface adhesins with the abiotic surface, thus avoiding the biofilm formation.

Therefore, all approaches used showed a reduced capability of the HMW-EPS-producing strains to form biofilms upon abiotic surfaces, as was also observed in the biotic (HT29) surface. Our observation confirms that previously reported with the high molecular mass EPS synthesized by *L. rhamnosus* GG (38) and *L. johnsonii* FI9785 (Dertli et al., 2015). The molecular weight of the HMW-EPS synthesized by these lactobacilli as well as our strain S89L was equal or higher than 1×10^6 Da; whereas, the most abundant polymer fractions in the DSM10140 had lower molecular weight (less than 3×10^4 Da). Therefore, although it cannot be discarded that some specific EPS could form a biofilm layer on the gut surface, other mechanisms could be involved in the capability of EPS-producing bacteria to counteract the adhesion of pathogens. In this regard, our previous observations with polymers purified from lactobacilli and bifidobacteria suggest that these polymers could also act as analogs of the eukaryotic PRR for pathogens, i.e., having a "lectin-like" activity, and therefore reducing their adhesion to the gut mucosa (Ruas-Madiedo et al., 2006). In any case, the contribution of EPS to counteracting microbial dysbiosis caused by infections deserves future research (Reid et al., 2011).

To sum up, our results show that fluorescent labeling of *B. animalis* subsp. *lactis* can be achieved by using green and mCherry fluorescent proteins but that these genes need to be under the control of a promoter from this species. It was demonstrated that the introduction of Balat-1410 mutation into the chromosome of parental DSM10140 strain was linked to the production of a larger abundance of a HMW-EPS, which in turn confers a ropy phenotype. Tagging bifidobacteria with mCherry allowed us to determine that some relevant functional characteristics of the strains, such as the adhesion to human intestinal cells or the capacity to form biofilms, are associated with the presence/absence of this ropy phenotype. The novel recombinant strains obtained in this work are a valuable tool to study the cross-talk mechanisms between bifidobacteria and host cells, and can make possible the development of further approaches to elucidate the role of these bacteria in complex *in vivo* systems. Furthermore, similar methodological approaches are required to demonstrate the functional properties of NGP bacteria which must be used to decipher the role of surface molecules involved in the beneficial properties attributable to beneficial microorganisms.

AUTHOR CONTRIBUTIONS

CH-C, PR-M, and AM contributed with the conception, experimental design and results interpretation of this study. NC-B carried out all experiments, some of them performed with the collaboration of MR-C. PR-M was in charge of the statistical analyses. AM and PR-M were in charge of writing the drafted manuscript. All authors performed a critical revision of the manuscript and approved the final version.

FUNDING

This work was financed by the Spanish Ministry of Economy and Competitiveness (MINECO) and FEDER European Union funds through the project AGL2015-64901-R. NC-B acknowledges her FPI (BES-2013-063984) fellowship to MINECO.

ACKNOWLEDGMENTS

The authors are grateful to C. H. Riedel (University of Ulm, Germany) for the kind supply of pVG-GFP and pVG-mCherry plasmids. A. B. Campelo (IPLA-CSIC) as well as M. Alonso and A. Salas (STC-University of Oviedo) are acknowledged for their excellent technical assistance. We also thank the "Centro de Investigación, Tecnología e Innovación" (CITIUS) of the University of Seville for NMR facilities.

REFERENCES

Alvarez-Martín, P., Flórez, A. B., Margolles, A., del Solar, G., and Mayo, B. (2008). Improved cloning vectors for bifidobacteria, based on the *Bifidobacterium catenulatum* pBC1 replicon. *Appl. Environ. Microbiol.* 74, 4656–4665. doi: 10.1128/AEM.00074-08

Arigoni, F., and Delley, M. (2008). Genetic remodeling in *Bifidobacterium*. International patent WO 2008019886 A1. Washington, DC: U.S. Patent and Trademark Office.

Bogsan, C. S. B., Ferreira, L., Maldonado, C., Perdigon, G., Almeida, S. R., and Oliveira, M. N. (2014). Fermented or unfermented milk using *Bifidobacterium animalis* subsp. *lactis* HN019: technological approach determines the probiotic modulation of mucosal cellular immunity. *Food Res. Int.* 64, 283–288.

Chen, X. Y., Woodward, A., Zijlstra, R. T., and Gänzle, M. G. (2014). Exopolysaccharides synthesized by *Lactobacillus reuteri* protect against enterotoxigenic *Escherichia coli* in Piglets. *Appl. Environ. Microbiol.* 80, 5752–5760. doi: 10.1128/AEM.01782-14

Cronin, M., Sleator, R. D., Hill, C., Fitzgerald, G. F., and van Sinderen, D. (2008). Development of a luciferase-based reporter system to monitor Bifidobacterium breve UCC2003 persistence in mice. *BMC Microbiol.* 8:161. doi: 10.1186/1471-2180-8-161

Dertli, E., Mayer, M. J., and Narbad, A. (2015). Impact of the exopolysaccharide layer on biofilms, adhesion and resistance to stress in *Lactobacillus johnsonii* FI9785. *BMC Microbiol.* 15:8. doi: 10.1186/s12866-015-0347-2

Fanning, S., Hall, L. J., Cronin, M., Zomer, A., MacSharry, J., Goulding, D., et al. (2012). Bifidobacterial surface-exopolysaccharide facilitates commensal-host interaction through immune modulation and pathogen protection. *Proc. Natl. Acad. Sci. U.S.A.* 109, 2108–2113. doi: 10.1073/pnas.1115621109

Ferrario, C., Milani, C., Mancabelli, L., Lugli, G. A., Duranti, S., Mangifesta, M., et al. (2016). Modulation of the eps-ome transcription of bifidobacteria through simulation of human intestinal environment. *FEMS Microbiol. Ecol.* 92:fiw056. doi: 10.1093/femsec/fiw056

Food, and Agricultural Organization of the United Nations, and World Health Organization [FAO/WHO] (2002). *Joint FAO/WHO Working Group Report on Drafting Guidelines for the Evaluation of Probiotics in Food.* Rome: FAO.

Fukuda, S., Toh, H., Hase, K., Oshima, K., Nakanishi, Y., Yoshimura, K., et al. (2011). Bifidobacteria can protect from enteropathogenic infection through production of acetate. *Nature* 469, 543–547. doi: 10.1038/nature09646

Gareau, M. G., Sherman, P. M., and Walker, W. A. (2010). Probiotics and the gut microbiota in intestinal health and disease. *Nat. Rev. Gastroenterol. Hepatol.* 7, 503–514. doi: 10.1038/nrgastro.2010.117

Gottlieb, H. E., Kotlyar, V., and Nudelman, A. (1997). NMR chemical shifts of common laboratory solvents as trace impurities. *J. Org. Chem.* 62, 7512–7515.

Grimm, V., Gleinser, M., Neu, C., Zhurina, D., and Riedel, C. H. (2014). Expression of fluorescent proteins in bifidobacteria for analysis of host-microbe interactions. *Appl. Environ. Microbiol.* 80, 2842–2850. doi: 10.1128/AEM.04261-13

Gutiérrez, D., Hidalgo-Cantabrana, C., Rodríguez, A., García, P., and Ruas-Madiedo, P. (2016). Monitoring in real time the formation and removal of biofilms from clinical related pathogens using an impedance-based technology. *PLoS ONE* 11:e0163966. doi: 10.1371/journal.pone.0163966

Hidalgo-Cantabrana, C., Algieri, F., Rodriguez-Nogales, A., Vezza, T., Martínez-Camblor, P., Margolles, A., et al. (2016). Effect of a ropy exopolysaccharide-producing *Bifidobacterium animalis* subsp. *lactis* strain orally administered on DSS-induced colitis mice model. *Front. Microbiol.* 7:868. doi: 10.3389/fmicb.2016.00868

Hidalgo-Cantabrana, C., Sánchez, B., Álvarez-Martín, P., López, P., Martínez-Álvarez, N., Delley, M., et al. (2015). A single mutation in the gene responsible for the mucoid phenotype of *Bifidobacterium animalis* subsp. *lactis* confers surface and functional characteristics. *Appl. Environ. Microbiol.* 81, 7960–7968. doi: 10.1128/AEM.02095-15

Hidalgo-Cantabrana, C., Sánchez, B., Milani, C., Ventura, M., Margolles, A., and Ruas-Madiedo, P. (2014). Genomic overview and biological functions of exopolysaccharide biosynthesis in *Bifidobacterium* spp. *Appl. Environ. Microbiol.* 80, 9–18. doi: 10.1128/AEM.02977-13

Hill, C., Guarner, F., Reid, G., Gibson, G. R., Merenstein, D. J., Pot, B., et al. (2014). The international scientific association for probiotics and prebiotics consensus statement on the scope and appropriate use of the term probiotic. *Nat. Rev. Gastroenterol. Hepatol.* 11, 506–514. doi: 10.1038/nrgastro.2014.66

Hirayama, Y., Sakanaka, M., Fukuma, H., Murayama, H., Kano, Y., Fukiya, S., et al. (2012). Development of a double-crossover markerless gene deletion system in *Bifidobacterium longum*: functional analysis of the -galactosidase gene for raffinose assimilation. *Appl. Environ. Microbiol.* 78, 4984–4994. doi: 10.1128/AEM.00588-12

Horn, N., Wegmann, U., Dertli, E., Mulholland, F., Collins, S. R. A., Waldron, K. W., et al. (2014). Spontaneous mutation reveals influence of exopolysaccharide on *Lactobacillus johnsonii* surface characteristics. *PLoS ONE* 8:e59957. doi: 10.1371/journal.pone.0059957

Ksonzeková, P., Bystricky, P., Vlcková, S., Pätoprsty, V., Pulzová, L., Mudronová, D., et al. (2016). Exopolysaccharides of *Lactobacillus reuteri*: their influence ona dherence of E. *coli* to epithelial cells and inflammatory response. *Carbohydr. Polym.* 141, 10–19. doi: 10.1016/j.carbpol.2015.12.037

Landete, J. M., Medina, M., and Arqués, J. L. (2016). Fluorescent reporter systems for tracking probiotic lactic acid bacteria and bifidobacteria. *World J. Microbiol. Biotechnol.* 32, 119. doi: 10.1007/s11274-016-2077-5

Landete, J. M., Peirotén, Á, Rodríguez, E., Margolles, A., Medina, M., and Arqués, J. L. (2014). Anaerobic green fluorescent protein as a marker of *Bifidobacterium* strains. *Int. J. Food Microbiol.* 175, 6–13. doi: 10.1016/j.ijfoodmicro.2014.01.008

Lebeer, S., Claes, I., Tytgat, H. L. P., Verhoeven, T. L. A., Marien, E., von Ossowski, I., et al. (2012). Functional analysis of *Lactobacillus rhamnosus* GG pili in relation to adhesion and immunomodulatory interactions with intestinal epithelial cells. *Appl. Environ. Microbiol.* 78, 185–193. doi: 10.1128/AEM.06192-11

Lebeer, S., Claes, I. J. J., Verhoeven, T. L. A., Vanderleyden, J., and De Keersmaecker, S. C. J. (2010a). Exopolysaccharides of *Lactobacillus rhamnosus* GG form a protective shield against innate immune factors in the intestine. *Microb. Biotechnol.* 4, 368–374. doi: 10.1111/j.1751-7915.2010.00199.x

Lebeer, S., Vanderleyden, J., and De Keersmaecker, S. C. J. (2010b). Host interactions of probiotic bacterial surface molecules: comparison with commensals and pathogens. *Nat. Rev. Microbiol.* 8, 171–184. doi: 10.1038/nrmicro2297

Lebeer, S., Verhoeven, T. L. A., Francius, G., Schoofs, G., Lambrichts, I., Dufrêne, Y., et al. (2009). Identification of a gene Cluster for the biosynthesis of a long, galactose-rich exopolysaccharide in *Lactobacillus rhamnosus* GG and functional analysis of the priming glycosyltransferase. *Appl. Environ. Microbiol.* 75, 3554–3563. doi: 10.1128/AEM.02919-08

Leivers, S., Hidalgo-Cantabrana, C., Robinson, G., Margolles, A., Ruas-Madiedo, P., and Laws, A. P. (2011). Structure of the high molecular weight exopolysaccharide produced by *Bifidobacterium animalis* subsp. *lactis* IPLA-R1 and sequence analysis of its putative eps cluster. *Carbohyd. Res.* 346, 2710–2717. doi: 10.1016/j.carres.2011.09.010

López, P., Monteserín, D. C., Gueimonde, M., de los Reyes-Gavilán, C. G., Margolles, A., Suárez, A., et al. (2012). Exopolysaccharide-producing *Bifidobacterium* strains elicit different in vitro responses upon interaction with human cells. *Food Res. Int.* 46, 99–107.

Meira, Q. G. S., de Medeiros Barbosa, I., Alves Aguiar Athayde, A. J., de Siqueira-Junior, J. P., and de Souza, E. L. (2012). Influence of temperature and surface kind on biofilm formation by Staphylococcus aureus from food-contact surfaces and sensitivity to sanitizers. *Food Control* 25, 469–475.

Montenegro-Rodríguez, C., Peirotén, A., Sanchez-Jimenez, A., Arqués, J. L., and Landete, J. M. (2015). Analysis of gene expression of bifidobacteria using as the reporter an anaerobic fluorescent protein. *Biotechnol. Lett.* 37, 1405–1413. doi: 10.1007/s10529-015-1802-8

Nácher-Vázquez, M., Ballesteros, N., Canales, A., Rodríguez Saint-Jean, S., Pérez-Prieto, S. I., Prieto, A., et al. (2015). Dextrans produced by lactic acid bacteria exhibit antiviral and immunomodulatory activity against salmonid viruses. *Carbohydr. Polym.* 124, 292–301. doi: 10.1016/j.carbpol.2015.02.020

Nikolic, M., López, P., Strahinic, I., Suárez, A., Kojic, M., Fernández-García, M., et al. (2012). Characterisation of the exopolysaccharide (EPS)-producing *Lactobacillus paraplantarum* BGCG11 and its non-EPS producing derivative strains as potential probiotics. *Int. J. Food Microbiol.* 158, 155–162. doi: 10.1016/j.ijfoodmicro.2012.07.015

O'Toole, P. W., Marchesi, J. R., and Hill, C. (2017). Next-generation probiotics: the spectrum from probiotics to live biotherapeutics. *Nature Microbiol.* 2, 17057. doi: 10.1038/nmicrobiol.2017.57

Reid, G., Younes, J. A., Van der Mei, H. C., Gloor, G. B., Knight, R., and Busscher, H. J. (2011). Microbiota restoration: natural and supplemented recovery of human microbial communities. *Nat. Rev. Microbiol.* 9, 27–38. doi: 10.1038/nrmicro2473

Rossi, O., Khan, M. T., Schwarzer, M., Hudcovic, T., Srutkova, D., Duncan, S. H., et al. (2015). *Faecalibacterium prausnitzii* strain HTF-F and its extracellular pPolymeric matrix attenuate clinical parameters in DSS-induced colitis. *PLoS ONE* 10:e0123013. doi: 10.1371/journal.pone.0123013

Ruas-Madiedo, P., Gueimonde, M., Margolles, A., de los Reyes-Gavilán, C. G., and Salminen, S. (2006). Exopolysaccharides produced by probiotic strains modify the adhesion of probiotics and enteropathogens to human intestinal mucus. *J. Food Proct.* 69, 2011–2015.

Ruas-Madiedo, P., Medrano, M., Salazar, N., de los Reyes-Gavilán, C. G., Pérez, P. F., and Abraham, A. G. (2010). Exopolysaccharides produced by *Lactobacillus* and *Bifidobacterium* strains abrogate in vitro the cytotoxic effect of bacterial toxins on eukaryotic cells. *J. Appl. Microbiol.* 109, 2079–2086. doi: 10.1111/j.1365-2672.2010.04839.x

Ruiz, L., O'Connell-Motherway, M., Zomer, A., de los Reyes-Gavilán, C. G., Margolles, A., and van Sinderen, D. (2012). A bile-inducible membrane protein mediates bifidobacterial bile resistance. *Microb. Biotechnol.* 5, 523–535. doi: 10.1111/j.1751-7915.2011.00329.x

Sánchez, B., Champomier-Vergès, M. C., Anglade, P., Baraige, F., de Los Reyes-Gavilán, C. G., Margolles, A., et al. (2005). Proteomic analysis of global changes in protein expression during bile salt exposure of *Bifidobacterium longum* NCIMB 8809. *J. Bacteriol.* 187, 5799–5808.

Sánchez, B., Champomier-Vergès, M. C., Collado, M. D. C., Anglade, P., Baraige, F., Sanz, Y., et al. (2007). Low-pH adaptation and the acid tolerance response of *Bifidobacterium longum* biotype *longum*. *Appl. Environ. Microbiol.* 73, 6450–6459.

Schiavi, E., Gleinser, M., Molloy, E., Groeger, F., Frei, R., Ferstl, R., et al. (2016). The surface-associated exopolysaccharide of *Bifidobacterium longum* 35624 plays an essential role in dampening host proinflammatory responses and repressing local TH17 responses. *Appl. Environ. Microbiol.* 82, 7185–7196.

Tojo, R., Suárez, A., Clemente, M. G., de los Reyes-Gavilán, C. G., Margolles, A., Gueimonde, M., et al. (2014). Intestinal microbiota in health and disease: role of bifidobacteria in gut homeostasis. *World J. Gastroenterol.* 20, 15163–15176. doi: 10.3748/wjg.v20.i41.15163

Uemura, Y., and Matsumoto, M. (2014). Chemical structure of the cell wall-associated polysaccharide of *Bifidobacterium animalis* subsp. *lactis* LKM512. *Glycoconjugate J.* 31, 555–561. doi: 10.1007/s10719-014-9534-x

Vallejo, A. N., Pogulis, R. J., and Pease, L. R. (1994). In vitro synthesis of novel genes: mutagenesis and recombination by PCR. *Genome Res.* 4, S123–S130.

Wan, L. Y. M., Chen, Z. J., Shah, N. P., and El-Nezami, H. (2015). Modulation of intestinal epithelial defense responses by probiotic bacteria. *Crit. Rev. Food Sci. Nutr.* 56, 2628–2641. doi: 10.1080/10408398.2014.905450

Wei, X., Wang, S., Zhao, X., Wang, X., Li, H., Lin, W., et al. (2016). Proteomic profiling of *Bifidobacterium bifidum* S17 cultivated under in vitro conditions. *Front. Microbiol.* 7:97. doi: 10.3389/fmicb.2016.00097

Westermann, C., Gleinser, M., Corr, S. C., and Riedel, C. U. (2016). A critical evaluation of bifidobacterial adhesion to the host tissue. *Front. Microbiol.* 7:1220. doi: 10.3389/fmicb.2016.01220

Zivkovic, M., Miljkovi, M. S., Ruas-Madiedo, P., Markeli, M. B., Veljovic, K., Tolinacki, M., et al. (2016). EPS-SJ exopolysaccharide produced by the strain *Lactobacillus paracasei* subsp. *paracasei* BGSJ2-8 is involved in adhesion to epithelial intestinal cells and decrease on *E.coli* association to Caco-2 cells. *Front. Microbiol.* 7:286. doi: 10.3389/fmicb.2016.00286

11

Shaping the Metabolism of Intestinal *Bacteroides* Population through Diet to Improve Human Health

David Rios-Covian, Nuria Salazar, Miguel Gueimonde and Clara G. de los Reyes-Gavilan *

Department of Microbiology and Biochemistry of Dairy Products, Instituto de Productos Lácteos de Asturias, Consejo Superior de Investigaciones Científicas (IPLA-CSIC), Villaviciosa, Asturias, Spain

***Correspondence:**
Clara G. de los Reyes-Gavilan
greyes_gavilan@ipla.csic.es

Keywords: *Bacteroides*, propionate, branched-chain amino acids, short chain fatty acids, diet, human metabolism, intestinal microbiota

INTESTINAL MICROBIOTA AND THE CONTROL OF GLUCOSE HOMEOSTASIS AND LIPID METABOLISM IN THE HOST

The human intestinal microbiota is dominated by five phyla: Firmicutes, Bacteroidetes, Actinobacteria, Proteobacteria, and Verrucomicrobia. In adults, more than 80% of the species belong to just two phyla, Firmicutes and Bacteroidetes. Short chain fatty acids (SCFA) are catabolic end-products from intestinal microbial fermentation. Acetate, propionate and butyrate are the most abundant (Ríos-Covián et al., 2016a) whilst branched chain fatty acids (BCFA; isobutyrate, valerate, and isovalerate), the organic acids lactate, succinate, formate, and gases, can be also formed.

In humans, the main fermentable sources of SCFA are undigested dietary polysaccharides; amino acids and proteins may constitute additional substrates for colonic fermentation, whereas host-derived glycoproteins contribute to a limited extent. BCFA can be formed at considerably lower proportions than SCFA from branched-chain amino acids (BCAA; valine, leucine, and isoleucine). Threonine renders propionate and butyrate, whereas glutamate, histidine, lysine, arginine, and alanine give rise to acetate and butyrate formation; additionally, the intestinal microbiota contributes to the production of amino acids available to the host through *de novo* biosynthesis (Neis et al., 2015). Moreover, metabolic cross-feeding, that is the utilization of end products from the carbohydrate catabolism of a given microorganism by another one, strongly influences the final balance of intestinal SCFA. It occurs mainly for the formation of butyrate from acetate or lactate, is considerably lower for butyrate conversion to propionate, and very scarce between propionate and acetate (Den Besten et al., 2013).

Intestinal SCFA can incorporate into the enterohepatic circulation, being metabolized in the liver and reaching other extra-intestinal locations (Den Besten et al., 2014). Increasing evidence supports a regulatory role for SCFA in glucose homeostasis and lipid metabolism, in which intestinal SCFA ligands FFAR2 and FFAR3 and the glucagon-like peptide are involved. In the liver propionate is gluconeogenic whereas acetate and butyrate are lipogenic. Recent studies evidence that propionate and butyrate activate the intestinal gluconeogenesis (De Vadder et al., 2014), the glucose synthesized serving as a homeostatic signal in the portal system, to control hepatic gluconeogenesis (causal factor of insulin resistance and type 2 diabetes) and improving whole-body glucose homeostasis. Moreover, propionate flux through the liver reduces visceral and liver fat by decreasing intrahepatic triglycerides (Chambers et al., 2015). Propionate inhibits hepatic lipogenesis and cholesterogenesis promoted by acetate (Demigne et al., 1995) whereas propionate and butyrate inhibit lipolysis and lipogenesis and increase the incorporation of glucose mediated by insulin into the adipose tissue (Heimann et al., 2015). These observations prompt to the acetate/propionate ratio as an indicator for the potential contribution of intestinal SCFA to body lipid metabolism. Additionally, the improvement of glucose homeostasis promoted by dietary fiber seems to be associated with elevated fluxes of SCFA from the intestinal lumen to other organs rather than with the fecal SCFA concentrations (Den Besten et al., 2014).

Several metabolic disorders as obesity, insulin resistance, and metabolic syndrome are associated with impairment of the metabolism of carbohydrates and lipids by the host, and are accompanied by changes in the gut microbiota (Turnbaugh et al., 2009; Bervoets et al., 2013). Higher levels and altered patterns of SCFA (Fernandes et al., 2014; Salazar et al., 2015) and changes in the Firmicutes to Bacteroidetes ratio, have been repeatedly reported in obese individuals (Ley et al., 2006; Turnbaugh et al., 2006). Nonetheless, contradictory results published so far on the relative abundance of both phyla exclude its use as a broadly applicable marker.

Increases in plasma circulating BCAA and aromatic amino acids (phenylalanine and tyrosine) were related with higher risk of type 2 diabetes and insulin resistance (Utzschneider et al., 2016), having been suggested that the altered functionality of the intestinal microbiota (also affecting *de novo* biosynthesis of amino acids) determines these differential profiles of circulating amino acids (Neis et al., 2015).

Increasing protein intake (Pillot et al., 2009) and gastric surgery (Liou et al., 2013) have demonstrated efficacy for weight control and improvement of glucose homeostasis, partly related to the increase of propionate (De Vadder et al., 2014), and enrichment of intestinal Bacteroidetes/*Bacteroides* (Furet et al., 2010; Jumpertz et al., 2011; Liou et al., 2013). In contrast, a significant reduction in butyrate and certain butyrate-producing Firmicutes have been associated with diets containing low amounts of fiber and carbohydrates (Duncan et al., 2007, 2008; Walker et al., 2011). These suggest a microbiota unbalance in obese subjects, or under inadequate diets, which is partly restored following gastric surgery or by introducing weight-loss diets. However, some microbiome alterations seem to persist after dietary interventions, facilitating post-dieting weight regain (Thaiss et al., 2016). This stresses the importance of achieving a full restoration of the intestinal microbiota after dietary treatments, including proper balanced microbial metabolic products, to ensure durable effects.

A FOCUS ON THE GENUS *BACTEROIDES* AND THE PRODUCTION OF PROPIONATE IN THE INTESTINAL MICROBIAL ECOSYSTEM

The order Bacteroidales is the most abundant Gram-negative bacteria, colonizing the human gut at densities up to 5–8 $\times$ 10^{10} CFU per gram of feces (Zitomersky et al., 2011). Among the predominant genera are *Bacteroides* and *Prevotella*. These microorganisms can use a wide range of dietary soluble polysaccharides that are firstly released from vegetable fiber in the intestine by microbial primary degraders (Martens et al., 2011). The genus *Bacteroides* displays a high flexibility to adapt to the nutritional conditions of the intestinal environment (Comstock and Coyne, 2003), being able to use dietary or host-derived glycans according to the nutrient availability (Sonnenburg et al., 2005). *Bacteroides* can also incorporate amino acids from outside (Smith and MacFarlane, 1998) which could be used to maintain cell structures and as an energy source.

Three different biochemical pathways have been identified in colonic bacteria for propionate formation (Reichardt et al., 2014). The succinate pathway is the only one for propionate production from hexoses by Bacteroidetes, although some Negativicutes (family *Veillonellaceae,* phylum Firmicutes) can form propionate by utilizing succinate. The acrylate pathway is used for the conversion of lactate into propionate by very few bacterial genera within the phylum Firmicutes, whereas deoxy-sugars (fucose and rhamnose) are converted through the propanediol pathway by some Proteobacteria and members of the *Lachnospiraceae* family (phylum Firmicutes). *Akkermansia muciniphila* (phylum Verrucomicrobia) has been identified as a key propionate producing mucin-degrading species (Derrien et al., 2004).

Notably, several studies point to Bacteroidetes as the largest propionate producers in the human gut (Salonen et al., 2014; Aguirre et al., 2016). Interestingly, by modifying microbiota composition with antibiotic treatment in mice, Zhao et al. (2013) found a strong correlation between fecal levels of SCFA and the abundance of *Bacteroides* and other members of the phylum Bacteroidetes.

THE TYPE OF CARBOHYDRATES AND AVAILABILITY OF ORGANIC NITROGEN SOURCES MODIFY *IN VITRO* THE METABOLISM OF *BACTEROIDES*

SCFA and organic acids formed in cultures of *Bacteroides* (acetate, succinate, lactate, and propionate) depend on the type of fermentable substrates, generation time and incubation period (Kotarski and Salyers, 1981; Rios-Covian et al., 2013, 2015, 2016b). Propionate is generally favored at long generation times, with complex carbohydrates, and under carbon source limitation.

We have studied the metabolism of *Bacteroides fragilis* growing in media containing different carbohydrates and nitrogen sources. Catabolic end-products formed in the presence of carbohydrates in non-defined peptone and yeast extract containing medium (BM; Rios-Covian et al., 2015) with respect to a minimal medium without no organic nitrogen source (MM; Rios-Covian et al., 2016b) evidenced higher SCFA and organic acids production in the former medium, when it was supplemented with bacterial exopolysaccharides (EPS), which are complex structures synthesized by some bacteria (**Figure 1A**). Acetate accounted for 30–54% of the total products formed in any condition, constituting a fundamental way for obtaining energy by this bacterium. An inverse correlation was found between the production of propionate plus succinate and that of lactate (Rios-Covian et al., 2015, 2016b; **Figure 1A**), this last being favored in the absence of organic nitrogen sources and with rapid fermentable carbohydrates, as occurs in MM added with glucose. Conversely, a shift toward propionate formation appears to occur in the presence of organic nitrogen when EPS are present. This probably reflects a preferential use of the glucolytic

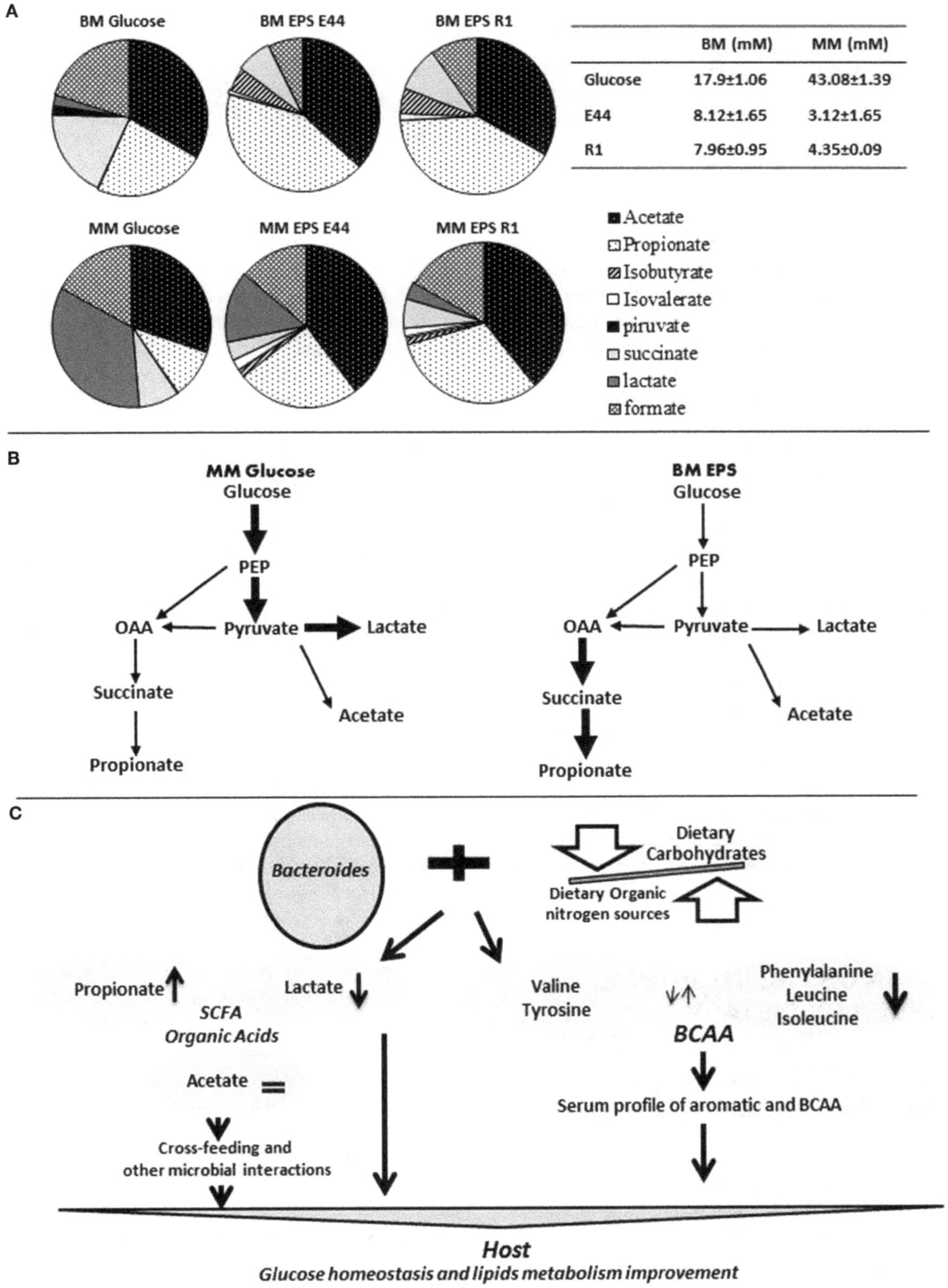

FIGURE 1 | The metabolic versatility of *Bacteroides* and the modulation of its metabolism through diet may impact human health. (A) The relative proportions of the different organic acids and SCFA produced by cultures of *Bacteroides fragilis* at 24 h of incubation in non-defined peptone and yeast extract containing medium (BM; Rios-Covian et al., 2015) and in minimal medium without no organic nitrogen source (MM; Rios-Covian et al., 2016b) and supplemented with glucose, or with exopolysaccharides produced by Bifidobacterium strains (EPS E44 and EPS R1), are represented in shaded circles. The table at the top right side indicates total concentration (mM) of SCFA plus organic acids produced by B. fragilis in the different culture conditions. **(B)** Schematic representation of

(Continued)

FIGURE 1 | Continued
catabolic routes for the formation of SCFA and organic acids by *B. fragilis*. Thick bold arrows indicate pathways probably favored in MM supplemented with glucose (left side) or in BM supplemented with bacterial EPS (right side). **(C)** Schematic representation of the general hypothesis on how re-shaping the intestinal Bacteroides metabolism through the adequate balance of dietary proteins and carbohydrates could influence human health. On the one hand, changes occurring in the profile of SCFA and organic acids produced by this bacterium could act on the host carbohydrates and lipids metabolism directly or through cross-feeding or other microbial interaction mechanisms. On the other hand, the metabolism of intestinal Bacteroides may modify blood circulating amino acids in the host, which have been related with some metabolic disorders. OAA, oxaloacetate; SCFA, short chain fatty acidis; BCAA, branched chain amino acids; PEP, phosphoenolpyruvate.

pathway and acetate formation for obtaining energy and keeping redox balance by *B. fragilis* in the presence of rapidly fermentable carbohydrates; in contrast, when complex/slowly fermentable carbohydrates are available and amino acids are present, carbon skeletons from amino acids could be incorporated at the level of pyruvate; in such conditions the propionate-succinate pathway seems to be potentiated as a way for energy obtaining whilst serving to restore cell redox balance (Rios-Covian et al., 2015; **Figure 1B**). Proteomics and gene expression analyses reinforced the hypothesis of the activation of amino acids catabolism and the succinate pathway in *B. fragilis* grown in BM with EPS (Rios-Covian et al., 2015). Therefore, the preferential metabolic route for energy production and redox maintaining, and the final metabolic products formed by *B. fragilis*, may be largely dependent on carbohydrates and nitrogen sources available. These results suggest the possibility of regulating the metabolism of *Bacteroides* by controlling dietary carbohydrate/protein balance.

Moreover, when analyzing the amino acids in cultures of *B. fragilis* added with different carbohydrates, we found a decrease in the concentration of leucine, isoleucine and phenylalanine after incubation in any condition, whereas valine and tyrosine showed much less increases or slight decreases in EPS as compared to glucose (Supplementary Material Table 2 in Rios-Covian et al., 2015). This points to a potential capacity of *B. fragilis* (as may probably occur with other Bacteroidetes) for regulating BCAA and aromatic amino acids levels in its growth environment.

MODULATION OF THE INTESTINAL *BACTEROIDES* BY DIETARY CARBON/NITROGEN SOURCES: A TOOL FOR RESTORING THE INTESTINAL MICROBIOTA METABOLIC BALANCE

Under sufficient organic nitrogen, the mildly acidic pH (5.5) stimulates butyrate producing species in the human colon curtailing the growth of *Bacteroides* that was however maximized at pH 6.5 (Walker et al., 2005). The pH in the caecum is about 5.7 but gradually increases to 6.7 in the rectum. Dietary fiber fermentation promotes a slight decrease of the luminal pH whereas high protein/amino acids fermentation, favored by low carbohydrate availability, causes slightly pH increases (Smith and MacFarlane, 1998). Interestingly, a recent study with mice demonstrated that diet-microbiome interactions are driven by the pattern of protein and carbohydrate intake (Holmes et al., 2017). Moreover, some experiments with gnotobiotic mice support shifts in *Bacteroides* metabolic functions as a response to dietary changes (McNulty et al., 2013; Wu et al., 2015).

The studies just commented support the interdependence between diet, gut microbiome and host metabolism, and allow to hypothesize that the combination of dietary organic nitrogen sources with appropriate carbohydrates may be used to modify the metabolic activity of colonic *Bacteroides* populations by modifying the profile of organic acids formed and enhancing propionate formation in some parts of the large intestine while promoting shifts toward healthier profiles of serum amino acids (**Figure 1C**).

Within this "scenario," the potential role that the functional control and metabolic reprogramming of *Bacteroides* through diet may play in the regulation of the host metabolism deserves more attention. It is essential to decipher to what extent organic nitrogen sources and carbohydrates could affect the different species of prominent intestinal bacteria, such as the genus *Bacteroides*. An important question raised is whether changes in SCFA and organic acids profile induced by remodeling the metabolic activity of *Bacteroides* through adequate dietary interventions would influence other less nutritionally versatile gut beneficial microbes through the enhancement of cross-feeding or other microbial interaction mechanisms. Omics, including metabolomics/metabonomics, applied to the analysis of microbial cultures, animal models, and human samples are necessary for understanding host and microbiota metabolic remodeling as a response to dietary combinations of organic nitrogen/carbohydrates.

The potential to re-shape the metabolism of *Bacteroides* with specific combinations of dietary carbohydrates-proteins based on their composition, structure and availability in the gut, merits further study. The final aim should be designing diets based on nutrient components targeted at modulating the metabolism of *Bacteroides,* which may interact with other intestinal beneficial microbes, in order to restore the metabolic balance of the microbiota to promote durable host's health effects.

AUTHOR CONTRIBUTIONS

DR, NS, MG, and Cd conceived the idea and designed the structure of the manuscript. All authors contributed significantly to the experimental data compared in the Figure 1A. Cd and DR drafted the manuscript and Figure. All authors have critically red, corrected, and approved the final version of the manuscript and agree with the opinions expressed here.

FUNDING

The work of the research group in the matter of this article is being currently financed by projects AGL2013-43770-R from Plan Estatal de I+D+I (Spanish Ministry of Economy and Competitiveness, MINECO) and by Grant GRUPIN14-043 from Plan Regional de Investigación del Principado de Asturias, Spain. Both national and regional grants received cofounding from European Union FEDER funds. DR-C was the recipient of a predoctoral FPI fellowship and NS benefits from a Juan de la Cierva post-doctoral contract, both granted by MINECO.

REFERENCES

Aguirre, M., Eck, A., Koenen, M. E., Svalkoul, P. H. M., Budding, A. E., and Venema, K. (2016). Diet drives quick changes in the metabolic activity and composition of human gut microbiota in a validated *in vitro* gut model. *Res. Microbiol.* 167, 114–125. doi: 10.1016/j.resmic.2015.09.006

Bervoets, L., Van Hoorenbeeck, K., Kortleven, I., Van Noten, C., Hens, N., Vael, C., et al. (2013). Differences in gut microbiota composition between obese and lean children: a cross-sectional study. *Gut Pathog.* 5:10. doi: 10.1186/1757-4749-5-10

Chambers, E. S., Viardot, A., Psichas, A., Morrison, D. J., Murphy, K. G., Zac-Varghese, S. E., et al. (2015). Effects of targeted delivery of propionate to the human colon on appetite regulation, body weight maintenance and adiposity in overweight adults. *Gut* 11, 1744–1754. doi: 10.1136/gutjnl-2014-307913

Comstock, L. E., and Coyne, M. J. (2003). Bacteroiades thetaiotaomicron: a dynamic, niche-adapted human symbiont. *Bioessays* 25, 926–929. doi: 10.1002/bies.10350

De Vadder, F., Kovatcheva-Datchary, P., Goncalves, D., Vinera, J., Zitoun, C., Duchampt, A., et al. (2014). Microbiota-generated metabolites promote metabolic benefits via gut-brain neural circuits. *Cell* 156, 84–96. doi: 10.1016/j.cell.2013.12.016

Demigne, C., Morand, C., Levrat, M. A., Besson, C., Moundras, C., and Remesy, C. (1995). Effect of propionate on fatty acid and cholesterol synthesis and on acetate metabolism in isolated rat hepatocytes. *Br. J. Nutr.* 74, 209–219. doi: 10.1079/BJN19950124

Den Besten, G., Havinga, R., Bleeker, A., Rao, S., Gerding, A., Van Eunen, K., et al. (2014). The short-chain fatty acid uptake fluxes by mice on a guar gum supplemented diet associate with amelioration of major biomarkers of the metabolic syndrome. *PLoS ONE* 9:e107392. doi: 10.1371/journal.pone.0107392

Den Besten, G., Lange, K., Havinga, R., Van Dijk, T. H., Gerding, A., Van Eunen, K., et al. (2013). Gut-derived short-chain fatty acids are vividly assimilated into host carbohydrates and lipids. *Am. J. Physiol. Gastrointest. Liver Physiol.* 305, G900–G910. doi: 10.1152/ajpgi.00265.2013

Derrien, M., Vaughan, E. E., Plugge, C. M., and de Vos, W. M. (2004). *Akkermansia muciniphila* gen. nov., sp nov., a human intestinal mucin-degrading bacterium. *Int. J. Syst. Evol. Microbiol.* 54, 1469–1476. doi: 10.1099/ijs.0.02873-0

Duncan, S. H., Belenguer, A., Holtrop, G., Johnstone, A. M., Flint, H. J., and Lobley, G. E. (2007). Reduced dietary intake of carbohydrates by obese subjects results in decreased concentrations of butyrate and butyrate-producing bacteria in feces. *Appl. Environ. Microbiol.* 73, 1073–1078. doi: 10.1128/AEM.02340-06

Duncan, S. H., Lobbley, G. E., Holtrop, G., Ince, J., Johnstone, A. M., Louis, P., et al. (2008). Human colonic microbiota associated with diet, obesity and weight loss. *Int. J. Obes.* 32, 1720–1724. doi: 10.1038/ijo.2008.155

Fernandes, J., Su, W., Rahat-Rozenbloom, S., Wolever, T. M., and Comelli, E. M. (2014). Adiposity, gut microbiota and faecal short chain fatty acids are linked in adult humans. *Nutr. Diabetes* 4, e121. doi: 10.1038/nutd.2014.23

Furet, J. P., Kong, L. C., Tap, J., Poitou, C., Basdevant, A., Bouillot, J. L., et al. (2010). Differential adaptation of human gut microbiota to bariatric surgery-induced weight loss links with metabolic and low-grade inflammation markers. *Diabetes* 59, 3049–3057. doi: 10.2337/db10-0253

Heimann, E., Nyman, M., and Degerman, E. (2015). Propionic acid and butyric acid inhibit lipolysis and *de novo* lipogenesis and increase insulin stimulated glucose uptake in primary rat adipocytes. *Adipocyte* 4, 81—88. doi: 10.4161/21623945.2014.960694

Holmes, A. J., Chew, Y. V., Colakoglu, F., Cliff, H. J., Klaassens, E., Read, M. N., et al. (2017). Diet-microbiome interactions in health are controlled by intestinal nitrogen source constraints. *Cell Metab.* 25, 140–151. doi: 10.1016/j.cmet.2016.10.021

Jumpertz, R., Le, D. S., Turnbaugh, P. J., Trinidad, C., Bogardus, C., Gordon, J. I., et al. (2011). Energy-balance studies reveal associations between gut microbes, caloric load, and nutrient absorption in humans. *Am. J. Clin. Nutr.* 94, 58–65. doi: 10.3945/ajcn.110.010132

Kotarski, S. F., and Salyers, A. A. (1981). Effect of long generation times on growth of *Bacteroides thetaiotaomicron* in carbohydrate-induced continuous culture. *J. Bacteriol.* 146, 853–860

Ley, R., Turnbaugh, P. J., Klein, S., and Gordon, J. (2006). Microbial ecology: human gut microbes associated with obesity. *Nature* 444, 1022–1023. doi: 10.1038/4441022a

Liou, A. P., Paziuk, M., Luevano, J. M., MacHineni, S., Turnbaugh, P. J., and Kaplan, L. M. (2013). Conserved shifts in the gut microbiota due to gastric bypass reduce host weight and adiposity. *Sci. Transl. Med.* 5, 178ra41. doi: 10.1126/scitranslmed.3005687

Martens, E. C., Lowe, E. C., Chiang, H., Pudlo, N. A., Wu, M., McNulty, N. P., et al. (2011). Recognition and degradation of plant cell wall polysaccharides by two human gut symbionts. *PLoS Biol.* 9:1001221. doi: 10.1371/journal.pbio.1001221

McNulty, N., Wu, M., Erickson, A., Pan, C., Erickson, B., Martens, E., et al. (2013). Effects of diet on resource utilization by a model human gut microbiota containing Bacteroides cellulosilyticus WH2, a symbiont with an extensive glycobiome. *PLoS Biol.* 11:e1001637. doi: 10.1371/journal.pbio.1001637

Neis, E. P. J. G., Dejong, C. H. C., and Rensen, S. S. (2015). The role of microbial amino acid metabolism in host metabolism. *Nutrients* 7, 2930–2946. doi: 10.3390/nu7042930

Pillot, B., Soty, M., Gautier-Stein, A., Zitoun, C., and Mithieux, G. (2009). Protein feeding promotes redistribution of endogenous glucose production to the kidney and potentiates its suppression by insulin. *Endocronology* 150, 616–624. doi: 10.1210/en.2008-0601

Reichardt, N., Duncan, S. H., Young, P., Belenguer, A., McWilliam Leitch, C., Scott, K. P., et al. (2014). Phylogenetic distribution of three pathways for propionate production within the human gut microbiota. *ISME J.* 8, 1323–1335. doi: 10.1038/ismej.2014.14

Rios-Covian, D., Arboleya, S., Hernandez-Barranco, A. M., Alvarez-Buylla, J. R., Ruas-Madiedo, P., Gueimonde, M., et al. (2013). Interactions between Bifidobacterium and Bacteroides species in cofermentations are affected by carbon sources, including exopolysaccharides produced by bifidobacteria. *Appl. Environ. Microbiol.* 79, 7518–7524. doi: 10.1128/AEM.02545-13

Rios-Covian, D., Cuesta, I., Alvarez-Buylla, J. R., Ruas-Madiedo, P., Gueimonde, M., and de los Reyes-Gavilan, C. G. (2016b). *Bacteroides fragilis* metabolises exopolysaccharides produced by bifidobacteria. *BMC Microbiol.* 16:150. doi: 10.1186/s12866-016-0773-9

Ríos-Covián, D., Ruas-Madiedo, P., Margolles, A., Gueimonde, M., de los Reyes-Gavilan, C. G., and Salazar, N. (2016a). Intestinal short chain fatty acids and their link with diet and human health. *Front. Microbiol.* 7:185. doi: 10.3389/fmicb.2016.00185

Rios-Covian, D., Sanchez, B., Salazar, N., Martinez, N., Redruello, B., Gueimonde, M., et al. (2015). Different metabolic features of *Bacteroides fragilis* growing in the presence of glucose and exopolysaccharides of bifidobacteria. *Front. Microbiol.* 6:825. doi: 10.3389/fmicb.2015.00825

Salazar, N., Dewulf, E. M., Neyrinck, A. M., Bindels, L. B., Cani, P. D., Mahillon, J., et al. (2015). Inulin-type fructans modulate intestinal Bifidobacterium species populations and decrease fecal short-chain fatty acids in obese women. *Clin. Nutr.* 34, 501–507. doi: 10.1016/j.clnu.2014.06.001

Salonen, A., Lahti, L., Salojarvi, J., Holtrop, G., Korpela, K., Duncan, S. H., et al. (2014). Impact of diet and individual variation on intestinal microbiota composition and fermentation products in obese men. *ISME J.* 8, 2218–2230. doi: 10.1038/ismej.2014.63

Smith, E. A., and MacFarlane, G. T. (1998). Enumeration of amino acid fermenting bacteria in the human large intestine: effects of pH and starch on peptide metabolism and dissimilation of amino acids. *FEMS Microbiol. Ecol.* 25, 355–368. doi: 10.1111/j.1574-6941.1998.tb00487.x

Sonnenburg, J. L., Xu, J., Leip, D. D., Chen, C. H., Westover, B. P., Weatherford, J., et al. (2005). Glycan foraging *in vivo* by an intestine-adapted bacterial symbiont. *Science* 307, 1955–1959. doi: 10.1126/science.1109051

Thaiss, C. A., Itav, S., Rothschild, D., Meijer, M., Levy, M., Moresi, C., et al. (2016). Persistent microbiome alterations modulate the rate of post-dieting weight regain. *Nature.* doi: 10.1038/nature20796

Turnbaugh, P. J., Hamady, M., Yatsunenko, T., Cantarel, B. L., Duncan, A., Ley, R. E., et al. (2009). A core gut microbiome in obese and lean twins. *Nature* 457, 480–484. doi: 10.1038/nature07540

Turnbaugh, P. J., Ley, R. E., Mahowald, M. A., Magrini, V., Mardis, E. R., and Gordon, J. I. (2006). An obesity-associated gut microbiome with increased capacity for energy harvest. *Nature* 444, 1027–1031. doi: 10.1038/nature05414

Utzschneider, K. M., Kratz, M., Damman, C. J., and Hullar, M. (2016). Mechanisms linking the gut microbiome and glucose metabolism. *J. Clin. Endocrinol. Metab.* 101, 2622–2622. doi: 10.1210/jc.2015-4251

Walker, A. W., Ince, J., Duncan, S. H., Webster, L. M., Holtrop, G., Ze, X. L., et al. (2011). Dominant and diet-responsive groups of bacteria within the human colonic microbiota. *ISME J.* 5, 220–230. doi: 10.1038/ismej.2010.118

Walker, A. W., Walker, A. W., Duncan, S. H., Leitch, E. C. M., Child, M. W., and Flint, H. J. (2005). pH and peptide supply can radically alter bacterial populations and short-chain fatty acid ratios within microbial communities from the human colon. *Appl. Environ. Microbiol.* 71, 3692–3700. doi: 10.1128/AEM.71.7.3692-3700.2005

Wu, M., McNulty, N., Rodionov, D., Khoroshkin, M., Griffin, N., Chen, J., et al. (2015). Genetic determinants of *in vivo* fitness and diet responsiveness in multiple human gut Bacteroides. *Science* 350:aac5992. doi: 10.1126/science.aac5992

Zhao, Y., Wu, J., Li, J. V., Zhou, N. Y., Tang, H., and Wang, Y. (2013). Gut microbiota composition modifies fecal metabolic profiles in mice. *J. Proteome Res.* 12, 2987–2999. doi: 10.1021/pr400263n

Zitomersky, N. L., Coyne, M. J., and Comstock, L. E. (2011). Longitudinal analysis of the prevalence, maintenance, and IgA response to species of the order Bacteroidales in the human gut. *Infect. Immun.* 79, 2012–2020. doi: 10.1128/IAI.01348-10

12

Development of a Synbiotic Beverage Enriched with Bifidobacteria Strains and Fortified with Whey Proteins

Federico Baruzzi[1]*, *Silvia de Candia*[1], *Laura Quintieri*[1], *Leonardo Caputo*[1] *and Francesca De Leo*[2]

[1] *Institute of Sciences of Food Production, National Research Council of Italy (ISPA-CNR), Bari, Italy,* [2] *Institute of Biomembranes, Bioenergetic and Molecular Biotechnologies, National Research Council of Italy (IBIOM-CNR), Bari, Italy*

***Correspondence:**
Federico Baruzzi
federico.baruzzi@ispa.cnr.it

The objective of this study was to develop a new synbiotic beverage evaluating the ability of some bifidobacteria strains to grow in this beverage which was fortified with whey proteins up to 20 g L^{-1}, and enriched with 10 g L^{-1} of prebiotic inulin or resistant starch. The ability of *Bifidobacterium* strains to survive for 30 days at 4°C was evaluated in two synbiotic whey protein fortified beverages formulated with 2% of whey proteins and 1% of inulin or resistant starch. Microbial growth was significantly affected by the whey protein amount as well as by the kind of prebiotic fiber. Resistant starch promoted the growth of the *Bifidobacterium pseudocatenulatum* strain and its viability under cold storage, also conferring higher sensory scores. The development of this new functional beverage will allow to carry out *in vivo* trials in order to validate its pre- and probiotic effects.

Keywords: *Bifidobacterium*, inulin, resistant starch, whey proteins, fortified beverage

INTRODUCTION

Functional foods are defined as foods or food ingredients that may provide a health benefit beyond the basic nutrition (IOM/NAS, 1994; Gibson and Williams, 2000). In the last century, a huge amount of research describes the role of *Bifidobacterium* genus in promoting human and animal health (Preising et al., 2010; Fukuda et al., 2011; Russell et al., 2011). Bifidobacteria have been also proposed to promote the correct microbial equilibrium of the intestinal microbiota in preterm infants (Szajewska et al., 2010) due to their beneficial effects on human health and predominance in the intestinal microflora. Furthermore, it has been demonstrated that the consumption of indigestible carbohydrates, such as resistant starch (RS), can enhance positive biological effects induced by natural occurring bifidobacteria in the human gastrointestinal tract and usually defined as prebiosis (Saulnier et al., 2009).

Indeed, bifidobacteria, exploiting their unique glycosidases, transporters, and metabolic enzymes for sugar fermentation, are able to activate fermentable molecules in an environment poor in nutrition and oxygen (Fushinobu, 2010).

Resistant starch, naturally present in many vegetables (e.g., plantains, green bananas, roots, and legumes) or obtained from processed cereals (Quintieri et al., 2012b), withstand the upper gastrointestinal digestive enzymes; in the distal colon, RS, can be preferentially and specifically hydrolyzed by bifidobacteria displaying bifidogenic effects (Nugent, 2005; Queiroz-Monici et al., 2005; Regmi et al., 2011).

Inulin, a linear D-fructose polymer containing small amounts of branched fructose by β(2-1)-glycosidic bonds with a terminal glucose moiety, is naturally present in several plants (Van Loo et al., 1995); it is partially fermented in the distal colon by bifidobacteria with a consequent increase in their population (De Vuyst and Leroy, 2011).

The microbial fermentation of both inulin and RS in the colon produces short chain fatty acids (SCFA; acetate, propionate, and butyrate, lactate), succinate, hydrogen and carbon dioxide; these metabolites, and in particular butyrate, are considered to improve water absorption in the large bowel, to modulate colonic muscular activity, to inhibit the growth of cancer cells, to stimulate the growth of normal cells, and to promote DNA repair in damaged cells, as recently reviewed by Topping et al. (2008). Based on these studies, World Health Organization (WHO) recommends to supplement the diet with low-carb fiber-rich meals in order to maximize colonic disease prevention and reduce body weight (WHO, 2015); thus, inulin and RS are commonly used to enrich different kinds of foods (Crittenden R.G. et al., 2001; Brown, 2004; Topping et al., 2008; Fushinobu, 2010; Pokusaeva et al., 2011). In addition to indigestible fibers, milk proteins also showed bifidogenic effects. In particular, α-lactalbumin was found to promote the growth of *Bifidobacterium breve*, *Bifidobacterium bifidum*, *Bifidobacterium infantis*, as well as caseinomacropeptide, isolated from whey protein concentrates, and supplemented in milk was reported to increase *Bifidobacterium lactis* counts in probiotic fermented milks (Pihlanto-Leppälä et al., 1999; Janer et al., 2004). The hydrolysates of whey proteins also boosted the growth of *Bifidobacterium animalis* subsp. *lactis* BB12 in yogurt preparation (Tian et al., 2015). Moreover, whey protein hydrolysates are rich in peptides endowed with hypotensive, anticancer, opioid antagonistic, and immunomodulatory properties (Morris and Fitzgerald, 2009). Antimicrobial peptides released from many whey proteins (Naidu, 2000) were also found useful for improving food safety and quality (Quintieri et al., 2012a, 2013; Baruzzi et al., 2015; Caputo et al., 2015). The nutritional and physiological aspects of whey protein based foods are well known as previously reported (Walzem et al., 2002; Morris and Fitzgerald, 2009) and, due to their high amount of digestible proteins and branched amino acids, they are usually consumed by sportsmen to strengthen the muscle anabolism (Walzem et al., 2002; Tang et al., 2009; Pennings et al., 2011; Deutz et al., 2014). Moreover, whey proteins could be also useful for debilitated subjects or people under restrictive diets (such as elderly people, gastrectomized or immunocompromised patients). The consumer demand for a daily intake of fibers and molecules with high nutritional value (as reported by WHO, 2003; National Health and Medical Research Council [NHMRC] and New Zealand Ministry of Health, 2006; Fungwe et al., 2007; EFSA Panel on Dietetic Products, Nutrition, and Allergies (NDA), 2010) has driven this work toward the optimization of a beverage endowed with these features.

Therefore, in this work three bifidobacteria strains (*B. animalis* subsp. *lactis* BI1 and BB12 and *B. breve* BBR8) also applied from the production of probiotic dairy foods (such as BB12) and the *Bifidobacterium pseudocatenulatum* M115 endowed with promising pro-healthy features were chosen in order to develop a new synbiotic beverage. Firstly, the influence of inulin and RS on the viability of bifidobacteria in a fermented whey protein medium was evaluated under laboratory conditions. Then, a synbiotic whey protein beverage enriched with prebiotic fibers was set up and characterized for microbial viability, residual fiber content, and organoleptic properties throughout cold storage period.

MATERIALS AND METHODS

Experimental plan was arranged on three levels (**Figure 1**) that included the optimization of a whey based medium (WBM) able to sustain bifidobacteria growth (1), the selection of bifidobacteria strains fermenting fibers in WBM (2), then the set up of the synbiotic beverage (3) which was evaluated for its shelf life and sensory profile over 30 days of cold storage.

Microorganisms and Media

The strains *B. animalis* subsp. *lactis* BI1 and *B. breve* BBR8 were a gift of the Centro Sperimentale del Latte S.r.l. (Lodi, Italy), the *B. pseudocatenulatum* M115 was from the Dairy Research Institute of Asturias (IPLA, Villaviciosa, Spain, Department of Science and Food Technology of the Spanish National Research Council, CSIC) and *B. animalis* subsp. *lactis* BB12 was previously isolated and included in the ISPA-CNR bacterial collection.

Fresh microbial cultures of bifidobacteria strains from frozen cultures (−80°C) were routinely grown in MRS (MRS Agar ISO Formulation, Biolife Italiana srl, Milan, Italy) amended with 0.5 g L^{-1} of L-cysteine (MRSC) for 48h at 37°C under anaerobic conditions (ANAEROGEN, AN0025, Oxoid S.p.A., Milan, Italy).

Growth of Bifidobacterium Strains in Whey-Based Medium (WBM)

Bifidobacteria strains were evaluated for their ability to grow in whey-based media (WBM). Whey protein isolate (WPI, Mirabol® Whey Protein Natural 97, Volchem s.r.l., Grossa di Gazzo, Italy), containing *ca.* 97 g of whey proteins on 100 g of powder, was diluted in distilled water in order to obtain two WBM at 10 and 20 g L^{-1} of total protein (WBM10 and WBM20). Based on Mirabol®'s nutritional fact, the raw composition per liter of WBM10 included 5 g of β-lactoglobulin, 1.7 g of α-lactalbumin, 1.8 g of other whey proteins, 0.02 g of simple sugars, 0.04 g of lipids; the protein concentration in WBM10 allowed to estimate a content 2.3 and 0.5 g L^{-1} of branched chain and sulfur-containing amino acids, respectively. In the case of WBM20 the concentration of nutrients doubled. In addition, WBM were supplemented with 0.5 g L^{-1} of L-cysteine and 10 g L^{-1} of lactose. Fresh bifidobacteria cultures were diluted in sterile saline solution in order to read an absorbance at 600 nm of 0.4 ± 0.05 (*ca.* 8 log cfu mL^{-1}), further diluted 1000 times in WBM10 and WBM20 and incubated as above described; MRSC was used as positive control. Then, bifidobacteria were enumerated on Bifidus Selective Medium (BSM) agar plates (Sigma–Aldrich SRL, Milan, Italy) recording pink-purple colored colonies. WBMs were also enriched with prebiotic fiber by the addition of 10 g L^{-1} of

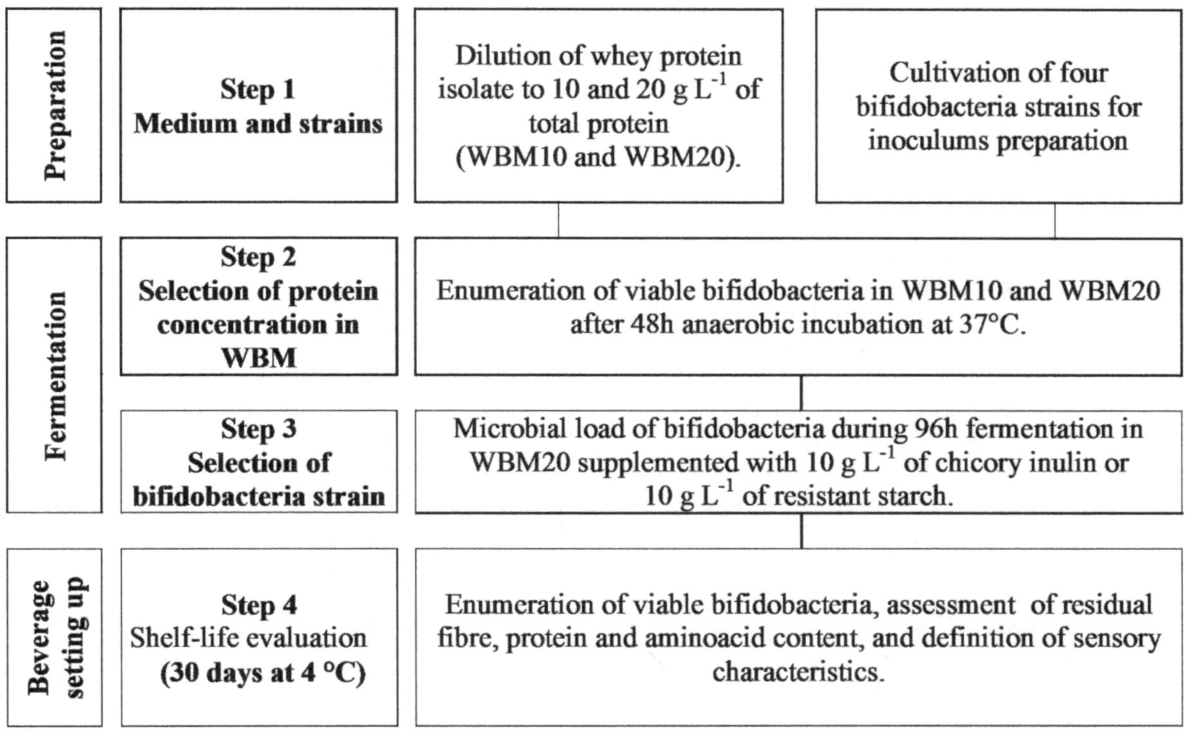

FIGURE 1 | Graphical scheme of the experimental plan carried out in the present work.

chicory inulin with a degree of polymerization > 23 (Orafti HP, BENEO-Orafti, Tienen, Belgium) or 10 g L^{-1} of retrograded RS (Novelose® 330, Ingredion Incorporated, Westchester, IL, USA) and then pasteurized at 110°C × 5 min. In order to reduce whey protein precipitation, thermal treatment parameters were set up by preliminary assays; however, the efficacy of pasteurization was preserved. Prebiotic WBMs were cooled at room temperature and then inoculated with fresh cultures of bifidobacteria, as described above. Strains were incubated under anaerobic conditions at 37°C up to 96 h. Viable cell evaluations were carried out in triplicate every 24 h, as described above.

Set Up of a Whey Protein Fortified Beverage Enriched with Prebiotic Fibers (WPF Beverage)

Two synbiotic whey protein fortified beverages enriched with prebiotic fiber (500 ml) were obtained, in triplicate, by supplementing WBM, at the protein concentration selected in the section "Growth of Bifidobacterium Strains in Whey-based Medium (WBM)," with inulin or with RS (1%). Glass bottles were filled with WPF beverages leaving less than 5 ml empty space on the top of the fluid, under the cork. After pasteurization and cooling, WPF beverages were inoculated with the bifidobacteria strains M115 or BBR8 (**Figure 1**, Step 3) at approximately 4 log cfu mL^{-1} by using a fresh bifidobacteria culture.

WPF beverages were incubated at 37°C under anaerobic conditions in order to obtain a concentration of bifidobacteria of at least 8 log cfu mL^{-1}; depending on the results achieved in the fermentation assays, the incubation ranged from 48 to 72 h. After fermentation, WPF beverages were refrigerated at 4°C for 30 days. WPF beverages without bifidobacteria were also prepared as negative controls.

Chemical and Microbiological Analyses of WPF Beverage

During cold storage (at days 0, 15, and 30), each WPF beverage was evaluated for pH (Model pH50 Lab pHMeter XS-Instrument, Concordia, Italy), concentration of viable bifidobacteria, residual fiber, protein and aminoacid content, and sensory characteristics. The percentage of resistant starches and inulin were determined with the KR-STAR kit and with the K-FRUCHK kit (Megazyme International Ltd., Wicklow, Ireland), respectively, following the manufacturer's instructions.

Protein concentration was determined by the Bradford Method whereas small peptide and aminoacid concentrations were determined after derivatization with *o*-phthaldialdehyde as previously described (Baruzzi et al., 2012).

Sensory Evaluation of WPF Beverage

Sensory evaluation was performed recruiting three groups of five habitual consumers of milk beverages. The samples (30 mL) of the different beverages, stored at 4°C for 0, 15, and 30 days, were served at 12 + 1°C in white plastic cups coded with random three-digit numbers, and mineral water at room temperature was provided for mouth-rising. The overall acceptability of each sample was calculated using a 9-point hedonic scale ranging from 1 ("dislike extremely") to 9 ("like extremely") and the level of suitability of taste, sweetness, milky appearance, flavor, and mouthfeel, using a 5-point just about right (JAR) scale (1 = too weak, 3 = just about right; 5 = too strong), was followed for each sample, according to Villegas et al. (2010).

Statistical Analysis

The concentration of viable cells in samples was calculated as the average number of colonies found for each decimal dilution, corrected by the dilution factor and expressed as the log cfu mL^{-1} ± standard deviation. Bifidobacteria viable cell counts, RS and inulin content were analyzed by one-way analysis of variance (ANOVA) carried out using IBM SPSS Statistics 22 (IBM Corporation, Armonk, NY, USA). Tukey's test and Fisher LSD *post hoc* test were applied in order to evaluate significant differences ($P \leq 0.05$) among means of viable cell counts and dietary fibers, respectively. In order to compare inoculum levels as well as viable cell load recorded after the same period of incubation among different experiments, the Mann–Whitney non-parametric test was applied.

The independent effects and interactions of the main factors (times of storage, beverages and sensory attributes) on sensory scores were evaluated applying a three- and two-way ANOVA ($P \leq 0.05$); multiple comparisons among individual means of the same strain were made by Fisher's LSD *post hoc* test after rejecting the homogeneity of their variances with the Levene's test ($P \leq 0.05$).

RESULTS AND DISCUSSION

Effect of Whey Proteins on Bifidobacteria Growth

The viable cell counts of Bifidobacteria, grown for 48 h at 37°C, in MRSC and in WBM supplemented with different amount of whey proteins (10 or 20 g L^{-1}; WBM10, WBM20), were reported in **Table 1**. WBM20 cultures of M115, BBR8, and BI1 showed cell counts significantly higher ($P < 0.05$) than those retrieved in WBM10, although all cultures reached the highest load values in MRSC (9.08 log cfu mL^{-1} on average). This result was in accordance with preliminary experiments carried out using different amounts of whey protein concentrate at 80% of proteins (Baruzzi et al., 2014). Furthermore, BB12 cell counts (7.75 log cfu mL^{-1}, on average) in WBM10 and WBM20 were consistent with results of Matijević et al. (2008), who also reported no significant difference in cultures of this strain grown in medium containing 1.5 or 3% of whey protein concentrate. On the basis of these results, the 20 g L^{-1} concentration was chosen for the subsequent analyses.

TABLE 1 | Viable cell counts (mean values ± standard deviation of three independent experiments, expressed as log cfu mL^{-1}) of *Bifidobacterium* strains in MRSC and WBM at 10 and 20 g L^{-1} protein concentration after 48h of anaerobic fermentation at 37°C.

Strain	MRSC	WBM10	WBM20
B. animalis ssp. *lactis* BB12	9.37 ± 0.38^a	7.40 ± 0.27^b	8.09 ± 0.27^b
B. animalis ssp. *lactis* BI1	8.61 ± 0.34^a	4.37 ± 0.31^c	6.73 ± 0.33^b
B. breve BBR8	9.55 ± 0.08^a	4.65 ± 0.19^c	7.43 ± 0.22^b
B. pseudocatenulatum M115	8.80 ± 0.73^a	4.50 ± 0.46^c	7.40 ± 0.38^b

Initial average microbial log cfu mL^{-1} 4.57 ± 0.05. Different letters indicate significant differences ($P < 0.05$) for a least significant difference (LSD) of: BB12, 0.97; BI1, 1.03; BBR8, 0.56; M115, 1.69.

Effect of Dietary Fibers on Bifidobacteria Growth

Aimed at promoting bifidobacteria growth at the similar levels of MRSC, used as a reference medium, within the same period of incubation, WBM enriched with total whey proteins to 20 g L^{-1} (WBM20) was amended with additional carbon sources different from lactose.

Therefore, the WBM20 was supplemented with 10 g L^{-1} of inulin (WBM20-I) or RS (WBM20-RS), as already assayed by Crittenden R. et al. (2001) and Rossi et al. (2005). Inulin and RS were selected as indigestible for humans but favor bifidobacteria growth. **Figure 2** showed that the addition of 10 g L^{-1} of inulin or the addition of 10 g L^{-1} of RS to WBM20 (containing 10 g L^{-1} of lactose) allowed to obtain microbial growth values similar to those occurred in MRS containing 20 g L^{-1} of glucose only when time of incubation was extended.

However, bifidobacteria growth kinetics demonstrated to be different after WBM20 was supplemented with inulin or RS; in particular, BI1 was negatively affected by both probiotic fibers, whilst M115 was favored by RS. Inulin caused a significant and faster growth increase of both M115 and BBR8 strains. Mann–Whitney analysis also showed the viable cell concentrations of all strains at T0 and T48 throughout the experiments of steps 2 and 3 were similar ($P > 0.05$) at experimental steps 2 and 3 (**Table 1** and **Figure 1**).

In accordance with previous studies, our results showed the bifidobacteria growth in presence of glucose (herein included in MRS) or other monosaccharides was improved in presence of complex carbohydrates (Palframan et al., 2003; Rossi et al., 2005; Rada et al., 2008).

Since amylolytic activity is present in approximately 60% of bifidobacteria species (Crittenden R. et al., 2001) only BB12 and M115 strains increased their viable cell loads after the addition of 10 g L^{-1} of RS to WBM20. This finding agrees with Wronkowska et al. (2006) demonstrating either a good growth and an acidifying activity of bifidobacteria in fermented heat-treated starch. With regards to inulin supplementation, the higher cell loads were found only for the M115 and BBR8 strains in WBM20-I, compared to WBM20, and results were in accordance with Selak et al. (2016) reporting the heterogeneously inulin hydrolysis spread among Bifidobacteria species.

Moreover, in this work the growth of *B. pseudocatenulatum* M115 was favored by inulin-type fructans at each time of sampling over 72 h incubation suggesting the presence and expression of β-fructofuranosidase genes as already reported (Janer et al., 2004; Omori et al., 2010). In addition, M115 was the only strain able to grow better also in presence of RS; this behavior could be attributed to the occurrence of glycosyl transferase, starch, and glycoside hydrolase genes generally found in the

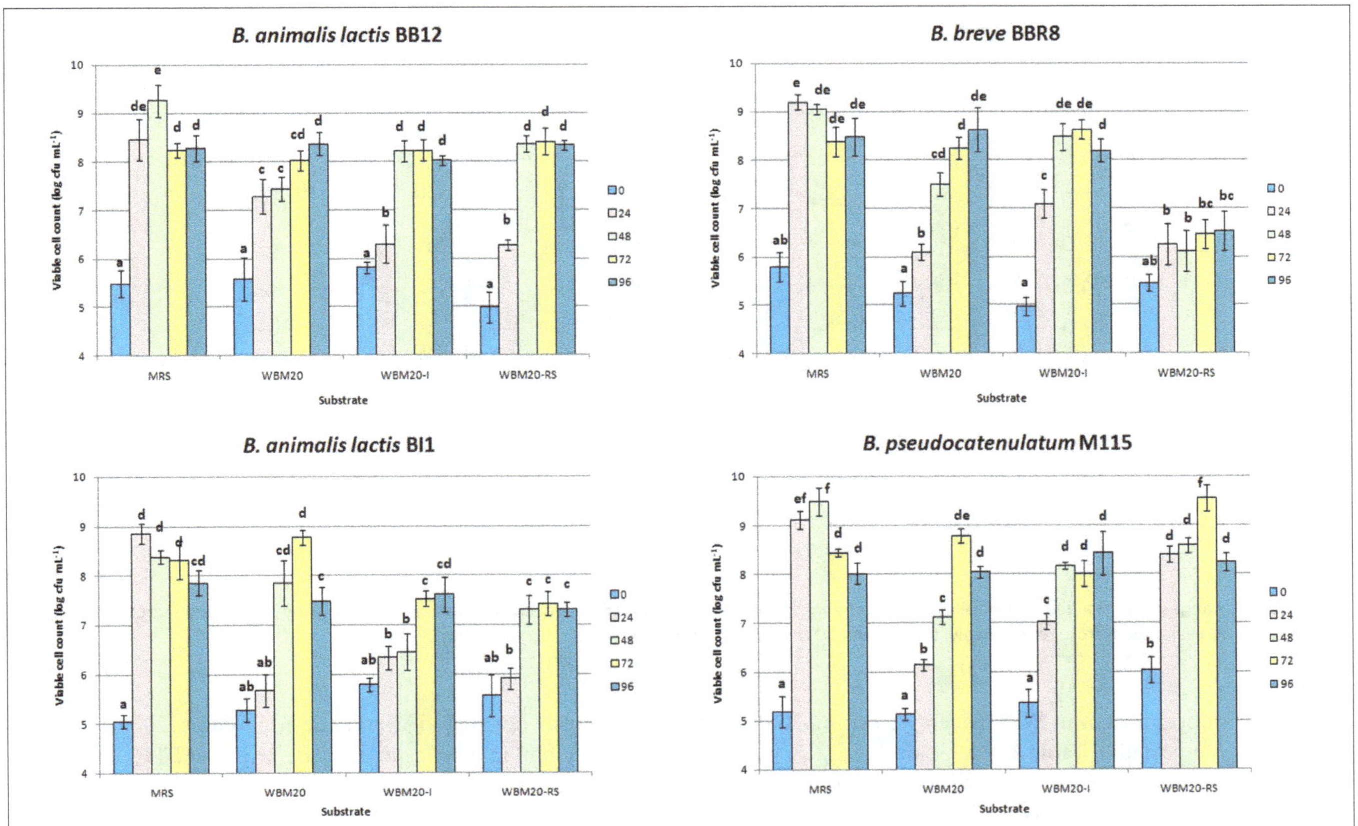

FIGURE 2 | Viable cell concentration of bifidobacteria strains throughout 96 h of anaerobic incubation at 37°C in MRS and in medium containing 20 g L^{-1} of whey proteins (WBM20), in WBM20 supplemented with 10 g L^{-1} of chicory inulin (WBM20-I) or 10 g L^{-1} of resistant starch (WBM20-RS). Bars represent mean value of viable cell count of three independent experiments (± standard deviation); values with different lowercase letters are significantly different ($P < 0.05$) according Tukey's test, within the same strain comparison.

genome of bifidobacteria (Liu et al., 2015) and particularly in the genome of the probiotic strain *B. pseudocatenulatum* IPLA 36007 (Alegría et al., 2014). These results increase the knowledge about the *B. pseudocatenulatum* M115 already proposed as a powerful probiotic strain thanks to its interesting pro-healthy features (Delgado et al., 2008; Losurdo et al., 2013).

Effect of Cold Storage on Viability of Bifidobacteria in WPF Beverages

In the light of previous results, the strain BI1 was excluded as both fibers reduced its viable cell load, conversely, the BBR8 was considered for beverage production only when WBM20 was supplemented with inulin as this fiber promoted its growth within 48 h.

As concerns BB12 and M115, the viable cell loads of both strains increased in WBM20-RS in comparison with WBM20 after 48 and 72 h, respectively. However, due to higher value reached by M115, this strain was selected and BB12 was excluded.

Thus, two synbiotic beverages fortified with whey proteins (at 20 g L^{-1}; WPF) were manufactured: the first beverage contained inulin and the strain BBR8, whilst the second one contained RS and it was fermented with the strain M115. After fermentation (48 h for the BBR8 and 72 h for the M115), WPF beverages were stored at 4°C evaluating viable cell count and pH (**Figure 3**) until day 30.

Confirming the results of preliminary fermentation assays, bifidobacteria reached a load by means of 8.5 log cfu mL^{-1}; then a reduction of *ca.* 2 log cycles was found in beverages within 15 days of cold storage. Subsequently, cell concentration remained stable for *B. pseudocatenulatum* M115, whereas a further reduction was observed in *B. breve* BBR8 reaching *ca.* 4.9 log cfu mL^{-1} (**Figure 3**).

TABLE 2 | Fiber content in WPF beverages calculated before and after fermentation and throughout 30 days of cold storage.

	Inulin (g L^{-1})[1]	RS (g L^{-1})[2]
Pre-pasteurization	6.77 ± 0.36^{a}	6.53 ± 1.08
Post-pasteurization	5.77 ± 0.53^{ab}	5.10 ± 0.83
T0f	6.52 ± 0.42^{a}	6.73 ± 0.75
T48f/T0cs	4.74 ± 0.43^{b}	5.46 ± 1.99
T15cs	3.24 ± 0.51^{c}	5.16 ± 0.94
T30cs	2.65 ± 0.43^{c}	7.26 ± 1.55

f, fermentation; cs, cold storage. Different letters represent average values statistically different ($P < 0.05$) according to Tukey's test within column. [1]*WPF beverage fermented with B. breve BBR8.* [2]*WPF beverage fermented with B. pseudocatenulatum M115.*

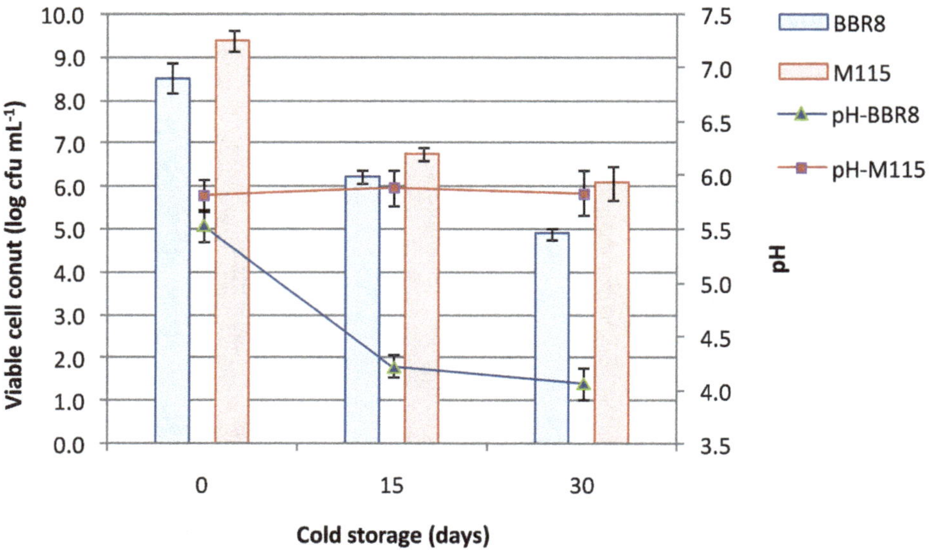

FIGURE 3 | Changes in pH values and viability of *Bifidobacterium breve* BBR8 and *B. pseudocatenulatum* M115 in whey beverages supplemented with inulin and resistant starch, respectively, throughout 30 days of cold storage.

The fiber concentration in WPF beverages during 30 days of cold storage is reported in **Table 2**.

In the case of inulin, after its supplementation in WPF beverage, its concentration was 6.77 ± 0.36 g L^{-1}, far below the estimated amount reported on the product label (10 g L^{-1} of Orafti® HP, corresponding to *ca.* 9.9 g of pure inulin); this difference could be attributed to the different methods used to determine fructans, AOAC 997.08, as stated by the BENEO-Orafti, and the AOAC 999.03 of the Megazyme kit used in this work. At the end of cold storage inulin concentration halved (**Table 2**).

At contrary, the amount of RS remained quite stable (*ca.* 6 g L^{-1}) during both the manufacturing process and the first 15 days of cold storage (**Table 2**). The large standard deviation found in the concentration of RS could be ascribed to their low solubility in water phase; in addition, as reported by the K-RSTAR kit manufacturers, higher errors are expected for samples with RS content lower than 2%.

Since the concentration of RS did not change during preparation, fermentation, and cold storage, it is possible to argue that the growth improvement recorded for M115 (**Figure 2**) could be due to non-resistant polysaccharides supplied with Novelose® 330.

At the end of fermentation, the total protein content of BBR8- or M115-fermented beverages, did not change significantly ($P < 0.05$) remaining stable at their initial average value of 4.19 ± 0.13 mg mL^{-1}. Conversely, the concentrations of small peptides and amino acids dropped from 161.6 ± 4.8 (control samples) to 11.99 ± 0.36 and 8.58 ± 0.26 μg mL^{-1} for BBR8 and M115 strains, respectively. No changes in total protein content as well as in small peptide and amino acid contents were found in both WPF beverages during cold storage (data not shown).

As concerns the reduction of viability of BBR8 and MM115 strains during refrigerate period, our result agreed with those of Donkor et al. (2006) and Jayamanne and Adams (2009) reporting the reduction in viable cells of *B. lactis* LAFTI® B94 or of *B. longum* and *B. animalis* ssp. *lactis* strains in yogurt over cold storage, respectively. Part of this decrease could be also attributed to the absence of L-cysteine that did not protect bifidobacteria cells against deleterious effects of cold storage, as demonstrated in refrigerated milk by Bolduc et al. (2006). We removed L-cysteine to avoid a negative influence on flavor. Refrigeration temperature hampered the increase in microbial load; in addition, cell viability was negatively affected by the post-acidification phenomenon as recently reported for six bifidobacteria cold stored for 21 days in milk (Djelled et al., 2016).

In our beverages the survival of bifidobacteria reached the same levels reported by Kailasapathy (2006) after cell microencapsulation, and was higher than that found by Antunes et al. (2005) in a probiotic yogurt containing a *B. longum* strain and enriched with both whey protein concentrate and skim milk powder. It is possible to argue that the occurrence of fibers in WPF beverages helped the survival of bifidobacteria as demonstrated by Crittenden R.G. et al. (2001) in yogurt supplemented with both RS and inulin, throughout 5 weeks of cold storage period. The inulin supplementation (40 mg g^{-1} of reconstituted skim milk) has been already reported by de Souza Oliveira et al. (2011, 2012), to cause an increase in the viable cell load of a *B. animalis* subsp. *lactis* strain or in the biomass of lactic acid bacteria; however, no data were produced about potential inulin consumption. The decrease in the inulin content found during 30 days of cold storage (to about 40% of the initial amount) suggests that inulin was consumed by the strain. The reduction in the inulin content together with the drop in pH values could be consistent with the production of SCFA from this fiber as already demonstrated either by single strains (Marx et al., 2000) and fecal cultures (Pompei et al., 2008; De Vuyst and Leroy, 2011).

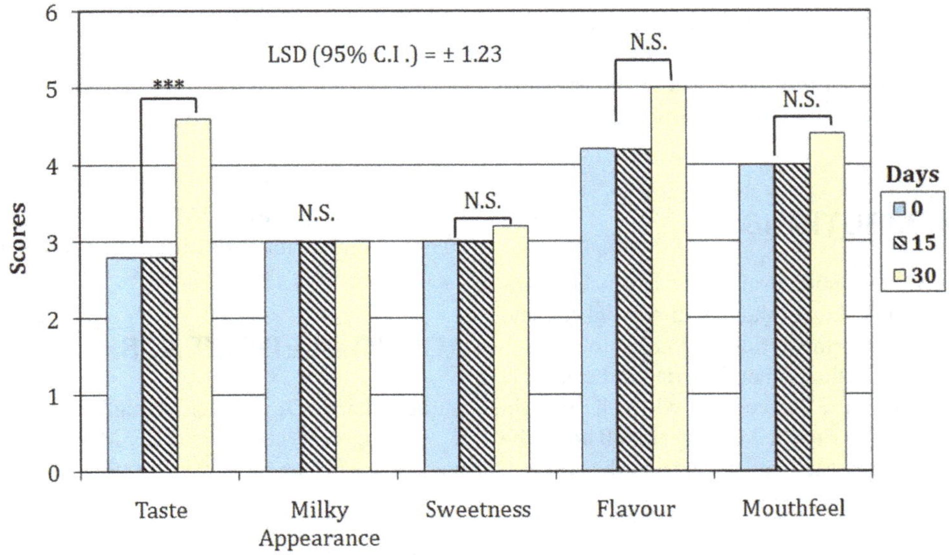

FIGURE 4 | Sensory attributes of WPF beverages fermented by bifidobacteria throughout the cold storage. Scores attributed with a 5-point just about right (JAR) scale (1 = too weak, 3 = just about right; 5 = too strong). NS, values are not significantly different; ***values were found significanlty different for $P < 0.01$.

The bifidogenic effect of RS has been widely reported (Wang et al., 2002; Bouhnik et al., 2004; Lesmes et al., 2008); however, to the best of our knowledge, no studies were reported about the effect of RS on the growth of bifidobacteria monocolture and their fate in milk-based beverage under the experimental conditions reported in this work. It is interesting to note that the M115 strain reached a viable cell load in WPF amended with RS close to that found in different milk based foods and considered sufficient to provide therapeutic benefits (Shin et al., 2000; Pérez-Conesa et al., 2005). Differently from the WPF beverage amended with inulin, the stable content of RS during storage suggests that this WPF beverage could contribute to the adult dietary fiber daily intake.

As concerns protein content, the results of this work confirm the well known low proteolytic activity of *Bifidobacterium* strains, in particular when compared with that of lactic acid bacteria (Klaver et al., 1993), that in our case assimilated preferentially free amino acids for their metabolisms during fermentation.

Sensory Evaluation of WPF Beverages

Sensory evaluation showed the overall acceptability decreased from 7.8 to 4.6 and from 6.8 to 4.2 for WPF with inulin and RS, respectively. As concerns sensory descriptors, the three-way interaction between beverage, time of storage and sensory attributes was not statistically significant ($p = 0.657$); thus, the scores of attributes changed only in relation to the beverage and throughout the time of cold storage. Therefore, in order to examine the effect of the attributes in relations to the time on sensory score only two-way ANOVA analyses were statistically allowed ($P < 0.00001$) for each beverage. Indeed, the simple main effect analysis showed the sensory scores of the beverage M115 were significantly ($P < 0.00001$) higher than those registered by BBR8 only in relation to the mouthfeel notes (data not shown). By contrast, both beverages showed, on average, a highly significant ($P < 0.01$) increase in the taste score only after 30 days of cold storage (**Figure 4**).

The overall acceptability of WPF beverages, at the early stage of cold storage, showed values similar to those previously found in a probiotic yogurt containing skim milk powder and WPC (Antunes et al., 2005). The worsening in sensory attributes was previously found in a yogurt containing microencapsulated bifidobacteria cells (Kailasapathy, 2006). The sensory scores registered for the WPF beverages including RS and fermented with the M115 strain could be partially attributed to the positive influence of RS in accordance with results of Kailasapathy (2006) suggested as positive effect of capsulant and filler materials (alginate and Hi-Maize^{TM} Starch) in masking the grittiness (mouthfeel) of the yogurt fermented with bifidobacteria.

CONCLUSION

The present work demonstrates that a whey-based substrate sustains the growth of bifidobacteria monocultures allowing to obtain a fermented beverage containing 20 g L^{-1} of whey proteins that are rich in branched chain and sulfur-containing amino acids.

The supplementation with prebiotic fibers improves the growth rate of some *Bifidobacterium* strains leading to set up a synbiotic food. In addition, after fermentation, the strains assayed resulted able to survive in these beverages under cold storage without being freeze dried, spray dried, or microencapsulated (McMaster and Kokott, 2005; Kailasapathy, 2006; Yeung et al., 2016).

Under the experimental conditions used in this study, the best result was obtained fermenting a whey protein medium, made up with 20 g L^{-1} of whey proteins and 10 g L^{-1} of RS, with the *B. pseudocatenulatum* M115. Further work will be addressed to improve sensory attributes of this new synbiotic whey protein fortified beverage.

AUTHOR CONTRIBUTIONS

SdC carried out experiments and evaluated viable cell loads of all Bifidobacteria strains; LQ evaluated dietary fibers and protein content throughout fermentation and cold storage; LC was responsible for sensory evaluation and carried out statistical analysis for all experiments; FDL cooperated with SdC in particular for experiment related to the M115 strain; FB being the lead investigator, designed the study and supervised the research team, drafted the manuscript and final proofreading. All authors contributed to the manuscript draft.

FUNDING

This work was supported by the Italian Ministry of Education, University and Research (MIUR) through the project PON-01-00851 "Bioinnovation for high healthy value dairy production."

ACKNOWLEDGMENTS

Authors thanks Dr. Sabino Formiglio for his technical assistance in realizing experiments and Dr. Maria Morea for her valuable suggestions for the improvement of this paper.

REFERENCES

Alegría, Á., Delgado, S., Guadamuro, L., Flórez, A. B., Felis, G. E., Torriani, S., et al. (2014). The genome of *Bifidobacterium pseudocatenulatum* IPLA 36007, a human intestinal strain with isoflavone-activation activity. *Gut pathog.* 6:31. doi: 10.1186/1757-4749-6-31

Antunes, A. E., Cazetto, T. F., and Bolini, H. (2005). Viability of probiotic micro-organisms during storage, postacidification and sensory analysis of fat-free yogurts with added whey protein concentrate. *Int. J. Dairy Technol.* 58, 169–173. doi: 10.1111/j.1471-0307.2005.00203.x

Baruzzi, F., de Candia, S., Quintieri, L., and Caputo, L. (2014). "Viability of *Bifidobacteria* strains in a whey protein fortified beverage," in *Proceedings of the 7th International Whey Conference, 7–9 September 2014*, Rotterdam.

Baruzzi, F., Lagonigro, R., Quintieri, L., Morea, M., and Caputo, L. (2012). Occurrence of non-lactic acid bacteria populations involved in protein hydrolysis of cold-stored high moisture Mozzarella cheese. *Food Microbiol.* 30, 37–44. doi: 10.1016/j.fm.2011.10.009

Baruzzi, F., Pinto, L., Quintieri, L., Carito, A., Calabrese, N., and Caputo, L. (2015). Efficacy of lactoferricin B in controlling ready-to-eat vegetable spoilage caused by *Pseudomonas* spp. *Int. J. Food Microbiol.* 215, 179–186. doi: 10.1016/j.ijfoodmicro.2015.09.017

Bolduc, M. P., Raymond, Y., Fustier, P., Champagne, C., and Vuillemard, J. C. (2006). Sensitivity of bifidobacteria to oxygen and redox potential in non-fermented pasteurized milk. *Int. Dairy J.* 16, 1038–1048. doi: 10.1016/j.idairyj.2005.10.030

Bouhnik, Y., Raskine, L., Simoneau, G., Vicaut, E., Neut, C., Flourié, B., et al. (2004). The capacity of nondigestible carbohydrates to stimulate fecal bifidobacteria in healthy humans: a double-blind, randomized, placebo-controlled, parallel-group, dose-response relation study. *Am. J. Clin. Nutr.* 80, 1658–1664.

Brown, I. L. (2004). Applications and uses of resistant starch. *J. AOAC Int.* 87, 727–732.

Caputo, L., Quintieri, L., Bianchi, D. M., Decastelli, L., Monaci, L., Visconti, A., et al. (2015). Pepsin-digested bovine lactoferrin prevents Mozzarella cheese blue discoloration caused by *Pseudomonas fluorescens*. *Food Microbiol.* 46, 15–24. doi: 10.1016/j.fm.2014.06.021

Crittenden, R., Laitila, A., Forssell, P., Mättö, J., Saarela, M., Mattila-Sandholm, T., et al. (2001). Adhesion of bifidobacteria to granular starch and its implications in probiotic technologies. *Appl. Environ. Microbiol.* 67, 3469–3475. doi: 10.1128/AEM.67.8.3469-3475.2001

Crittenden, R. G., Morris, L. F., Harvey, M. L., Tran, L. T., Mitchell, H. L., and Playne, M. J. (2001). Selection of a *Bifidobacterium* strain to complement resistant starch in a synbiotic yoghurt. *J. Appl. Microbiol.* 90, 268–278. doi: 10.1046/j.1365-2672.2001.01240.x

de Souza Oliveira, R. P., Perego, P., de Oliveira, M. N., and Converti, A. (2011). Effect of inulin as prebiotic and synbiotic interactions between probiotics to improve fermented milk firmness. *J. Food Eng.* 107, 36–40. doi: 10.1016/j.jfoodeng.2011.06.005

de Souza Oliveira, R. P., Torres, B. R., Perego, P., de Oliveira, M. N., and Converti, A. (2012). Co-metabolic models of *Streptococcus thermophilus* in co-culture with *Lactobacillus bulgaricus* or *Lactobacillus acidophilus*. *Biochem. Eng. J.* 62, 62–69. doi: 10.1016/j.bej.2012.01.004

De Vuyst, L., and Leroy, F. (2011). Cross-feeding between bifidobacteria and butyrate-producing colon bacteria explains bifdobacterial competitiveness, butyrate production, and gas production. *Int. J. Food Microbiol.* 149, 73–80. doi: 10.1016/j.ijfoodmicro.2011.03.003

Delgado, S., O'Sullivan, E., Fitzgerald, G., and Mayo, B. (2008). In vitro evaluation of the probiotic properties of human intestinal *Bifidobacterium* species and selection of new probiotic candidates. *J. Appl. Microbiol.* 104, 1119–1127. doi: 10.1111/j.1365-2672.2007.03642.x

Deutz, N. E., Bauer, J. M., Barazzoni, R., Biolo, G., Boirie, Y., Bosy-Westphal, A., et al. (2014). Protein intake and exercise for optimal muscle function with aging: recommendations from the ESPEN Expert Group. *Clin. Nutr.* 33, 929–936. doi: 10.1016/j.clnu.2014.04.007

Djelled, Y., Miloud, H., Eddine, M. A., and Mebrouk, K. (2016). Effect of cold storage and industrial aromas on the viability of bifidobacteria in fermented dairy products. *World J. Dairy Food Sci.* 11, 18–23.

Donkor, O. N., Henriksson, A., Vasiljevic, T., and Shah, N. P. (2006). Effect of acidification on the activity of probiotics in yoghurt during cold storage. *Int. Dairy J.* 16, 1181–1189. doi: 10.1016/j.idairyj.2005.10.008

EFSA Panel on Dietetic Products, Nutrition, and Allergies (NDA) (2010). Scientific opinion on dietary reference values for carbohydrates and dietary fibre. *EFSA J.* 8:1462.

Fukuda, S., Toh, H., Hase, K., Oshima, K., Nakanishi, Y., Yoshimura, K., et al. (2011). Bifidobacteria can protect from enteropathogenic infection through production of acetate. *Nature* 469, 543–547. doi: 10.1038/nature09646

Fungwe, T. V., Bente, L., and Hiza, H. (2007). *The Food Supply and Dietary Fiber: Its Availability and Effect on Health.* Available at: http://www.cnpp.usda.gov/sites/default/files/nutrition_insights_uploads/Insight36.pdf [accessed January 23, 2017].

Fushinobu, S. (2010). Unique sugar metabolic pathways of bifidobacteria. *Biosci. Biotechnol. Biochem.* 74, 2374–2384. doi: 10.1271/bbb.100494

Gibson, G. R., and Williams, C. M. (2000). *Functional Foods: Concept to Product.* Cambridge: Woodhead Publishing, 374. doi: 10.1533/9781855736436

IOM/NAS (1994). *Opportunities in the Nutrition and Food Sciences*, eds P. R. Thomas and R. Earl. Washington, D.C: National Academies Press, 109.

Janer, C., Rohr, L. M., Pelaez, C., Laloi, M., Cleusix, V., Requena, T., et al. (2004). Hydrolysis of oligofructoses by the recombinant beta-fructofuranosidase from *Bifidobacterium lactis*. *Syst. Appl. Microbiol.* 27, 279–285. doi: 10.1078/0723-2020-00274

Jayamanne, V. S., and Adams, M. R. (2009). Modelling the effects of pH, storage temperature and redox potential (Eh) on the survival of bifidobacteria in fermented milk. *Int. J. Food Sci. Technol.* 44, 1131–1138. doi: 10.1111/j.1365-2621.2009.01931.x

Kailasapathy, K. (2006). Survival of free and encapsulated probiotic bacteria and their effect on the sensory properties of yoghurt. *LWT Food Sci. Technol.* 39, 1221–1227. doi: 10.3168/jds.2012-5710

Klaver, F. A. M., Kingma, F., and Weerkamp, A. H. (1993). Growth and survival of bifidobacteria in milk. *Neth. Milk Dairy J.* 47, 151–164.

Lesmes, U., Beards, E. J., Gibson, G. R., Tuohy, K. M., and Shimoni, E. (2008). Effects of resistant starch type III polymorphs on human colon microbiota and short chain fatty acids in human gut models. *J. Agric. Food Chem.* 56, 5415–5421. doi: 10.1021/jf800284d

Liu, S., Ren, F., Zhao, L., Jiang, L., Hao, Y., Jin, J., et al. (2015). Starch and starch hydrolysates are favorable carbon sources for Bifidobacteria in the human gut. *BMC Microbiol.* 15, 54. doi: 10.1186/s12866-015-0362-3

Losurdo, L., Quintieri, L., Caputo, L., Gallerani, R., Mayo, B., and De Leo, F. (2013). Cloning and expression of synthetic genes encoding angiotensin-I converting enzyme (ACE)-inhibitory bioactive peptides in *Bifidobacterium pseudocatenulatum*. *FEMS Microbiol. Lett.* 340, 24–32. doi: 10.1111/1574-6968.12068

Marx, S. P., Winkler, S., and Hartmeier, W. (2000). Metabolization of β-(2, 6)-linked fructose-oligosaccharides by different bifidobacteria. *FEMS Microbiol. Lett.* 182, 163–169. doi: 10.1016/s0378-1097(99)00584-4

Matijević, B., Božanić, R., Tratnik, L., and Jeličić, I. (2008). "Fermentation of whey enriched with whey protein concentrate by bifidobacteria," in *Proceedings of the 3rd International Probiotic Conference, Probiotics for the 3rd Millennium*, ed. E. Ochabová (Bratislava: SAMEDI), 44s–44s.

McMaster, L. D., and Kokott, S. A. (2005). Micro-encapsulation of *Bifidobacterium lactis* for incorporation into soft foods. *World J. Microbiol. Biotechnol.* 21, 723–728. doi: 10.1007/s11274-004-4798-0

Morris, P. E., and Fitzgerald, R. J. (2009). "Whey proteins and peptides in human health," in *Whey Processing, Functionality and Health Benefits*, eds C. Onwulata and P. Huth (Ames, IA: John Wiley & Sons), 285–384.

Naidu, A. S. (2000). "Lactoferrin," in *Natural food Antimicrobial Systems*, ed. A. S. Naidu (Boca Raton, FL: CRC Press), 17–102. doi: 10.1201/9781420039368

National Health and Medical Research Council [NHMRC] and New Zealand Ministry of Health (2006). *Nutrient Reference Values for Australia and New Zealand including recommended dietary intakes*. Canberra, ACT: National Health and Medical Research Council.

Nugent, A. P. (2005). Health properties of resistant starch. *Nutr. Bull.* 30, 27–54. doi: 10.1111/j.1467-3010.2005.00481.x

Omori, T., Ueno, K., Muramatsu, K., Kikuchi, M., Onodera, S., and Shiomi, N. (2010). Characterization of recombinant β-fructofuranosidase from *Bifidobacterium adolescentis* G1. *Chem. Cent. J.* 4, 1–10. doi: 10.1186/1752-153X-4-9

Palframan, R. J., Gibson, G. R., and Rastall, R. A. (2003). Carbohydrate preferences of *Bifidobacterium* species isolated from the human gut. *Curr. Issues Intest. Microbiol.* 4, 71–75.

Pennings, B., Boirie, Y., Senden, J. M., Gijsen, A. P., Kuipers, H., and van Loon, L. J. (2011). Whey protein stimulates postprandial muscle protein accretion more effectively than do casein and casein hydrolysate in older men. *Am. J. Clin. Nutr.* 93, 997–1005. doi: 10.3945/ajcn.110.008102

Pérez-Conesa, D., López, G., and Rosau, G. (2005). Fermentation capabilities of bifidobacteria using nondigestible oligosaccharides, and their viability as probiotics in commercial powder infant formula. *J. Food Sci.* 70, m279–m285. doi: 10.1111/j.1365-2621.2005.tb11447.x

Pihlanto-Leppälä, A., Marnila, P., Hubert, L., Rokka, T., Korhonen, H. J. T., and Karp, M. (1999). The effect of α-lactalbumin and β-lactoglobulin hydrolysates on the metabolic activity of *Escherichia coli* JM103. *J. Appl. Microbiol.* 87, 540–545. doi: 10.1046/j.1365-2672.1999.00849.x

Pokusaeva, K., Fitzgerald, G. F., and van Sinderen, D. (2011). Carbohydrate metabolism in Bifidobacteria. *Genes Nutr.* 6, 285–306. doi: 10.1007/s12263-010-0206-6

Pompei, A., Cordisco, L., Raimondi, S., Amaretti, A., Pagnoni, U. M., Matteuzzi, D., et al. (2008). In vitro comparison of the prebiotic effects of two inulin-type fructans. *Anaerobe* 14, 280–286. doi: 10.1016/j.anaerobe.2008.07.002

Preising, J., Philippe, D., Gleinser, M., Wei, H., Blum, S., Eikmanns, B. J., et al. (2010). Selection of bifidobacteria based on adhesion and anti-inflammatory capacity in vitro for amelioration of murine colitis. *Appl. Environ. Microbiol.* 76, 3048–3051. doi: 10.1128/AEM.03127-09

Queiroz-Monici, K. D. S., Costa, G. E., da Silva, N., Reis, S. M., and de Oliveira, A. C. (2005). Bifidogenic effect of dietary fiber and resistant starch from leguminous on the intestinal microbiota of rats. *Nutrition* 21, 602–608. doi: 10.1016/j.nut.2004.09.019

Quintieri, L., Caputo, L., Monaci, L., Deserio, D., Morea, M., and Baruzzi, F. (2012a). Antimicrobial efficacy of pepsin-digested bovine lactoferrin on spoilage bacteria contaminating traditional Mozzarella cheese. *Food Microbiol.* 31, 64–71. doi: 10.1016/j.fm.2012.02.015

Quintieri, L., Monteverde, A., and Caputo, L. (2012b). Changes in prolamin and high resistant starch composition during the production process of Boza, a traditional cereal-based beverage. *Eur. Food Res. Technol.* 235, 699–709.

Quintieri, L., Pistillo, B. R., Caputo, L., Favia, P., and Baruzzi, F. (2013). Bovine lactoferrin and lactoferricin on plasma-deposited coating against spoilage *Pseudomonas* spp. *Innov. Food Sci. Emerg. Technol.* 20, 215–222. doi: 10.1016/j.ifset.2013.04.013

Rada, V., Nevoral, J., Trojanová, I., Tománková, E., Šmehilová, M., and Killer, J. (2008). Growth of infant faecal bifidobacteria and clostridia on prebiotic oligosaccharides in in vitro conditions. *Anaerobe* 14, 205–208. doi: 10.1016/j.anaerobe.2008.05.003

Regmi, P. R., Metzler-Zebeli, B. U., Gänzle, M. G., van Kempen, T. A., and Zijlstra, R. T. (2011). Starch with high amylose content and low in vitro digestibility increases intestinal nutrient flow and microbial fermentation and selectively promotes bifidobacteria in pigs. *J. Nutr.* 141, 1273–1280. doi: 10.3945/jn.111.140509

Rossi, M., Corradini, C., Amaretti, A., Nicolini, M., Pompei, A., Zanoni, S., et al. (2005). Fermentation of fructooligosaccharides and inulin by bifidobacteria: a comparative study of pure and fecal cultures. *Appl. Environ. Microbiol.* 71, 6150–6158. doi: 10.1128/AEM.71.10.6150-6158.2005

Russell, D. A., Ross, R. P., Fitzgerald, G. F., and Stanton, C. (2011). Metabolic activities and probiotic potential of bifidobacteria. *Int. J. Food Microbiol.* 149, 88–105. doi: 10.1016/j.ijfoodmicro.2011.06.003

Saulnier, D. M., Spinler, J. K., Gibson, G. R., and Versalovic, J. (2009). Mechanisms of probiosis and prebiosis: considerations for enhanced functional foods. *Curr. Opin. Biotechnol.* 20, 135–141. doi: 10.1016/j.copbio.2009.01.002

Selak, M., Rivière, A., Moens, F., Van den Abbeele, P., Geirnaert, A., Rogelj, I., et al. (2016). Inulin-type fructan fermentation by bifidobacteria depends on the strain rather than the species and region in the human intestine. *Appl. Microbiol. Biotechnol.* 100, 4097–4107. doi: 10.1007/s00253-016-7351-9

Shin, H. S., Jong-Hwa, L., Pestka, J., and Ustunol, Z. (2000). Viability of bifidobacteria in commercial dairy products during refrigerated storage. *J. Food Protect.* 63, 327–331. doi: 10.4315/0362-028X-63.3.327

Szajewska, H., Guandalini, S., Morelli, L., Van Goudoever, J. B., and Walker, A. (2010). Effect of *Bifidobacterium animalis* subsp *lactis* supplementation in preterm infants: a systematic review of randomized controlled trials. *J. Pediatr. Gastroenterol. Nutr.* 51, 203–209. doi: 10.1097/MPG.0b013e3181dc0d93

Tang, J. E., Moore, D. R., Kujbida, G. W., Tarnopolsky, M. A., and Phillips, S. M. (2009). Ingestion of whey hydrolysate, casein, or soy protein isolate: effects on mixed muscle protein synthesis at rest and following resistance exercise in young men. *J. Appl. Physiol.* 107, 987–992. doi: 10.1152/japplphysiol.00076.2009

Tian, Q., Wang, T. T., Tang, X., Han, M. Z., Leng, X. J., and Mao, X. Y. (2015). Developing a potential prebiotic of yogurt: growth of *Bifidobacterium* and yogurt cultures with addition of glycomacropeptide hydrolysate. *Int. J. Food Sci. Technol.* 50, 120–127. doi: 10.1111/ijfs.12611

Topping, D. L., Bajka, B. H., Bird, A. R., Clarke, J. M., Cobiac, L., Conlon, M. A., et al. (2008). Resistant starches as a vehicle for delivering health benefits to the human large bowel. *Microb. Ecol. Health Dis.* 20, 103–108. doi: 10.1080/08910600802106541

Van Loo, J., Coussement, P., De Leenheer, L., Hoebregs, H., and Smits, G. (1995). On the presence of inulin and oligofructose as natural ingredients in the western diet. *Crit. Rev. Food Sci. Nutr.* 35, 525–552. doi: 10.1080/10408399509527714

Villegas, B., Tárrega, A., Carbonell, I., and Costell, E. (2010). Optimising acceptability of new prebiotic low-fat milk beverages. *Food Qual. Prefer.* 21, 234–242. doi: 10.1016/j.foodqual.2009.03.001

Walzem, R. L., Dillard, C. J., and German, J. B. (2002). Whey components: millennia of evolution create functionalities for mammalian nutrition: what we know and what we may be overlooking. *Crit. Rev. Food Sci. Nutr.* 42, 353–375. doi: 10.1080/10408690290825574

Wang, X., Brown, I. L., Khaled, D., Mahoney, M. C., Evans, A. J., and Conway, P. L. (2002). Manipulation of colonic bacteria and volatile fatty acid production by dietary high amylose maize (amylomaize) starch granules. *J. Appl. Microbiol.* 93, 390–397. doi: 10.1046/j.1365-2672.2002.01704.x

World Health Organization [WHO] (2003). *Report of a Joint WHO/FAO Expert Consultation. Diet Nutrition and the Prevention of Chronic Diseases.* WHO Technical Report Series No. 916. Geneva: WHO.

World Health Organization [WHO] (2015). *Healthy diet. Fact sheet N° 394.* Geneva: WHO.

Wronkowska, M., Soral-Śmietana, M., Krupa, U., and Biedrzycka, E. (2006). In vitro fermentation of new modified starch preparations–changes of microstructure and bacterial end-products. *Enzyme Microb. Technol.* 40, 93–99. doi: 10.1016/j.enzmictec.2005.10.039

Yeung, T. W., Üçok, E. F., Tiani, K. A., McClements, D. J., and Sela, D. A. (2016). Microencapsulation in alginate and chitosan microgels to enhance viability of *Bifidobacterium longum* for oral delivery. *Front. Microbiol.* 7:494. doi: 10.3389/fmicb.2016.00494

13

Enhanced Probiotic Potential of *Lactobacillus reuteri* When Delivered as a Biofilm on Dextranomer Microspheres that Contain Beneficial Cargo

Jason B. Navarro[1], *Lauren Mashburn-Warren*[1], *Lauren O. Bakaletz*[1], *Michael T. Bailey*[1,2] *and Steven D. Goodman*[1*]

[1] *Center for Microbial Pathogenesis, The Research Institute at Nationwide Children's Hospital, Columbus, OH, USA,* [2] *Wexner Medical Center, Institute for Behavioral Medicine Research, The Ohio State University, Columbus, OH, USA*

Correspondence:
Steven D. Goodman
steven.goodman@
nationwidechildrens.org

As with all orally consumed probiotics, the Gram-positive bacterium *Lactobacillus reuteri* encounters numerous challenges as it transits through the gastrointestinal tract of the host, including low pH, effectors of the host immune system, as well as competition with commensal and pathogenic bacteria, all of which can greatly reduce the availability of live bacteria for therapeutic purposes. Recently we showed that *L. reuteri*, when adhered in the form of a biofilm to a semi-permeable biocompatible dextranomer microsphere, reduces the incidence of necrotizing enterocolitis by 50% in a well-defined animal model following delivery of a single prophylactic dose. Herein, using the same semi-permeable microspheres, we showed that providing compounds beneficial to *L. reuteri* as diffusible cargo within the microsphere lumen resulted in further advantageous effects including glucosyltransferase-dependent bacterial adherence to the microsphere surface, resistance of bound bacteria against acidic conditions, enhanced adherence of *L. reuteri* to human intestinal epithelial cells *in vitro*, and facilitated production of the antimicrobial compound reuterin and the anti-inflammatory molecule histamine. These data support continued development of this novel probiotic formulation as an adaptable and effective means for targeted delivery of cargo beneficial to the probiotic bacterium.

Keywords: *Lactobacillus reuteri*, microsphere, reuterin, glucosyltransferase, maltose, dextranomer

INTRODUCTION

Probiotic bacteria are "live microorganisms that, when administered in adequate amounts, confer a health benefit on the host" (Araya et al., 2006). Commercially, probiotics can be diverse genera of bacteria both alone and in combination are utilized for the treatment of numerous ailments and diseases, such as diarrheal diseases (McFarland, 2006; Johnston et al., 2012), infant colic (Savino et al., 2010; Sung et al., 2014), allergies (Soh et al., 2009; Stefka et al., 2014), and elevated LDL-cholesterol (Agerholm-Larsen et al., 2000; Nguyen et al., 2007).

Orally consumed beneficial bacteria face a gauntlet of challenges in the host, such as low pH in the stomach, effectors of the host immune system and competition with commensal and pathogenic bacteria (Ding and Shah, 2007). All of these factors negatively impact the ability of ingested probiotic bacteria to be sufficiently sustained within the host and thus reduce the potentially beneficial effects conferred. Commercially, encapsulation of lyophilized probiotics is used as the primary means to protect bacterial viability (Cook et al., 2012; Kailasapathy, 2014), however there is no evidence of improved probiotic persistence within the host.

We have devised a novel delivery method that utilizes hollow semi-permeable, biocompatible and biodegradable microspheres comprised of cross-linked dextran (dextranomer microspheres or DMs). We have previously shown that allowing the probiotic bacterium *Lactobacillus reuteri* to adhere to DMs prior to oral delivery reduces the incidence of experimental necrotizing enterocolitis (NEC) (a disease of high mortality in premature infants born under 1,500 g, Neu and Walker, 2011) by 50% with a single dose in a rat model of the disease (Olson et al., 2016). Importantly, in the same study, a single dose of planktonic *L. reuteri* showed no prophylactic effect. We surmised that it was delivery of the probiotic bacteria in the biofilm state that facilitated the significantly increased therapeutic value of *L. reuteri* in this model system. According to our model (as shown in **Figure 1**), bacteria on the surface of the DMs in the form of a biofilm (i.e., an adhered community of bacteria that produces a self-forming protective matrix to resist adverse environmental conditions, Hall-Stoodley et al., 2004), would also have ready access to any beneficial compounds that diffused from the lumen of the DMs.

The choice to pair the Gram-positive bacterium *L. reuteri* with DMs is many fold. *L. reuteri* is a popular choice for commercialization due to its production of lactic acid and the antimicrobial compound reuterin, a metabolite of glycerol metabolism known chemically as 3-hydroxypropionaldehyde (3-HPA), which typically exists in equilibrium with other downstream products such as 3-HPA hydrate and acrolein (Talarico et al., 1988; Engels et al., 2016). Reuterin induces oxidative stress in a broad range of microorganisms (Schaefer et al., 2010), and is highly effective at inhibiting growth of many gastrointestinal pathogens (el-Ziney and Debevere, 1998; Arques et al., 2004; Spinler et al., 2008; De Weirdt et al., 2012). In addition to the antimicrobial reuterin, *L. reuteri* also produces anti-inflammatory factors including histamine that modulate cytokine production *in vitro* (Jones and Versalovic, 2009) and ameliorate the symptoms of inflammatory bowel disease (Ghouri et al., 2014). Indeed, in animal models, *L. reuteri* can prevent the exacerbating effects of the physiological stress response on colonic inflammation. However, once administration of *L. reuteri* is terminated, colonic inflammation is again exacerbated (Mackos et al., 2016). Thus, strategies to enhance the ability of *L. reuteri* to better persist in the GI tract may have more impactful therapeutic value.

Integral to our probiotic formulation strategy is *L. reuteri*'s extracellular glucosyltransferase (GTF) protein, which in the strain of *L. reuteri* used in this study (DSM 20016, containing GTFW encoded by *gtfW*) (Leemhuis et al., 2013; Bai et al., 2015) catalyzes the formation of exopolysaccharides of glucose (glucans) from its sole known substrate maltose. Importantly,

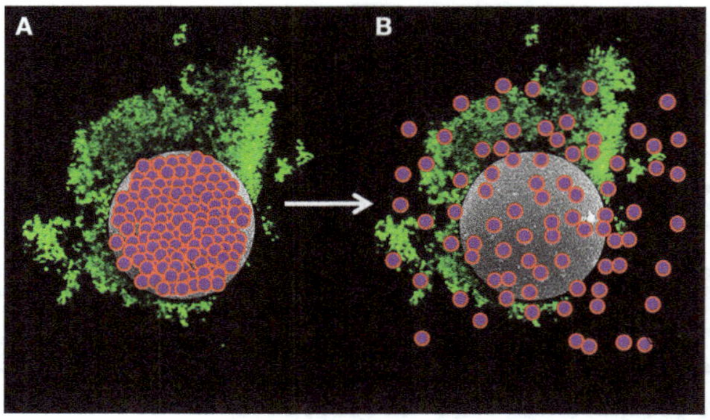

FIGURE 1 | Model of novel probiotic delivery formulation. (A) A biofilm of *L. reuteri* (green) adhered to the surface of a dextranomer microsphere (gray) that contained beneficial compounds as cargo (purple and pink spheres) within the lumen of the microsphere. **(B)** Over time, the cargo will diffuse out of the porous microsphere thereby facilitating ready access by the adhered bacteria.

GTF proteins typically have a glucan binding domain that recognizes its own produced exopolysaccharide (Monchois et al., 1999; Kralj et al., 2004). The GTF protein, its substrate, and resulting glucan product are highly strain-specific in *L. reuteri*; some are characterized as producing dextran (primarily α-1,6 linkages), mutan (primarily α-1,3 linkages), or the aptly named reuteran (primarily α-1,4 linkages) (Kralj et al., 2002, 2004). Cell aggregation, biofilm formation, and gut colonization are directly linked to the activity of GTFA in *L. reuteri* strain TMW1.106; inactivating *gtfA* significantly diminishes the ability of *L. reuteri* to aggregate, form biofilms, and colonize the GI tract *in vivo* (Walter et al., 2008).

Our novel approach was to choose DMs (a macroscopic porous microsphere that is sold commercially for size exclusion chromatography, Porath and Flodin, 1959) as a biocompatible surface so as to take advantage of *L. reuteri*'s GTFW native ability to bind to this cross-linked dextran (Tieking et al., 2005; Schwab et al., 2007; Walter et al., 2008). Our strategy is based on concurrent research which shows that the highly similar GTFs of *Streptococccus mutans*, an oral pathogen that contributes to tooth decay, binds to DMs with high affinity (Mooser et al., 1985) and, as a consequence of GTF being cell-associated, results in strong binding of *S. mutans* to DMs (Mashburn-Warren et al., submitted). Here in we show that GTFW-dependent binding of *L. reuteri* to DMs results in: one, selectivity of binding to DMs and as a result better binding of *L. reuteri* to colonic epithelial cells; two, protection against low pH and three, the ability of *L. reuteri* to acquire the luminal contents of the DMs at sufficiently high concentrations to enhance *L. reuteri*'s probiotic effects.

MATERIALS AND METHODS

Strains and Culturing Conditions

Bacterial strains, plasmids and oligonucleotides used are listed in **Table 1**. *L. reuteri* (ATCC 23272) and *Lactobacillus rhamnosus* GG (ATCC 53103) were grown in MRS (de Man, Rogosa, Sharpe) medium (De Man et al., 1960) (BD, Franklin Lakes, NJ) for

TABLE 1 | Bacterial strains, cell lines, plasmids, and oligos used in this study.

Bacterial strains	Description	Source/Reference
Lactobacillus reuteri ATCC 23272	Wild type (GTFW)	American Type Culture Collection
LMW500	*L. reuteri* 23272 Δ*gtfW*; Cm^R	This study
LMW501	*L. reuteri* 23272 + pWAR501 Cm^R	This study
LMW502	*E. coli* ER2566 + pWAR502	This study
LMW503	*L. reuteri* 23272 + pWAR503 Cm^R	This study
Lactobacillus rhamnosus GG ATCC 53102	Wild type (non-dextran forming GTF)	G. Rajashekara J.S. Gunn
Salmonella enterica serovar typhi TY2 ATCC 700931	Wild type (non-dextran forming GTF)	
Citrobacter rodentium ATCC 51459	Wild type (non-dextran forming GTF)	American Type Culture Collection
Clostridium difficile R20291 (BI/NAP1/027)	Wild type (non-dextran forming GTF)	J.K. Spinier
Human cell lines	**Description**	**Source/Reference**
DLD-1 ATCC CCL-221	Human colonic epithelial cells (colorectal adenocarcinoma)	G.E. Besner
FHs 74 Int ATCC CCL-241	Human fetal small intestinal epithelial cells	G.E. Besner
Plasmids	**Description**	**Source/Reference**
pWAR500	pFED760 (Mashburn-Warren et al., 2012) derivative containing *cat* and DNA fragments flanking *gtfW* to create insertion mutant; see Materials and Methods; Cm^R, Erm^R	This study
pWAR501	pJC156 (Mashburn-Warren et al., 2012) derivative containing the promoter region of *gtfW* upstream of the click beetle luciferase; see Materials and Methods; Cm^R	This study
pWAR502	pTXB1 derivative containing *gtfW* (with its stop codon); see Materials and Methods; Amp^R	
pWAR503	pJC156 (Mashburn-Warren et al., 2012) derivative containing the promoter region of elongation factor Tu (EF-Tu) upstream of the click beetle luciferase; see Materials and Methods; Cm^R	This study
Oligos	**DNA sequence***	**Source/Reference**
oSG1082	GCGTG**GCGGCCGC**CATTATTTTCATGTAGTGTATT T	This study
oSG1083	GCGTG**GTCGAC**CTTTTTTATGTCCATAATCTATT	This study
oSG1084	GCGTG**GTCGAC**GAAAATATTTAATATGAAAATGA	This study
oSG1085	GCGTG**CTCGAG**CCAAGCACTATTTCACGAGAAT	This study
LMW34	GCGTG**GTCGAC**GATGAAAATTTGTTTGATTT	Mashburn-Warren et al., 2012
LMW35	GCGTG**GTCGAC**TTATAAAAGCCAGTCATTAG	Mashburn-Warren et al., 2012
oSG1102	GCGTG**CTCGAG**CAACAAGAGTATCAGGGTAAAGC	This study
oSG1103	GCGTG**GTCGAC**TCCTTCCCAATAGATGATTGATT	This study
oSG1067	GCGTG**GTCGAC**ATGGTAAAACGTGAAAAAAATGT	This study
oSG1068	**GCGGCCGC**TCCGCCAGCTTTTTCTAATAACT	This study
oSG1120	GCGTG**GCTAGC**ATGAACCTGCCAACAATTCCTAA	This study
oSG1126	GCGTG**GCTCTTCCGCA**TTAAATATTTTCTTGGTTT	This study
oSG1069	GCGTG**CTCGAG**CGCAACAAATACAGTTTCTAATA	This study
oSG1070	GCGTG**GTCGAC**AAACCTCCTGATAATTTACAAGT	This study

Cm^R, chloramphenicol resistant; Erm^R, Erythromycin resistant; Amp^R, Ampicillin resistant.
Sequences in bold indicate restriction enzyme sequences.

16 h at 37°C, 5% CO_2. *Salmonella typhi* (strain JSG698) and *Citrobacter rodentium* (ATCC 51459) were grown in Lysogeny broth (LB) at 37°C, 5% CO_2. *Clostridium difficile* (strain R20291) was grown in degassed brain-heart infusion (BHI) medium (BD, Franklin Lakes, NJ) at 37°C in an anaerobic chamber (Thermo Forma Scientific, 1025 Anaerobic System, Hampton, NJ) established with an atmosphere of 5% H_2, 85% N_2, and 10% CO_2. DLD-1 (ATCC CCL-221) human colonic cells were grown in RPMI medium supplemented with 10% fetal bovine serum at 37°C, 5% CO_2. FHs 74 Int (ATCC CCL-241) human

fetal small intestinal cells were grown in Hybri-Care medium (ATCC 46-X) supplemented with 30 ng/ml epidermal growth factor (EGF) and 10% fetal bovine serum at 37°C, 5% CO_2. The *gtfW* deletion strain (LMW500) was constructed by insertion of a chloramphenicol resistance cassette (cat) into the *gtfW* open reading frame by allelic exchange as described previously (Mashburn-Warren et al., 2012). Briefly, 1kb fragments upstream and downstream of *gtfW* were amplified by PCR using oligos oSG1082-1083 and oSG1084-1085, followed by cloning into pFED760 (Mashburn-Warren et al., 2012) using NotI/SalI and SalI/XhoI restriction sites, respectively. The *cat* cassette was amplified from pEVP3 (Mashburn-Warren et al., 2012) using oligos LMW34-35, followed by cloning into pFED760 that contained the upstream and downstream fragments of *gtfW* using the SalI restriction site. The resulting *gtfW* knock-out construct plasmid (pWAR500) was then introduced into *L. reuteri* ATCC 23272 by electroporation. *L. reuteri* electrocompetent cells were prepared by growing 5 ml of culture in MRS at 37°C with 5% CO_2 until OD_{600nm} of ~1.0. Cells were then pelleted and resuspended in 10 ml of sterile cold 0.5 M sucrose and 10% glycerol twice, followed by a final resuspension in100 μl sterile cold 0.5 M sucrose and 10% glycerol. To this resuspension 1 μg of pWAR500 was added and the cell/DNA mixture was placed into an ice cold 2 mm electroporation cuvette (BioRad, Hercules, CA). Cells were electroporated at 2500V, 25 μF and 400 Ω using a BioRad Gene Pulser Xcell (BioRad, Hercules, CA). Immediately after electroporation, cells were resuspended in 1 mL of MRS and incubated at 30°C for 2 h, followed by serial dilution and plating onto MRS agar containing 5 μg/ml chloramphenicol and incubated at 30°C. The mutant was selected and confirmed as previously described (Chang et al., 2011).

To estimate transcription from the *gtfW* promoter (P_{gtfW}), the P_{gtfW}-*CBluc* reporter plasmid was constructed by amplifying the promoter region 350 bp upstream of the *gtfW* start codon (including the native ribosome binding site) by PCR using oligos oSG1102-1103. The resulting DNA fragment was inserted into pJC156 using the XhoI/SalI restriction sites. The click beetle luciferase (CBluc) gene was amplified from the *Streptococcus mutans strain* ldhCBGSm (Merritt et al., 2016) using oligos oSG1067-1068 and inserted downstream of the *gtfW* promoter region in pJC156 using SalI/NotI restriction sites. The resulting reporter plasmid pWAR501 was transformed into *L. reuteri* 23272 as described above to create the reporter strain LMW501.

The *E. coli gtfW* overexpression strain (LMW 502) was created by amplifying the *L. reuteri gtfW* open reading frame (including the stop codon) using primers oSG1120-1126. The resulting DNA fragment was inserted into pTXB1 (New England BioLabs, Ipswich, MA) using NheI/SapI restriction sites. The resulting plasmid, pWAR502 was then transformed into the *E. coli* expression strain ER2566 (New England BioLabs, Ipswich, MA) and selected on LB agar containing 100 μg/ml ampicillin and confirmed by DNA sequencing. This strain allows the overexpression of tagless GTFW protein.

To produce a *L. reuteri* strain constitutively expressing click beetle luciferase, a reporter plasmid was constructed by amplifying the promoter region 250 bp upstream of the elongation factor Tu (EF-Tu) start codon (including the native ribosome binding site) by PCR using oligos oSG1069-1070. The resulting DNA fragment was inserted into pJC156 using the XhoI/SalI restriction sites. The click beetle luciferase (CBluc) gene was amplified from the *S. mutans strain* ldhCBGSm (Merritt et al., 2016) using oligos oSG1067-1068 and inserted downstream of the EF-Tu promoter region in pJC156 using SalI/NotI restriction sites. The resulting reporter plasmid pWAR503 was transformed into *L. reuteri* 23272 as described above to create LMW503.

Microsphere Preparation and Application

Anhydrous dextranomer microspheres (DMs; Sephadex® G-25 Superfine) were purchased from GE Healthcare Life Sciences (Pittsburgh, PA). Anhydrous cellulose microspheres (CMs; Cellulobeads D50) were obtained from Kobo Products, Inc. (South Plainfield, NJ). Anhydrous microspheres were hydrated in growth medium or water at 50 mg/ml then autoclaved for 20 min. For conditions with microspheres that contained maltose, sucrose, fructose, or glucose only, microspheres previously autoclaved in water were removed from solution on a vacuum filter apparatus and approximately 50 mg were collected via sterile loop into 1ml of filter-sterilized 1M solution of the sugar (see Figure S1). The microsphere mixture was then vortexed vigorously and incubated for 24 h at room temperature to reach equilibrium.

For application with *L. reuteri*, microspheres loaded with water, 1M maltose, 1M sucrose, 1M glucose, or 1M fructose were removed from solution on a vacuum filter apparatus and collected via a 10 μl sterile loop. Approximately 5 mg of hydrated microspheres were then added to 1 ml of 2×10^9 CFU *L. reuteri* from an overnight culture that had previously been pelleted by centrifugation at 3220 × g for 10 min, washed twice with sterile 0.9% saline, and resuspended in 1 ml sterile saline. For experiments involving eukaryotic cell lines, 2×10^9 CFU of bacteria were resuspended in 1 ml RPMI instead of saline. For experiments with no microspheres but equivalent volume of cargo, 10 μl of cargo was added to 1 ml of bacteria either in sterile saline or RPMI. For all experiments, the bacteria and microsphere mixture were incubated together at room temperature for 30 min (unless otherwise stated) to facilitate bacterial adherence and biofilm formation on the microsphere surface prior to use in assays.

Microsphere Adherence Assay

L. reuteri culture was grown and prepared as described above and incubated with microspheres filled with either: water, 1M maltose, 1M sucrose, 1M fructose, or 1M glucose. To examine bacterial adherence to the microspheres, 300 μl of bacteria (from an overnight culture containing $\sim 2 \times 10^9$ CFU) in sterile saline and 5 mg of microspheres were combined and incubated for 5 min in a Micro Bio-Spin column (BioRad, Hercules, CA) (see Figure S2). The columns were then centrifuged (100 × g) for 1 min. The flow-through was serially diluted and plated to calculate the total number of non-adhered bacteria, and this value was subtracted from the total number of starting bacteria to derive the total number of adhered bacteria. For all experiments, a control preparation that consisted of bacteria with no microspheres was used.

Reporter Assay

The reporter strain LMW501 was grown at 37°C with 5% CO_2in MRS or MRS containing 3% glucose, sucrose, fructose, or maltose and optical densities (OD_{600nm}) of the cultures were measured throughout growth using an Epoch Microplate Spectrophotometer (BioTek Instruments Inc., Winooski, VT). At the indicated times, 80 μl aliquots of the bacterial cultures were mixed with 20 μl 2 mM D-luciferin in 0.1M citrate buffer, pH 6.0 and placed in a Falcon white flat-bottom 96-well plate (Becton, Dickinson Labware, Franklin Lakes, NJ), followed by luminescence detection using a Veritas Microplate Luminometer (Turner BioSystems Inc., Sunnyvale, CA).

GTF Enzymatic Assay

S. mutans was grown in Todd Hewitt Broth at 37°C with 5% CO_2 until early log phase (OD_{600nm} ~0.3), *L. reuteri* WT and the Δ*gtfW* mutant were grown in MRS at 37°C with 5% CO_2 until late log phase ($OD_{600\ nm}$ ~1.0) for optimal *gtf* expression, and the *E. coli gtfW* overexpression strain was grown in LB broth at 37°C shaking (200 rpm) until mid-log phase ($OD_{600\ nm}$ ~0.4) followed by the addition of 1 mM IPTG to induce *gtfW* expression and was then grown at 37°C shaking for an additional 2 h. Whole cells of *S. mutans*, *L. reuteri* WT, *L. reuteri* Δ*gtfW*, and the *E. coli gtfW* overexpression strain were assayed for GTF activity as previously described (Bai et al., 2015) using Periodic acid-Schiff staining of SDS-PAGE gels.

Cargo Diffusion Assay

The rate of cargo diffusion out of the microspheres was determined by tracking crystal violet, a small molecular weight dye (407.979 g/mol) (Fisher Scientific, Hampton, NJ). The microspheres were loaded with a 0.1% solution of crystal violet by incubating 20 mg of microspheres in 1 ml of 0.1% crystal violet solution either with or without added glycerol (40 or 80% v/v) overnight to reduce the diffusion rate by increasing viscosity. After 16 h, excess crystal violet solution was removed from the microspheres as described above using a vacuum filter apparatus. The crystal violet-loaded microspheres were then placed into 1 ml of water, and aliquots of water were removed and analyzed for diffusion of crystal violet into solution using an Epoch Microplate Spectrophotometer (BioTek, Winooski, VT) at OD_{590nm} every hour for 16 h. Percent diffusion was calculated using the equivalent amount of crystal violet within the microspheres (10 μl) in water as a control equivalent to 100% cargo diffusion.

Reuterin Assay

Production of reuterin by *L. reuteri* was measured via a quantitative colorimetric assay (Cadieux et al., 2008). As this assay did not differentiate between similar aldehyde products, measurements included 3-HPA and any potential derivatives, such as acrolein and 3-HPA hydrate. *L. reuteri* was grown overnight in MRS as described above, 1 ml aliquots of 2×10^9 CFU were pelleted at 3,220 × g for 10 min, washed twice with sterile saline, and resuspended in either 1 ml of sterile saline or 1 ml sterile saline containing 2% v/v glycerol. DM containing 0, 2, 10, 20, 30, 40, 50, 60, 70, or 80% glycerol were prepared as described above for other cargo, and added to the resuspended *L. reuteri* in saline (so that the only source of glycerol available for reuterin production was via the microsphere cargo) for 1 h at 37°C. Cells were then pelleted again and the reuterin-containing supernatant was removed, filtered through a 0.45 μm filter, and assayed for reuterin as described in Cadieux et al. (2008) without modification. A standard curve using reuterin at known concentrations was used to extrapolate bacterial-produced reuterin concentrations from DM-glycerol and the 2% v/v glycerol control experimental conditions.

L. reuteri Survival with DM-80% Glycerol

Overnight cultures of WT *L. reuteri* were aliquoted into microcentrifuge tubes, centrifuged, washed twice with sterile saline, and resuspended in either 1 ml saline or 1 ml MRS medium. Five mg of either DM-water or DM-80% glycerol were then added to the tubes and incubated at 37°C. At hourly intervals the tubes were mixed thoroughly and aliquots were taken for subsequent serial dilution and plating for viable CFU of bacteria.

Histamine Assay

Production of histamine from L-histidine by *L. reuteri* was measured via ELISA (Enzo Life Sciences, Inc., Farmingdale, NY). *L. reuteri* was grown overnight in MRS as described above, 1 ml aliquots of 2×10^9 CFU were pelleted at 3220 × g for 10 min, washed twice with sterile saline, and resuspended in one of the following conditions: sterile saline, saline with 3% maltose, saline with 2% v/v glycerol, 4 mg/ml L-histidine (Sigma-Aldrich, St. Louis, MO), 4 mg/ml L-histidine with 3% maltose, or 4 mg/ml L-histidine with 2% v/v glycerol. 5 mg of DM containing either 4 mg/ml or 30 mg/ml L-histidine were added to media lacking L-histidine, so that the only source of L-histidine for *L. reuteri* was as cargo diffusing out of the DMs. Each condition was then incubated at 37°C for 2 h, after which time the contents were pelleted and the supernatant was removed for histamine quantification via a histamine ELISA kit (Enzo Life Sciences, Inc., Farmingdale, NY) following the manufacturer's instructions without modifications. All conditions were done in at least triplicate.

pH Survivability Assay

Bacteria were exposed to a synthetic gastric acid equivalent to determine survival at pH 2. Gastric acid equivalent is a modified version of synthetic gastric fluid (Cotter et al., 2001), composed of 0.1M HCl, 0.1M NaCl, and 0.01M KCl, with pH adjusted to 2 using 0.1M NaOH. For the assay, 1 ml of 2×10^9 CFU of *L. reuteri* from a fresh overnight culture were pelleted at 3,220 × g for 10 min, washed twice with sterile saline, and resuspended in 1 ml 0.9% sterile saline. The cells were incubated for 30 min with approximately 5 mg of loaded or unloaded microspheres as described above, and the bacteria-microsphere mixture was diluted 1:100 directly into gastric acid equivalent. Aliquots of the inoculated acid solution were mixed, serially diluted, and plated at hourly time points for 4 h to determine the number of viable bacteria. Bacteria without microspheres were used as a control.

Adherence to Intestinal Epithelial Cells

DLD-1 colonic cells and FHs 74 small intestinal cells were cultured as described above. When the adherent epithelial cells reached confluence, the growth medium was removed, cells were washed twice with sterile phosphate buffered saline (PBS), and trypsin-EDTA (0.25%) was added for 10 min at 37°C to dislodge the cells from the culture flask surface. Total epithelial cells were counted using a hemacytometer (Hausser Scientific, Horsham, PA). Cells were then diluted to a concentration of 5×10^5 cells/ml and 1 ml per well was seeded into a 24-well plate and incubated at 37°C, 5% CO_2. After either 48 h (for DLD-1 cells) or 120 h (for FHs 74 cells) of growth, the spent medium was removed and replaced with 1 ml of RPMI or Hybri-Care medium containing 2×10^9 CFU of *L. reuteri* alone, *L. reuteri* with 5 mg water-filled DMs, *L. reuteri* with 5 mg sucrose-filled DMs, or *L. reuteri* with 5 mg maltose-filled DMs. After a 1 h incubation, the spent medium was removed and the well was washed with 1 ml of sterile PBS 3 times to remove non-adhered bacteria. The remaining epithelial cells, with adhered bacteria, were then trypsinized as described above, serially diluted, and plated onto solid MRS medium for enumeration of total adhered bacteria. For confocal microscopy experiments with DLD-1, Nunc Lab-Tek 8-well borosilicate chamber slides (Fisher Scientific, Hampton, NJ) were used in place of 24-well plates. The chamber slides were treated with collagen prior to DLD-1 seeding to improve cellular adherence using the following protocol: a mixture of 100 μl of 7.5% BSA (Sigma-Aldrich, St. Louis, MO), 50 μl of 3.79 mg/ml collagen (Millipore, Temecula, CA), 100 μl of 1 mg/ml rat fibronectin (Biomedical Technologies, Stoughton, MA), and 9.75 ml of PBS was prepared, and 200 μl of this solution was added per chamber slide well. After incubation for 1 h at 37°C, the solution was removed from the well, and epithelial cells were seeded and grown as described above.

Mucin Adherence Assay

Mucin agar plates were created using porcine stomach mucin (Sigma-Aldrich, St. Louis, MO). Mucin agar plates contained 2% mucin and 0.8% agar to simulate the consistency of the mucus layer found *in vivo* (Macfarlane et al., 2005; Van den Abbeele et al., 2009). To assess *L. reuteri*'s ability to bind mucin, 2×10^9 CFU of *L. reuteri* that contained a plasmid that encoded expression of the click beetle luciferase enzyme either planktonically or bound to 5 mg DM-water, DM-sucrose, or DM-maltose were incubated on both mucin agar and agar without mucin stationary at room temperature. After 60 min, the non-adhered *L. reuteri* were removed by washing the plates twice with sterile saline. The luciferase substrate D-luciferin (Sigma-Aldrich, St. Louis, MO) was then added to the plates at a concentration of 0.4 mM to visualize the remaining adhered bacteria. Relative luminosity generated from the bacteria on the plates was measured using a FluorChem E system (ProteinSimple, San Jose, CA) with a 20 min exposure setting. To assess the number of bacteria bound to the mucin within the plate (and not any background binding that may occur to the agar within the plate), the amount of luminescent signal from the agar-only plates was subtracted from the mucin agar plates.

Confocal Microscopy

All confocal laser scanning microscopy (CLSM) was performed using a Zeiss LSM 510 confocal microscope (Ziess AG, Oberkochen, Germany). For fluorescent staining, dextranomer and cellulose microspheres were pre-stained with Congo Red (Fisher Scientific, Hampton, NJ) prior to incubation with the cargo (e.g., sucrose) and experiments with bacteria. *L. reuteri* was stained with SYTO 9 (Life Technologies, Carlsbad, CA). Differential fluorescent visualization was performed using the following settings: Congo Red excitation 554 nm/emission 568 nm, and SYTO 9 excitation 490 nm/emission 525 nm. Samples were fixed using a custom biofilm fixative containing 1.5% paraformaldehyde, 0.025% glutaraldehyde, 4.0% acetic acid, and 0.1M phosphate buffer at pH 7.4 (Devaraj et al., 2015). All microscopy was performed on samples in Nunc Lab-Tek 8-well borosilicate chamber slides (Fisher Scientific, Hampton, NJ). For CLSM experiments with DLD-1 epithelial cells, DLD-1 was stained with 4′,6-Diamidino-2-Phenylindole (DAPI, Life Technologies, Carlsbad, CA), *L. reuteri* was stained with carboxyfluorescein succinimidyl ester (CFSE, Life Technologies, Carlsbad, CA). AxioVision software (Ziess AG, Oberkochen, Germany) and ICY (de Chaumont et al., 2012) were used to analyze images and create figures from CLSM images. COMSTAT (Heydorn et al., 2000) software was used to quantify bacterial biomass in CLSM images.

For *in vitro* biofilm assays, overnight cultures of WT and Δ*gtfW L. reuteri* were diluted into fresh MRS growth medium to 0.01 OD_{600nm}, incubated at 37°C 5% CO_2 for 2.5 h until reaching 0.65 $OD_{600\ nm}$, diluted 1:2,500 into either MRS, MRS + 3% sucrose, or MRS + 3% maltose, seeded into 8-well borosilicate chamber slides and incubated for 1, 3, or 6 h at 37°C 5% CO_2. At the designated time intervals, the bacteria were stained for viability with LIVE/DEAD stain, fixed, visualized via confocal microscopy, and quantified via COMSTAT analysis of the fluorescent signal.

Scanning Electron Microscopy

All scanning electron microscopy (SEM) was performed using a Hitachi S-4800 field emission SEM (Hitachi, Tokyo, Japan). Samples were prepared as described in "Adherence to colonic cells," with the exception that DLD-1 human colonic epithelial cells were grown on 15 mm diameter thermanox coverslips (Electron Microscopy Sciences, Hatfield, PA) placed within the well of a 12-well plate. Samples of DLD-1 cells and adhered bacteria were fixed overnight at 4°C in a solution of 2.5% glutaraldehyde in 0.1M phosphate buffer (pH 7.2). Samples were then washed with double distilled water and stained with a 1% solution of osmium tetroxide (Sigma-Aldrich, St. Louis, MO) in 0.1M phosphate buffer (pH 7.2) for 1 h, washed for 5 min, stained with a 1% solution of thiocarbohydrazide (Sigma-Aldrich, St. Louis, MO), washed for 5 min, and further stained with 1% osmium tetroxide for 30 min. Samples were then dehydrated using a graded series of ethanol: 25% ethanol for 15 min, 50% ethanol for 15 min, 70% ethanol for 30 min, 95% ethanol for 15 min (twice), 100% ethanol (twice), a 1:1 mixture of 100% ethanol to 100% hexamethyldisilazane (HMDS, Sigma-Aldrich, St. Louis, MO) for 100 min, 100% HMDS for 15 min, and a final immersion in 100% HMDS that was allowed to air dry overnight. Dehydrated sample coverslips were then mounted onto 15 mm diameter metal SEM specimen stubs (Electron Microscopy Sciences, Hatfield, PA) using colloidal silver (Electron Microscopy Sciences, Hatfield, PA). The outer edge, where the stub and coverslip meet, was then coated with a light layer of colloidal silver, and allowed to dry overnight. Samples were sputter coated with gold and palladium for 2 min at 25 mA using an Emitech K550X sputter coater (Quorum Technologies Ltd., Laughton, United Kingdom).

Statistical Analysis

All experiments were conducted a minimum of three times and statistical analysis was performed via a Student's *t*-test using GraphPad Prism software (GraphPad Software, Inc., La Jolla, CA), wherein a *P*-value less than 0.05 was accepted as significant.

RESULTS

Maltose or Sucrose within the Lumen of DMs Improved *L. reuteri* Adherence to DMs in a GTF-Dependent Manner

Our strategy was to have probiotic bacteria adhere to a biocompatible surface to induce the formation of a biofilm (**Figure 1**). To investigate this, we differentially stained DMs with Congo Red and *L. reuteri* with SYTO 9, and examined binding via confocal laser scanning microscopy (CLSM). As shown in **Figure 2**, aggregates of bacteria were associated with the surface of numerous DMs which indicated that *L. reuteri* was able to adhere to the DM surface within the time allotted. Since DMs are cross-linked glucan similar to the native reuteran produced by *L. reuteri,* we hypothesized that either an increase in GTFW (for enhanced binding to DMs) or production of glucan to stimulate aggregation and biofilm formation would facilitate the adhered state of *L. reuteri.* To this end, we compared adherence of *L. reuteri* to DMs that contained luminal cargo of either sucrose (an inducer of *gtfW* expression but not a substrate for GTFW; see Figure S3) or maltose (the sole substrate of GTFW). As shown in **Figures 2B,C**, compared to DMs that contained only water within the lumen (**Figure 2A**) there were greater numbers of *L. reuteri* adhered to DMs with either sugar as cargo.

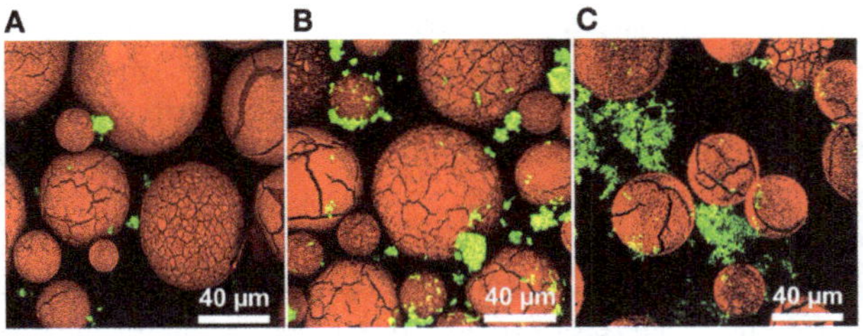

FIGURE 2 | *L. reuteri* binds to dextranomer microspheres. Confocal laser scanning microscopy (CLSM) of *L. reuteri* adhered to DMs. **(A)** Water-filled DMs, **(B)** sucrose-filled DMs, and **(C)** maltose-filled DMs after incubation with *L. reuteri* for 30 min showed that *L. reuteri* adherence to DMs can be enhanced to incorporate biofilm-promoting cargo within the DM lumen (green: bacteria stained with SYTO 9, red: DMs stained with Congo Red).

To further investigate *L. reuteri*'s ability to bind DMs, we tested other DM lumen compounds that we hypothesized should not affect GTFW protein mediated binding and thus unlikely to support increased adherence to DMs. For this assay we chose the monosaccharide subunits of maltose and sucrose (e.g., glucose for maltose, glucose and fructose for sucrose), which the GTF enzyme cannot utilize to catalyze glucan polymers. Interestingly, fructose (and not glucose) was shown to induce *gtfW* expression at a rate similar to sucrose, but did not result in enhanced binding to DMs as was found with sucrose (Figure S3A, **Figure 3A**).

To determine if this GTFW-dependent binding is specific to the glycosyl linkages of DMs, we compared *L. reuteri* binding to cellulose microspheres (CMs), as DMs are composed of polymers of glucose with α-linkages while CMs possess β-linkages between the glucose units (Updegraff, 1969; Kralj et al., 2002). As shown in **Figure 3A**, only ~10% of *L. reuteri* adhered to CMs regardless of luminal contents. Collectively the data in **Figure 3** indicated that *L. reuteri* does not bind to CMs, binding to DMs was GTFW-dependent and further, that inclusion of maltose or sucrose significantly enhanced the binding of *L reuteri* to DMs. We hypothesized that the predicted glucan binding domain of GTFW is a necessary component of *L. reuteri's* ability to adhere to DMs. To further test if the adherence to DM is GTF-dependent, we created a mutant strain of *L. reuteri* (LMW500) with a chloramphenicol resistance gene inserted in place of the *gtfW* gene. As shown in **Figure 3B**, the Δ*gtfW* strain was not able to bind to DMs as effectively as the wild type (WT) in our spin column assay, regardless of the cargo within the DM lumen. To further demonstrate the difference between the WT and Δ*gtfW*, we examined biofilm formation on glass chamber slides in media supplemented with sucrose or maltose (Figure S4). After a 1 h incubation, the WT had more bacteria present and noticeably more bacterial aggregation when sucrose or maltose was added to the growth medium (Figures S4A,B). After 3 and 6 h with sucrose or maltose supplemented media, the WT displayed a significantly more robust biofilm with greater biomass compared to the *gtfW* mutant under every condition, with significantly more cells present when sucrose or maltose was in the growth medium (Figures S4A,C,D).

We next tested whether bacteria that do not express a similar GTF would lack the adherent phenotype shown in **Figures 3A,B**. To examine this, we performed our DM adherence assay with another probiotic bacterium and three enteric pathogens that *L. reuteri* would likely encounter within the gastrointestinal tract: *Lactobacillus rhamnosus* GG, a Gram-positive bacterium commonly found in the genitourinary system and sold commercially as a probiotic; *Salmonella typhi*, a Gram-negative bacterium responsible for typhoid fever in humans; *Citrobacter rodentium*, a Gram-negative bacterium that causes colitis in rodents; and *Clostridium difficile*, a Gram-positive spore-forming bacterium that can cause severe colitis and recurring infections in humans. As shown in **Figure 3C**, all of

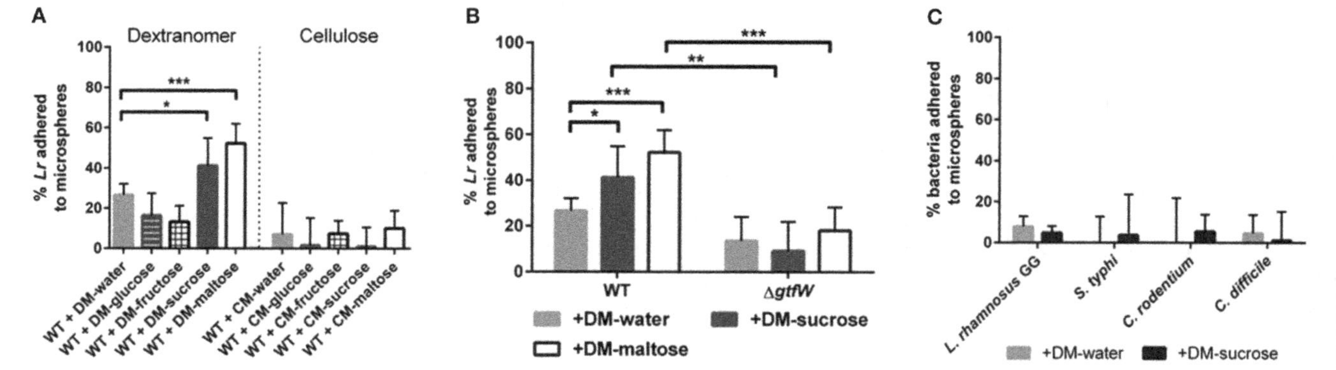

FIGURE 3 | Microsphere composition and lumen cargo affected *L. reuteri* adherence, *L. reuteri* adhered to DMs in GTFW-dependent manner, and bacteria lacking GTF did not bind to DMs. A spin column assay was performed to assess relative bacterial adherence to microspheres. Bacteria were incubated for 5 min with 5 mg of microspheres, centrifuged at 100 × g to separate bound and unbound bacteria, then CFU of non-adhered bacteria were quantified in the flow-through of the spin column. **(A)** Microspheres composed of either cross-linked dextran (DM) or cross-linked cellulose (CM) were filled with water or various sugars at a concentration of 1M to determine which microsphere type supported greatest adherence of *L. reuteri*. **(B)** Relative WT and Δ*gtfW* *L. reuteri* adherence to DM showed that *L. reuteri* adhered to DMs in a GTF-dependent manner. **(C)** Non-GTF expressing bacteria were similarly tested for microsphere adherence with water-loaded and sucrose-loaded DMs. Error bars represent standard error of the mean. Statistical significance is indicated by the following: **P* < 0.05, ***P* < 0.01, ****P* < 0.0005.

the non-GTF expressing bacteria showed minimal adherence to DMs, regardless of cargo present within the DM lumen.

Diffusion of Cargo from DMs

Initial binding of bacteria to DMs is a critical component of our formulation, however equally important is the ability to co-deliver beneficial luminal cargo needed by the adherent bacteria during transit of DMs through the gastrointestinal tract. Targeted delivery of maltose (or any other beneficial compound) via diffusion out of the DMs directly to the probiotic bacterium over time was a desired feature of our system (**Figure 1**). However, since the method of cargo delivery would be diffusion through the porous surface of the microsphere and not its degradation, such as occurs in poly(lactic-co-glycolic) acid (PLGA) microspheres (Danhier et al., 2012), the rate of diffusion is dependent upon the size of the microsphere, the mass of the solute, and the viscosity of the diluent. As proof of concept, we filled the DMs with crystal violet, a small molecular weight stain (407.979 g/mol), and tested the diffusion rate of the dye out of the DMs with and without changing the viscosity of the solution in the DM lumen. As shown in **Figure 4**, the crystal violet diffused out of the DM lumen with a half-life of ~6 h. When the viscosity was increased by adding 40% glycerol, the half-life of release was increased to ~8 h. At 80% glycerol, the half-life of crystal violet release was further enhanced to 12 h. By 16 h >95% of all of the crystal violet had been released under all tested conditions.

L. reuteri Produced Reuterin From Glycerol-Loaded Microspheres

An important feature of *L. reuteri*'s function as a probiotic bacterium is its ability to compete with pathogenic bacteria within the host potentially via production of antimicrobials e.g., extracellular reuterin (Cleusix et al., 2007; Spinler et al., 2008). Due to limited glycerol availability, suboptimal endogenous concentrations of glycerol in the GI tract would likely limit adequate reuterin production. In order to obviate the need to provide high levels of glycerol to satisfy *L. reuteri*'s optimal needs, we provided targeted delivery of glycerol directly to the bacteria attached to the surface of DMs. To test this *in vitro*, we utilized a colorimetric assay for reuterin production (Cadieux et al., 2008). As shown in Figure S5, DMs filled with glycerol concentrations ranging from 10 to 80% were able to induce reuterin production. Compared to the 2% glycerol solution control, DMs filled with 80% glycerol produced on average 53% more reuterin in 1 h (average concentration of reuterin produced: 2% glycerol = 40 mM, DM-80% glycerol = 61 mM). To determine if the 80% glycerol or the resulting reuterin/downstream metabolites of glycerol fermentation produced by *L. reuteri* is toxic to *L. reuteri*, we compared hourly colony forming units (CFU) of *L. reuteri* incubated with either DM-water or DM-80% glycerol, in either sterile saline or MRS growth medium. As shown in Figure S6, there was no loss of CFU regardless of DM cargo when *L. reuteri* was incubated in MRS. Incubating *L. reuteri* in saline did result in a steady loss of viable CFU over time, though there was no difference in viability between the DM-water and DM-80% glycerol over this time, suggesting the loss of CFU was not due to any potentially toxic compounds, such as reuterin or acrolein, from glycerol fermentation (Figure S6). As acrolein in particular is known to be toxic to humans and is a byproduct of reuterin production, we next calculated the maximum possible amount of acrolein that could be produced from the dosage of *L. reuteri* and volume of glycerol provided via DMs in our formulation, assuming all available glycerol was converted 1:1 into acrolein. As shown in Figure S7, the amount of acrolein that could possibly be produced via our formulation is a nominal ~6 μg (for reference, the World Health Organization recommends less than 7.5 μg/kg body weight per day) (Gomes et al., 2002). From these results and the data presented in **Figure 4**, we hypothesized that DMs loaded

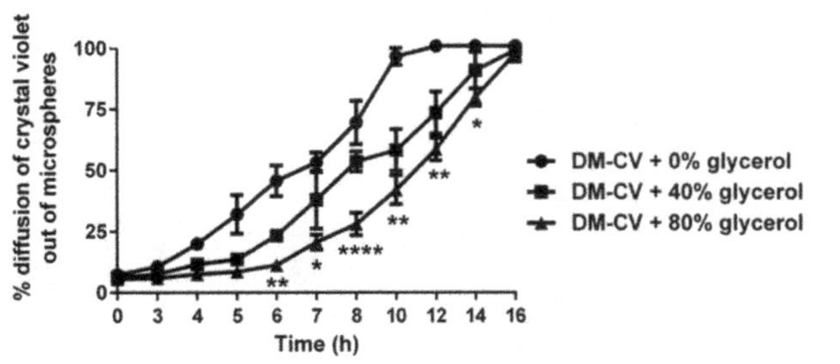

FIGURE 4 | Diffusion of cargo out of microspheres over time. Crystal violet (CV)-loaded DMs with and without glycerol (added to increase viscosity) were assayed to determine the relative rate of CV diffusion from the microspheres. With 0% added glycerol, CV diffused at a higher rate (100% diffusion after 10 h) compared to DMs that contained 40 or 80% glycerol. We observed 100% diffusion from DMs after 16 h regardless of viscosity. Error bars represent standard error of the mean. Statistical significance from DMs with 0% added glycerol is indicated by the following: $^{*}P < 0.05$, $^{**}P < 0.01$, $^{****}P < 0.0001$.

with glycerol would have two beneficial effects *in vivo*, namely slowing the release of beneficial cargo and providing a substrate for reuterin production.

L. reuteri Produced Histamine from L-Histidine-Loaded Microspheres

Histamine produced by *L. reuteri* has previously been shown to inhibit pro-inflammatory cytokines such as TNF via H_2 receptors and reduce colitis in an animal model (Thomas et al., 2012; Gao et al., 2015). Our microsphere-based approach provides a unique method for delivery of the histamine precursor substrate L-histidine to *L. reuteri*. To test this *in vitro*, we filled DMs with 30 mg/ml and 4 mg/ml L-histidine and measured the amount of histamine produced by the bacteria when the only source of L-histidine was via diffusion out of the DMs. As shown in **Figure 5**, DM- L-histidine (4 mg/ml) resulted in histamine levels only slightly lower than those produced when bacteria were incubated in 4 mg/ml L-histidine solution without DMs. When the DMs were loaded with a higher concentration of L-histidine, the amount of histamine produced was 6–7 times greater than the lower 4 mg/ml concentration, consistent with the DM-L-histidine (30 mg/ml) providing ~7 times more L-histidine than the DM-L-histidine (4 mg/ml) (**Figure 5**). In addition, we tested whether other cargo relevant DM cargo substrates, such as maltose and glycerol, would negatively affect histamine production. Addition of glycerol did not result in reduced histamine production, regardless of whether the L-histidine was in solution or provided via DMs (**Figure 5**). With addition of maltose, histamine production actually increased when L-histidine was provided in solution, but statistically unchanged when L-histidine was provided via DMs (**Figure 5**).

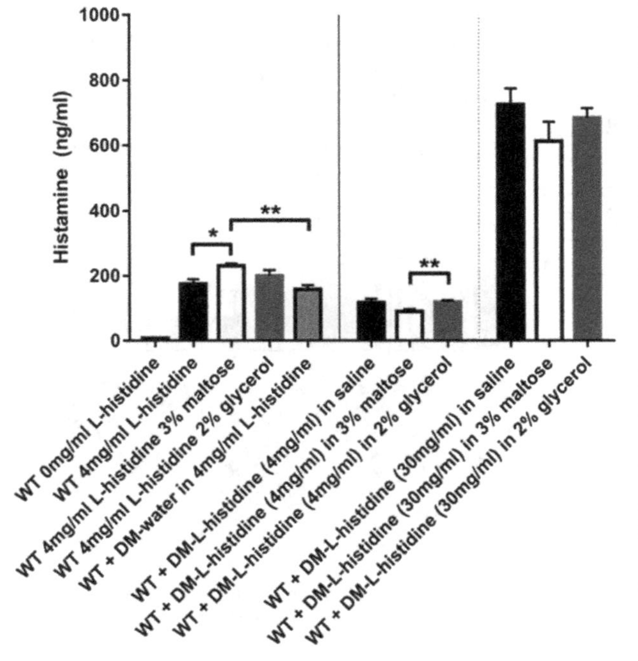

FIGURE 5 | Histamine can be produced by *L. reuteri* from L-histidine delivered via DM. Stationary phase WT *L. reuteri* was incubated for 2 h in either saline with and without 3% maltose or 2% glycerol, or 4 mg/ml L-histidine with and without 3% maltose or 2% glycerol. Histamine production was increased with addition of 3% maltose to 4 mg/ml L-histidine solution (white bar black border) compared to just 4 mg/ml L-histidine (black bar and gray bar black border). When L-histidine at 4 mg/ml was provided via DM the overall levels of histamine produced were significantly lower (middle 3 bars) compared to L-histidine provided in solution (left 4 bars), likely due to less immediate availability of L-histidine to the bacteria. However, when the concentration of L-histidine loaded into DM was increased to 30 mg/ml, significantly more histamine was produced (right 3 bars) despite any caveats related to slower access to L-histidine due to availability only via diffusion out of DM. Error bars represent standard error of the mean. Statistical significance is indicated by the following: $^{*}P < 0.05$, $^{**}P < 0.01$.

Microspheres Filled with Sucrose or Maltose Improved *L. reuteri* Survival at Low pH

Orally consumed probiotics face a significant pH challenge upon reaching the stomach, where pH values are as low as 1.5 when the stomach is empty (Dressman et al., 1990). Enhancing the ability to deliver a maximal number of viable *L. reuteri* to the colon is crucial to its sustainability and effectiveness as a probiotic. We thereby hypothesized that *L. reuteri* bound to the surface of DMs in the form of a biofilm would increase survival upon exposure to acid, and that DMs filled with sucrose or maltose would result in even greater survival in a GTFW-dependent manner. As shown in **Figure 6**, less than 0.1% of WT *L. reuteri* without DMs survived in synthetic gastric acid after 4 h at pH 2, which resulted in a nearly 3 log loss of viable probiotic. Addition of water-filled DMs did not significantly alter the survival rate of WT *L. reuteri* in gastric acid; however, when either DM-sucrose or DM-maltose was delivered with WT, nearly 1 log more survived the acid stress (**Figure 6**). To show that the protective effect is dependent on the microspheres and not the cargo within the DM lumen, we also incubated *L. reuteri* with the equivalent amount of diffusible cargo without the DMs. Acid survival in the presence of cargo only was no different than *L. reuteri* alone (**Figure 6**), which strongly indicated the importance of the bacterial biofilm-on-DM delivery system for the observed protective effect.

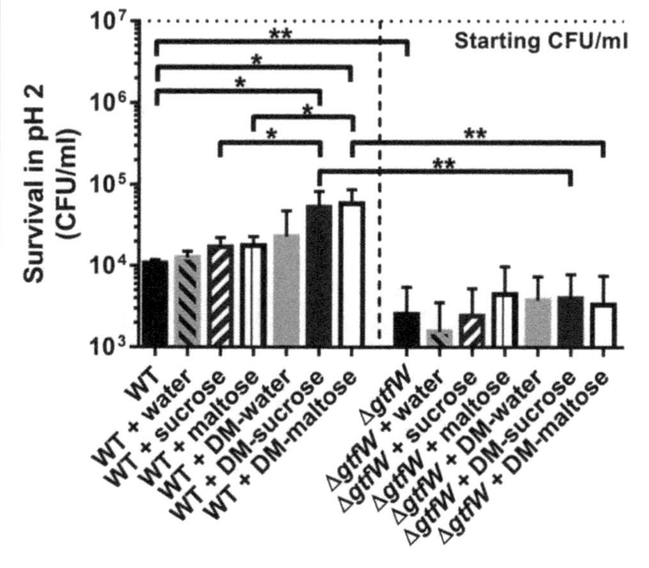

FIGURE 6 | Gastric acid survival. WT and Δ*gtfW* *L. reuteri* (10^7 CFU/ml) viability after 4 h in pH 2 synthetic gastric acid in the absence or presence of 5 mg of DMs that contained water, sucrose (1 M), or maltose (1 M) as cargo, or 10 μl of the cargo alone without DMs. Relative survival in acid was enhanced when WT *L. reuteri* was adhered as a biofilm on DMs that contained sucrose or maltose compared to equivalent volumes of the same cargo delivered without DMs, which indicated that the biofilm phenotype contributed to better survival during exposure to low pH. Δ*gtfW* showed decreased resistance to acid compared to the WT, regardless of the presence or absence of either DMs or sugar alone. Error bars represent standard error of the mean. Statistical significance is indicated by the following: *$P < 0.05$, **$P < 0.01$.

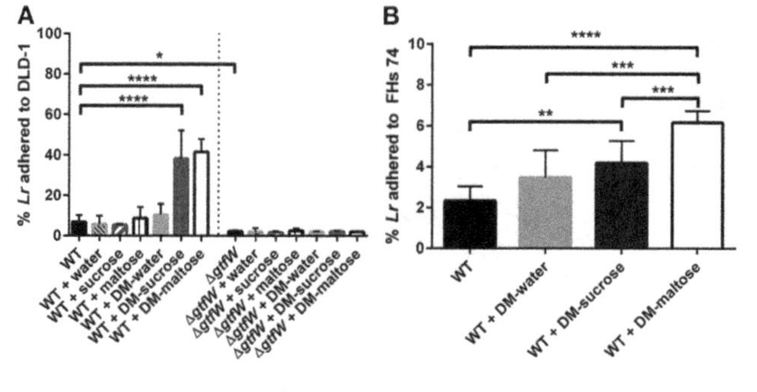

FIGURE 7 | Delivery of *L. reuteri* adhered to DMs as a biofilm supported increased adherence to intestinal epithelial cells. (A) *L. reuteri* WT and Δ*gtfW* adhered as a biofilm on DMs that contained either water, sucrose (1 M), or maltose (1 M), or the equivalent volume of sugar alone (without DMs), were examined for relative adherence to human colonic DLD-1 cells after incubation for 60 min. Significantly more WT adhered to DLD-1 cells when delivered as a biofilm on the surface of DMs that contained sucrose or maltose, compared to water-filled DMs or the equivalent volume of sugar alone. Significantly fewer Δ*gtfW* mutant cells adhered to DLD-1 cells, regardless of cargo, which indicated that the GTFW protein contributes to *L. reuteri* adherence. **(B)** Adherence of WT to fetal small intestinal FHs 74 cells after 60 min incubation showed that providing *L. reuteri* adherent on the DM surface as a biofilm with either sucrose or maltose as cargo resulted in greater adherence to intestinal cells. Error bars represent standard error of the mean. Statistical significance is indicated by the following: *$P < 0.05$, **$P < 0.01$, ***$P < 0.001$, ****$P < 0.0001$.

To investigate whether this phenotype is GTFW-dependent, we also tested synthetic gastric acid survival using the Δ*gtfW* strain of *L. reuteri* and found that the beneficial effect of DM-sucrose and DM-maltose was lost (**Figure 6**). Interestingly, the mutant also showed deficiency in acid survival without DMs compared to WT, which indicated that GTFW's role in cellular aggregation and biofilm formation (Figure S4) may contribute significantly to survival in synthetic gastric acid.

Microspheres Promote *L. reuteri* Adherence to Human Intestinal Epithelial Cells

Next, we examined what effect the DMs, the DM luminal cargo and the product of the *gtfW* gene have on the relative adherence of *L. reuteri* when delivered as planktonic cells or as biofilms on DMs to the human intestinal cell lines DLD-1 (adult human colonic epithelial cells) and FHs 74 Int (3–4 months gestation, small intestine epithelial cells) *in vitro*. As shown in **Figure 7A**, after a 1 h incubation on DLD-1 cells, significantly more WT *L. reuteri* (without DMs) adhered to the colonic cells compared to Δ*gtfW* either with or without DMs, which indicated that GTFW contributed to host cell adherence. When *L. reuteri* adhered to DMs that contained sucrose or maltose were added to colonic cells, relative adherence of WT *L. reuteri* to the colonic cells was increased by 4.7-fold for DMs that contained sucrose and by 5.2-fold for DMs that contained maltose (**Figure 7A**). Although overall fewer WT *L. reuteri* adhered to the FHs 74 cells than to DLD-1 cells, delivering the bacteria with either DM-sucrose or DM-maltose resulted in 1.8-fold (DM-sucrose) or 2.7-fold (DM-maltose) more adhered bacteria compared to WT bacteria without DM (**Figure 7B**).

To further show that DM luminal cargo of maltose and sucrose improved relative adherence of *L. reuteri* to epithelial cells *in vitro*, we analyzed WT and Δ*gtfW* *L. reuteri* adherence after 1 h incubation on DLD-1 cells visually, using CSLM (**Figure 8**). As with the CFU data presented in **Figure 7**, delivery of WT *L. reuteri* as a biofilm on maltose or sucrose-loaded DMs supported greater adherence to the DLD-1 cells than those delivered on water-loaded DMs or with no DMs, both by visual inspection (**Figure 8A**) and when analyzed by quantification of bacterial biomass using COMSTAT analysis of CSLM images (**Figure 8B**). The observed adherence was significantly diminished in the Δ*gtfW* mutant compared to the wild type, consistent with measured CFUs (**Figure 7A**).

Finally, we tested the effect of DM adhered WT *L. reuteri*'s ability to bind to mucin. While cellular binding of probiotics likely plays a role in colonization, a healthy GI tract has a mucus layer on the apical surface of epithelial cells, of which the primary constituent is mucin (Turner, 2009). Indeed it is believed that healthy commensals are found primarily within this layer so it is imperative that our formulation maintains it enhanced probiotic effects in the presence of mucin. As mucin adherence is not GTF-dependent, but rather controlled by specific mucin-binding proteins (Miyoshi et al., 2006; Lukic et al., 2012), we hypothesized that being bound to DMs would not have an effect on the ability

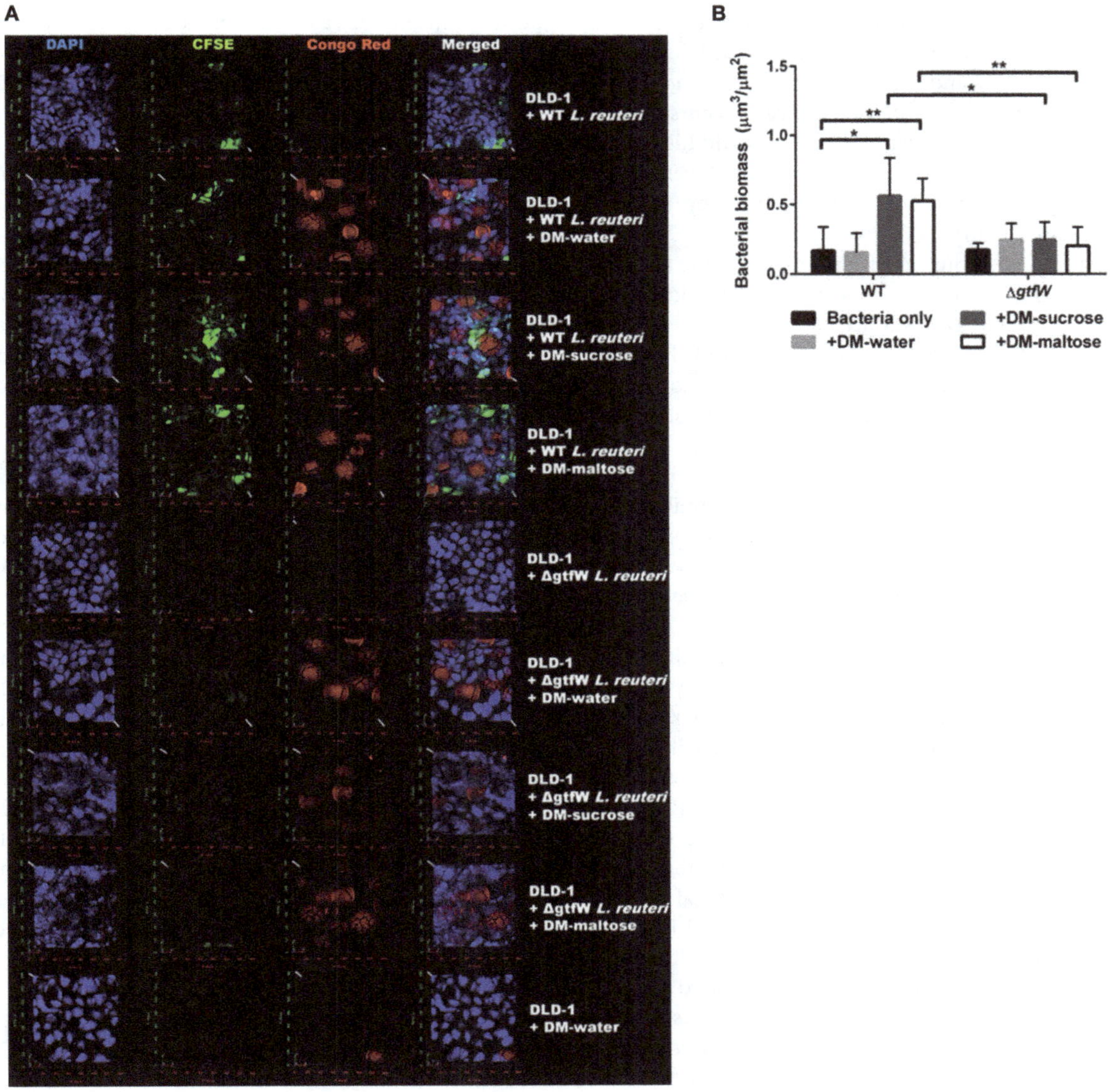

FIGURE 8 | Increased adherence to DLD-1 colonic epithelial cells is observed when *L. reuteri* was delivered as a biofilm attached to DMs. (A) *In vitro* CLSM of DLD-1 epithelial cells (blue, DAPI), *L. reuteri* (green, CFSE), and DMs (red, Congo Red). WT *L. reuteri* (top four rows) compared to Δ*gtfW L. reuteri* (middle four rows) and no *L. reuteri* (bottom row). Bacteria and DMs were pre-stained, incubated for 1 h on pre-stained DLD-1 epithelial cells, washed three times, and fixed for CLSM analysis. **(B)** Comparison of bacterial biomass quantified via COMSTAT analysis of the green channel of CLSM images of WT and Δ*gtfW L. reuteri*. WT without DMs ($n = 10$) resulted in less total bacterial signal compared to either WT + DM-sucrose ($n = 10$) or WT + DM-maltose ($n = 10$). Δ*gtfW* showed no difference in relative number of bacteria adhered to DLD-1 cells, regardless of the presence of DMs. Error bars represent standard error of the mean. Statistical significance is indicated by the following: **P* < 0.05, ***P* < 0.01.

of *L. reuteri* to adhere to mucin. As shown in Figure S8, there is no significant difference in relative adherence of WT *L. reuteri* to mucin when delivered as either a planktonic bacterial suspension or as a biofilm adhered to DMs after a 60 min incubation on mucin agar plates.

DISCUSSION

We have previously shown that a single dose of *L. reuteri* delivered as a biofilm adhered to DMs reduces the incidence of necrotizing enterocolitis (NEC) by 50% (Olson et al., 2016) in a rat pup model. Here we showed that *L. reuteri* bound to DMs with appropriate luminal cargo promoted significantly increased survival at low pH and supported increased adherence to human epithelial cells *in vitro*. Importantly *L. reuteri* and DMs are considered "generally recognized as safe" (GRAS) by the FDA. In fact, DMs have been used in medical products that are left in the body for long periods of time (years) with no ill effects (Hoy, 2012), such as with Debrisan®, a cicatrizant wound dressing (Jacobsson et al., 1976), Deflux®, a bulking gel used to treat vesicoureteral reflux (VUR) in children (Stenberg and Lackgren, 1995), and Solesta™, a bulking gel injected submucosaly into the anal canal to treat fecal incontinence (Hoy, 2012). The scope of the research presented here shows a small subset of possible beneficial cargos that can be placed into the DM lumen for utilization by *L. reuteri,* and for many applications it may be as simple as matching the correct lumen cargo precursor to the desired *L. reuteri*-produced effect (e.g., reuterin and histamine). Moreover, this formulation obviates recombinant versions of probiotics, an approach not currently approved by the FDA (Venugopalan et al., 2010).

An exciting feature of our novel formulation is the ability to directly deliver beneficial compounds to the probiotic bacteria that are adhered to the DM surface as a biofilm (**Figure 1**). To combine beneficial compounds (prebiotics) with beneficial bacteria to stimulate growth is a well-established concept in probiotic research and commercial applications (Collins and Gibson, 1999; de Vrese and Schrezenmeir, 2008). There is significant evidence to show that synergism between probiotics and prebiotics effectively increases the overall population of probiotic bacteria (de Vrese and Schrezenmeir, 2008; van Zanten et al., 2014) and promotes effective treatments of diseases such as inflammatory bowel disease (Geier et al., 2007) and necrotizing enterocolitis (Asmerom et al., 2015). However, a major drawback of traditional prebiotics is that they are typically limited to carbohydrates that are non-digestible or absorbable by the host to ensure sufficient availability to the probiotic bacteria in the gut. Our delivery system effectively solves this problem in that the probiotic bacterium *L. reuteri* is now delivered: (1) in association with DMs to which it adheres in greater numbers; (2) in the form of a biofilm which confers resistance to clearance; (3) along with a cargo of nutrients that promotes bacterial growth; (4) with cargos that promote production of the antimicrobial reuterin or histamine; (5) in a format that is resistant to acid-mediated killing thus promoting improved survival during transit through the acidic stomach, and (6) in a manner that appeared to better support adherence to intestinal epithelial cells and thus likely to promote persistence in the gut. With regard to *L. reuteri*-induced release of substance potentially beneficial to the host, reuterin has been suggested to inhibit competition by other gut flora, and histamine has been shown to have anti-inflammatory effects. Although the secondary metabolites produced from glycerol metabolism to generate reuterin (e.g., acrolein) and histamine could result in adverse effects at high levels, the maximum quantities generated with our formulations are <1% and < 40% less than what is thought to be problematic in humans for acrolein (Figure S7) and histamine, respectively (Maintz and Novak, 2007; Thomas et al., 2012; Engels et al., 2016). Ongoing and future experiments utilizing *L. reuteri* adhered to DMs will test the putative aforementioned beneficial cargos in an *in vivo* animal model (Olson et al., in preparation) to demonstrate both safety and efficacy. Concurrently we are also investigating strategies for long-term storage and downstream application and delivery of our DM-based formulation.

Using maltose as cargo have particular value for several reasons; it is the substrate for this strain of *L. reuteri*'s glucosyltransferase (GTFW) (Leemhuis et al., 2013; Bai et al., 2015), induces *L. reuteri* to aggregate in a GTF-dependent manner (Walter et al., 2008), and causes *L. reuteri* to grow significantly faster and to a higher cell density (CFU/ml). In this study, we show that both maltose and sucrose have a positive effect on *L. reuteri* adherence to microspheres, promote adherence of *L. reuteri* to human intestinal epithelial cells, and improves bacterial survival in gastric acid (**Figures 2**, **3**, **6**, **7**, **8**). We have demonstrated in concurrent work that *S. mutans* binds rapidly and with high affinity to DMs, and the effect is increased in the presence of sucrose in a GTF-dependent manner (Mashburn-Warren et al., submitted). *S. mutans* and *L. reuteri* GTF proteins are very similar in sequence and structure. Sucrose is the sole substrate for *S. mutans* and most *L. reuteri* GTF proteins (Tieking et al., 2005; Walter et al., 2008), and sucrose has previously been shown to cause *L. reuteri* cultures to aggregate rapidly in a GTF-dependent manner (Walter et al., 2008). The positive effect of sucrose to induce GTFW dependent adhesion is likely due to GTFW acting as an adhesin to DMs (via the glucan binding domain) and sucrose's ability to induce *gtfW* expression (Figure S3A). Indeed, failure of sucrose to affect *L. reuteri* adherence to CMs (cross-linked glucan with variant glycosidic linkages) supports this notion. Sucrose-dependent biofilm formation has previously been linked to two-component regulatory systems in the rodent strain 100-23 of *L. reuteri* (Frese et al., 2011; Su and Ganzle, 2014); however, the genes necessary for this phenomenon appear to be absent in the human-derived strain of *L. reuteri* used in this study (23272/DSM 20016). Since sucrose is a preferred carbon source of the *L. reuteri* used in this study via its sucrose phophorylase mediated metabolism (Ganzle and Follador, 2012) it was not surprising that sucrose had a positive impact on biofilm formation and increased adherence to DMs and is likely due to the increased doubling time of *L. reuteri* in the presence of sucrose. The failure of glucose (a carbon source but not a *gtfW* inducer or GTFW substrate) and fructose [an inducer of *gtfW*, but not a carbon source (Figure S3 and data not shown), or substrate for GTFW] to enhance adherence to DMs suggests that understanding bacterial physiology will be critical in selecting beneficial luminal cargos.

Although we describe *L. reuteri* adhered to DMs as a biofilm, we have yet to characterize this physiologic state. We have demonstrated in previous work with the dental pathogen *Aggregatibacter actinomycetemcomitans*, that challenging a host with an already-established pathogenic biofilm results in greater ability of the pathogen to establish disease in an animal model of oral infection (Freire et al., 2011, 2017). While it is clear that being bound to DMs offers multiple advantages in terms of survivability and relative adherence to an epithelial target cell, the actual state of the DM-adhered *L. reuteri* and its phenotype has yet to be determined. There is evidence that microbes such as *L. reuteri* exist naturally as biofilms in the gastrointestinal tract (Macfarlane and Dillon, 2007), but there has thus far been a lack of research as to the composition and dynamics of biofilm communities of the gut (Hall-Stoodley et al., 2004; de Vos, 2015). *L. reuteri* adhered to DMs in our experiments are biofilms by definition and via our observations in **Figure 6**, which showed that bacteria adhered to DMs resisted low pH challenge better than planktonic bacteria. In experiments where *L. reuteri* bound to DMs are incubated with colonic cells we observed both aggregates of bacteria surrounding the DMs as well as those that were adhered to the confluent eukaryotic cell surface (Figure S9). Future work on the biofilm state will include the dlt operon that encodes proteins involved in D-alanylation of teichoic acid, and shown to be important in biofilm formation, adherence, and host colonization (Walter et al., 2007).

In this study we show that many parameters important to *L. reuteri*'s survivability and sustainability within the host can be improved by delivering *L. reuteri* as a biofilm on the surface of DMs that contain beneficial cargo. With more viable bacteria available after low pH challenge and supporting increased adherence to intestinal epithelial cells, the resulting expansion of probiotic bacteria available within the host should have an increased potentially beneficial effect. Further, we are able to deliver targeted nutrients and substrates directly to the bacteria adhered on the DM surface, which has broad-reaching implications for the type of compounds that can be co-delivered with orally consumed *L. reuteri,* which to date have been limited to carbohydrates that are indigestible by the host. Taken together, our novel delivery system provides an exciting framework for future probiotic development and deployment.

AUTHOR CONTRIBUTIONS

SG, LM, and JN designed the study. JN and LM performed the experimental work. JN, LM, and SG analyzed the data. JN prepared the manuscript; and LM, SG, MB, and LB contributed to the final manuscript.

FUNDING

This work was conducted utilizing discretionary funds.

ACKNOWLEDGMENTS

We would like to thank the following collaborators for providing strains used in this work: Dr. John S. Gunn (Ohio State University) for providing *S. typhi*, Dr. Jennifer K. Spinler (Texas Children's Hospital) for providing *C. difficile* and a reuterin standard, Dr. Gireesh Rajashekara (Ohio State University) for providing *L. rhamnosus* GG, Jens Kreth (Oregon Health and Science University) for providing the Click Beetle luciferase, and Dr. Gail E. Besner (Nationwide Children's Hospital) for providing DLD-1 human colonic cells and FHs 74 Int human fetal small intestinal epithelial cells. Additional thanks to Dr. Aishwarya Devaraj (Nationwide Children's Hospital), Joe Jurcisek (Nationwide Children's Hospital), and Cindy McAllister (Nationwide Children's Hospital) for CLSM and SEM advice and assistance.

REFERENCES

Agerholm-Larsen, L., Bell, M. L., Grunwald, G. K., and Astrup, A. (2000). The effect of a probiotic milk product on plasma cholesterol: a meta-analysis of short-term intervention studies. *Eur. J. Clin. Nutr.* 54, 856–860. doi: 10.1038/sj.ejcn.1601104

Araya, M., Morelli, L., Reid, G., Sanders, M. E., and Stanton, C. (2006). *Probiotics in Food: Health and Nutritional Properties and Guidelines for Evaluation.* Rome: Food and Agriculture Organization of the United Nations, World Health Organization.

Arques, J. L., Fernandez, J., Gaya, P., Nunez, M., Rodriguez, E., and Medina, M. (2004). Antimicrobial activity of reuterin in combination with nisin against food-borne pathogens. *Int. J. Food Microbiol.* 95, 225–229. doi: 10.1016/j.ijfoodmicro.2004.03.009

Asmerom, M., Crowe, L., and Marin, T. (2015). Understanding the biologic therapies of probiotics, prebiotics, and synbiotics: exploring current evidence for use in premature infants for the prevention of necrotizing enterocolitis. *J. Perinat. Neonatal Nurs.* 29, 240–247. doi: 10.1097/JPN.0000000000000120

Bai, Y., van der Kaaij, R. M., Leemhuis, H., Pijning, T., van Leeuwen, S. S., Jin, Z., et al. (2015). Biochemical characterization of the *Lactobacillus reuteri* glycoside hydrolase family 70 GTFB type of 4,6-alpha-glucanotransferase enzymes that synthesize soluble dietary starch fibers. *Appl. Environ. Microbiol.* 81, 7223–7232. doi: 10.1128/AEM.01860-15

Cadieux, P., Wind, A., Sommer, P., Schaefer, L., Crowley, K., Britton, R. A., et al. (2008). Evaluation of reuterin production in urogenital probiotic *Lactobacillus reuteri* RC-14. *Appl. Environ. Microbiol.* 74, 4645–4649. doi: 10.1128/AEM.00139-08

Chang, J. C., LaSarre, B., Jimenez, J. C., Aggarwal, C., and Federle, M. J. (2011). Two group A streptococcal peptide pheromones act through opposing Rgg regulators to control biofilm development. *PLoS Pathog.* 7:e1002190. doi: 10.1371/journal.ppat.1002190

Cleusix, V., Lacroix, C., Vollenweider, S., Duboux, M., and Le Blay, G. (2007). Inhibitory activity spectrum of reuterin produced by *Lactobacillus reuteri* against intestinal bacteria. *BMC Microbiol.* 7:101. doi: 10.1186/1471-2180-7-101

Collins, M. D., and Gibson, G. R. (1999). Probiotics, prebiotics, and synbiotics: approaches for modulating the microbial ecology of the gut. *Am. J. Clin. Nutr.* 69, 1052S–1057S.

Cook, M. T., Tzortzis, G., Charalampopoulos, D., and Khutoryanskiy, V. V. (2012). Microencapsulation of probiotics for gastrointestinal delivery. *J. Control. Release* 162, 56–67. doi: 10.1016/j.jconrel.2012.06.003

Cotter, P. D., Gahan, C. G., and Hill, C. (2001). A glutamate decarboxylase system protects Listeria monocytogenes in gastric fluid. *Mol. Microbiol.* 40, 465–475. doi: 10.1046/j.1365-2958.2001.02398.x

Danhier, F., Ansorena, E., Silva, J. M., Coco, R., Le Breton, A., and Preat, V. (2012). PLGA-based nanoparticles: an overview of biomedical applications. *J. Control. Release* 161, 505–522. doi: 10.1016/j.jconrel.2012.01.043

de Chaumont, F., Dallongeville, S., Chenouard, N., Herve, N., Pop, S., Provoost, T., et al. (2012). Icy: an open bioimage informatics platform for extended reproducible research. *Nat. Methods* 9, 690–696. doi: 10.1038/nmeth.2075

De Man, J. C., Rogosa, M., and Sharpe, M. E. (1960). A medium for the cultivation of Lactobacilli. *J. Appl. Bact.* 23:6. doi: 10.1111/j.1365-2672.1960.tb00188.x

Devaraj, A., Justice, S. S., Bakaletz, L. O., and Goodman, S. D. (2015). DNABII proteins play a central role in UPEC biofilm structure. *Mol. Microbiol.* 96, 1119–1135. doi: 10.1111/mmi.12994

de Vos, W. M. (2015). Microbial biofilms and the human intestinal microbiome. *Npj Biofilms Microbio.* 1:15005. doi: 10.1038/npjbiofilms.2015.5

de Vrese, M., and Schrezenmeir, J. (2008). Probiotics, prebiotics, and synbiotics. *Adv. Biochem. Eng. Biotechnol.* 111, 1–66. doi: 10.1007/10_2008_097

De Weirdt, R., Crabbé, A., Roos, S., Vollenweider, S., Lacroix, C., van Pijkeren, J. P., et al. (2012). Glycerol supplementation enhances *L. reuteri's* protective effect against *S. Typhimurium* colonization in a 3-D model of colonic epithelium. *PLoS ONE* 7:e37116. doi: 10.1371/journal.pone.0037116

Ding, W. K., and Shah, N. P. (2007). Acid, bile, and heat tolerance of free and microencapsulated probiotic bacteria. *J. Food Sci.* 72, M446–M450. doi: 10.1111/j.1750-3841.2007.00565.x

Dressman, J. B., Berardi, R. R., Dermentzoglou, L. C., Russell, T. L., Schmaltz, S. P., Barnett, J. L., et al. (1990). Upper gastrointestinal (GI) pH in young, healthy men and women. *Pharm. Res.* 7, 756–761. doi: 10.1023/A:1015827908309 el-Ziney, M. G., and Debevere, J. M. (1998). The effect of Reuterin on Listeria monocytogenes and *Escherichia coli* O157:H7 in milk and cottage cheese. *J. Food Prot.* 61, 1275–1280. doi: 10.4315/0362-028X-61.10.1275

Engels, C., Schwab, C., Zhang, J., Stevens, M. J., Bieri, C., Ebert, M. O., et al. (2016). Acrolein contributes strongly to antimicrobial and heterocyclic amine transformation activities of reuterin. *Sci. Rep.* 6:36246. doi: 10.1038/srep36246

Freire, M. O., Devaraj, A., Young, A., Navarro, J. B., Downey, J. S., Chen, C., et al. (2017). A bacterial biofilm induced oral osteolytic infection can be successfully treated by immuno-targeting an extracellular nucleoid associated protein. *Mol. Oral Microbiol.* 32, 74–88. doi: 10.1111/omi.12155

Freire, M. O., Sedghizadeh, P. P., Schaudinn, C., Gorur, A., Downey, J. S., Choi, J. H., et al. (2011). Development of an animal model for Aggregatibacter actinomycetemcomitans biofilm-mediated oral osteolytic infection: a preliminary study. *J. Periodontol.* 82, 778–789. doi: 10.1902/jop.2010.100263

Frese, S. A., Benson, A. K., Tannock, G. W., Loach, D. M., Kim, J., Zhang, M., et al. (2011). The evolution of host specialization in the vertebrate gut symbiont *Lactobacillus reuteri*. *PLoS Genet.* 7:e1001314. doi: 10.1371/journal.pgen.1001314

Ganzle, M. G., and Follador, R. (2012). Metabolism of oligosaccharides and starch in lactobacilli: a review. *Front. Microbiol.* 3:340. doi: 10.3389/fmicb.2012.00340

Gao, C., Major, A., Rendon, D., Lugo, M., Jackson, V., Shi, Z., et al. (2015). Histamine H2 receptor-mediated suppression of intestinal inflammation by probiotic *Lactobacillus reuteri*. *MBio* 6, e01358–e01315. doi: 10.1128/mBio.01358-15

Geier, M. S., Butler, R. N., and Howarth, G. S. (2007). Inflammatory bowel disease: current insights into pathogenesis and new therapeutic options; probiotics, prebiotics and synbiotics. *Int. J. Food Microbiol.* 115, 1–11. doi: 10.1016/j.ijfoodmicro.2006.10.006

Ghouri, Y. A., Richards, D. M., Rahimi, E. F., Krill, J. T., Jelinek, K. A., and DuPont, A. W. (2014). Systematic review of randomized controlled trials of probiotics, prebiotics, and synbiotics in inflammatory bowel disease. *Clin. Exp. Gastroenterol.* 7, 473–487. doi: 10.2147/CEG.S27530

Gomes, R., Meek, M. E., and Eggleton, M. (2002). *Acrolein*. Geneva: World Health Organization.

Hall-Stoodley, L., Costerton, J. W., and Stoodley, P. (2004). Bacterial biofilms: from the natural environment to infectious diseases. *Nat. Rev. Microbiol.* 2, 95–108. doi: 10.1038/nrmicro821

Heydorn, A., Nielsen, A. T., Hentzer, M., Sternberg, C., Givskov, M., Ersboll, B. K., et al. (2000). Quantification of biofilm structures by the novel computer program COMSTAT. *Microbiology* 146, 2395–2407. doi: 10.1099/00221287-146-10-2395

Hoy, S. M. (2012). Dextranomer in stabilized sodium hyaluronate (Solesta(R)): in adults with faecal incontinence. *Drugs* 72, 1671–1678. doi: 10.2165/11209030-000000000-00000

Jacobsson, S., Jonsson, L., Rank, F., and Rothman, U. (1976). Studies on healing of Debrisan-treated wounds. *Scand. J. Plast. Reconstr. Surg.* 10, 97–101. doi: 10.3109/02844317609105196

Johnston, B. C., Ma, S. S. Y., Goldenberg, J. Z., Thorlund, K., Vandvik, P. O., Loeb, M., et al. (2012). Probiotics for the prevention of clostridium difficile-associated diarrhea a systematic review and meta-analysis. *Ann. Intern. Med.* 157, 878–U225. doi: 10.7326/0003-4819-157-12-201212180-00563

Jones, S. E., and Versalovic, J. (2009). Probiotic *Lactobacillus reuteri* biofilms produce antimicrobial and anti-inflammatory factors. *BMC Microbiol.* 9:35. doi: 10.1186/1471-2180-9-35

Kailasapathy, K. (2014). "Microencapsulation for gastrointestinal delivery of probiotic bacteria," in *Nano Microencapsulation Foods*, ed H.-S. Kwak (Wiley-Blackwell), 167–197. doi: 10.1002/9781118292327.ch7

Kralj, S., van Geel-Schutten, G. H., Dondorff, M. M. G., Kirsanovs, S., van der Maarel, M. J. E. C., and Dijkhuizen, L. (2004). Glucan synthesis in the genus Lactobacillus: isolation and characterization of glucansucrase genes, enzymes and glucan products from six different strains. *Microbiology* 150, 3681–3690. doi: 10.1099/mic.0.27321-0

Kralj, S., van Geel-Schutten, G. H., Rahaoui, H., Leer, R. J., Faber, E. J., van der Maarel, M. J., et al. (2002). Molecular characterization of a novel glucosyltransferase from *Lactobacillus reuteri* strain 121 synthesizing a unique, highly branched glucan with alpha-(1->4) and alpha-(1->6) glucosidic bonds. *Appl. Environ. Microbiol.* 68, 4283–4291. doi: 10.1128/AEM.68.9.4283-4291.2002

Leemhuis, H., Dijkman, W. P., Dobruchowska, J. M., Pijning, T., Grijpstra, P., Kralj, S., et al. (2013). 4,6-alpha-Glucanotransferase activity occurs more widespread in Lactobacillus strains and constitutes a separate GH70 subfamily. *Appl. Microbiol. Biotechnol.* 97, 181–193. doi: 10.1007/s00253-012-3943-1

Lukic, J., Strahinic, I., Jovcic, B., Filipic, B., Topisirovic, L., Kojic, M., et al. (2012). Different roles for lactococcal aggregation factor and mucin binding protein in adhesion to gastrointestinal mucosa. *Appl. Environ. Microbiol.* 78, 7993–8000. doi: 10.1128/AEM.02141-12

Macfarlane, S., and Dillon, J. F. (2007). Microbial biofilms in the human gastrointestinal tract. *J. Appl. Microbiol.* 102, 1187–1196. doi: 10.1111/j.1365-2672.2007.03287.x

Macfarlane, S., Woodmansey, E. J., and Macfarlane, G. T. (2005). Colonization of mucin by human intestinal bacteria and establishment of biofilm communities in a two-stage continuous culture system. *Appl. Environ. Microbiol.* 71, 7483–7492. doi: 10.1128/AEM.71.11.7483-7492.2005

Mackos, A. R., Galley, J. D., Eubank, T. D., Easterling, R. S., Parry, N. M., Fox, J. G., et al. (2016). Social stress-enhanced severity of *Citrobacter rodentium*-induced colitis is CCL2-dependent and attenuated by probiotic *Lactobacillus reuteri*. *Mucosal Immunol.* 9, 515–526. doi: 10.1038/mi.2015.81

Maintz, L., and Novak, N. (2007). Histamine and histamine intolerance. *Am. J. Clin. Nutr.* 85, 1185–1196.

Mashburn-Warren, L., Morrison, D. A., and Federle, M. J. (2012). The cryptic competence pathway in Streptococcus pyogenes is controlled by a peptide pheromone. *J. Bacteriol.* 194, 4589–4600. doi: 10.1128/JB.00830-12

McFarland, L. V. (2006). Meta-analysis of probiotics for the prevention of antibiotic associated diarrhea and the treatment of Clostridium difficile disease. *Am. J. Gastroenterol.* 101, 812–822. doi: 10.1111/j.1572-0241.2006.00465.x

Merritt, J., Senpuku, H., and Kreth, J. (2016). Let there be bioluminescence: development of a biophotonic imaging platform for *in situ* analyses of oral biofilms in animal models. *Environ. Microbiol.* 18, 174–190. doi: 10.1111/1462-2920.12953

Miyoshi, Y., Okada, S., Uchimura, T., and Satoh, E. (2006). A mucus adhesion promoting protein, MapA, mediates the adhesion of *Lactobacillus reuteri* to Caco-2 human intestinal epithelial cells. *Biosci. Biotechnol. Biochem.* 70, 1622–1628. doi: 10.1271/bbb.50688

Monchois, V., Willemot, R. M., and Monsan, P. (1999). Glucansucrases: mechanism of action and structure-function relationships. *FEMS Microbiol. Rev.* 23, 131–151. doi: 10.1111/j.1574-6976.1999.tb00394.x

Mooser, G., Shur, D., Lyou, M., and Watanabe, C. (1985). Kinetic-studies on dextransucrase from the cariogenic oral bacterium streptococcus-mutans. *J. Biol. Chem.* 260, 6907–6915.

Neu, J., and Walker, W. A. (2011). Necrotizing enterocolitis. *N. Engl. J. Med.* 364, 255–264. doi: 10.1056/NEJMra1005408

Nguyen, T. D. T., Kang, J. H., and Lee, M. S. (2007). Characterization of Lactobacillus plantarum PH04, a potential probiotic bacterium with cholesterol-lowering effects. *Int. J. Food Microbiol.* 113, 358–361. doi: 10.1016/j.ijfoodmicro.2006.08.015

Olson, J. K., Rager, T. M., Navarro, J. B., Mashburn-Warren, L., Goodman, S. D., and Besner, G. E. (2016). Harvesting the benefits of biofilms: a novel probiotic delivery system for the prevention of necrotizing enterocolitis. *J. Pediatr. Surg.* 51, 936–941. doi: 10.1016/j.jpedsurg.2016.02.062

Porath, J., and Flodin, P. (1959). Gel filtration: a method for desalting and group separation. *Nature* 183, 1657–1659. doi: 10.1038/1831657a0

Savino, F., Cordisco, L., Tarasco, V., Palumeri, E., Calabrese, R., Oggero, R., et al. (2010). *Lactobacillus reuteri* DSM 17938 in infantile colic: a randomized, double-blind, placebo-controlled trial. *Pediatrics* 126, e526–e533. doi: 10.1542/peds.2010-0433

Schaefer, L., Auchtung, T. A., Hermans, K. E., Whitehead, D., Borhan, B., and Britton, R. A. (2010). The antimicrobial compound reuterin (3-hydroxypropionaldehyde) induces oxidative stress via interaction with thiol groups. *Microbiology* 156(Pt 6), 1589–1599. doi: 10.1099/mic.0.035642-0

Schwab, C., Walter, J., Tannock, G. W., Vogel, R. F., and Ganzle, M. G. (2007). Sucrose utilization and impact of sucrose on glycosyltransferase expression in *Lactobacillus reuteri*. *Syst. Appl. Microbiol.* 30, 433–443. doi: 10.1016/j.syapm.2007.03.007

Soh, S. E., Aw, M., Gerez, I., Chong, Y. S., Rauff, M., Ng, Y. P. M., et al. (2009). Probiotic supplementation in the first 6 months of life in at risk Asian infants - effects on eczema and atopic sensitization at the age of 1 year. *Clin. Exp. Allergy* 39, 571–578. doi: 10.1111/j.1365-2222.2008.03133.x

Spinler, J. K., Taweechotipatr, M., Rognerud, C. L., Ou, C. N., Tumwasorn, S., and Versalovic, J. (2008). Human-derived probiotic *Lactobacillus reuteri* demonstrate antimicrobial activities targeting diverse enteric bacterial pathogens. *Anaerobe* 14, 166–171. doi: 10.1016/j.anaerobe.2008.02.001

Stefka, A. T., Feehley, T., Tripathi, P., Qiu, J., McCoy, K., Mazmanian, S. K., et al. (2014). Commensal bacteria protect against food allergen sensitization. *Proc. Natl. Acad. Sci. U.S.A.* 111, 13145–13150. doi: 10.1073/pnas.1412008111

Stenberg, A., and Lackgren, G. (1995). A new bioimplant for the endoscopic treatment of vesicoureteral reflux - experimental and short-term clinical-results. *J. Urol.* 154, 800–803. doi: 10.1016/S0022-5347(01)67168-4

Su, M. S., and Ganzle, M. G. (2014). Novel two-component regulatory systems play a role in biofilm formation of *Lactobacillus reuteri* rodent isolate 100-23. *Microbiology* 160(Pt 4), 795–806. doi: 10.1099/mic.0.071399-0

Sung, V., Hiscock, H., Tang, M. L. K., Mensah, F. K., Nation, M. L., Satzke, C., et al. (2014). Treating infant colic with the probiotic *Lactobacillus reuteri*: double blind, placebo controlled randomised trial. *Br. Med. J.* 348:g2107. doi: 10.1136/bmj.g2107

Talarico, T. L., Casas, I. A., Chung, T. C., and Dobrogosz, W. J. (1988). Production and isolation of reuterin, a growth inhibitor produced by *Lactobacillus reuteri*. *Antimicrob. Agents Chemother.* 32, 1854–1858. doi: 10.1128/AAC.32.12.1854

Thomas, C. M., Hong, T., van Pijkeren, J. P., Hemarajata, P., Trinh, D. V., Hu, W., et al. (2012). Histamine derived from probiotic *Lactobacillus reuteri* suppresses TNF via modulation of PKA and ERK signaling. *PLoS ONE* 7:e31951. doi: 10.1371/journal.pone.0031951

Tieking, M., Kaditzky, S., Valcheva, R., Korakli, M., Vogel, R. F., and Ganzle, M. G. (2005). Extracellular homopolysaccharides and oligosaccharides from intestinal lactobacilli. *J. Appl. Microbiol.* 99, 692–702. doi: 10.1111/j.1365-2672.2005.02638.x

Turner, J. R. (2009). Intestinal mucosal barrier function in health and disease. *Nat. Rev. Immunol.* 9, 799–809. doi: 10.1038/nri2653

Updegraff, D. M. (1969). Semimicro determination of cellulose in biological materials. *Anal. Biochem.* 32, 420–424. doi: 10.1016/S0003-2697(69)80009-6

Van den Abbeele, P., Grootaert, C., Possemiers, S., Verstraete, W., Verbeken, K., and Van de Wiele, T. (2009). *In vitro* model to study the modulation of the mucin-adhered bacterial community. *Appl. Microbiol. Biotechnol.* 83, 349–359. doi: 10.1007/s00253-009-1947-2

van Zanten, G. C., Krych, L., Roytio, H., Forssten, S., Lahtinen, S. J., Abu Al-Soud, W., et al. (2014). Synbiotic Lactobacillus acidophilus NCFM and cellobiose does not affect human gut bacterial diversity but increases abundance of lactobacilli, bifidobacteria and branched-chain fatty acids: a randomized, double-blinded cross-over trial. *FEMS Microbiol. Ecol.* 90, 225–236. doi: 10.1111/1574-6941.12397

Venugopalan, V., Shriner, K. A., and Wong-Beringer, A. (2010). Regulatory oversight and safety of probiotic use. *Emerging Infect. Dis.* 16, 1661–1665. doi: 10.3201/eid1611.100574

Walter, J., Loach, D. M., Alqumber, M., Rockel, C., Hermann, C., Pfitzenmaier, M., et al. (2007). D-alanyl ester depletion of teichoic acids in *Lactobacillus reuteri* 100-23 results in impaired colonization of the mouse gastrointestinal tract. *Environ. Microbiol.* 9, 1750–1760. doi: 10.1111/j.1462-2920.2007.01292.x

Walter, J., Schwab, C., Loach, D. M., Ganzle, M. G., and Tannock, G. W. (2008). Glucosyltransferase A (GtfA) and inulosucrase (Inu) of *Lactobacillus reuteri* TMW1.106 contribute to cell aggregation, *in vitro* biofilm formation, and colonization of the mouse gastrointestinal tract. *Microbiology* 154(Pt 1), 72–80. doi: 10.1099/mic.0.2007/010637-0

14

Intra-Species Genomic and Physiological Variability Impact Stress Resistance in Strains of Probiotic Potential

*Jason W. Arnold[1], Joshua B. Simpson[2], Jeffrey Roach[3], Jakub Kwintkiewicz[1] and M. Andrea Azcarate-Peril[1]**

[1] Division of Gastroenterology and Hepatology, Department of Medicine, Microbiome Core Facility, Center for Gastrointestinal Biology and Disease, School of Medicine, University of North Carolina, Chapel Hill, NC, United States, [2] Department of Chemistry, College of Arts and Sciences, University of North Carolina, Chapel Hill, NC, United States, [3] Research Computing, University of North Carolina, Chapel Hill, NC, United States

Correspondence:
M. Andrea Azcarate-Peril
azcarate@med.unc.edu

Large-scale microbiome studies have established that most of the diversity contained in the gastrointestinal tract is represented at the strain level; however, exhaustive genomic and physiological characterization of human isolates is still lacking. With increased use of probiotics as interventions for gastrointestinal disorders, genomic and functional characterization of novel microorganisms becomes essential. In this study, we explored the impact of strain-level genomic variability on bacterial physiology of two novel human *Lactobacillus rhamnosus* strains (AMC143 and AMC010) of probiotic potential in relation to stress resistance. The strains showed differences with known probiotic strains (*L. rhamnosus* GG, Lc705, and HN001) at the genomic level, including nucleotide polymorphisms, mutations in non-coding regulatory regions, and rearrangements of genomic architecture. Transcriptomics analysis revealed that gene expression profiles differed between strains when exposed to simulated gastrointestinal stresses, suggesting the presence of unique regulatory systems in each strain. *In vitro* physiological assays to test resistance to conditions mimicking the gut environment (acid, alkali, and bile stress) showed that growth of *L. rhamnosus* AMC143 was inhibited upon exposure to alkaline pH, while AMC010 and control strain LGG were unaffected. AMC143 also showed a significant survival advantage compared to the other strains upon bile exposure. Reverse transcription qPCR targeting the bile salt hydrolase gene (*bsh*) revealed that AMC143 expressed *bsh* poorly (a consequence of a deletion in the *bsh* promoter and truncation of *bsh* gene in AMC143), while AMC010 had significantly higher expression levels than AMC143 or LGG. Insertional inactivation of the *bsh* gene in AMC010 suggested that *bsh* could be detrimental to bacterial survival during bile stress. Together, these findings show that coupling of classical microbiology with functional genomics methods for the characterization of bacterial strains is critical for the development of novel probiotics, as variability between strains can dramatically alter bacterial physiology and functionality.

Keywords: probiotics, intra-Species variability, bacterial stress, *Lactobacillus rhamnosus*, bile salt hydrolase (BSH)

INTRODUCTION

The gastrointestinal tract is host to one of the densest and most diverse microbial communities on the planet (Gill et al., 2006; Li et al., 2012). The composition and function of the gut microbiota is critical to maintenance of host gastrointestinal health (Jones, 2016). In fact, diseases including diabetes (Tilg and Moschen, 2014), obesity (Carding et al., 2015), and colorectal cancer (Sobhani et al., 2011; Borges-Canha et al., 2015) have been shown to have gut dysbioses associated with progression. Conversely, modulation of the gut microbiota can alleviate or even eliminate disorders like *Clostridium difficile* infections (Petrof et al., 2013; Allegretti et al., 2014), inflammatory bowel disease (D'Haens et al., 2014), and lactose intolerance (Azcarate-Peril et al., 2017).

Intra-species genetic polymorphisms constitute the majority of the diversity within the microbiota of the human gut (Greenblum et al., 2015; Zhang and Zhao, 2016). Coupling classical microbiology approaches with next generation sequencing provides an opportunity to study physiological characteristics of individual microbial strains, and to identify unique genomic elements associated with those phenotypes. Moreover, advances in cultivation technologies have improved isolation of novel microorganisms from human subjects, provided the ability to study physiology of difficult to grow microbes (Faith et al., 2010), and ultimately develop advanced microbiota-derived treatments for gastrointestinal diseases (Forster and Lawley, 2015).

Use of probiotics, live microbes that convey a benefit to their host when administered in adequate amounts, as interventions for gastrointestinal disorders has gained increasing support (Grover et al., 2012; Vandenplas et al., 2015); however, intra-species variations can impact their functionality as effective probiotics (Chapman et al., 2012). Isolation and characterization of novel intestinal organisms are important steps toward the development of new and improved probiotics. Moreover, high throughput sequencing technology allow for cost-effective whole genome sequencing of bacterial isolates, providing a wealth of genomic data. Nevertheless, identification and characterization of novel probiotics also require careful examination of microbial physiology (Papadimitriou et al., 2015).

One essential physiological characteristic of probiotics is their ability to survive the environmental conditions of the gastrointestinal tract. Gut microorganisms have evolved highly conserved mechanisms for tolerance to gastrointestinal stresses, which include variations in pH and the antimicrobial effects of bile (Azcarate-Peril et al., 2004; Bruno-Bárcena et al., 2004). These mechanisms are controlled by well-regulated genetic systems (Azcarate-Peril et al., 2004), often with rapid response times to acute stresses, allowing for immediate resistance to environmental changes (Anderson et al., 2010; Bove et al., 2013). Bacterial responses to environmental stress occur in a highly regulated manner. First, stress-specific genes aim to aleviate the immediate stress (maintenance of cytoplasmic pH homeostasis, transport/degradation of toxic compounds, and others), followed by universal stress response systems aimed to repair DNA, protein, membrane, and cell wall damage.

If exposed to an acidic environment, H^+ pump of ATPases (F_0F_1-ATPases) maintain pH homeostasis within the cytoplasm by pumping excess H^+ ions back into the environment (Wang et al., 2013; Cusumano and Caparon, 2015). Other mechanisms involved in resistance to acid stress in *Lactobacillus* are arginine deiminases (ArcABC) (Fulde et al., 2014) that synthesize ammonia from arginine and free H^+ within the cytoplasm (Casiano-Colón and Marquis, 1988) and amino acid decarboxylases coupled with amino acid/biogenic amines antiporter systems (Azcarate-Peril et al., 2004; Papadimitriou et al., 2016). Upon surviving the acidic conditions in the stomach and passing into the duodenum, the pH of the environment shifts from highly acidic to alkaline. Alkaline Shock Proteins (Asp) are encoded by lactic acid bacteria including *Lactobacillus rhamnosus* (Arnold et al., 2017), and have been implicated in resistance to sudden pH shifts (Kuroda et al., 1995; Seetharaaman, 2008; Anderson et al., 2010).

Entry into the duodenum not only involves a change in pH, but also exposes microorganisms to bile salts, which act as detergents, causing cell damage and cytotoxicity (Andreichin, 1980; Begley et al., 2005). Lactic acid bacteria including *Lactobacillus* and *Bifidobacterium* species encode bile salt hydrolases (*bsh*), which have been shown in some cases to provide resistance to bile toxicity (Grill et al., 2000; Patel et al., 2010; Lin et al., 2014). *Lactobacillus acidophilus* and *Bifidobacterium* encode multiple *bsh* genes, which exhibit substrate specificity for different conjugated bile salt targets (McAuliffe et al., 2005; Jarocki and Targonski, 2013). As different bile salts have varying toxicity, individual *bsh* genes may or may not provide survival advantages against bile (Fang et al., 2009). In addition to providing survival advantages in the gastrointestinal environment, bile salt hydrolases encoded by lactic acid bacteria (Jarocki and Targonski, 2013; Jarocki et al., 2014; Pithva et al., 2014) have been implicated in modulation of host cholesterol and lipid metabolism (Patel et al., 2010; Joyce et al., 2014), and as a mechanism for microbe-host signaling (Ridlon et al., 2006).

Universal bacterial stress-response systems encode mechanisms to cope with the deleterious consequences of exposure to environmental stresses, including DNA damage, protein misfolding, and loss of cell wall/membrane integrity. Bacterial DNA damage is repaired by MutS and RecA-like recombinases (Lee and Pi, 2010; Rossi et al., 2016; Calderini et al., 2017; Overbeck et al., 2017). Protein misfolding is reduced and repaired by molecular chaperones including heat-shock proteins (Ruiz et al., 2013; Calderini et al., 2017). Cell wall integrity of gram positive bacteria is maintained through lipoteichoic acid (LTA), exopolysaccharide, and fatty acid metabolism/synthesis genes (Koskenniemi et al., 2011). Membrane proteins including metalloproteases provide additional stress resistance in lactic acid bacteria (Bove et al., 2012). *Lactobacillus* also encodes two component regulatory systems (2CRS) that promote rapid responses to environmental stresses. These systems usually consist of a histidine kinase and a response regulator gene that work to sense and react to changes in the environment (Yu et al., 2014; Monedero et al., 2017), facilitating stress resistance (Morel-Deville et al., 1998; Alcántara et al., 2011). Together, universal stress-response genes work with specific stress resistance systems to ensure bacterial survival to gastrointestinal conditions.

Douillard et al. (2013) in their analysis of 100 *L. rhamnosus* genomes, showed that strains had unique genomic elements coupled with physiological traits that were influenced by the strain origin. In particular, bile resistance was higher in *L. rhamnosus* isolates derived from the gastrointestinal tract as opposed to dairy, oral, or vaginal isolates. In this study we analyzed genomic, transcriptomic, and physiological characteristics of two novel human *L. rhamnosus* strains of probiotic potential for which our group recently generated genomic sequence information (Thompson et al., 2015; Arnold et al., 2017), and compared them with an established probiotic strain of human origin (LGG). *Lactobacillus rhamnosus* GG (LGG) is a well-characterized probiotic lactic acid bacteria isolated from a healthy human host in 1983. The strain provides a number of benefits to its host including immunomodulation (Lebeer et al., 2012; Segers and Lebeer, 2014), pathogen exclusion (De Keersmaecker et al., 2006; Makras et al., 2006), and modulation of host gene expression (Kankainen et al., 2009; Yan et al., 2013; Segers and Lebeer, 2014). LGG sets a precedent for *L. rhamnosus* as a functional probiotic as well as for the isolation and identification of novel probiotics from healthy human hosts. Additionally, the strains were compared with *L. rhamnosus* of dairy origin (Lc705, HN001; Ceapa et al., 2015) to demonstrate the impact of intra-species genetic polymorphisms on tolerance to gastrointestinal stress.

MATERIALS AND METHODS

Strains and Culture Media

Bacterial strains used in this study are presented in **Table 1**. Strains were propagated in MRS broth (Pronadisa, Madrid) at 37°C without agitation, or on MRS agar plates containing 1.5% agar. For growth assays, MRS supplemented with 0.1–1.0% Oxgall was used to test resistance to bile. MRS was titrated with HCl–pH 4 to test growth in acidic conditions, and titrated with NaOH to pH 8 to test growth under alkaline stress.

Bacterial Growth Assays

Lactobacillus rhamnosus strains were grown statically for 16 h in MRS broth at 37°C. Freshly harvested cells were washed with MRS without glucose and diluted 1:100 in MRS (pH 6.6) containing either bile (0, 0.1, 0.3, 0.5, and 1.0% w/v oxgall), or adjusted to pH 4 (HCl) or pH 8 (NaOH). 200 μl of bacterial suspensions were placed into each well of a 96 well plate, sealed and placed into Tecan Infinite 200 Pro spectrophotometer (Tecan, Switzerland), where they were grown for 24 h at 37°C. Measurements of optical density at 600 nm ($OD_{600\,nm}$) were taken every 15 min during this 24-h period. Maximum specific growth rates (μ_{max}) were then calculated for each treatment type and plotted in Origin2016 (OriginLab, Northampton, MA).

Bacterial Survival Assays

Bacterial cells grown to mid-log growth phase ($OD_{600\,nm}$ = ~0.6) were centrifuged, washed twice with sterile PBS and diluted 1:10,000 in simulated gastric juice (0.5% pepsin, 0.5% NaCl, pH3), simulated intestinal juice (0.3% pancreatin, 0.5% NaCl, pH8), or bile (0.5% Oxgall in MRS + 0% Glucose). Cell suspensions were incubated for 2 h at 37°C and then plated onto MRS agar plates by WASP Spiral Plater (Don Whitley Scientific, West Yorkshire, UK) at 1 and 2 h post inoculation. Plates were incubated at 37°C for 48 h. Survival was measured using ProtoCOL colony counter (Synbiosis, Frederick, MD) to count colonies present on MRS plates of treated and untreated cells. Three biological replicates with three technical replicates were included in survival experiments. Pairwise comparisons using a two-tailed Student's *t*-test were performed to determine statistically significant differences between treatments.

TABLE 1 | Bacterial strains used in this study.

Strain	Origin	References
L. rhamnosus GG	Healthy human isolate	Kankainen et al., 2009
L. rhamnosus Lc705	Fermented dairy product	Kankainen et al., 2009
L. rhamnosus HN001	Fermented dairy product	Tannock et al., 2014
L. rhamnosus AMC010	Human infant stool	Arnold et al., 2017
L. rhamnosus AMC010::*bsh*		This study
L. rhamnosus AMC143	Human infant stool	Arnold et al., 2017

RNA Isolation

AMC010, AMC143, and LGG were grown to early log phase ($OD_{600\,nm}$ = ~0.4) in MRS prior to harvesting. Cells were then washed twice with sterile PBS and re-suspended in simulated gastric juice, simulated intestinal juice, or bile (0.5% w/v Oxgall in sterile PBS) and incubated for 10 min at 37°C. Three biological replicates were included in expression experiments. After incubation, cells were centrifuged, flash frozen in RNAlater (Thermo Fisher Scientific, Waltham, MA), and stored in −80°C until RNA isolation was performed. RNA isolation was performed using the Qiagen RNeasy PowerMicrobiome kit (Qiagen, Valencia, CA) as directed. RNA was eluted in 50 μl RNase free water and quantified using the 2200TapeStation (Agilent Technologies, Santa Clara, CA).

Real Time Quantitative PCR

Five ng of total RNA isolated from bacterial cultures exposed to bile (0.5% w/v Oxgall in sterile PBS for 30 min at 37°C) were reverse transcribed using qScript cDNA SuperMix (Quanta BioSciences, Gaithersburg, MD). To generate a standard curve, genomic DNA from AMC010 was amplified using primer set BSHqPCR-F (TTGGCGCTGACGACTTGC), BSHqPCR-R (AATCTTGACGCCTTGACC) (this study) and purified via gel extraction in 1.5% agarose gel. The purified PCR product was serially diluted and used in RT–qPCR experiments. The qPCR master mix included 10 μl of Power SYBR® Green 2x PCR Master Mix (Applied Biosystems, Foster City, CA), 2 μl of each primer (BSHqPCR-F, BSHqPCR-R) (1 μM stock), 1 μl PCR grade water, and 5 μl of template cDNA (1 ng/μl). The reaction was run for 40 cycles of melting (95°C) 15 s, annealing/extension (65°C) 45 s followed by SYBR detection was carried out on the 7,500 Fast Real Time PCR System (Applied Biosystems, Foster City, CA) after 10 min denaturation step at 95°C. Samples and standards were run in triplicate.

mRNA Sequencing

Ribosomal RNA was depleted from total RNA using the Ribo-Zero Gold Bacterial rRNA Removal Reagent (Epidemiology Kit) (Illumina, San Diego, CA) according to manufacturer's instructions. Briefly, the rRNA-specific magnetic beads were removed from storage buffer and mixed with 500 ng of total sample RNA. Subsequently, rRNA removal solution was added and samples were incubated for 10 min at 65°C. Finally, samples were placed on magnetic stand for 15 min at 22°C and mRNA was removed and immediately processed with TruSeq Stranded mRNA HT kit (Illumina, San Diego, CA) according to manufacturer's instructions. Briefly, RNA was mixed with Fragment-Prime mix and incubated at 94°C for 8 min. Samples were immediately subject to first strand and second strand cDNA synthesis reactions, respectively, followed by 3′ end repair, adenylation and adapter ligation. After adapter ligation, the libraries were enriched by PCR using the following thermal cycling conditions: 98°C for 30 s followed by 15 cycles of 98°C for 10 s, 60°C for 30 s and 72°C for 30 s. Final extension step of 70°C for 5 min was carried out following the last cycle. After enrichment, libraries were purified with Beckman Coulter magnetic beads (Brea, CA), washed with 80% ethanol and eluted in Tris pH 8.5. Following enrichment, cDNA was barcoded for multiplexing via PCR, using dual-index barcodes [index 1(i7) and index 2(i5)] (Illumina, San Diego, CA) in a combination unique to each sample. Final ds cDNA was purified with Beckman Coulter magnetic beads (Brea, CA). Library concentrations and quality were measured via TapeStation2200 (Agilent Technologies, Santa Clara, CA). Barcoded libraries were pooled at equimolar concentrations and sequenced on the Illumina HiSeq platform (Illumina, San Diego, CA).

mRNA Sequencing Data Analysis

Sequencing output from the Illumina HiSeq platform was converted to FASTQ format and demultiplexed using Illumina BclFastq 2.18.0.12 (Illumina, San Diego, CA). Quality control was performed via FastQC on both raw and processed sequencing reads (Babrahm Institute, Cambridge, UK). Demultiplexed FASTQ sequence files were uploaded to Geneious software (Biomatters, New Zealand). Sequencing reads from each treatment were mapped against LGG genome in Geneious software using "Geneious for RNA Seq" mapper, a minimum mapping quality of 30 (99.9% confidence), allowing gaps with a maximum of 10% per read, 20% maximum mismatches per read, with word length of 20 bases. Expression levels were calculated in Geneious and compared between treatment types. Genes identified as significantly differentially regulated between treatments ($p \leq 0.05$) were further filtered to include only genes with 2-fold expression differences. Genes identified as significantly differentially regulated at ≥2-fold in at least one treatment type for each isolate were plotted as heat maps in OriginLab software (Origin Lab, Northampton, MA), and compared between strains to show differences.

Preparation of Electrocompetent Cells of *L. rhamnosus*

Electrocompetent *L. rhamnosus* cells were generated using a combination of previously described methods (Kim et al., 2005; Welker et al., 2015), with minor adjustments. Briefly, an overnight culture of *L. rhamnosus* AMC010 was diluted to 10^6 cells/ml in pre-warmed MRS broth supplemented with 2% glycine and was incubated overnight at 37°C without agitation. After incubation, 5 ml of culture was inoculated in 100 ml of freshly prepared, pre-warmed MRS medium supplemented with 2% glycine. The culture was incubated at 37°C without agitation until it reached and $OD_{600\,nm}$ of 0.2. Ampicillin was then added to the culture at a final concentration of 10 μg/ml, and incubation at 37°C continued until the culture reached an $OD_{600\,nm}$ of 0.4. Cells were then harvested by centrifugation at room temperature (10 min at 6,000 g), washed twice at room temperature with electroporation buffer (0.5 M sucrose, 7 mM potassium phosphate pH7.4, 1 mM $MgCl_2$), resuspended in 1 ml of the same buffer, and placed on ice. The electrocompetent cells were used immediately for electroporation.

Generation of the *bsh* Insertional Mutant Strain

Insertional inactivation of the *bsh* gene in *L. rhamnosus* AMC010 was done as described (Welker et al., 2015). Briefly, primers BshFHindIII (TATTAAGCTTTTCAGACAGAGGCGGCTTTG C) and BshREcoRI (AATAGAATTCAATCTTGACGCCTTGA CCAC) were designed to amplify a 652 bp region of the *bsh* gene in AMC010. The primers included EcoR1 and HindIII restriction sites for cloning into the pFAJ-5301 vector (Lebeer et al., 2012). The resulting vector (pFAJ-BSHi) was used to transform AMC010 by electroporation using an Bio-Rad Gene Pulser (peak voltage, 1.7 kV; capacitance, 25 μF; resistance, 200 Ω with time constant of 2–4 ms). Electroporated AMC010 cells were allowed to recover for 24 h in MRS at 37°C without agitation, and subsequently plated on MRS containing erythromycin at a final concentration of 2 μg/ml. Individual erythromycin resistant colonies were selected after 48 h of growth at 37°C and sub-cultured in MRS containing 2 μg/ml erythromycin overnight without agitation at 37°C. Disruption of the *bsh* genes was verified by PCR amplification using primers Bsh1753F (AT TGCCTGACCTAGATGCAGG) and Bsh1753R (AACACCGGC GACAGGTCCATC). Genomic integration of the erythromycin resistance cassette was also verified by PCR amplification with the primers Ery625F (CTACTTAATCTGATAAGTGAGC) and Ery625R (TCAGCACAGTTCATTATCAACC). AMC010::*bsh* mutants were cultivated in MRS broth containing 2 μg/ml erythromycin and stored at −80°C in 15% glycerol.

RESULTS

Comparative Analysis of the *L. rhamnosus* Stress Genomic Complement

The genomes of *L. rhamnosus* AMC 143 and AMC010 isolated from infant stools (Thompson et al., 2015; Arnold et al., 2017) were aligned to the genome of the well-characterized probiotic

L. rhamnosus GG (Segers and Lebeer, 2014) for comparison (**Figure 1A**). Our study focused on stress genes and systems encoded by AMC143 and AMC010 in comparison with other *L. rhamnosus* strains of dairy and human origin.

When exposed to environmental pH fluctuations, proton translocating F_0F_1-ATPases are the primary genes responsible for maintaining cytoplasmic pH homeostasis (Azcarate-Peril et al., 2004). Each strain in this study encoded ATPase genes with high nucleotide identity to one another (>98%), however the genomic architecture surrounding the ABC-F Family ATPase varied between strains (**Figure 1B**). In addition to ATPases, cytoplasmic pH homeostasis can be maintained by amino acid decarboxylases and their corresponding antiporters (Azcarate-Peril et al., 2004). Both AMC010 and AMC143 encoded the arginine/ornithine antiporter *arcD* gene; however, the 12 kb region that included this unique *arc*D gene was absent in LGG and HN001 (**Figure 1C**). This region encompassed *arc*D as well as an NADH oxidase, two diguanylate cyclases, cellulose synthase, glycosyl transferase, glycosyl hydrolase and a hypothetical protein. An ornithine decarboxylase was identified in all strains with over 97% nucleotide identity with no architectural deviations between strains. Another amino acid decarboxylase and antiporter system, the glutamate decarboxylase/glutamate gamma-aminobutyrate antiporter (*gad*C) has been shown to reduce the impact of acid stress in *Lactobacillus* (Azcarate-Peril et al., 2004); however, the *gad*C gene, as well as the corresponding decarboxylase gene were absent in both AMC010 and AMC143. Finally, an uncharacterized amino acid decarboxylase gene was present in LGG (LGG_RS12751) with 97.2% nucleotide identity to its homolog in AMC010, but this gene was absent in AMC143.

Similarly to acid exposure, cytoplasmic pH homeostasis is critical to maintain when cells are exposed to alkaline stress. Sodium-proton antiporters and potassium-proton antiporters maintain cytoplasmic pH in alkaline extracellular environments (Lee et al., 2011; Nyanga-Koumou et al., 2012). The strains in this study encoded 3 sodium-proton antiporters (98.2, 98, and 97.1% nucleotide identity). LGG encoded a unique sodium-proton antiporter absent in AMC010 and AMC143. Each strain also encoded a single potassium transporter, with 97.3% nucleotide identity between strains. Alkaline shock proteins (Asp) have been implicated in providing protection from damage caused by increases in extracellular pH change (Kuroda et al., 1995; Seetharaaman, 2008; Anderson et al., 2010). Each of the strains in this study encoded 4 *asp* genes including *asp23*, each with minimum of 98.3% nucleotide identity between strains.

The anti-microbial/detergent properties of bile salts require cells to respond upon exposure in order to resist cytotoxic effects. Each strain in this study encoded a single copy of a bile salt hydrolase (*bsh*). This gene has been implicated in bile-stress tolerance in other lactobacilli (McAuliffe et al., 2005). The sequence identity of the *bsh* gene exceeded 98.2% between strains, however AMC143 contained a deletion of 208 base pairs upstream of the *bsh* gene, eliminating a putative promoter, ribosome binding site, and inducing a 38 bp truncation of the *bsh*

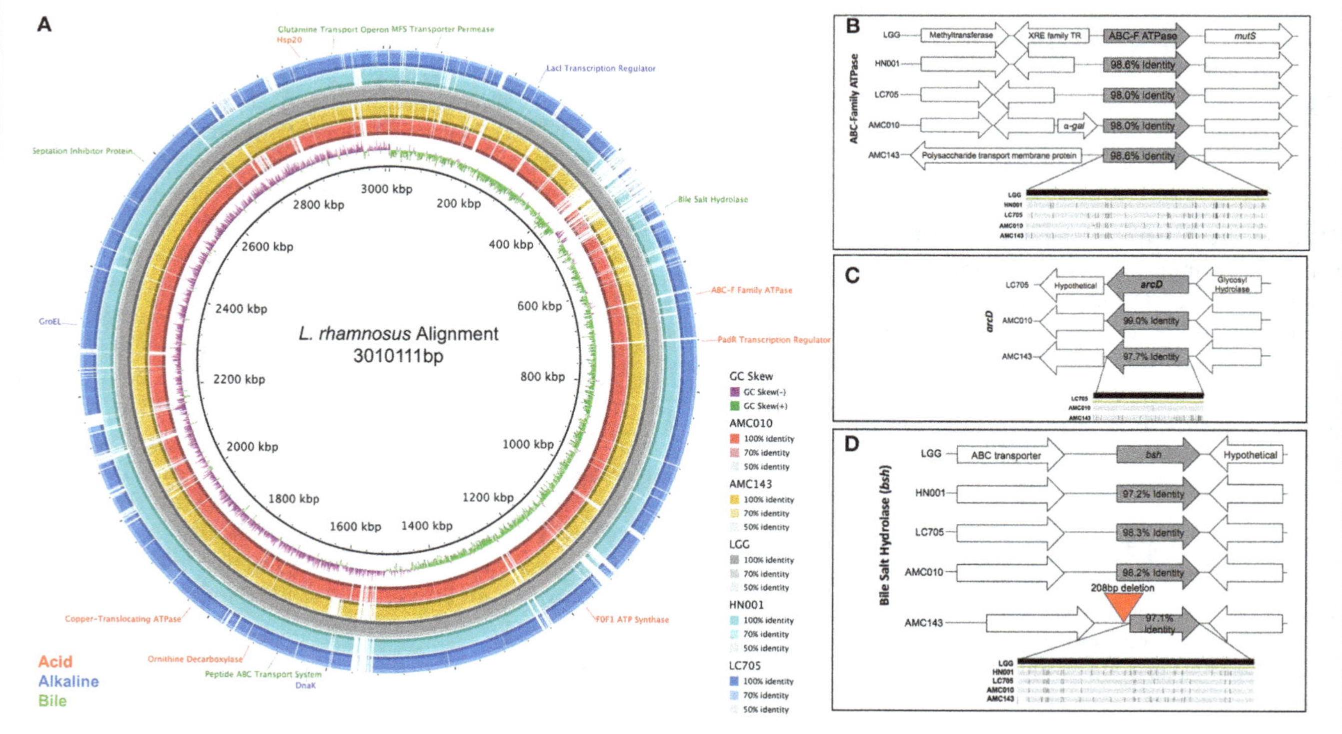

FIGURE 1 | Comparative genomic analysis of *Lactobacillus rhamnosus* isolates. **(A)** Genome alignment of *L. rhamnosus* strains. Strains AMC43, AMC010, Lc705, and HN001 were compared to LGG using BRIG genome alignment software. Relevant stress-response genes are annotated. Comparison of relevant stress-response genes in *L. rhamnosus*, **(B)** ABC-F ATPase, **(C)** *arc*D, **(D)** *bsh* were aligned and compared in Geneious 10.1.3 software. The bottom figure in each graph represents single nucleotide polymorphisms within the compared gene.

gene itself (**Figures 1D, 5B**). Aside from the deletion in AMC143, the *bsh* upstream non-coding region has 93% nucleotide identity between strains. Each strain also encoded cell wall synthesis/repair pathways including DltABCD (Koskenniemi et al., 2011).

In addition to specific stress-response mechanisms, universal stress response systems were present in AMC143 and AMC010. Genes associated with DNA repair were highly conserved, including *radA*, *recN*, *recO*, *recU*, *radC*, *recA*, and *mutS*, each of which had over 96.5% nucleotide identity between strains. Additionally, each strain encoded a suite of highly conserved molecular chaperones, which mitigate stress-associated protein misfolding. These genes included *dnaK*, *groEL*, *groES*, *HSP20*, *HSP33*, *dnaI*, and *clpB*, each exhibiting 98.2% nucleotide identity or higher between strains. Finally, bacteria membrane integrity is often compromised as a result of environmental stress, allowing metal ions otherwise excluded from the cytoplasm to permeate through the membrane, causing further DNA damage and cell death (Pratviel, 2012; Qiao and Ma, 2013). One mechanism that bacteria have to survive declines in membrane integrity is to actively pump cytotoxic metal ions out of their cytoplasm utilizing metal translocating ATPases (Chien et al., 2013). Each strain encoded three different non-specific metal transporting ATPases each with 97.6% nucleotide identity between strains, as well as specific ATPases for transport of copper (97.0% nucleotide identity between strains) and magnesium (97.5% nucleotide identity between strains).

Gene Expression Analysis under Stress Conditions

Differential transcription profiles were generated for AMC010 and AMC143 from mRNA sequencing data obtained from cells exposed to acid (pH 3 adjusted with HCl), alkaline (pH8 adjusted with NaOH), or bile (0.5% w/v oxgall in PBS) stress, and compared to untreated cells. A total 216 genes were identified as differentially regulated (>2-fold change, $p < 0.05$) for AMC010 in response to all treatments, while 79 genes were identified in AMC143. **Figure 2** shows a heatmap indicating genes that were up or down regulated in each strain. We mapped our strains to *L. rhamnosus* GG to provide gene homolog references. Our data confirmed differential regulation of universal stress-response genes and specific stress response genes, although most specific genes were differentially regulated below either the statistical or fold change cutoffs (**Supplementary Table 1**).

Exposure to pH 3 increased expression of a copper-translocating P-type ATPase homologous to LGG_RS08675 by approximately 4-fold in both strains. F_0F_1-ATPases were not differentially regulated between strains, however a metal transporting ATPase homologous to LGG_RS00670 was up-regulated approximately 1.5-fold in both AMC010 and AMC143 upon acid exposure. Amino acid decarboxylases were not differentially regulated between strains. All treatments induced expression of a gene encoding a small heat shock protein Hsp20 homologous to LGG_RS13420 in both AMC143 and AMC010. Exposure of AMC010 to acid induced expression of an additional uncharacterized Hsp20-like molecular chaperone (LGG_RS03170, 11.3-fold), the *padR* transcription regulator (LGG_RS03330, 7.5-fold), and two hypothetical proteins (uncharacterized, *Lactobacillus*-specific LGG_RS11075, 9.2-fold, and *fliK*-like LGG_RS13395, 6-fold). Conversely, a gene cluster including 5 genes involved in purine biosynthesis (LGG_RS08715, LGG_RS08720, LGG_RS08725, LGG_RS08730, and LGG_RS08735) was inhibited in AMC010 across all conditions.

Exposure to alkaline conditions induced expression of the alkaline-shock protein Asp23/Gls24 family envelope stress response protein homologous to LGG_RS01130 in AMC010 by 2.3-fold. This gene also showed a non-statistically significant 2-fold induction in AMC143. Other alkaline shock proteins homologous to LGG_RS01125 and LGG_RS08100 were induced by at least 2-fold in both strains, while the putative alkaline shock protein homologous to LGG_RS01130 was repressed by approximately 2-fold under the same condition, though *p*-values for each of these genes fell below the significance cutoffs set for this study. Alkaline stress also induced the *lacI* transcription regulator (homologous to LGG_RS01785) in both AMC010 (6.1-fold) and AMC143 (12.1-fold), the Hsp20-like molecular chaperone (LGG_RS03170, 19.7-fold in AMC143), which was also induced by exposure to acid in AMC010, and uncharacterized hypothetical proteins homologous to LGG_RS00635 (7-fold) and LGG_RS01080 (5.7-fold) in AMC010. Additionally, exposure to pH 8 resulted in decreased expression of the translation initiation factor IF-3 (LGG_RS08400) and a ribosomal-processing cysteine protease (Prp) homologous to LGG_RS08120, reducing expression levels by 2.6-fold and 4.3-fold respectively in AMC143. Alkaline challenge of AMC010 resulted in reduced expression of the septation inhibitor protein similar to *divIC* (Bennett et al., 2007) (LGG_RS12050) by 3.7-fold, and *minC/ftsL*, genes associated with inhibition of cell division (LGG_RS06095 by 2-fold and LGG_RS06140 by −3.5-fold) ABC transport ATP binding protein (LGG_RS09570) by 4.3-fold and a YbjQ_1 domain-containing hypothetical protein homologous to LGG_RS02955 by 42.2-fold. The galactose-6-phosphate isomerase operon (LGG_RS03135, LGG_RS03140, LGG_RS03145, and LGG_RS03150) was specifically up regulated in AMC143 exposed to pH 8, while the Rpml/translation initiation factor gene cluster (LGG_RS08400 and LGG_RS08395) was down regulated in the same strain by approximately 3-fold.

Exposure to bile resulted in the differential expression of 52 genes in AMC143 and 111 genes in AMC010 with considerable overlap with alkaline treatment. Although the *bsh* gene has been shown to be induced by exposure to bile in *Lactobacillus* (Koskenniemi et al., 2011), in our study, *bsh* (similar to LGG_RS02395) showed a non-statistically significant ($p = 0.2$) 1.2-fold induction in AMC010 while AMC143 showed a marginal repression. The genes more impacted by bile exposure in AMC143 were a HU-family transcription regulator homologous to LGG_RS06660 (induced 2-fold), a septation inhibitor protein (LGG_RS12050), which was down regulated 9-fold, the glutamine ABC transport system operon composed of genes homologus to LGG_RS13875, LGG_RS13880, and LGG_RS13885, which were down regulated

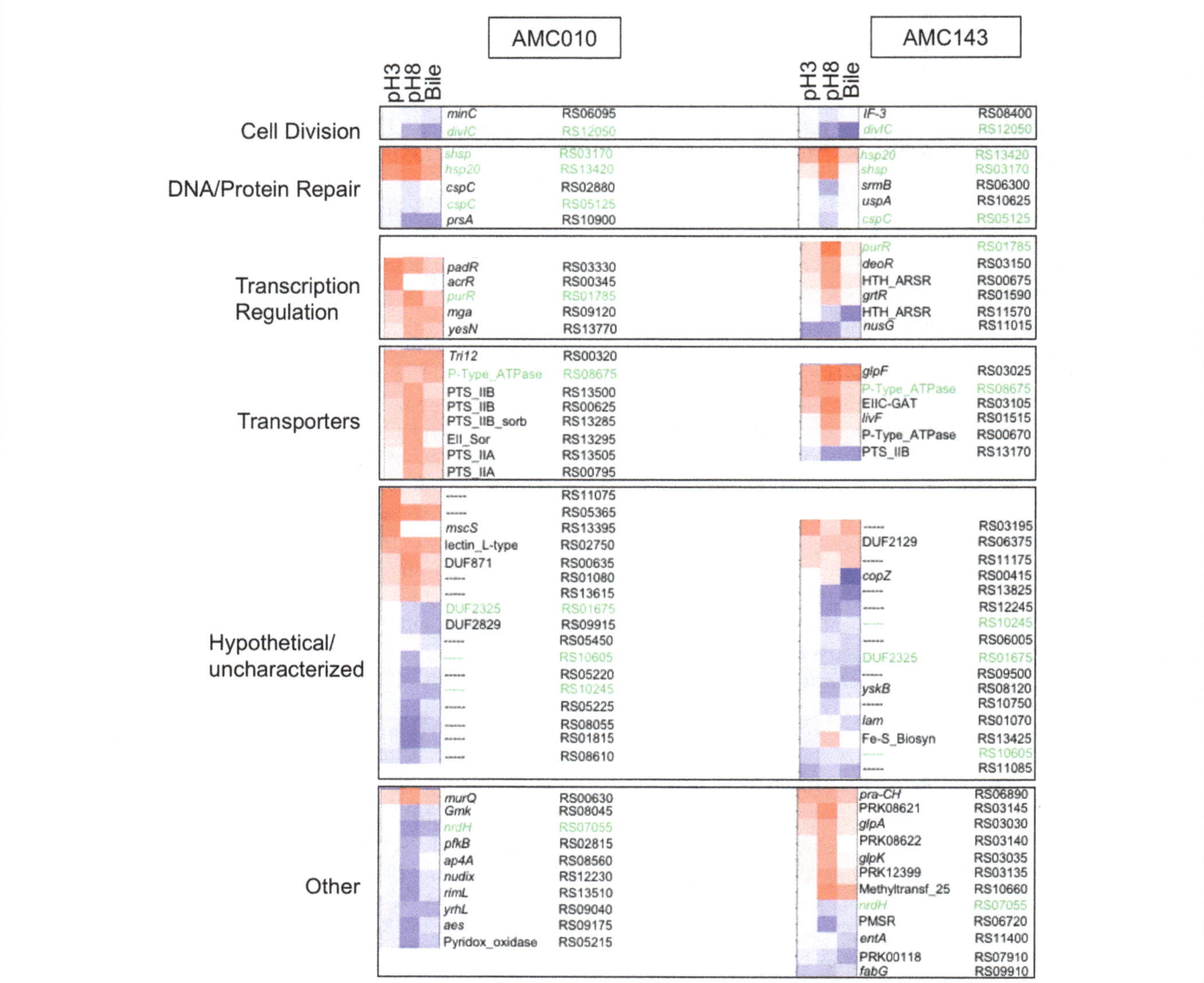

FIGURE 2 | Transcriptomics analysis. mRNA sequencing data from each treatment (pH3, pH8, 0.5%, w/v Bile) was mapped to LGG genome and compared to untreated cells to calculate Log2 differential expression ratio and *p*-value. The 50 genes with the highest differential expression ratio (FDR corrected $p \leq 0.05$) from each strain were categorized by function (cell division, DNA/protein repair, transcription regulation, and molecular transport) and plotted in OriginLab software. Highly differentially expressed hypothetical genes and genes with functions that did not fit into a defined category were also included. Green text highlights genes differentially regulated in both AMC010 and AMC143.

2-fold, and hypothetical proteins homologous to LGG_RS01070, LGG_RS09500, and LGG_RS00415, down regulated 2.8-, 4-, and 13.9-fold respectively.

Exposure of AMC010 to Oxgall resulted in a 2.8-fold induction of a 2CRS response regulator (RR), *dcu*R (homologous to LGG_RS13770), similar to the RR involved in regulation of the anaerobic fumarate respiratory system in *E. coli* (Janausch et al., 2004), as well as a 5.3-fold induction of a major facilitator superfamily (MFS) transporter permease (LGG_RS00320) and 4.3-fold induction of the Hsp20-like molecular chaperone (LGG_RS03170). Conversely, a septation inhibitor protein (LGG_RS12050), *prsA* similar to LGG_RS10900, a molecular chaperone potentially involved in a late stage of protein export (Jakob et al., 2015; Jousselin et al., 2015), the NrdH-redoxin (LGG_RS07055), uracil transport (LGG_RS06995, LGG_RS07000, and LGG_RS07005) and peptide ABC transport system operon (LGG_RS07940, LGG_RS07945, LGG_RS07950, LGG_RS07955, and LGG_RS07960 were down regulated in AMC010 exposed to bile.

In Vitro Growth and Survival of *L. rhamnosus* Exposed to Simulated Gastrointestinal Conditions

Under normal growth conditions (MRS broth, pH 6.6 at 37°C) LGG showed the highest growth rate among strains (0.63 h^{-1}), while AMC143 had the lowest growth rate (0.48 h^{-1}) with no significant differences between AMC010, Lc705, and HN001 (**Figure 3A**). While growth rates between strains were similar under normal conditions, there were distinct differences in growth phenotypes between strains when exposed to simulated gastrointestinal conditions. Growth rates of all strains were reduced approximately 5-fold at pH 4 (adjusted with HCl); however the strains isolated from dairy products, HN001 and Lc705, showed further reduced rates than the human-derived strains, AMC010, AMC143, and LGG (**Figure 3A**). As expected, survival of early-log cells exposed to simulated gastric juice (pepsin, NaCl, HCl pH3) was minimally impacted. No decrease in survival was observed for LGG, Lc705, or AMC143 after 1 h of exposure, while an approximately 15% decrease was observed for HN001 and AMC010 strains. After 2 h, Lc705 showed close to 100% survival, LGG and HN001 were reduced by approximately 20%, and AMC010 and AMC143 populations were reduced by 40% (**Figure 3B**).

Exposure of *L. rhamnosus* strains to MRS adjusted to pH 8 with NaOH showed nearly a 50% decline in growth rate only in AMC143. HN001 and Lc705 showed increased growth rates when grown in media at higher pH 8, while AMC010 and LGG showed no significant differences in growth rates compared to pH 6.6 (**Figure 3A**). When early-log cells were exposed to simulated intestinal juice (pancreatin, NaCl, NaOH pH8) (Charteris et al., 1998) cell numbers increased after 1 h to then decrease in all strains, except HN001 where survival was stable (**Figure 3C**).

Finally, we sought to evaluate growth and survival of *L. rhamnosus* strains in the presence of bile. At sub-physiological concentrations of bile (0.1% w/v), the only strain that showed growth inhibition was Lc705 (60% growth rate reduction). As the concentration of bile in the growth medium increased to physiological levels (0.3% w/v), growth rates decreased by approximately 50% for AMC010, AMC143, and LGG, while HN001 and Lc705 were further inhibited (58 and 80% respectively) (**Figure 4A**). Lc705 showed significant decreased growth rates in all bile concentrations tested. As bile concentrations exceeded physiological levels (0.5% bile) growth rates decreased by over 60%. The growth inhibition observed at 1.0% w/v bile was greater for HN001 and Lc705 (83–92%) than for the strains of human origin (71–78%).

Exposure of *L. rhamnosus* to 0.5% bile resulted in a significant decrease in survival in all strains except AMC143. AMC143 exhibited nearly 20-fold higher survival rates compared to all other strains after 1 h of exposure to 0.5% bile. After 2 h, no HN001 colonies were detected, and the LGG and AMC010 populations were reduced by >95%. AMC143 however remained resistant to the antimicrobial effects of bile, with over 15% of cells surviving after 2 h of exposure (**Figure 4B**).

The Bile Salt Hydrolase (*bsh*) Gene from *L. rhamnosus* AMC010 and AMC143

Despite a highly conserved chromosomal architecture and gene sequence, the region upstream of the *bsh* gene in AMC143

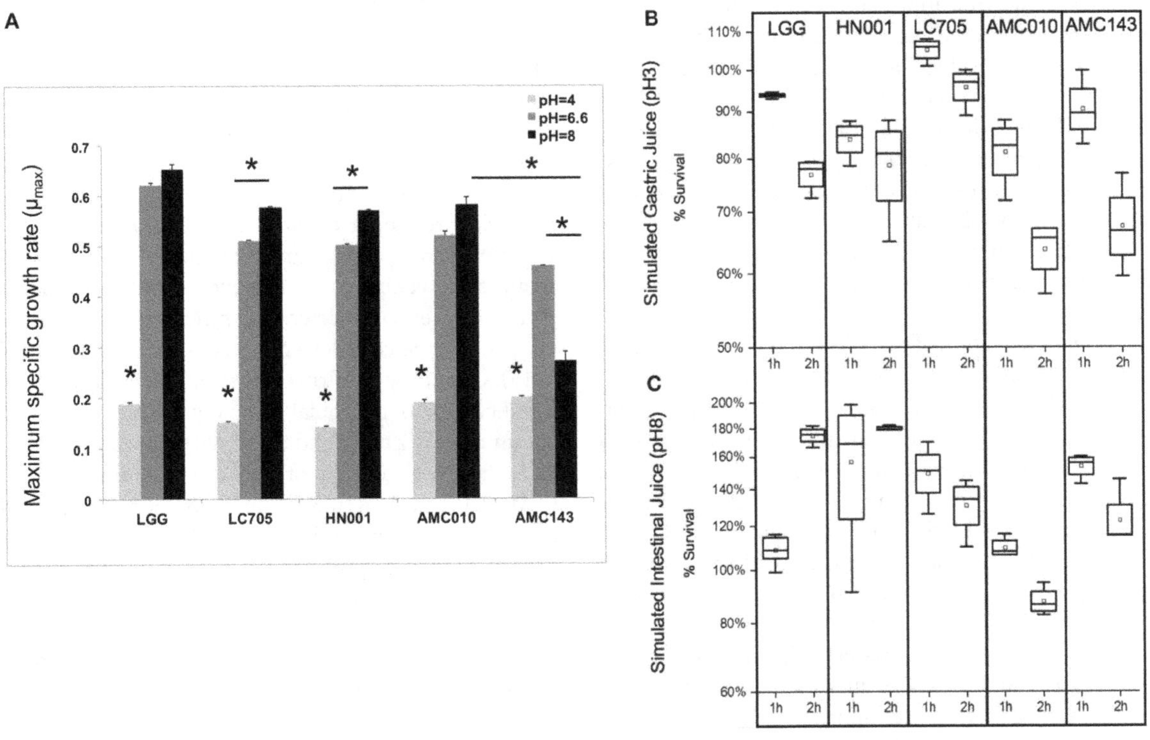

FIGURE 3 | Growth and survival of *L. rhamnosus* under pH-stress conditions. **(A)** Growth rates were calculated for cells grown at pH 6.6 (MRS) pH4 (adjusted with HCl), or pH8 (adjusted with NaOH). (*$p < 0.01$). **(B,C)** Bacterial survival was assayed by plating and enumerating cells exposed to simulated gastric juice (NaCl, HCl, Pepsin pH3) or simulated intestinal juice (NaCl, HCl, Pancreatin pH8) for 1 or 2 h.

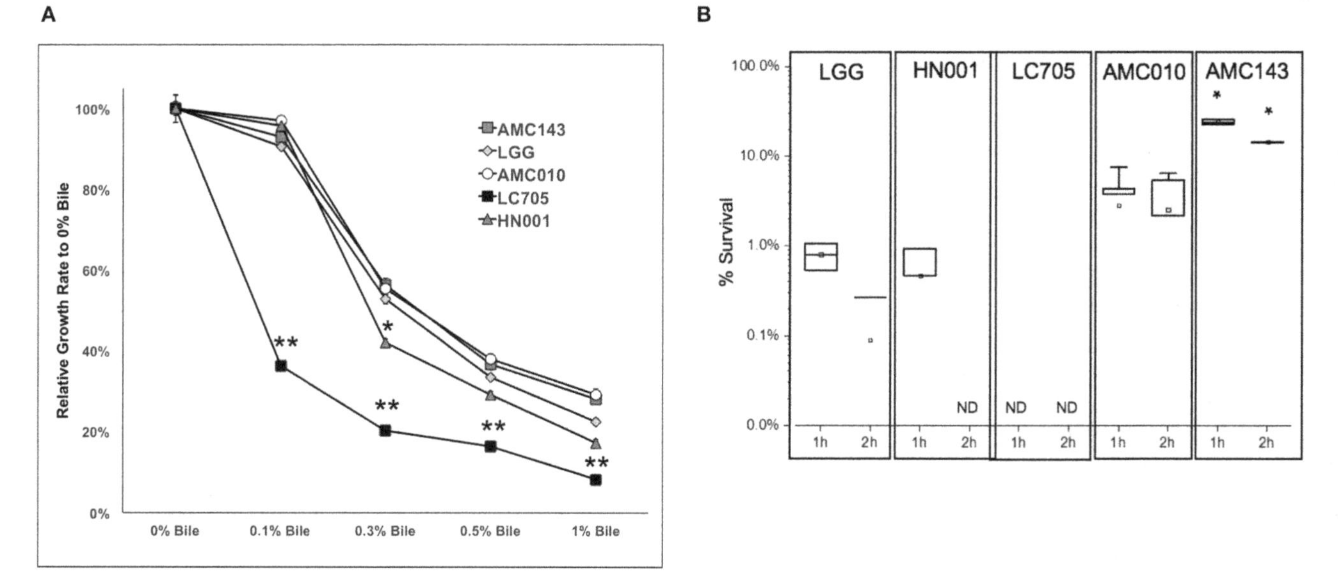

FIGURE 4 | Growth and survival of *L. rhamnosus* under bile-stress conditions. **(A)** Growth rates relative to 0% bile were calculated for cells grown in MRS containing 0.1, 0.3 0.5, and 1.0% w/v oxgall. ($^*p > 0.05$, $^{**}p > 0.01$). **(B)** Bacterial survival was determined by plating and enumerating colonies post exposure to 0.5% w/v oxgall in MRS devoid of any carbohydrate source for 2 h. *Indicates significant difference between AMC143 and each other strain tested. ($^*p > 0.01$, *ND* = No detected growth).

contained a 208 bp deletion, eliminating a putative promoter region and ribosome binding site that is highly conserved in the other strains in the study (**Figure 5B**). Additionally, this deletion resulted in a truncation of the *bsh* gene. AMC143 showed significantly increased resistance to bile. To investigate if the deletion was responsible for the increased resistance of the strain to bile, we first assessed *bsh* expression levels in *L. rhamnosus* AMC143, AMC010, and LGG by RT-qPCR. Data showed variable expression of the gene in absence of bile. Upon bile exposure the *bsh* gene in AMC010 was induced approximately 4-fold, while expression of *bsh* homologs in AMC143 and LGG did not vary. Moreover, *bsh* expression was significantly lower in the presence or absence of bile in AMC143 (**Figure 5A**).

To determine if inactivation of the *bsh* gene in AMC010 would replicate the bile resistant phenotype observed in AMC143, *bsh* was disrupted by insertion of the pFAJ-BSHi vector. Growth of the AMC010::*bsh* mutant under normal growth conditions was indistinguishable from the wild type strain. Survival and growth rates of the mutant were assayed under each stress condition previously performed in this study and compared to the wild type strain. When exposed to acid stress conditions, growth and survival of AMC010::*bsh* was identical to AMC010. Similarly, growth and survival at high pH was identical between the two strains (**Supplementary Figure 1A**). Growth rates of AMC010::*bsh* and AMC010 in varying concentrations of bile (0–1.0% w/v Oxgall) were similar in the presence of glucose (**Supplementary Figure 1B**); however, when exposed to high concentrations of bile (0.5% w/v Oxgall) without a carbohydrate source, survival of AMC010::*bsh* was enhanced 4–6-fold compared to the wild type strain (**Figure 6**), further suggesting a link between *bsh* expression and bile resistance in *L. rhamnosus*.

DISCUSSION

The future of personalized medicine will employ defined bacterial consortia to treat or prevent diseases according to host genotype, diet, and life stage, and the essential first step to develop such consortia is the extensive characterization of gastrointestinal organisms (Faith et al., 2010).

High-throughput *in silico* and *in vitro* analyses of gene-level variation across a large array of species in the human gut are useful as screening tools; however, detailed characterization of strains is essential to determine functional implications of strain variation in the complex ecosystem of the gut (Greenblum et al., 2015). Our study confirms that strain-level variability contribute significantly to microbial diversity within complex microbial communities (Zhang and Zhao, 2016). We compared genomic and physiological data of two novel strains of *L. rhamnosus* (AMC010 and AMC143) (Thompson et al., 2015; Arnold et al., 2017) to three characterized strains (LGG, Lc705, and HN001) to determine their response to simulated gastrointestinal stress.

One of the most striking physiological differences between the strains in our study was the growth inhibition of AMC143 exposed to alkaline conditions. Comparative genomic analysis revealed no major differences between genes previously identified as alkaline-stress response genes, with nucleotide identities ranging from 98.5 to 99.6% between strains. Despite this growth defect, the strain had comparable survival rates when exposed to simulated intestinal juice, suggesting that the growth defect is caused by arrest of cell division as opposed to cell death. Upon

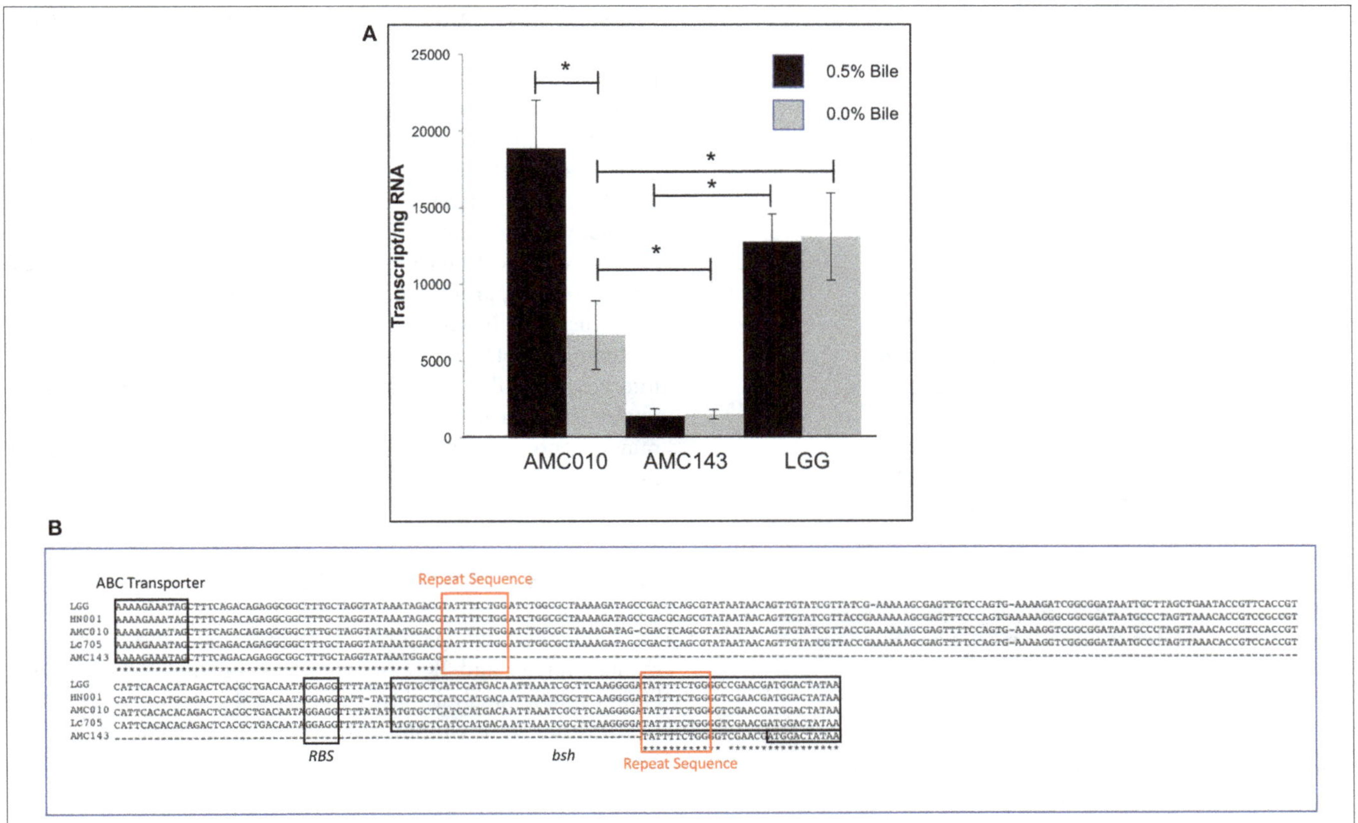

FIGURE 5 | Bile salt hydrolase (*bsh*) expression and sequence analysis. **(A)** RTqPCR targeting *bsh* was performed on AMC010, AMC143, and LGG with and without acute bile treatment, ($^*p > 0.05$). **(B)** Sequence alignment of *bsh* performed in CLUSTAL including annotations of coding regions and ribosome binding site.

exposure to alkaline stress, expression levels of genes associated with growth inhibition (*divIC*, *ftsL*, and *minC*) were repressed in AMC010, while expression of the same genes in AMC143 was unaffected. Conversely, expression of the translation initiation factor *IF-3* was downregulated in AMC143 when exposed to alkaline conditions. We could speculate that this differential expression plays a role in the growth inhibition observed for AMC143. A previous study in *Lactobacillus plantarum* showed that expression of two endopeptidases (Accession numbers Q52071 and Q048X8) was reduced under alkaline conditions (Lee et al., 2011); however we failed to identify homologus genes significantly downregulated in AMC143. Further study of cellular response to alkaline pH is required to better understand the reasons for a growth defect in AMC143.

Analysis of genome sequencing data revealed a 208 bp deletion upstream of the *bsh* gene in AMC143 (**Figure 1D**). Sequence comparison between strains identified a repeat of 10 base pairs flanking the deleted region, suggesting that this deletion may have occurred in AMC143 through homologous recombination. Physiological assays showed that AMC143 was more resistant to bile-induced toxicity than the other strains tested, which led us to investigate the impact of *bsh* expression on bile toxicity. RTqPCR expression data showed a significantly lower *bsh* transcript count in AMC143 compared to LGG or AMC010, both in absence or presence of bile. A non significant induction of the *bsh* gene in AMC010 was also observed by mRNA sequencing data. Bile salt hydrolases have been associated to bile stress resistance in *Lactobacillus* and *Bifidobacterium* (Grill et al., 2000; McAuliffe et al., 2005; Lin et al., 2014) and implicated as a mechanism for host-microbe signaling (Zhou and Hylemon, 2014; Song et al., 2015; McMillin et al., 2016). These enzymes hydrolyze conjugated bile salts generating unconjugated bile acids, which often function as a signaling molecules to host cells and have strong anti-microbial effects (Sytnik et al., 1978; Grill et al., 2000; Schmidt et al., 2001; Kong et al., 2011), and an amino acid, which can be utilized by both host and microorganisms for protein synthesis (Ridlon et al., 2006, 2014; Patel et al., 2010). Studies have shown that BSHs do not always provide a survival advantage to bacteria exposed to bile (Fang et al., 2009), suggesting that BSH activity differs between microorganisms. In fact, lactobacilli encode variable *bsh* genes, each with unique substrates and activities (McAuliffe et al., 2005; Ren et al., 2011). To determine if *bsh* expression was correlated to lower survival upon bile exposure in our strains, we generated a mutant strain of AMC010 containing a disrupted *bsh* gene by site directed insertion (Lebeer et al., 2012). AMC010::*bsh* recapitulated the physiological phenotype observed in AMC143. These findings suggest that the unconjugated products of BSH activity were cytotoxic to the strains used in this study. Our survival assays were performed in MRS broth devoided of a carbohydrate

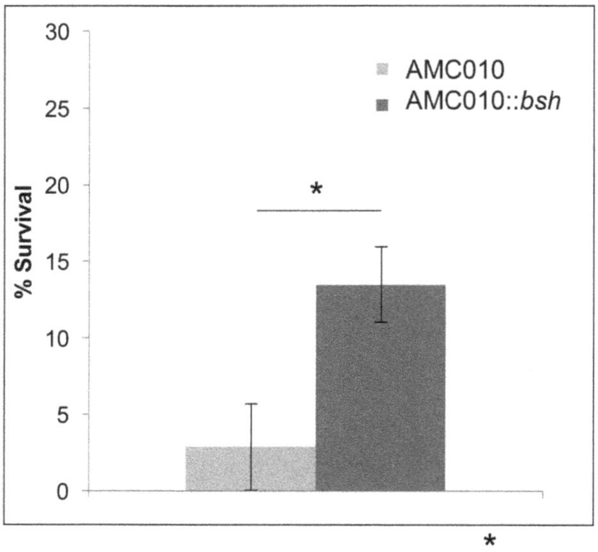

FIGURE 6 | Survival of AMC010::*bsh* under bile-stress. Survival of AMC010::*bsh* was compared to wild type AMC010 by plating and enumerating colonies post exposure to 0.5% w/v oxgall (*$p < 0.01$).

source. In accordance to a previous report (Ziar et al., 2014), when survival experiments were performed in the presence of a carbohydrate source, bile cytotoxity was almost completely abolished for all strains (data not shown).

Strains of the same species derived from different environments are likely to have evolved different abilities to tolerate environmental stress (Douillard et al., 2013). Our data shows distinct physiological differences between strains isolated from human hosts (LGG, AMC010, and AMC143) and strains isolated from fermented dairy products (Lc705, HN001). When grown in alkaline conditions, dairy-derived strains exhibited accelerated growth, which correlates with studies done with other dairy-derived lactobacillus strains (Mojgani et al., 2015), while intestinal strains were either inhibited (AMC143) or unaffected (LGG, AMC010). Additionally, we found that while strains isolated from human hosts were able to grow with limited inhibition at sub-physiological levels of bile, the dairy isolate Lc705 was significantly inhibited even at very low bile concentrations (0.1%w/v). Moreover, survival of dairy-derived strains exposed to high bile concentrations was lower than intestinal strains, suggesting that the strain environmental origin may have driven evolution of their stress response pathways. Strains evolving in environments devoid of bile have no selective pressure to retain bile resistance genes, and these molecular mechanisms are lost over time. This phenomenon has been observed in dairy derived samples as well as in the oral microbiota (Douillard et al., 2013; de Barros et al., 2016).

Analysis of 16S rRNA sequencing data is unable to accurately resolve taxonomy at the species/sub-species level (Janda and Abbott, 2007) as single gene sequencing is insufficient to differentiate between similar species, especially in highly diverse and complex communities. Even with the best of what next generation sequencing has to offer, classical microbiology approaches are absolutely critical in understanding how microbial behavior and physiology correlate to genomic, proteomic, and transcriptomic data. As novel microbiota-derived interventions like new probiotics are being developed, it is important to keep in mind the magnitude to which seemingly minor genomic variability can result in changes to cellular physiology and thus probiotics efficacy.

AUTHOR CONTRIBUTIONS

JA Designed and performed experiments, and wrote the manuscript; JS and JK Performed experiments; JR Performed bioinformatics analysis; MA Designed the experiments, advised JA, contributed to bioinformatic and statistical analyses of data and wrote the manuscript; All authors read and approved the final manuscript.

ACKNOWLEDGMENTS

We would like to thank Dr. Sarah Lebeer from the Department of Bioscience Engineering at University of Antwerp for generously supplying us with the pFAJ-5301 suicide vector for use in this study. We would also like to thank Dr. Rodolphe Barrangou from the Department of Food, Bioprocessing and Nutrition Sciences at North Carolina State University for his help with optimization of electroporation protocols. The Microbiome Core is supported in part by the NIH/National Institute of Diabetes and Digestive and Kidney Diseases grant P30 DK34987.

SUPPLEMENTARY MATERIAL

Supplementary Figure 1 | (A) Growth rates of AMC010::*bsh* in MRS at pH 4, 6.6, and 8. **(B)** Relative growth rate of AMC010::*bsh* in bile (0, 0.1, 0.3, 0.5, and 1.0% w/v oxgall).

Supplementary Table 1 | Expression fold change of Lactobacillus rhamnosus genes under stress conditions.

REFERENCES

Alcántara, C., Revilla-Guarinos, A., and Zúñiga, M. (2011). Influence of two-component signal transduction systems of *Lactobacillus casei* BL23 on tolerance to stress conditions. *Appl. Environ. Microbiol.* 77, 1516–1519. doi: 10.1128/AEM.02176-10

Allegretti, J. R., Korzenik, J. R., and Hamilton, M. J. (2014). Fecal Microbiota Transplantation via Colonoscopy for Recurrent, C. difficile Infection. *J. Vis. Exp.* doi: 10.3791/52154

Anderson, K. L., Roux, C. M., Olson, M. W., Luong, T. T., Lee, C. Y., Olson, R., et al. (2010). Characterizing the effects of inorganic acid and Alkaline Shock on the Staphylococcus aureus transcriptome and messenger RNA turnover.

FEMS Immunol. Med. Microbiol. 60, 208–250. doi: 10.1111/j.1574-695X.2010.00736.x

Andreichin, M. A. (1980). [Antimicrobial properties of bile and bile acids]. *Antibiotiki* 25, 936–939.

Arnold, J. W., Monteagudo-Mera, A., Altermann, E., Cadenas, M. B., Thompson, A. L., and Azcarate-Peril, M. A. (2017). Genome sequences of potential probiotic *Lactobacillus rhamnosus* isolates from human infants. *Genome Announc.* 5:e00107-17. doi: 10.1128/genomeA.00107-17

Azcarate-Peril, M. A., Altermann, E., Hoover-Fitzula, R. L., Cano, R. J., and Klaenhammer, T. R. (2004). Identification and inactivation of genetic loci involved with *Lactobacillus acidophilus* acid tolerance. *Appl. Environ. Microbiol.* 70, 5315–5322. doi: 10.1128/AEM.70.9.5315-5322.2004

Azcarate-Peril, M. A., Ritter, A. J., Savaiano, D., Monteagudo-Mera, A., Anderson, C., Magness, S. T., et al. (2017). Impact of short-chain galactooligosaccharides on the gut microbiome of lactose-intolerant individuals. *Proc. Natl. Acad. Sci. U.S.A.* 114, E367–e375. doi: 10.1073/pnas.1606722113

Begley, M., Gahan, C. G., and Hill, C. (2005). The interaction between bacteria and bile. *FEMS Microbiol. Rev.* 29, 625–651. doi: 10.1016/j.femsre.2004.09.003

Bennett, J. A., Aimino, R. M., and McCormick, J. R. (2007). Streptomyces coelicolor genes ftsL and divIC play a role in cell division but are dispensable for colony formation. *J. Bacteriol.* 189, 8982–8992. doi: 10.1128/JB.01303-07

Borges-Canha, M., Portela-Cidade, J. P., Dinis-Ribeiro, M., Leite-Moreira, A., F., and Pimentel-Nunes (2015). Role of colonic microbiota in colorectal carcinogenesis: a systematic review. *Rev. Esp. Enferm. Dig.* 107, 659-671. doi: 10.17235/reed.2015.3830/2015

Bove, P., Capozzi, V., Garofalo, C., Rieu, A., Spano, G., and Fiocco, D. (2012). Inactivation of the ftsH gene of *Lactobacillus plantarum* WCFS1: effects on growth, stress tolerance, cell surface properties and biofilm formation. *Microbiol. Res.* 167, 187–193. doi: 10.1016/j.micres.2011.07.001

Bove, P., Russo, P., Capozzi, V., Gallone, A., Spano, G., and Fiocco, D. (2013). *Lactobacillus plantarum* passage through an oro-gastro-intestinal tract simulator: carrier matrix effect and transcriptional analysis of genes associated to stress and probiosis. *Microbiol. Res.* 168, 351–359. doi: 10.1016/j.micres.2013.01.004

Bruno-Bárcena, J. M., Andrus, J. M., Libby, S. L., Klaenhammer, T. R., and Hassan, H. M. (2004). Expression of a heterologous manganese superoxide dismutase gene in intestinal lactobacilli provides protection against hydrogen peroxide toxicity. *Appl. Environ. Microbiol.* 70, 4702–4710. doi: 10.1128/AEM.70.8.4702-4710.2004

Calderini, E., Celebioglu, H. U., Villarroel, J., Jacobsen, S., Svensson, B., and Pessione, E. (2017). Comparative proteomics of oxidative stress response of *Lactobacillus acidophilus* NCFM reveals effects on DNA repair and cysteine de novo synthesis. *Proteomics* 17:1600178. doi: 10.1002/pmic.201600178

Carding, S., Verbeke, K., Vipond, D. T., Corfe, B. M., and Owen, L. J. (2015). Dysbiosis of the gut microbiota in disease. *Microb. Ecol. Health Dis.* 26:26191. doi: 10.3402/mehd.v26.26191

Casiano-Colón, A., and Marquis, R. E. (1988). Role of the arginine deiminase system in protecting oral bacteria and an enzymatic basis for acid tolerance. *Appl. Environ. Microbiol.* 54, 1318–1324.

Ceapa, C., Lambert, J., van Limpt, K., Wels, M., Smokvina, T., Knol, J., et al. (2015). Phenotype profiling links genotype to carbohydrate utilization signatures in the species *Lactobacillus rhamnosus*. *Appl. Environ. Microbiol.* 81, 5458–5470. doi: 10.1128/AEM.00851-15

Chapman, C. M., Gibson, G. R., and Rowland, I. (2012). *In vitro* evaluation of single- and multi-strain probiotics: inter-species inhibition between probiotic strains, and inhibition of pathogens. *Anaerobe* 18, 405–413. doi: 10.1016/j.anaerobe.2012.05.004

Charteris, W. P., Kelly, P. M., Morelli, L., and Collins, J. K. (1998). Development and application of an *in vitro* methodology to determine the transit tolerance of potentially probiotic *Lactobacillus* and *Bifidobacterium* species in the upper human gastrointestinal tract. *J. Appl. Microbiol.* 84, 759–768. doi: 10.1046/j.1365-2672.1998.00407.x

Chien, C. C., Huang, C. H., and Lin, Y. W. (2013). Characterization of a heavy metal translocating P-type ATPase gene from an environmental heavy metal resistance *Enterobacter* sp. *isolate*. *Appl. Biochem. Biotechnol.* 169, 1837–1846. doi: 10.1007/s12010-012-0047-4

Cusumano, Z. T., and Caparon, M. G. (2015). Citrulline protects Streptococcus pyogenes from acid stress using the arginine deiminase pathway and the F1Fo-ATPase. *J. Bacteriol.* 197, 1288–1296. doi: 10.1128/JB.02517-14

de Barros, J. M., Costabile, A., Charalampopoulos, D., Khutoryanskiy, V. V., and Edwards, A. D. (2016). Evaluating and optimizing oral formulations of live bacterial vaccines using a gastro-small intestine model. *Eur. J. Pharm. Biopharm.* 102, 115–122. doi: 10.1016/j.ejpb.2016.03.010

De Keersmaecker, S. C., Verhoeven, T. L., Desair, J., Marchal, K., Vanderleyden, J., and Nagy, I. (2006). Strong antimicrobial activity of *Lactobacillus rhamnosus* GG against *Salmonella typhimurium* is due to accumulation of lactic acid. *FEMS Microbiol. Lett.* 259, 89–96. doi: 10.1111/j.1574-6968.2006.00250.x

D'Haens, G. R., Sartor, R. B., Silverberg, M. S., Petersson, J., and Rutgeerts, P. (2014). Future directions in inflammatory bowel disease management. *J. Crohns Colitis* 8, 726–734. doi: 10.1016/j.crohns.2014.02.025

Douillard, F. P., Ribbera, A., Kant, R., Pietilä, T. E., Järvinen, H. M., Messing, M., et al. (2013). Comparative genomic and functional analysis of 100 *Lactobacillus rhamnosus* strains and their comparison with strain GG. *PLoS Genet.* 9:e1003683. doi: 10.1371/journal.pgen.1003683

Faith, J. J., Rey, F. E., O'Donnell, D., Karlsson, M., McNulty, N. P., Kallstrom, G., et al. (2010). Creating and characterizing communities of human gut microbes in gnotobiotic mice. *ISME J.* 4, 1094–1098. doi: 10.1038/ismej.2010.110

Fang, F., Li, Y., Bumann, M., Raftis, E. J., Casey, P. G., Cooney, J. C., et al. (2009). Allelic variation of bile salt hydrolase genes in Lactobacillus salivarius does not determine bile resistance levels. *J. Bacteriol.* 191, 5743–5757. doi: 10.1128/JB.00506-09

Forster, S. C., and Lawley, T. D. (2015). Systematic discovery of probiotics. *Nat. Biotechnol.* 33, 47–49. doi: 10.1038/nbt.3111

Fulde, M., Willenborg, J., Huber, C., Hitzmann, A., Willms, D., Seitz, M., et al. (2014). The arginine-ornithine antiporter ArcD contributes to biological fitness of Streptococcus suis. *Front. Cell. Infect. Microbiol.* 4:107. doi: 10.3389/fcimb.2014.00107

Gill, S. R., Pop, M., Deboy, R. T., Eckburg, P. B., Turnbaugh, P. J., Samuel, B. S., et al. (2006). Metagenomic analysis of the human distal gut microbiome. *Science* 312, 1355–1359. doi: 10.1126/science.1124234

Greenblum, S., Carr, R., and Borenstein, E. (2015). Extensive strain-level copy-number variation across human gut microbiome species. *Cell* 160, 583–594. doi: 10.1016/j.cell.2014.12.038

Grill, J. P., Perrin, S., and Schneider, F. (2000). Bile salt toxicity to some bifidobacteria strains: role of conjugated bile salt hydrolase and pH. *Can. J. Microbiol.* 46, 878–884. doi: 10.1139/w00-066

Grover, S., Rashmi, H. M., Srivastava, A. K., and Batish, V. K. (2012). Probiotics for human health -new innovations and emerging trends. *Gut Pathog.* 4:15. doi: 10.1186/1757-4749-4-15

Jakob, R. P., Koch, J. R., Burmann, B. M., Schmidpeter, P. A., Hunkeler, M., Hiller, S., et al. (2015). Dimeric structure of the bacterial extracellular foldase PrsA. *J. Biol. Chem.* 290, 3278–3292. doi: 10.1074/jbc.M114.622910

Janausch, I. G., Garcia-Moreno, I., Lehnen, D., Zeuner, Y., and Unden, G. (2004). Phosphorylation and DNA binding of the regulator DcuR of the fumarate-responsive two-component system DcuSR of Escherichia coli. *Microbiology* 150 (Pt 4), 877–883. doi: 10.1099/mic.0.26900-0

Janda, J. M., and Abbott, S. L. (2007). 16S rRNA gene sequencing for bacterial identification in the diagnostic laboratory: pluses, perils, and pitfalls. *J. Clin. Microbiol.* 45, 2761–2764. doi: 10.1128/JCM.01228-07

Jarocki, P., Podleśny, M., Glibowski, P., and Targonski, Z. (2014). A new insight into the physiological role of bile salt hydrolase among intestinal bacteria from the genus Bifidobacterium. *PLoS ONE* 9:e114379. doi: 10.1371/journal.pone.0114379

Jarocki, P., and Targonski, Z. (2013). Genetic diversity of bile salt hydrolases among human intestinal bifidobacteria. *Curr. Microbiol.* 67, 286–292. doi: 10.1007/s00284-013-0362-1

Jones, R. M. (2016). The Influence of the Gut Microbiota on Host Physiology: in pursuit of mechanisms. *Yale J. Biol. Med.* 89, 285–297.

Jousselin, A., Manzano, C., Biette, A., Reed, P., Pinho, M. G., Rosato, A. E., et al. (2015). The *Staphylococcus aureus* chaperone PrsA is a new auxiliary factor of oxacillin resistance affecting penicillin-binding protein 2A. *Antimicrob. Agents Chemother.* 60, 1656–1666. doi: 10.1128/AAC.02333-15

Joyce, S. A., Shanahan, F., Hill, C., and Gahan, C. G. (2014). Bacterial bile salt hydrolase in host metabolism: potential for influencing gastrointestinal microbe-host crosstalk. *Gut Microbes* 5, 669–674. doi: 10.4161/19490976.2014.969986

Kankainen, M., Paulin, L., Tynkkynen, S., von Ossowski, I., Reunanen, J., Partanen, P., et al. (2009). Comparative genomic analysis of *Lactobacillus rhamnosus* GG reveals pili containing a human- mucus binding protein. *Proc. Natl. Acad. Sci. U.S.A.* 106, 17193–17198. doi: 10.1073/pnas.0908876106

Kim, Y. H., Han, K. S., Oh, S., You, S., and Kim, S. H. (2005). Optimization of technical conditions for the transformation of *Lactobacillus acidophilus* strains by electroporation. *J. Appl. Microbiol.* 99, 167–174. doi: 10.1111/j.1365-2672.2005.02563.x

Kong, W., Wang, J., Xing, X., Xiao, X., Zhao, Y., Zang, Q., et al. (2011). Antifungal evaluation of cholic acid and its derivatives on *Candida albicans* by microcalorimetry and chemometrics. *Anal. Chim. Acta* 689, 250–256. doi: 10.1016/j.aca.2011.01.050

Koskenniemi, K., Laakso, K., Koponen, J., Kankainen, M., Greco, D., Auvinen, P., et al. (2011). Proteomics and transcriptomics characterization of bile stress response in probiotic *Lactobacillus rhamnosus* GG. *Mol. Cell. Proteomics* 10:M110.002741. doi: 10.1074/mcp.M110.002741

Kuroda, M., Ohta, T., and Hayashi, H. (1995). Isolation and the gene cloning of an alkaline shock protein in methicillin resistant *Staphylococcus aureus. Biochem. Biophys. Res. Commun.* 207, 978–984. doi: 10.1006/bbrc.1995.1281

Lebeer, S., Claes, I., Tytgat, H. L., Verhoeven, T. L., Marien, E., von Ossowski, I., et al. (2012). Functional analysis of *Lactobacillus rhamnosus* GG pili in relation to adhesion and immunomodulatory interactions with intestinal epithelial cells. *Appl. Environ. Microbiol.* 78, 185–193. doi: 10.1128/AEM.06192-11

Lee, K., and Pi, K. (2010). Effect of transient acid stress on the proteome of intestinal probiotic *Lactobacillus reuteri. Biochemistry* 75, 460–465. doi: 10.1134/S0006297910040097

Lee, K., Rho, B. S., Pi, K., Kim, H. J., and Choi, Y. J. (2011). Proteomic analysis of protein expression in *Lactobacillus plantarum* in response to alkaline stress. *J. Biotechnol.* 153, 1–7. doi: 10.1016/j.jbiotec.2011.02.008

Li, K., Bihan, M., Yooseph, S., and Methé, B. A. (2012). Analyses of the microbial diversity across the human microbiome. *PLoS ONE* 7:e32118. doi: 10.1371/journal.pone.0032118

Lin, J., Negga, R., Zeng, X., and Smith, K. (2014). Effect of bile salt hydrolase inhibitors on a bile salt hydrolase from *Lactobacillus acidophilus. Pathogens* 3, 947–956. doi: 10.3390/pathogens3040947

Makras, L., Triantafyllou, V., Fayol-Messaoudi, D., Adriany, T., Zoumpopoulou, G., Tsakalidou, E., et al. (2006). Kinetic analysis of the antibacterial activity of probiotic lactobacilli towards *Salmonella enterica* serovar Typhimurium reveals a role for lactic acid and other inhibitory compounds. *Res. Microbiol.* 157, 241–247. doi: 10.1016/j.resmic.2005.09.002

McAuliffe, O., Cano, R. J., and Klaenhammer, T. R. (2005). Genetic analysis of two bile salt hydrolase activities in *Lactobacillus acidophilus* NCFM. *Appl. Environ. Microbiol.* 71, 4925–4929. doi: 10.1128/AEM.71.8.4925-4929.2005

McMillin, M., Frampton, G., Quinn, M., Ashfaq, S., de los Santos, M. III., Grant, S., et al. (2016). Bile acid signaling is involved in the neurological decline in a murine model of acute liver failure. *Am. J. Pathol.* 186, 312–323. doi: 10.1016/j.ajpath.2015.10.005

Mojgani, N., Hussaini, F., and Vaseji, N. (2015). Characterization of indigenous Lactobacillus Strains for probiotic properties. *Jundishapur J. Microbiol.* 8:e17523. doi: 10.5812/jjm.17523

Monedero, V., Revilla-Guarinos, A., and Zúñiga, M. (2017). Physiological role of two-component signal transduction systems in food-associated lactic acid bacteria. *Adv. Appl. Microbiol.* 99, 1–51. doi: 10.1016/bs.aambs.2016.12.002

Morel-Deville, F., Fauvel, F., and Morel, P. (1998). Two-component signal-transducing systems involved in stress responses and vancomycin susceptibility in *Lactobacillus sakei. Microbiology* 144 (Pt 10), 2873–2883. doi: 10.1099/00221287-144-10-2873

Nyanga-Koumou, A. P., Ouoba, L. I., Kobawila, S. C., and Louembe, D. (2012). Response mechanisms of lactic acid bacteria to alkaline environments: a review. *Crit. Rev. Microbiol.* 38, 185–190. doi: 10.3109/1040841X.2011.640978

Overbeck, T. J., Welker, D. L., Hughes, J. E., Steele, J. L., and Broadbent, J. R. (2017). Transient MutS-Based hypermutation system for adaptive evolution of *Lactobacillus casei* to low pH. *Appl. Environ. Microbiol.* 83:e01120-17. doi: 10.1128/AEM.01120-17

Papadimitriou, K., Alegría Á, A., Bron, P. A., de Angelis, M., Gobbetti, M., Kleerebezem, M., et al. (2016). Stress physiology of lactic acid bacteria. *Microbiol. Mol. Biol. Rev.* 80, 837–890. doi: 10.1128/MMBR.00076-15

Papadimitriou, K., Zoumpopoulou, G., Foligné, B., Alexandraki, V., Kazou, M., Pot, B., et al. (2015). Discovering probiotic microorganisms: in vitro, in vivo, genetic and omics approaches. *Front. Microbiol.* 6:58. doi: 10.3389/fmicb.2015.00058

Patel, A. K., Singhania, R. R., Pandey, A., and Chincholkar, S. B. (2010). Probiotic bile salt hydrolase: current developments and perspectives. *Appl. Biochem. Biotechnol.* 162, 166–180. doi: 10.1007/s12010-009-8738-1

Petrof, E. O., Gloor, G. B., Vanner, S. J., Weese, S. J., Carter, D., Daigneault, M. C., et al. (2013). Stool substitute transplant therapy for the eradication of Clostridium difficile infection: 'RePOOPulating' the gut. *Microbiome* 1:3. doi: 10.1186/2049-2618-1-3

Pithva, S., Shekh, S., Dave, J., and Vyas, B. R. (2014). Probiotic attributes of autochthonous *Lactobacillus rhamnosus* strains of human origin. *Appl. Biochem. Biotechnol.* 173, 259–277. doi: 10.1007/s12010-014-0839-9

Pratviel, G. (2012). Oxidative DNA damage mediated by transition metal ions and their complexes. *Met. Ions Life Sci.* 10, 201–216. doi: 10.1007/978-94-007-2172-2_7

Qiao, Y., and Ma, L. (2013). Quantification of metal ion induced DNA damage with single cell array based assay. *Analyst* 138, 5713–5718. doi: 10.1039/c3an00967j

Ren, J., Sun, K., Wu, Z., Yao, J., and Guo, B. (2011). All 4 bile salt hydrolase proteins are responsible for the hydrolysis activity in *Lactobacillus plantarum* ST-III. *J. Food Sci.* 76, M622–628. doi: 10.1111/j.1750-3841.2011.02431.x

Ridlon, J. M., Kang, D. J., and Hylemon, P. B. (2006). Bile salt biotransformations by human intestinal bacteria. *J. Lipid Res.* 47, 241–259. doi: 10.1194/jlr.R500013-JLR200

Ridlon, J. M., Kang, D. J., Hylemon, P. B., and Bajaj, J. S. (2014). Bile Acids and the Gut Microbiome. *Curr. Opin. Gastroenterol.* 30, 332–338. doi: 10.1097/MOG.0000000000000057

Rossi, F., Zotta, T., Iacumin, L., and Reale, A. (2016). Theoretical insight into the heat shock response (HSR) regulation in *Lactobacillus casei* and *L. rhamnosus. J. Theor. Biol.* 402, 21–37. doi: 10.1016/j.jtbi.2016.04.029

Ruiz, L., Margolles, A., and Sánchez, B. (2013). Bile resistance mechanisms in Lactobacillus and Bifidobacterium. *Front. Microbiol.* 4:396. doi: 10.3389/fmicb.2013.00396

Schmidt, E. J., Boswell, J. S., Walsh, J. P., Schellenberg, M. M., Winter, T. W., Li, C., et al. (2001). Activities of cholic acid-derived antimicrobial agents against multidrug-resistant bacteria. *J. Antimicrob. Chemother.* 47, 671–674. doi: 10.1093/jac/47.5.671

Seetharaaman, B. K. V. (2008). In Silico analysis of Alkaline Shock proteins in Enterobacteria. *J. Proteomics Bioinform.* S1, S021–S037. doi: 10.4172/jpb.s1000005

Segers, M. E., and Lebeer, S. (2014). Towards a better understanding of *Lactobacillus rhamnosus* GG–host interactions. *Microb. Cell Fact.* 13(Suppl. 1):S7. doi: 10.1186/1475-2859-13-S1-S7

Sobhani, I., Tap, J., Roudot-Thoraval, F., Roperch, J. P., Letulle, S., Langella, P., et al. (2011). Microbial dysbiosis in colorectal cancer (CRC) patients. *PLoS ONE* 6:e16393. doi: 10.1371/journal.pone.0016393

Song, P., Rockwell, C. E., Cui, J. Y., and Klaassen, C. D. (2015). Individual bile acids have differential effects on bile acid signaling in mice. *Toxicol. Appl. Pharmacol.* 283, 57–64. doi: 10.1016/j.taap.2014.12.005

Sytnik, I. A., Andreichin, M. A., and Kalashnik, S. A. (1978). [Bacteriostatic and bactericidal action of bile acids and antibiotics on staphylococci]. *Antibiotiki* 23, 600–605.

Tannock, G. W., Taylor, C., Lawley, B., Loach, D., Gould, M., Dunn, A. C., et al. (2014). Altered transcription of murine genes induced in the small bowel by administration of probiotic strain Lactobacillus rhamnosus HN001. *Appl. Environ. Microbiol.* 80, 2851–2859. doi: 10.1128/AEM.00336-14

Thompson, A. L., Monteagudo-Mera, A. Cadenas, M. B., Lampl, M. L., and Azcarate-Peril, M. A. (2015). Milk-and solid-feeding practices and daycare attendance are associated with differences in bacterial diversity, predominant communities, and metabolic and immune function of the infant gut microbiome. *Front. Cell Infect. Microbiol.* 5:3. doi: 10.3389/fcimb.2015.00003

Tilg, H., and Moschen, A. R. (2014). Microbiota and diabetes: an evolving relationship. *Gut* 63, 1513-1521. doi: 10.1136/gutjnl-2014-306928

Vandenplas, Y., Huys, G., and Daube, G. (2015). Probiotics: an update. *J. Pediatr. (Rio. J).* 91, 6–21. doi: 10.1016/j.jped.2014.08.005

Wang, X., Ren, H., Liu, D., Wang, B., Zhu, W., and Wang, W. (2013). H(+) -ATPase-defective variants of Lactobacillus delbrueckii subsp. bulgaricus contribute to inhibition of postacidification of yogurt during chilled storage. *J. Food Sci.* 78, M297–302. doi: 10.1111/1750-3841.12038

Welker, D. L., Hughes, J. E., Steele, J. L., and Broadbent, J. R. (2015). High efficiency electrotransformation of *Lactobacillus casei*. *FEMS Microbiol. Lett.* 362, 1–6. doi: 10.1093/femsle/fnu033

Yan, F., Liu, L., Dempsey, P. J., Tsai, Y. H., Raines, E. W., Wilson, C. L., et al. (2013). A *Lactobacillus rhamnosus* GG-derived soluble protein, p40, stimulates ligand release from intestinal epithelial cells to transactivate epidermal growth factor receptor. *J. Biol. Chem.* 288, 30742–30751. doi: 10.1074/jbc.M113.492397

Yu, S., Peng, Y., Chen, W., Deng, Y., and Guo, Y. (2014). Comparative genomic analysis of two-component signal transduction systems in Probiotic *Lactobacillus casei*. *Indian J. Microbiol.* 54, 293–301. doi: 10.1007/s12088-014-0456-x

Zhang, C., and Zhao, L. (2016). Strain-level dissection of the contribution of the gut microbiome to human metabolic disease. *Genome Med.* 8:41. doi: 10.1186/s13073-016-0304-1

Zhou, H., and Hylemon, P. B. (2014). Bile acids are nutrient signaling hormones. *Steroids* 86, 62–68. doi: 10.1016/j.steroids.2014.04.016

Ziar, H., Gérard, P., and Riazi, A. (2014). Effect of prebiotic carbohydrates on growth, bile survival and cholesterol uptake abilities of dairy-related bacteria. *J. Sci. Food Agric.* 94, 1184–1190. doi: 10.1002/jsfa.6395

15

Next-Generation Beneficial Microbes: The Case of *Akkermansia muciniphila*

Patrice D. Cani[1] and Willem M. de Vos[2,3]*

[1] Walloon Excellence in Life Sciences and Biotechnology (WELBIO), Metabolism and Nutrition Research Group, Louvain Drug Research Institute, Université catholique de Louvain, Brussels, Belgium, [2] Laboratory of Microbiology, Wageningen University, Wageningen, Netherlands, [3] Immunobiology Research Program, Research Programs Unit, Department of Bacteriology and Immunology, University of Helsinki, Helsinki, Finland

***Correspondence:**
Patrice D. Cani
patrice.cani@uclouvain.be

Metabolic disorders associated with obesity and cardiometabolic disorders are worldwide epidemic. Among the different environmental factors, the gut microbiota is now considered as a key player interfering with energy metabolism and host susceptibility to several non-communicable diseases. Among the next-generation beneficial microbes that have been identified, *Akkermansia muciniphila* is a promising candidate. Indeed, *A. muciniphila* is inversely associated with obesity, diabetes, cardiometabolic diseases and low-grade inflammation. Besides the numerous correlations observed, a large body of evidence has demonstrated the causal beneficial impact of this bacterium in a variety of preclinical models. Translating these exciting observations to human would be the next logic step and it now appears that several obstacles that would prevent the use of *A. muciniphila* administration in humans have been overcome. Moreover, several lines of evidence indicate that pasteurization of *A. muciniphila* not only increases its stability but more importantly increases its efficacy. This strongly positions *A. muciniphila* in the forefront of next-generation candidates for developing novel food or pharma supplements with beneficial effects. Finally, a specific protein present on the outer membrane of *A. muciniphila*, termed Amuc_1100, could be strong candidate for future drug development. In conclusion, as plants and its related knowledge, known as pharmacognosy, have been the source for designing drugs over the last century, we propose that microbes and microbiomegnosy, or knowledge of our gut microbiome, can become a novel source of future therapies.

Keywords: *Akkermansia muciniphila*, obesity, diabetes mellitus, type 2, probiotics and prebiotics, gut barrier function

INTRODUCTION

Overweight and obesity have reached epidemic proportions with more than 600 million of adults and 100 million children of the world's population suffering from obesity (GBD 2015 Obesity Collaborators et al., 2017). Obesity predisposes to the development of type 2 diabetes and cardiovascular diseases. These two pathologies are part of the metabolic syndrome that is also becoming major problem in public health (Abdelaal et al., 2017; Ajala et al., 2017). Gut microbes play an important role in the regulation of host metabolism and low-grade inflammation (Hartstra et al., 2015; Marchesi et al., 2016; Cani, 2017). The perturbation of the composition and the activity of the gut microbiota, also known as dysbiosis, is thought to be involved in the emergence of the metabolic syndrome (Wen and Duffy, 2017). Nowadays, numerous studies have demonstrated that our dietary habits strongly influence the composition and function of the gut microbiota and eventually may contribute to the onset or the protection against metabolic disorders (David et al., 2014; Korpela et al., 2014; Salonen et al., 2014; Carmody et al., 2015; Zeevi et al., 2015; Cani and Everard, 2016; Thaiss et al., 2016).

Well documented among the potential ways to affect the gut microbiota, is the consumption of selected microbes that are marketed as probiotics defined as "live microorganisms that when administered in adequate amounts confer a health benefit on the host" (Hill et al., 2014). It is worth noting that the current majority of probiotics sold on the market include mainly microorganisms from the genera *Lactobacillus* and *Bifidobacterium* (Douillard and de Vos, 2014). However, other ways such as the consumption of prebiotics have gained considerable attention over the last 20 years (Roberfroid et al., 2010). The prebiotic concept, discovered in Gibson and Roberfroid (1995), has led to a great number of dietary supplements that is an important growth market. The definition of prebiotic is now widely used and has been recently revised as "a substrate that is selectively utilized by host microorganisms conferring a health benefit" (Gibson et al., 2017). Thus, nutritional components that escape the digestion in the upper alimentary tract may have an impact on the gut microbiota by modulating some members of the gut microbiota its composition and its activity. However, the concept of prebiotic has not yet revealed all its secrets. In spite of numerous discoveries of molecular mechanisms explaining how prebiotics and the gut microbiota interact with the host, it remains difficult to identify the bacterial candidate(s) involved in the beneficial effects observed on the energy, glucose, lipid metabolism and immunity.

FROM PREBIOTIC TO NEXT-GENERATION BENEFICIAL MICROBE: FOCUS ON THE IDENTIFICATION OF *Akkermansia muciniphila*

Akkermansia muciniphila is one of the most abundant single species in the human intestinal microbiota (0.5–5% of the total bacteria) and has been isolated and characterized as a mucin-utilizing specialist in 2004 by Muriel Derrien in her Ph.D. research at Wageningen University (Derrien et al., 2004; Collado et al., 2007). This discovery was initiated by the notion that the human body produces its own "prebiotics" or microbial substrates, namely mucus, an abundant glycoprotein that is specifically produced and degraded in the colon (Ouwehand et al., 2005). While germ-free mouse experiments showed that *A. muciniphila* showed immune and metabolic signaling, specifically in the colon, the exact functions of this unusual microbe remained enigmatic (Derrien et al., 2008, 2011).

Further indications for the function of *A. muciniphila* were subsequently determined in other prebiotic studies using inulin-type fructans that were initially characterized as bifidogenic compounds able to increase the abundance of *Bifidobacterium* spp. (Gibson and Roberfroid, 1995). Thanks to the development of novel culture-independent techniques, we decided to revise in depth the impact of such kind of prebiotics on the overall microbial community in mice. Therefore, in search of potential novel bacterial candidates, we combined different techniques (phylogenetic microarray, high-throughput sequencing, gradient denaturation gel and qPCR), which allowed us to analyze and to compare all the bacteria that were present in the intestinal microbiota. The first surprise was to discover that more than 100 different taxa were affected by prebiotics (Everard et al., 2011; Everard et al., 2014). Among these bacteria, we found that the relative abundance of *A. muciniphila* increased more than 100-fold following the ingestion of prebiotics thereby reaching the abundance of up to 4.5% under high-fat diet (Everard et al., 2014), whereas this effect was lower under normal chow diet (0.09–2.5%) depending on the model (Everard et al., 2011, 2014). It is worth noting that these findings are confirmed in different set of experiments (Everard et al., 2013; Liu et al., 2016; Reid et al., 2016; Catry et al., 2017; Zhu et al., 2017). Interestingly, we and others discovered that *A. muciniphila* was less abundant in the intestinal microbiota of both genetic and diet-induced obese and diabetic mice (Everard et al., 2011, 2013, 2014; Schneeberger et al., 2015; Leal-Diaz et al., 2016; Ojo et al., 2016; Song et al., 2016; Singh et al., 2017), however, few studies reported in mice an increased abundance of *A. muciniphila* upon the ingestion of a high-fat high sucrose diet (Anhe et al., 2015; Carmody et al., 2015). It has also been largely demonstrated that inulin-type fructans feeding improves metabolic disorders associated with obesity, including a decreased fat mass, insulin resistance, lower liver steatosis and a reinforcement of the gut barrier (**Figure 1**) (Cani et al., 2004, 2006, 2009; Maurer et al., 2010; Everard et al., 2011; Pachikian et al., 2012; Greer et al., 2016). Importantly, in humans the abundance of *A. muciniphila* was decreased in several pathological situations such as obesity, type 2 diabetes, inflammatory bowel diseases, hypertension and liver diseases (Png et al., 2010; Belzer and de Vos, 2012; Zhang et al., 2013; Dao et al., 2015; Yassour et al., 2016; Grander et al., 2017; Li et al., 2017). Conversely, antidiabetic treatments, such as metformin administration and bariatric surgery were both found to be associated with a marked increase in the abundance of *A. muciniphila* (**Figure 1**) (Shin et al., 2014; Forslund et al., 2015; de la Cuesta-Zuluaga et al., 2017). Therefore, a large body of evidence suggested that *A. muciniphila* may contribute to protect from specific metabolic disorders and cardiometabolic risk factors associated with a low-grade inflammatory tone.

ADMINISTRATION OF *Akkermansia muciniphila*: MULTIPLE EFFECTS ON THE GUT AND BEYOND

Inspired by the numerous indications that the relative levels of *A. muciniphila* decreased during obesity and metabolic disorders

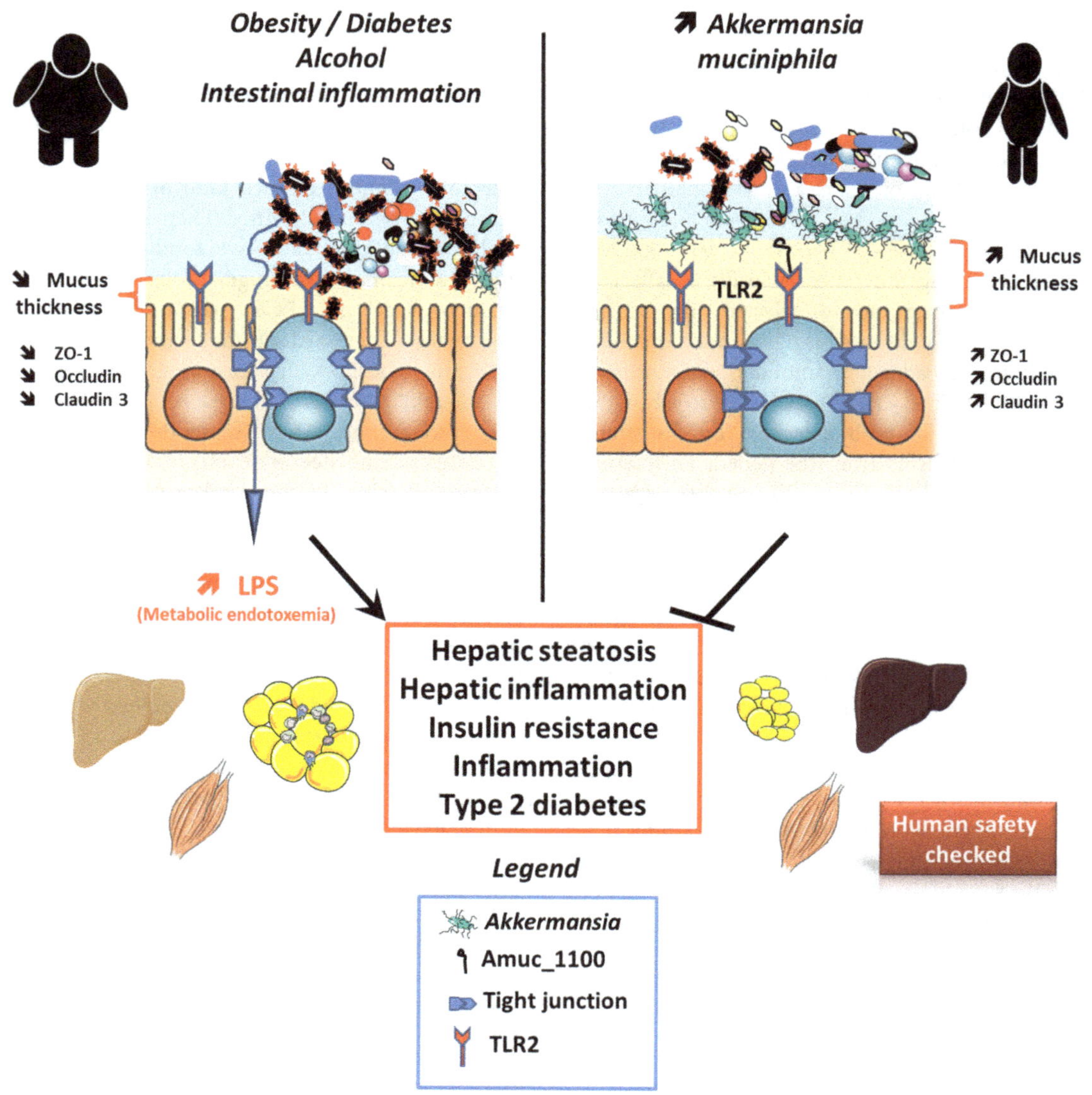

FIGURE 1 | Effects of *A. muciniphila* and derived products on host metabolism. *A. muciniphila* has been found to be lower in several conditions such as during obesity, diabetes, intestinal inflammation, liver diseases, or chronic alcohol consumption. This is associated with an altered gut barrier function leading to an increased plasma LPS levels and eventually triggering low grade inflammation and metabolic disorders. *A. muciniphila* alive or pasteurized as well as Amuc_1100 has been shown to restore gut barrier function likely by acting on TLR2 and restoring appropriate tight junction expression. All these results are associated with an increased mucus later thickness and an improvement of metabolic disorders. It is worth noting that an exploratory human investigation has shown that *A. muciniphila* is apparently safe.

in mouse and man, we decided to study the causal link between *A. muciniphila* and improvements in metabolism. This was done by investigating the impact of a daily oral supplementation with live *A. muciniphila* on the onset of obesity, diabetes and gut barrier dysfunction in mice. We found that the administration of live *A. muciniphila* at the dose of 2.10^8 bacterial cells per day was partly protecting against diet-induced obesity in mice (Everard et al., 2013). Indeed, mice showed a 50% lower body weight gain when treated with live *A. muciniphila* without altering neither their dietary food intake nor the elimination of dietary fats in fecal matter. This protection was mirrored by two times less visceral and subcutaneous fat mass (**Figure 1**), but also by increased markers of fatty acid oxidation in the adipose tissue (Everard et al., 2013). In addition, animals receiving live *A. muciniphila* did no longer exhibited insulin resistance, nor infiltration of inflammatory cells (CD11c) in the adipose tissue, which is a key characteristic of obesity and associated low-grade inflammation (Everard et al., 2013). Interestingly, most of all the metabolic improvements observed following treatment with live *A. muciniphila* were in the range as those observed following oligofructose or inulin treatment (Cani et al., 2009; Dewulf et al., 2011; Everard et al., 2011, 2014), although live *A. muciniphila* was not affecting food intake behavior as do prebiotics like inulin and oligofructose.

Knowing that these metabolic features can be caused by an increased plasma LPS level (i.e., metabolic endotoxemia) or bacterial translocation (Cani et al., 2007; Amar et al., 2011), we next investigated the gut barrier function by measuring several markers. We observed that live *A. muciniphila* prevented the development of metabolic endotoxemia, an effect associated with the restoration of a normal mucus layer thickness (**Figure 1**) (Everard et al., 2013). We also found that administration of live *A. muciniphila* restored the endogenous production of antimicrobial peptides. We then discovered that live *A. muciniphila* increased the endogenous production of specific bioactive lipids that belongs to the endocannabinoid family and are known to have anti-inflammatory activities and regulating the endogenous production of gut peptides involved in glucose regulation and gut barrier, respectively, glucagon-like peptide-1 and 2 (GLP-1 and GLP-2) (Cani et al., 2016). It is worth noting that all these findings have subsequently been confirmed by different groups and extended to other specific disorders such as atherosclerosis, hepatic inflammation and hypercholesterolemia (Shin et al., 2014; Li et al., 2016; Shen et al., 2016; Grander et al., 2017; Plovier et al., 2017).

Collectively all these data reinforce the assumption that live *A. muciniphila* can be considered as a next-generation beneficial microbe with the exceptional particularity that this bacterium can act on numerous facets of the metabolic syndrome and cardiometabolic disorders. Still, these discoveries have raised different fundamental questions that will still have to be studied in humans with the aim to generate new therapeutic tools.

CROSSING THE BARRIER OF SPECIES: FROM MICE TO MAN

Akkermansia muciniphila requires specific culture conditions and complex animal-based medium (i.e., mucin from animal source) and although it may respire under microaerophilic conditions, the cells are relatively sensitive to oxygen (Ouwerkerk et al., 2016). These properties complicate the administration of *A. muciniphila* to human as to evaluate its potential, hence limiting its therapeutic perspectives. In order to solve this problem, a synthetic medium was developed in order to allow the culture of *A. muciniphila* with a high yield and devoid of compounds incompatible with administration in humans (Plovier et al., 2017; Van der Ark et al., unpublished data). Besides the successful development of this synthetic medium, the previous assessment of the efficacy of *A. muciniphila* were performed with cells grown on a mucin-based medium. Therefore, the bacteria cultured on the different media were tested and compared. Interestingly, *A. muciniphila* retains its effectiveness independently of the medium used, and as previously observed, mice treated with the bacterium gained less weight, exhibited an improved glucose tolerance, and insulin resistance under hyperlipidic diet (**Figure 1**) (Plovier et al., 2017).

SERENDIPITY: THE UNEXPECTED ADVANTAGE OF PASTEURIZATION

In 2013, it was showed that the protective effects of *A. muciniphila* disappeared when the bacterium was destroyed by using autoclaving, a heat treatment that destroyes all the constituents of bacteria and spores (Everard et al., 2013). As *A. muciniphila* is a Gram-negative bacterium and hence no spore-former, we were interested what the effects would be of pasteurization, a milder heat inactivation method than autoclaving. Therefore, we tested the impact of administrating pasteurized *A. muciniphila* (30 min at 70°C) cells on diet-induced metabolic disorders in mice. Unexpectedly, this method of inactivation did not abolish the effect of *A. muciniphila* but even exacerbated its beneficial impact. Specifically, mice receiving the pasteurized bacterium and the high-fat diet had a similar body weight gain and fat mass than those observed in mice fed a control diet. Again, these effects were independent of the food intake but pasteurized *A. muciniphila* increased the loss of energy in the feces of the treated mice, indicating a decrease in energy absorption that could contribute to explain the lower weight gain. Pasteurized *A. muciniphila* also strongly improved glucose tolerance, hepatic insulin sensitivity, and completely blocked the diet-induced metabolic endotoxemia. Although, the mechanisms of action of the bacteria are not yet fully elucidated, it is known that *A. muciniphila* express numerous highly abundant protein on its outer membrane (Ottman et al., 2017). Among these proteins, Amuc_1100, implicated in the formation of pili by *A. muciniphila*, was one of the most abundant (Plovier et al., 2017).

Akkermansia muciniphila: A GATE KEEPER THAT DIALOGS WITH THE INNATE IMMUNE SYSTEM

We previously found that *A. muciniphila* was able to restore the expression of specific antimicrobial peptides (Everard et al., 2013). However, Nucleotide oligomerization domain (NOD)-like receptors (NLRs) and Toll-Like Receptors (TLRs) are a specialized group of membrane and intracellular proteins that play a critical role in the regulation of immunity and are directly involved in the recognition of bacterial constituents by the immune system. Therefore, we evaluated the potential of *A. muciniphila* to activate different NOD and TLRs. Strikingly, we found that the bacteria specifically interact with TLR2. TLR2 has been shown to modulate intestinal homeostasis and host metabolism (Caricilli et al., 2011; Brun et al., 2013), thereby participating in the interactions between microbes and host. In addition, to better characterize the interaction between *A. muciniphila* and this receptor, we took advantage of genomic and proteomic analyzes of the external membrane of the bacterium, which may be exposed to host receptors (Ottman et al., 2016). Among these proteins, Amuc_1100 was one of the most abundant. This protein is implicated in the formation of pili by *A. muciniphila* and thus could participate in the interaction between the bacterium and TLR2. This hypothesis was further confirmed by showing that a version of the genetically engineered protein (called Amuc_1100*) was effectively activating TLR2 and with the same magnitude as *A. muciniphila*. In addition, Amuc_1100* remained stable at the temperature used during pasteurization, and could therefore contribute to the effects of the pasteurized bacterium. Amuc_1100* was also able to replicate almost all the effects of *A. muciniphila* alive or pasteurized in high-fat diet fed mice. *A. muciniphila*, whether live or pasteurized, and Amuc_1100* also decreased high cholesterol levels induced by the high-fat diet. Conversely, the pasteurized bacterium specifically also reduced the triglyceridemia of the treated mice, reinforcing the idea that the pasteurization of *A. muciniphila* reinforces its protective effects. A potential mechanism explaining this could be the exposure of active molecules by the heat treatments, including Amuc_1100, or the inactivation of inhibitory compounds, or combinations thereof.

FIRST ASSESSMENT OF *Akkermansia muciniphila* IN HUMANS WITH METABOLIC SYNDROME

As discussed earlier, *A. muciniphila* has various advantages as compared to other beneficial microbes and specific probiotics, at least in the context of the metabolic syndrome. *A. muciniphila* is present in the human milk, is highly abundant in lean and non-diabetic subjects, and is even highly increased upon metformin treatment of gastric bypass surgery, and this without obvious deleterious impact. This unique character does not preclude the fact the human investigations and safety assessment must be done. Hence, to become a putative future food supplement, the safety must be tested. We evaluated the toxicity and the emergence of possible side effects related to the administration of *A. muciniphila* in humans (20 subjects) as part of an ongoing clinical trial of individuals with metabolic syndrome (Plovier et al., 2017). To this end, we analyzed relevant clinical parameters related to liver, muscles and renal functions as well as markers of immunity and inflammation in individuals who received *A. muciniphila* daily for 2 weeks and then extended to 3 months. Whatever the formulation of *A. muciniphila* (live at 10^9 and 10^{10} bacteria per day or pasteurized at 10^{10} bacteria per day), no changes were observed for the markers tested after 2 weeks or 3 months of daily administration. In addition, the frequency of side effects reported by patients were similar in the different groups. These first data indicate that *A. muciniphila* (active or pasteurized) is tolerated in individuals with metabolic syndrome and is likely not toxic.

While *A. muciniphila* is one of the handful of core microbes identified in the intestinal microbiota of over 1000 human adults (Shetty et al., 2017), the administration of its cells, either in live or pasteurized form, in a dietary supplement may be subject to regulatory frameworks that aim to safeguard the consumer. The regulatory requirements relating to the use of live *A. muciniphila* have recently been addressed (Gomez-Gallego et al., 2016). This review summarized the recent comprehensive studies related to *A. muciniphila* and its safety properties and provided criteria be addressed when *A. muciniphila* cells are to be considered as a novel food by the European Food Safety Authority in Europe. One aspect that is relevant here and applies to other core intestinal microbes as well, is the fact that most if not all healthy subjects carry these anaerobes. So these have to be consumed at some stage and in this context it is important to note that *A. muciniphila* is present in early life microbiota and has been detected in mothers' milk (Collado et al., 2007, 2012; Derrien et al., 2008; Jeurink et al., 2013; Ward et al., 2013). Another aspect relates to the antibiotic resistance of *A. muciniphila* that has been studied to some extent in healthy human subjects that carried high levels of *A. muciniphila*-like bacteria and apparently were sensitive to penicillin and tetracycline derivatives but resistant to vancomycin (Dubourg et al., 2013). This was confirmed in *in vitro* studies on the antibiotic resistance profile with the type strain Amuc^T (Ouwerkerk Ph.D. Thesis Wageningen University 2016). Moreover, inspection of the genome sequence did not reveal antibiotic resistance genes that are linked to known genetically transferrable elements (Gomez-Gallego et al., 2016).

CONCLUSION

Since its discovery in 2004, numerous studies have mostly linked the abundance of *A. muciniphila* with beneficial effects, and this although very few exceptions exist in specific non-physiological models (i.e., gnotobiotic models, specific immune double knock-out models) (Seregin et al., 2017).

Nowadays, *A. muciniphila* is widely considered as a novel potential candidate to improve metabolic disorders associated with obesity, diabetes, liver diseases and cardiometabolic disorders. Indeed, its administration has been shown to profoundly reduce the development of such diseases.

Other important steps toward the development of *A. muciniphila* as a next-generation beneficial microbe have been successfully reached. First, the discovery that *A. muciniphila* remained effective by being grown on a synthetic medium compatible with administration in humans. Second, the discovery that inactivation of the bacteria by pasteurization improved its effects, and thus its stability and potential shelf life. Third, the identification of a key mechanisms of interaction between *A. muciniphila* and its host via the identification of Amuc_1100, and last but not least; fourth, the demonstration that *A. muciniphila* may be safely administered in the human targeted population.

Finally, the pasteurized bacteria and the identification and the isolation of bacterial constituents such as the relatively small 30-kDa Amuc_1100 open the door to putative development of drugs based on *A. muciniphila*-related product that could also target pathologies such as type 1 diabetes, inflammatory bowel diseases or diseases where the intestinal barrier function is compromised.

AUTHOR CONTRIBUTIONS

PC and WdV: Conceptualized the review content.

FUNDING

PC is senior research associate at FRS-FNRS (Fonds de la Recherche Scientifique). PC is recipient of grants from FNRS (Project de Recherche, convention: T.0138.14) and Walloon region DG06-FSO project (Microbes 1510053). This work was supported by the FRFS-WELBIO under grant: WELBIO-CR-2012S-02R. This work is supported in part by the Funds Baillet Latour (Grant for Medical Research 2015). PC is a recipient of POC ERC grant 2016 (European Research Council, Microbes4U_713547) and ERC Starting Grant 2013 (Starting grant 336452-ENIGMO). WdV is partially supported by ERC Advanced Grant 250172 (Microbes Inside), the SIAM Gravity Grant 024.002.002 and Spinoza Award of the Netherlands Organization for Scientific Research, and Grants 137389, 141140 and 1272870 of the Academy of Finland.

ACKNOWLEDGMENT

We thank all the collaborators who have contributed to 10 years of *Akkermansia* discoveries, Dr. M. Derrien, Dr. C. Belzer, Dr. A. Everard, and Dr. H. Plovier.

REFERENCES

Abdelaal, M., le Roux, C. W., and Docherty, N. G. (2017). Morbidity and mortality associated with obesity. *Ann. Transl. Med.* 5:161. doi: 10.21037/atm.2017.03.107

Ajala, O., Mold, F., Boughton, C., Cooke, D., and Whyte, M. (2017). Childhood predictors of cardiovascular disease in adulthood. A systematic review and meta-analysis. *Obes. Rev.* 18, 1061–1070. doi: 10.1111/obr.12561

Amar, J., Chabo, C., Waget, A., Klopp, P., Vachoux, C., Bermudez-Humaran, L. G., et al. (2011). Intestinal mucosal adherence and translocation of commensal bacteria at the early onset of type 2 diabetes: molecular mechanisms and probiotic treatment. *EMBO Mol. Med.* 3, 559–572. doi: 10.1002/emmm.201100159

Anhe, F. F., Roy, D., Pilon, G., Dudonne, S., Matamoros, S., Varin, T. V., et al. (2015). A polyphenol-rich cranberry extract protects from diet-induced obesity, insulin resistance and intestinal inflammation in association with increased Akkermansia spp. population in the gut microbiota of mice. *Gut* 64, 872–883. doi: 10.1136/gutjnl-2014-307142

Belzer, C., and de Vos, W. M. (2012). Microbes inside-from diversity to function: the case of Akkermansia. *ISME J.* 6, 1449–1458. doi: 10.1038/ismej.2012.6

Brun, P., Giron, M. C., Qesari, M., Porzionato, A., Caputi, V., Zoppellaro, C., et al. (2013). Toll-like receptor 2 regulates intestinal inflammation by controlling integrity of the enteric nervous system. *Gastroenterology* 145, 1323–1333. doi: 10.1053/j.gastro.2013.08.047

Cani, P. D. (2017). Gut microbiota - at the intersection of everything? *Nat. Rev. Gastroenterol. Hepatol.* 14, 321–322. doi: 10.1038/nrgastro.2017.54

Cani, P. D., Amar, J., Iglesias, M. A., Poggi, M., Knauf, C., Bastelica, D., et al. (2007). Metabolic endotoxemia initiates obesity and insulin resistance. *Diabetes Metab. Res. Rev.* 56, 1761–1772. doi: 10.2337/db06-1491

Cani, P. D., Dewever, C., and Delzenne, N. M. (2004). Inulin-type fructans modulate gastrointestinal peptides involved in appetite regulation (glucagon-like peptide-1 and ghrelin) in rats. *Br. J. Nutr.* 92, 521–526. doi: 10.1079/BJN20041225

Cani, P. D., and Everard, A. (2016). Talking microbes: when gut bacteria interact with diet and host organs. *Mol. Nutr. Food Res.* 60, 58–66. doi: 10.1002/mnfr.201500406

Cani, P. D., Knauf, C., Iglesias, M. A., Drucker, D. J., Delzenne, N. M., and Burcelin, R. (2006). Improvement of glucose tolerance and hepatic insulin sensitivity by oligofructose requires a functional glucagon-like peptide 1 receptor. *Diabetes Metab. Res. Rev.* 55, 1484–1490. doi: 10.2337/db05-1360

Cani, P. D., Plovier, H., Van Hul, M., Geurts, L., Delzenne, N. M., Druart, C., et al. (2016). Endocannabinoids - at the crossroads between the gut microbiota and host metabolism. *Nat. Rev. Endocrinol.* 12, 133–143. doi: 10.1038/nrendo.2015.211

Cani, P. D., Possemiers, S., Van de, W. T., Guiot, Y., Everard, A., Rottier, O., et al. (2009). Changes in gut microbiota control inflammation in obese mice through a mechanism involving GLP-2-driven improvement of gut permeability. *Gut* 58, 1091–1103. doi: 10.1136/gut.2008.165886

Caricilli, A. M., Picardi, P. K., de Abreu, L. L., Ueno, M., Prada, P. O., Ropelle, E. R., et al. (2011). Gut microbiota is a key modulator of insulin resistance in TLR 2 knockout mice. *PLOS Biol.* 9:e1001212. doi: 10.1371/journal.pbio.1001212

Carmody, R. N., Gerber, G. K., Luevano, JM Jr, Gatti, D. M., Somes, L., Svenson, K. L., et al. (2015). Diet dominates host genotype in shaping the murine gut microbiota. *Cell Host Microbe* 17, 72–84. doi: 10.1016/j.chom.2014.11.010

Catry, E., Bindels, L. B., Tailleux, A., Lestavel, S., Neyrinck, A. M., Goossens, J. F., et al. (2017). Targeting the gut microbiota with inulin-type fructans: preclinical demonstration of a novel approach in the management of endothelial dysfunction. *Gut* doi: 10.1136/gutjnl-2016-313316 [Epub ahead of print].

Collado, M. C., Derrien, M., Isolauri, E., de Vos, W. M., and Salminen, S. (2007). Intestinal integrity and *Akkermansia muciniphila*, a mucin-degrading member of the intestinal microbiota present in infants, adults, and the elderly. *Appl. Environ. Microbiol.* 73, 7767–7770. doi: 10.1128/AEM.01477-07

Collado, M. C., Laitinen, K., Salminen, S., and Isolauri, E. (2012). Maternal weight and excessive weight gain during pregnancy modify the immunomodulatory potential of breast milk. *Pediatr. Res.* 72, 77–85. doi: 10.1038/pr.2012.42

Dao, M. C., Everard, A., Aron-Wisnewsky, J., Sokolovska, N., Prifti, E., Verger, E. O., et al. (2015). *Akkermansia muciniphila* and improved metabolic health during a dietary intervention in obesity: relationship with gut microbiome richness and ecology. *Gut* 65, 426–436. doi: 10.1136/gutjnl-2014-308778

David, L. A., Maurice, C. F., Carmody, R. N., Gootenberg, D. B., Button, J. E., Wolfe, B. E., et al. (2014). Diet rapidly and reproducibly alters the human gut microbiome. *Nature* 505, 559–563. doi: 10.1038/nature12820

de la Cuesta-Zuluaga, J., Mueller, N. T., Corrales-Agudelo, V., Velasquez-Mejia, E. P., Carmona, J. A., Abad, J. M., et al. (2017). Metformin is associated with higher relative abundance of mucin-degrading *Akkermansia muciniphila* and several short-chain fatty acid-producing microbiota in the gut. *Diabetes Care* 40, 54–62. doi: 10.2337/dc16-1324

Derrien, M., Collado, M. C., Ben-Amor, K., Salminen, S., and de Vos, W. M. (2008). The Mucin degrader *Akkermansia muciniphila* is an abundant resident of the human intestinal tract. *Appl. Environ. Microbiol.* 74, 1646–1648. doi: 10.1128/AEM.01226-07

Derrien, M., Van Baarlen, P., Hooiveld, G., Norin, E., Muller, M., and de Vos, W. M. (2011). Modulation of mucosal immune response, tolerance, and proliferation in mice colonized by the mucin-degrader *Akkermansia muciniphila*. *Front. Microbiol.* 2:166. doi: 10.3389/fmicb.2011.00166

Derrien, M., Vaughan, E. E., Plugge, C. M., and de Vos, W. M. (2004). *Akkermansia muciniphila* gen. nov., sp. nov., a human intestinal mucin-degrading bacterium. *Int. J. Syst. Evol. Microbiol.* 54(Pt 5), 1469–1476. doi: 10.1099/ijs.0.02873-0

Dewulf, E. M., Cani, P. D., Neyrinck, A. M., Possemiers, S., Holle, A. V., Muccioli, G. G., et al. (2011). Inulin-type fructans with prebiotic properties counteract GPR43 overexpression and PPARgamma-related adipogenesis in the white adipose tissue of high-fat diet-fed mice. *J. Nutr. Biochem.* 22, 712–722. doi: 10.1016/j.jnutbio.2010.05.009

Douillard, F. P., and de Vos, W. M. (2014). Functional genomics of lactic acid bacteria: from food to health. *Microb. Cell Fact.* 13(Suppl. 1), S8. doi: 10.1186/1475-2859-13-S1-S8

Dubourg, G., Lagier, J. C., Armougom, F., Robert, C., Audoly, G., Papazian, L., et al. (2013). High-level colonisation of the human gut by Verrucomicrobia following broad-spectrum antibiotic treatment. *Int. J. Antimicrob. Agents* 41, 149–155. doi: 10.1016/j.ijantimicag.2012.10.012

Everard, A., Belzer, C., Geurts, L., Ouwerkerk, J. P., Druart, C., Bindels, L. B., et al. (2013). Cross-talk between *Akkermansia muciniphila* and intestinal epithelium controls diet-induced obesity. *Proc. Natl. Acad. Sci. U.S.A.* 110, 9066–9071. doi: 10.1073/pnas.1219451110

Everard, A., Lazarevic, V., Derrien, M., Girard, M., Muccioli, G. M., Neyrinck, A. M., et al. (2011). Responses of gut microbiota and glucose and lipid metabolism to prebiotics in genetic obese and diet-induced leptin-resistant mice. *Diabetes Metab. Res. Rev.* 60, 2775–2786. doi: 10.2337/db11-0227

Everard, A., Lazarevic, V., Gaia, N., Johansson, M., Stahlman, M., Backhed, F., et al. (2014). Microbiome of prebiotic-treated mice reveals novel targets involved in host response during obesity. *ISME J.* 8, 2116–2130. doi: 10.1038/ismej.2014.45

Forslund, K., Hildebrand, F., Nielsen, T., Falony, G., Le Chatelier, E., Sunagawa, S., et al. (2015). Disentangling type 2 diabetes and metformin treatment signatures in the human gut microbiota. *Nature* 528, 262–266. doi: 10.1038/nature15766

GBD 2015 Obesity Collaborators, Afshin, A., Forouzanfar, M. H., Reitsma, M. B., Sur, P., Estep, K., et al. (2017). Health effects of overweight and obesity in 195 countries over 25 Years. *N. Engl. J. Med.* 377, 13–27. doi: 10.1056/NEJMoa1614362

Gibson, G. R., Hutkins, R., Sanders, M. E., Prescott, S. L., Reimer, R. A., Salminen, S. J., et al. (2017). Expert consensus document: the International Scientific Association for Probiotics and Prebiotics (ISAPP) consensus statement on the definition and scope of prebiotics. *Nat. Rev. Gastroenterol. Hepatol.* 14, 510–526. doi: 10.1038/nrgastro.2017.75

Gibson, G. R., and Roberfroid, M. B. (1995). Dietary modulation of the human colonic microbiota: introducing the concept of prebiotics. *J. Nutr.* 125, 1401–1412.

Gomez-Gallego, C., Pohl, S., Salminen, S., De Vos, W. M., and Kneifel, W. (2016). *Akkermansia muciniphila*: a novel functional microbe with probiotic properties. *Benef. Microbes* 7, 571–584. doi: 10.3920/BM2016.0009

Grander, C., Adolph, T. E., Wieser, V., Lowe, P., Wrzosek, L., Gyongyosi, B., et al. (2017). Recovery of ethanol-induced *Akkermansia muciniphila* depletion ameliorates alcoholic liver disease. *Gut* doi: 10.1136/gutjnl-2016-313432 [Epub ahead of print].

Greer, R. L., Dong, X., Moraes, A. C., Zielke, R. A., Fernandes, G. R., Peremyslova, E., et al. (2016). *Akkermansia muciniphila* mediates negative effects of IFNγ on glucose metabolism. *Nat. Commun.* 7:13329. doi: 10.1038/ncomms13329

Hartstra, A. V., Bouter, K. E., Backhed, F., and Nieuwdorp, M. (2015). Insights into the role of the microbiome in obesity and type 2 diabetes. *Diabetes Care* 38, 159–165. doi: 10.2337/dc14-0769

Hill, C., Guarner, F., Reid, G., Gibson, G. R., Merenstein, D. J., Pot, B., et al. (2014). Expert consensus document: the international scientific association for probiotics and prebiotics consensus statement on the scope and appropriate use of the term probiotic. *Nat. Rev. Gastroenterol. Hepatol.* 11, 506–514. doi: 10.1038/nrgastro.2014.66

Jeurink, P. V., van Bergenhenegouwen, J., Jimenez, E., Knippels, L. M., Fernandez, L., Garssen, J., et al. (2013). Human milk: a source of more life than we imagine. *Benef. Microbes* 4, 17–30. doi: 10.3920/BM2012.0040

Korpela, K., Flint, H. J., Johnstone, A. M., Lappi, J., Poutanen, K., Dewulf, E., et al. (2014). Gut microbiota signatures predict host and microbiota responses to dietary interventions in obese individuals. *PLOS ONE* 9:e90702. doi: 10.1371/journal.pone.0090702

Leal-Diaz, A. M., Noriega, L. G., Torre-Villalvazo, I., Torres, N., Aleman-Escondrillas, G., Lopez-Romero, P., et al. (2016). Aguamiel concentrate from *Agave salmiana* and its extracted saponins attenuated obesity and hepatic steatosis and increased *Akkermansia muciniphila* in C57BL6 mice. *Sci. Rep.* 6:34242. doi: 10.1038/srep34242

Li, J., Lin, S., Vanhoutte, P. M., Woo, C. W., and Xu, A. (2016). *Akkermansia muciniphila* protects against atherosclerosis by preventing metabolic endotoxemia-induced inflammation in apoe-/- mice. *Circulation* 133, 2434–2446. doi: 10.1161/CIRCULATIONAHA.115.019645

Li, J., Zhao, F., Wang, Y., Chen, J., Tao, J., Tian, G., et al. (2017). Gut microbiota dysbiosis contributes to the development of hypertension. *Microbiome* 5:14. doi: 10.1186/s40168-016-0222-x

Liu, T. W., Cephas, K. D., Holscher, H. D., Kerr, K. R., Mangian, H. F., Tappenden, K. A., et al. (2016). Nondigestible fructans alter gastrointestinal barrier function, gene expression, histomorphology, and the microbiota profiles of diet-induced obese C57BL/6J mice. *J. Nutr.* 146, 949–956. doi: 10.3945/jn.115.227504

Marchesi, J. R., Adams, D. H., Fava, F., Hermes, G. D., Hirschfield, G. M., Hold, G., et al. (2016). The gut microbiota and host health: a new clinical frontier. *Gut* 65, 330–339. doi: 10.1136/gutjnl-2015-309990

Maurer, A. D., Eller, L. K., Hallam, M. C., Taylor, K., and Reimer, R. A. (2010). Consumption of diets high in prebiotic fiber or protein during growth influences the response to a high fat and sucrose diet in adulthood in rats. *Nutr.Metab. (Lond)* 7:77. doi: 10.1186/1743-7075-7-77

Ojo, B., El-Rassi, G. D., Payton, M. E., Perkins-Veazie, P., Clarke, S., Smith, B. J., et al. (2016). Mango supplementation modulates gut microbial dysbiosis and short-chain fatty acid production independent of body weight reduction in C57BL/6 mice fed a high-fat diet. *J. Nutr.* 146, 1483–1491. doi: 10.3945/jn.115.226688

Ottman, N., Huuskonen, L., Reunanen, J., Boeren, S., Klievink, J., Smidt, H., et al. (2016). Characterization of outer membrane proteome of *Akkermansia muciniphila* reveals sets of novel proteins exposed to the human intestine. *Front. Microbiol.* 7:1157. doi: 10.3389/fmicb.2016.01157

Ottman, N., Reunanen, J., Meijerink, M., Pietila, T. E., Kainulainen, V., Klievink, J., et al. (2017). Pili-like proteins of *Akkermansia muciniphila* modulate host immune responses and gut barrier function. *PLOS ONE* 12:e0173004. doi: 10.1371/journal.pone.0173004

Ouwehand, A. C., Derrien, M., de Vos, W., Tiihonen, K., and Rautonen, N. (2005). Prebiotics and other microbial substrates for gut functionality. *Curr. Opin. Biotechnol.* 16, 212–217. doi: 10.1016/j.copbio.2005.01.007

Ouwerkerk, J. P., van der Ark, K. C., Davids, M., Claassens, N. J., Robert Finestra, T., de Vos, W. M., et al. (2016). Adaptation of *Akkermansia muciniphila* to the oxic-anoxic interface of the mucus layer. *Appl. Environ. Microbiol.* doi: 10.1128/AEM.01641-16 [Epub ahead of print].

Pachikian, B. D., Essaghir, A., Demoulin, J. B., Catry, E., Neyrinck, A. M., Dewulf, E. M., et al. (2012). Prebiotic approach alleviates hepatic steatosis: implication of fatty acid oxidative and cholesterol synthesis pathways. *Mol. Nutr. Food Res.* 57, 347–359. doi: 10.1002/mnfr.201200364

Plovier, H., Everard, A., Druart, C., Depommier, C., Van Hul, M., Geurts, L., et al. (2017). A purified membrane protein from *Akkermansia muciniphila* or the pasteurized bacterium improves metabolism in obese and diabetic mice. *Nat. Med.* 23, 107–113. doi: 10.1038/nm.4236

Png, C. W., Linden, S. K., Gilshenan, K. S., Zoetendal, E. G., McSweeney, C. S., Sly, L. I., et al. (2010). Mucolytic bacteria with increased prevalence in IBD mucosa augment in vitro utilization of mucin by other bacteria. *Am. J. Gastroenterol.* 105, 2420–2428. doi: 10.1038/ajg.2010.281

Reid, D. T., Eller, L. K., Nettleton, J. E., and Reimer, R. A. (2016). Postnatal prebiotic fibre intake mitigates some detrimental metabolic outcomes of early overnutrition in rats. *Eur. J. Nutr.* 55, 2399–2409. doi: 10.1007/s00394-015-1047-2

Roberfroid, M., Gibson, G. R., Hoyles, L., McCartney, A. L., Rastall, R., Rowland, I., et al. (2010). Prebiotic effects: metabolic and health benefits. *Br. J. Nutr.* 104, S1–S63. doi: 10.1017/S0007114510003363

Salonen, A., Lahti, L., Salojarvi, J., Holtrop, G., Korpela, K., Duncan, S. H., et al. (2014). Impact of diet and individual variation on intestinal microbiota composition and fermentation products in obese men. *ISME J.* 8, 2218–2230. doi: 10.1038/ismej.2014.63

Schneeberger, M., Everard, A., Gomez-Valades, A. G., Matamoros, S., Ramirez, S., Delzenne, N. M., et al. (2015). *Akkermansia muciniphila* inversely correlates with the onset of inflammation, altered adipose tissue metabolism and metabolic disorders during obesity in mice. *Sci. Rep.* 5:16643. doi: 10.1038/srep16643

Seregin, S. S., Golovchenko, N., Schaf, B., Chen, J., Pudlo, N. A., Mitchell, J., et al. (2017). NLRP6 protects Il10-/- mice from colitis by limiting colonization of *Akkermansia muciniphila*. *Cell Rep.* 19, 733–745. doi: 10.1016/j.celrep.2017.03.080

Shen, J., Tong, X., Sud, N., Khound, R., Song, Y., Maldonado-Gomez, M. X., et al. (2016). Low-density lipoprotein receptor signaling mediates the triglyceride-lowering action of *Akkermansia muciniphila* in genetic-induced hyperlipidemia. *Arterioscler. Thromb. Vasc. Biol.* 36, 1448–1456. doi: 10.1161/ATVBAHA.116.307597

Shetty, S. A., Hugenholtz, F., Lahti, L., Smidt, H., and de Vos, W. M. (2017). Intestinal microbiome landscaping: insight in community assemblage and implications for microbial modulation strategies. *FEMS Microbiol. Rev.* 41, 182–199. doi: 10.1093/femsre/fuw045

Shin, N. R., Lee, J. C., Lee, H. Y., Kim, M. S., Whon, T. W., Lee, M. S., et al. (2014). An increase in the Akkermansia spp. population induced by metformin treatment improves glucose homeostasis in diet-induced obese mice. *Gut* 63, 727–735. doi: 10.1136/gutjnl-2012-303839

Singh, D. P., Singh, J., Boparai, R. K., Zhu, J., Mantri, S., Khare, P., et al. (2017). Isomalto-oligosaccharides, a prebiotic, functionally augment green tea effects against high fat diet-induced metabolic alterations via preventing gut dysbacteriosis in mice. *Pharmacol. Res.* 123, 103–113. doi: 10.1016/j.phrs.2017.06.015

Song, H., Chu, Q., Yan, F., Yang, Y., Han, W., and Zheng, X. (2016). Red pitaya betacyanins protects from diet-induced obesity, liver steatosis and insulin resistance in association with modulation of gut microbiota in mice. *J. Gastroenterol. Hepatol.* 31, 1462–1469. doi: 10.1111/jgh.13278

Thaiss, C. A., Levy, M., Korem, T., Dohnalova, L., Shapiro, H., Jaitin, D. A., et al. (2016). Microbiota diurnal rhythmicity programs host transcriptome oscillations. *Cell* 167, 1495–1510.e12. doi: 10.1016/j.cell.2016.11.003

Ward, T. L., Hosid, S., Ioshikhes, I., and Altosaar, I. (2013). Human milk metagenome: a functional capacity analysis. *BMC Microbiol.* 13:116. doi: 10.1186/1471-2180-13-116

Wen, L., and Duffy, A. (2017). Factors influencing the gut microbiota, inflammation, and type 2 diabetes. *J. Nutr.* 147, 1468S–1475S. doi: 10.3945/jn.116.240754

Yassour, M., Lim, M. Y., Yun, H. S., Tickle, T. L., Sung, J., Song, Y. M., et al. (2016). Sub-clinical detection of gut microbial biomarkers of obesity and type 2 diabetes. *Genome Med.* 8:17. doi: 10.1186/s13073-016-0271-6

Zeevi, D., Korem, T., Zmora, N., Israeli, D., Rothschild, D., Weinberger, A., et al. (2015). Personalized nutrition by prediction of glycemic responses. *Cell* 163, 1079–1094. doi: 10.1016/j.cell.2015.11.001

Zhang, X., Shen, D., Fang, Z., Jie, Z., Qiu, X., Zhang, C., et al. (2013). Human gut microbiota changes reveal the progression of glucose intolerance. *PLOS ONE* 8:e71108. doi: 10.1371/journal.pone.0071108

Zhu, L., Qin, S., Zhai, S., Gao, Y., and Li, L. (2017). Inulin with different degrees of polymerization modulates composition of intestinal microbiota in mice. *FEMS Microbiol. Lett.* 364:fnx075. doi: 10.1093/femsle/fnx075

Novel Aggregation Promoting Factor AggE Contributes to the Probiotic Properties of *Enterococcus faecium* BGGO9-28

*Katarina Veljović, Nikola Popović, Marija Miljković, Maja Tolinački, Amarela Terzić-Vidojević and Milan Kojić**

Institute of Molecular Genetics and Genetic Engineering, University of Belgrade, Belgrade, Serbia

Correspondence:
Milan Kojić
mkojic@imgge.bg.ac.rs

The understanding of mechanisms of interactions between various bacterial cell surface proteins and host receptors has become imperative for the study of the health promoting features of probiotic enterococci. This study, for the first time, describes a novel enterococcal aggregation protein, AggE, from *Enterococcus faecium* BGGO9-28, selected from a laboratory collection of enterococcal isolates with auto-aggregation phenotypes. Among them, *En. faecium* BGGO9-28 showed the strongest auto-aggregation, adhesion to components of ECM and biofilm formation. Novel aggregation promoting factor AggE, a protein of 178.1 kDa, belongs to the collagen-binding superfamily of proteins and shares similar architecture with previously discovered aggregation factors from lactic acid bacteria (LAB). Its expression in heterologous enterococcal and lactococcal hosts demonstrates that the *aggE* gene is sufficient for cell aggregation. The derivatives carrying *aggE* exhibited the ten times higher adhesion ability to collagen and fibronectin, possess about two times higher adhesion to mucin and contribute to the increase of biofilm formation, comparing to the control strains. Analysis for the presence of virulence factors (cytolysin and gelatinase production), antibiotic resistance (antibiotic susceptibility) and genes (*cylA*, *agg*, *gelE*, *esp*, *hylN*, *ace*, *efaA*^{fs}, and *efaA*^{fm}) showed that BGGO9-28 was sensitive to all tested antibiotics, without hemolytic or gelatinase activity. This strain does not carry any of the tested genes encoding for known virulence factors. Results showed that BGGO9-28 was resistant to low pH and high concentrations of bile salts. Also, it adhered strongly to the Caco-2 human epithelial cell line. In conclusion, the results of this study indicate that the presence of AggE protein on the cell surface in enterococci is a desirable probiotic feature.

Keywords: enterococci, auto-aggregation, AggE, adhesion, biofilm, probiotic

INTRODUCTION

Enterococci are an important group of lactic acid bacteria (LAB) which have the ability to survive various environmental conditions, allowing them to inhabit different ecological niches, such as water, soil (Giraffa, 2003), human, and animal gastrointestinal (GI) tracts (Bhardwaj et al., 2011) and food products, especially fermented dairy products (Gomes et al., 2008; Martín-Platero et al., 2009). It has been shown that enterococci have positive properties, such as enterocin production and aroma producing components (Foulquié-Moreno et al., 2006). Many enterococci isolated from fermented dairy products have proven to be great natural probiotics and are generally considered to be beneficial and safe to the host (Eaton and Gasson, 2001; Pieniz et al., 2014).

To evaluate the microorganism as novel food constituent with a health claim, several essential characteristics should be considered, including the survival throughout the GI passage, adhesion, metabolic activities and its effect on intestinal homeostasis (Miquel et al., 2015).

One of the important criteria for probiotic selection is the capability to adhere to the host's intestinal epithelium, according to Guidelines for the Evaluation of Probiotics in Food published in 2006 by the FAO/WHO working group. It is believed that adherence ability of probiotic bacteria to intestinal cells is important for successful colonization and consequently may lead to exclusion of pathogens and/or immunomodulation; expected to provide long time lasting beneficial effects for health (McNaught and MacFie, 2001; Kravtsov et al., 2008). There are also scientists who have a controversial opinion on this issue (or that it is still questionable) because proximity to the intestinal mucosa and a long transit time in the gut are not sufficient to maximize the beneficial effects of a strain (Miquel et al., 2015). Moreover, microorganisms do not have to permanently colonize the system to be achieved the effect on the host. The mechanism by which the consortium of strains from fermented milk product elicit this response is still unclear, but it seems that the effect is rapid (occurring within the first 24 h after application) and it lasts regardless of whether the consortium was introduced during a 1 day period, or with subsequent repeated applications over a several weeks (McNulty et al., 2011).

The precise mechanisms of host-microbe interaction remain still unclear, although there is growing evidence that adherence to the components of the extracellular matrix (ECM) such as mucin, fibronectin, fibrinogen, collagen or laminin (Lorca et al., 2002; Yadav et al., 2013) depends on bacterial cell-surface composition. The expression of ECM-binding proteins on the surface of pathogenic bacteria provide adherence to distinct components of the ECM. The presence of enterococcal surface proteins has been shown to increase the persistence of bacteria in the urinary bladders of mice (Shankar et al., 2001). Collagen binding protein from *Enterococcus faecalis* has been shown to be a putative virulence factor involved in the colonization of renal tissue (Lebreton et al., 2009). On the other hand, probiotic microorganisms express cell-surface adhesins that mediate microbial adhesion to ECM components of host tissue. The expression of aggregation factors on the cell surface of bacteria could induce cell aggregation, visible as auto-aggregation, an important property for colonization of the oral cavity, human gut or urogenital tract.

In LAB and bifidobacteria strains, the ability of adhesion and auto-aggregation has been reported to be significantly related (Del Re et al., 2000). Correlations between the adhesion, aggregation and surface charges were observed among the *Lactobacillus fermentum* and *Lb. paracasei* strains (Piwat et al., 2015). Aggregation promoting factors from LAB differ in molecular weight and primary structure. The best characterized aggregation factors of high molecular weight (proteins of molecular mass >170 kDa), which are responsible for forming large cell aggregates, causing strong auto-aggregation and directly involved in adhesion to collagen and fibronectin, are from *Lactococcus lactis* subsp. *lactis* BGKP1 (Kojic et al., 2011), *Lb. paracasei* subsp. *paracasei* BGNJ1-64 (Miljkovic et al., 2015) and *Lb. paracasei* subsp. *paracasei* BGSJ2-8 (Lozo et al., 2007).

This paper, for the first time, describes the occurrence of novel enterococcal aggregation protein AggE from *En. faecium* BGGO9-28, selected from a laboratory collection as a strain, which belongs to a group with strong aggregation ability. The objectives of this study were to assess the adhesion and aggregation abilities of *En. faecium* BGGO9-28 and to determine a possible correlation between the adhesion of cells and aggregation ability. The novel plasmid-located *aggE* gene was cloned, sequenced and expressed in homologous and heterologous enterococcal and lactococcal hosts, showing that AggE protein is sufficient for cell aggregation in all tested hosts. AggE aggregation factor, protein of 178.1 kDa shares the highest identity with AggL protein from lactococci (81.4%). In addition to its adherence property, BGGO9-28 fulfills several essential criteria required to be considered as a potential probiotic strain: absence of genes coding for virulence factors, the ability to survive in the presence of gastric juices, bile salts and intestinal juices, and strong adhesion ability to host intestinal cells.

MATERIALS AND METHODS

Bacterial Strains, Media, and Growth Conditions

The *Enterococcus* and *Lactococcus* strains used in this study (**Table 1**) were grown in M17 broth (Merck, GmbH, Darmstadt, Germany) supplemented with glucose (0.5% w/v) (GM17) at 30°C. Enterococcal and lactococcal transformants were grown in GM17 medium supplemented with erythromycin (10 μg/ml). *Escherichia coli* DH5α was grown in Luria-Bertani broth (LB) at 37°C aerobically. Solid medium plates were prepared by adding 1.7% agar (Torlak, Belgrade, Serbia) into each medium broth.

Identification of Strains

Primary identification of enterococcal isolates was done by catalase testing, Gram staining and cell morphology, hydrolysis of arginine, CO_2 production from glucose and formation of black zones on bile esculin agar (Himedia, Mumbai, India). Sequencing of genes for 16S rRNA of BGGO9-28 was performed using primers: UNI16SF (5′-GAGAGTTTGATCCTGGC-3′) and UNI16SR (5′-AGGAGGTGATCCAGCCG-3′) (Jovcic et al., 2009).

The Polymerase Chain Reaction (PCR) amplicons were purified using a GeneJet PCR Purification Kit (Thermo Scientific, Lithuania) and sequenced (Macrogen Europe, Amsterdam, The Netherlands). The Basic Local Alignment Search Tool (BLAST) algorithm was used to determine the most related sequences in the NCBI nucleotide sequence database (http://www.ncbi.nlm.nih.gov/BLAST). Based on 16S rRNA gene sequencing results

TABLE 1 | Bacterial strains and plasmids used in this study.

Strains	Source	Strain characteristics	Source or references
***Enterococcus* sp.**			
BGGO9-27	Semi-fat 30 days artisanal old cheese	Agg^+	Terzic-Vidojevic et al., 2014
BGGO9-28		Agg^+	
BGGO9-30		Agg^+	
BGGO9-32		Agg^+	
BGGO9-33		Agg^+	
BGGO9-56		Agg^+	
BGGO10-37		Agg^+	
BGGO10-38		Agg^+	
BGGO11-27	Semi-fat 10 days artisanal old cheese	Agg^+	Golić et al., 2013
BGGO11-29		Agg^+	
BGGO11-33		Agg^+	
BGGO11-41		Agg^+	
BGDU4-1	Semi-had, semi-fat, 15 days old cheese	Agg^+	Laboratory collection
BGDB23-11	Semi-had, full-fat, 12 days old cheese	Agg^+	Laboratory collection
BGZLS10-27	Semi-fat 10 days artisanal old cheese	Agg^-	Valenzuela et al., 2009
BGZLS10-27/pAggES10	Derivative of BGZLS10-27 carrying pAggES10	Agg^+, Em^r	This study
BGZLS10-27/pAggEPX48	Derivative of BGZLS10-27 carrying pAggEPX48	Agg^+, Em^r	This study
Lactococcus lactis* subsp. *lactis			
BGKP1		Agg^+	Kojic et al., 2011
Lactococcus lactis* subsp. *cremoris			
MG7284	Derivative of MG1363	Fus^r, Spc^r, Agg^-	Gasson, 1983
MG7284/pAggES10	Derivative of MG7284 carrying pAggES10	Agg^+, Em^r	This study
MG7284/pAggEPX48	Derivative of MG7284 carrying pAggEPX48	Agg^+, Em^r	This study
Escherichia coli			
DH5α		*supE44 ΔlacU169 (ø80 lacZΔM15) hsdR17 recA1 endA1 gyrA96 thi-1 relA1*	Hanahan, 1983
PLASMIDS AND CONSTRUCTS			
pAZIL	Shuttle cloning vector	Em^r	Kojic et al., 2011
pAggES10	Derivative of pAZIL vector	Carrying *StuI* fragment of 8,944 bp from BGGO9-28	This study
pAggEPX48	Derivative of pAZIL vector	Carrying *PvuI-XbaI* fragment of 7,115 bp subcloned from pAggES10	This study

Agg^+, aggregation-positive; Agg^-, aggregation-negative; Em^r, resistance to erythromycin; Fus^r, resistance to fusaric acid; Spc^r, resistance to spectinomycin.

the BGGO9-28 strain was classified as *En. faecium* (submitted to the European Nucleotide Archive (ENA) under accession No: LT222049).

Auto-Aggregation Assay

The auto-aggregation ability of the selected enterococci strains was tested according to the method of García-Cayuela et al. (2014). Percentage of auto-aggregation was determined using the equation: $[1 - (At/A0) \times 100]$ where At represents the absorbance at different time points (1, 2, 3, 4, and 5 h) and A0 is absorbance at time 0 of three independent measurements.

In Vitro Adhesion Ability to Components of ECM

The collagen binding ability of all the selected enterococci strains and derivates was tested according to Miljkovic et al. (2015). The wells were coated with 100 μg/ml of type I collagen from rat tail (BD Bioscience, New Jersey, USA). The ability of the tested strains to bind to fibronectin was assessed as previously described by Ahmed et al. (2001). The wells were coated with 100 μg/ml human fibronectin (Serva, Heidelberg, Germany). The ability of the tested strains to bind to mucin was tested according to Muñoz-Provencio et al. (2009) with modification. The wells were coated with 100 μg/ml mucin from porcine stomach (Sigma,

St. Louis, USA). After coating with collagen/fibronectin/mucin, wells were washed with PBS and blocked with bovine serine albumin (BSA) (2% in PBS). Also, empty wells were coated with BSA (control wells). Upon removal of BSA solution and washing of wells with PBS, the test cultures (100 μl, 10^8 CFU/ml) were added and plates were incubated on an orbital platform shaker for 2 h at 37°C. Non-adhered cells were removed by washing of the wells three times with 200 μl of PBS. The adhered cells were fixed at 60°C for 20 min and stained with crystal violet (100 μl/well, 0.1% solution) for 45 min. Wells were subsequently washed tree times with PBS to remove the excess stain. The stain bounded to the cells was dissolved by 100 μl of citrate buffer (pH 4.3) and absorbance was measured at 570 nm. The results are presented as the average of absorbance values per each strain (normalized with respect to absorbance values of BSA-coated wells) from three independent experiments per strain.

Biofilm Formation Assay

The ability of the enterococci to form biofilm was assessed as previously described by Peter et al. (2013) with minor modifications. The culture (10^8 CFU/mL) was diluted to 1:40 in GM17 and 200 μl of dilution was used to inoculate sterile 96 well-polystyrene microtiter plates. After incubating for 24 h at 37°C, the excess bacterial cells were removed (the removal of "planktonic bacteria") and wells were gently washed tree times with PBS, dried in an inverted position and stained with crystal violet (100 μl/well, 0.1% solution) for 45 min. The wells were rinsed again with PBS and retained crystal violet was solubilized in 200 μl of ethanol - acetone (80:20) mixture. The absorbance was measured at 570 nm. The results were presented as average of absorbance values per each strain (normalized with respect to absorbance values of empty wells) from three independent experiments.

Southern Blot Hybridization

Transfer of DNA from agarose gel to membrane, labeling of probe and detection of hybrids was performed as recommended by the manufacturer of the DIG DNA Labeling and Detection Kit (Roche, Mannheim, Germany). Hybridizations were carried out at 65°C.

Cloning and Expression of Novel Enterococcal Aggregation Promoting Factor AggE

The procedure described by O'Sullivan and Klaenhammer (1993) was applied for plasmid isolation from enterococci and lactococci.

For preparation of plasmid libraries, plasmid DNA from *En. faecium* BGGO9-28 was digested separately with *Xba*I and *Stu*I restriction enzymes. The resulting DNA fragments were cloned into the pAZIL vector and plasmid libraries were screened in *E. coli* DH5α. All derivatives carrying different fragments were transferred into non-aggregating derivatives *Lc. lactis* subsp. *cremoris* MG7284 (Agg^-) and *En. faecalis* BGZLS10-27 (Agg^-).

All relevant constructs were sequenced (Macrogen, Amsterdam, The Netherlands). The BLAST program was used for sequence annotation and analysis of sequence similarities. ORF prediction was obtained by DNA Strider. Motif Scan (http://myhits.isb-sib.ch/cgi-bin/motif_scan), and Superfamily 1.75 (http://supfam.org/) programs were used to analyse AggE protein.

Comparative analyses of enterococcal (AggE) and lactococcal (AggL) aggregation factors were performed by PCR reactions. The primers used in PCR amplification were: AggE-1DF (5′-GAC TGCTAAGTCAACGGGGG-3′) and AggE-1DR (5′-GATAGGT AATATTTGCTGG-3′). Total DNA (1 ng) was mixed with 17.75 μl of bidistilled water, 2.5 μl of 10 × PCR buffer (Fermentas, Lithuania), 1 μl dNTP mix (10 mM), 1.5 μl of $MgCl_2$ (25 mM), 1 μl (10 pmole) of each primer and 0.25 μl of Taq polymerase (Fermentas, Lithuania). Performed using the GeneAmp 2700 PCR Cycler (Applied Biosystems, Foster City, California, USA), the PCR program consisted of 5 min at 96°C, 30 cycles of 96°C for 30 s, 40°C for 30 s and 72°C for 60 s, and an additional extension step of 5 min at 72°C.

Haemolytic and Gelatinase Activities

Haemolytic activity of enterococcal strain BGGO9-28 was tested on Columbia Blood Agar (Oxoid LTD, Basingstoke, Hampshire, England) containing 5% (v/v) defibrinated horse blood after 48 h of incubation at 37°C. Production of β-haemolysin was detected as the appearance of clear zones around colonies. Also, production of gelatinase of enterococcal strain BGGO9-28 was tested on agar plates containing 30 g of gelatine (Difco, Detroit, MI, USA) per liter as described by Lopes et al. (2006). After filling the Petri plate with 550 g/l ammonium sulfate, the appearance of clean zones around colonies indicated gelatinase production.

Susceptibility Testing

The antibiotic susceptibility of enterococcal strain BGGO9-28 was done by determining the minimum inhibitory concentrations (MICs) by microdilution testing following The Clinical and Laboratory Standards Institute (CLSI), 2015 criteria. Susceptibility was tested against: ampicillin (4–16 μg/ml), vancomycin (4–32 μg/ml), erythromycin (0.5–8 μg/ml), tetracycline (4–16 μg/ml), ciprofloxacin (1–4 μg/ml), nitrofurantoin (32–128 μg/ml), chloramphenicol (8–32 μg/ml), linezolid (2–8 μg/ml) and gentamicin (>500 μg/ml). After 24 h incubation at 30°C, cell density was determined spectrophotometrically by measuring absorbance at 595 nm using a Plate Reader Infinite 200 pro (MTX Lab Systems, Austria). MIC values were determined as the lowest concentration of antibiotic that inhibits visible growth of bacteria.

PCR Detection of Virulence Determinants

In order to test for the presence of genes which indicate virulence, determinants cytolysin (*cylA*), aggregation factor (*agg*), gelatinase (*gelE*), enterococcal surface protein (*esp*), cell wall adhesions ($efaA^{fs}$, and $efaA^{fm}$), collagen adhesin (*ace*), and hyaluronidase (*hylN*) (Eaton and Gasson, 2001; Vankerckhoven et al., 2004) the total DNA of *En. faecium* BGGO9-28 was used.

Survival in Simulated GI Tract

Survival of enterococcal strain BGGO9-28 in a simulated GI tract was performed according to Nikolic et al. (2012). Strain was grown in GM17 for 24 h and culture was harvested by centrifugation (10,000 g for 10 min), washed twice with 0.85% NaCl and concentrated 10-times in reconstituted (10%) sterile skimmed-milk (Difco, Becton Dickinson, Franklin Lakes, NJ, USA). Afterwards, bacterial suspensions were diluted 10-times with gastric juice (125 mM NaCl, 7 mM KCl, 45 mM NaHCO3, 0.3% pepsin (Sigma, St. Louis, MO, USA) adjusted to pH 2.0 with HCl), incubated for 90 min at 37°C in aerobic conditions under shaking. Then, bacterial suspensions were centrifuged (2,050 g, 15 min), resuspended in duodenal juice [1% bovine bile (Sigma, St. Louis, MO, USA) adjusted with 10 M NaOH to pH 8.0] and incubated for 10 min at 37°C in anaerobic conditions. Finally, harvested cell suspensions were resuspended in intestinal juice (0.3% bovine bile, 0.1% pancreas acetone powder porcine type I (Sigma, St. Louis, MO, USA), pH 8.0) and incubated for 120 min at 37°C in anaerobic conditions. Determination of viable counts was carried out in the initial cultures and after each of the challenges (gastric, bile salt, and intestinal juices). Serial dilutions of the samples were made and inoculated on the surface of GM17 agar using spread plate technique. Viable colony counts were determined and survival rate was presented as means of log units of BGGO9-28 growth. Experiments were carried out in triplicate.

Adhesion to Caco-2 Cell Lines

The colonocyte-like cell line Caco-2, was used to determine the adhesion ability of enterococcal strain BGGO9-28. A Caco-2 cell line was purchased from the European Collection of Cell Cultures (ECACC No. 86010202). Adhesion to the Caco-2 cell line was done according to Sánchez et al. (2010). The results of adhesion were expressed as percentage (%) (colony forming units (CFU) adhered bacteria/CFU added bacteria × 100) from two replicated plates. In each plate three wells were used per sample.

Statistical Analysis

Differences between treatments were examined for significance by a Student's *t*-test after analysis of variance (Kirkman, 1996).

RESULTS AND DISCUSSION

The important goals of this study were to investigate the aggregation ability of *Enterococcus* sp. in general, and to examine the possible role of *Enterococcus* aggregation factor as a potential probiotic feature.

Identification and Auto-Aggregation of Selected Enterococci

Considering the importance of aggregation phenomena for human health, the laboratory collection of enterococci was screened for strains exhibiting strong aggregation ability for further analysis. Fourteen *Enterococcus* strains were selected from among 636 examined enterococcal isolates (Terzić-Vidojević et al., 2015) from a laboratory collection, based on their ability to cause auto-aggregation of the cells, using an aggregation visual assay. All of them were isolated from artisanal homemade cow's milk cheeses, produced in households of the Golija and Valjevo mountain regions of the Republic of Serbia (**Table 1**). All enterococcal isolates were Gram positive and catalase negative cocci, in pairs or short chains. Hydrolysis of arginine and formation of black zones on bile esculin agar were positive. None of the enterococci chosen were able to produce CO_2 from glucose. It was found that aggregation ability is a rare phenotype among enterococci (2.2% in our laboratory collection) similarly as in other LAB (Miljkovic et al., 2015).

Some LAB, including enterococcal species, represent beneficial microbiota existing in the human and animal GI and urogenital tracts (Bhardwaj et al., 2011). One beneficial property of bacteria with auto-aggregation ability is the prevention of colonization of pathogenic bacteria by the formation of a barrier via auto-aggregation to intestinal mucosa (O'Toole and Cooney, 2008; Prince et al., 2012).

Based on a visual assay, auto-aggregation ability was further confirmed by monitoring the changes in absorbance (OD_{600}) of cultures during 5 h of sedimentation at 30°C. All analyzed enterococci strains showed varying levels (1 h: 5.34%–81.09%; 5 h: 29.825–89.86%) of auto-aggregation ability and can be classified in three groups: (*i*) strong auto-aggregation (strains BGGO9-27, BGGO9-28, BGGO9-32, BGGO9-33, BGGO9-56, BGGO10-37, BGGO11-27, BGGO11-41, BGDU4-1, and BGDB23-11; with more than 80% of precipitated cells for 5 h); (*ii*) medium auto-aggregation (strains BGGO10-38 and BGGO11-29; with about 60% of the precipitated cells for 5 h); and (*iii*) low auto-aggregation (strains BGGO9-30 and BGGO11-33; with about 40% of the precipitated cells for 5 h) (**Figure 1A**).

Adhesion of Selected Enterococci to Components of ECM

One of the important goals of this study was to investigate the possible role of *Enterococcus* aggregation factor in its adherence to the main components of ECM, such as collagen (**Figure 1B**), structural glycoprotein fibronectin (**Figure 1C**) and mucin (**Figure 1D**), in order to assess its probiotic potential. The strains most adhesive to all tested components of ECM were BGGO9-27, BGGO9-28, BGGO9-32, BGGO9-33, and BGGO9-56. The rest of the strains showed a difference in affinity for various components of ECM. Interestingly, strains BGGO11-29 and BGGO11-41 exhibited the ability to bind collagen (absorbance value 1.17 and 1.97, respectively), while binding to fibronectin and mucin was absent (absorbance value is less that 0.4). Also, it was noted that strain BGDB23-11 binds to collagen and fibronectin (absorbance value 2.82 to collagen and 2.16 to fibronectin), but binding to mucin was very poor (absorbance value 0.28).

The results obtained for auto-aggregation and adhesion to components of ECM among the selected enterococcal strains indicate that they possess a different kind of molecules present on their surface that are involved in cell-to-cell interaction. However, the selected enterococci can be classified into at least four groups: group I (consisting of strains BGGO9-27,

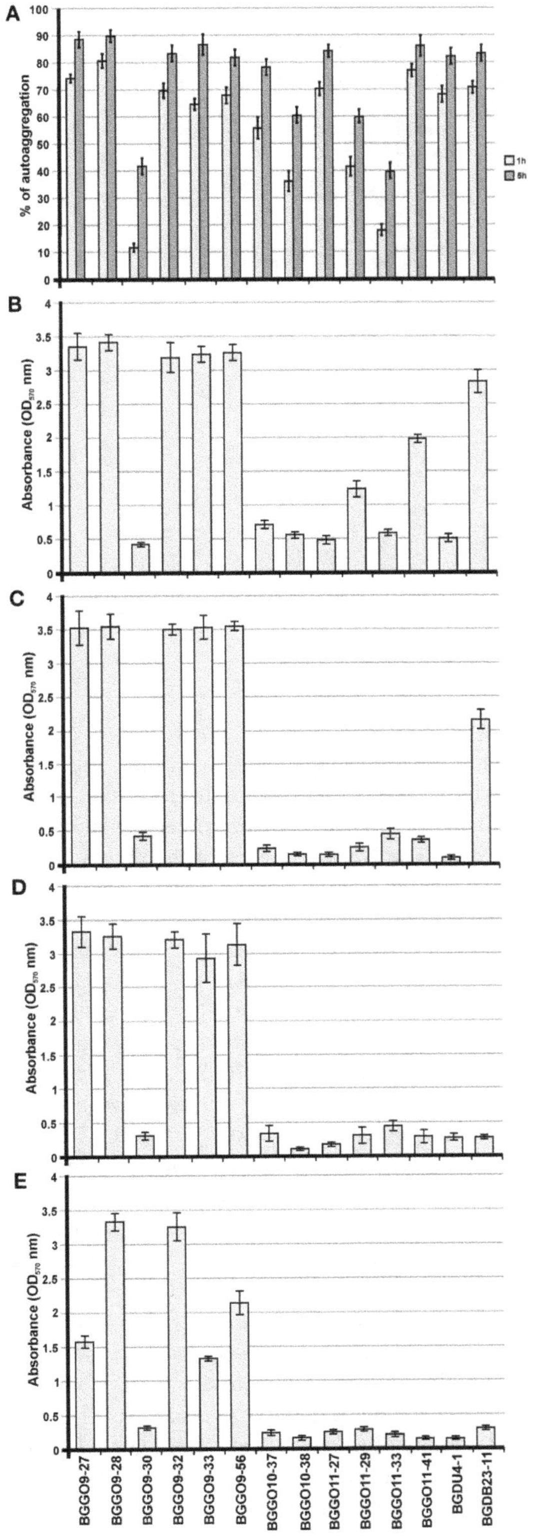

FIGURE 1 | Adhesion capability of selected enterococcal strains. Graphical presentation of results obtained in **(A)** auto-aggregation assay (auto-aggregation ability is expressed as percentages); **(B)** collagen-binding assay; **(C)** fibronectin-binding assay; **(D)** mucin-binding assay; **(E)** biofilm formation assay of selected strains (results were expressed as average of normalized A_{570} values). The error bars show the standard deviations.

BGGO9-28, BGGO9-32, BGGO9-33, and BGGO9-56) showed strong ability to bind to collagen, fibronectin and mucin, while at the same time exhibiting very powerful auto-aggregation ability; group II (consisting of strains BGGO9-30, BGGO10-37, BGGO10-38, BGGO11-27, BGGO11-33, and BGDU4-1) showed a moderate to high auto-aggregation ability, but poor adhesion to all ECM components; group III (consisting of strains BGGO11-29 and BGGO11-41) showed a moderate to high auto-aggregation ability and binding to collagen, but poor adhesion to other ECM components; and group IV (consisting of strain BGDB23-11) showed high auto-aggregation ability and binding to collagen and fibronectin, but poor adhesion to mucin.

Biofilm Formation of Selected Enterococci

Excluding many environmental factors, the number of genetic factors known to be involved in biofilm production has increased in recent years (Mohamed and Huang, 2007). Different surface molecules, such as polysaccharides, have been implicated in biofilm formation. An *En. faecalis* gene mutation which encodes a putative glycosyltransferase that is involved in polysaccharide synthesis showed a 73% reduction in biofilm formation (Xu et al., 2000). In this context, we evaluated biofilm formation by the selected enterococcal strains and investigated the possible correlation between the presence of aggregation factor on the cell surface and the ability to form biofilm.

Cells of the tested strains showed differing abilities to form biofilm. Among the tested enterococci, strains BGGO9-28 and BGGO9-32 showed the strongest ability to form biofilms on the plates (plastic surface), and three strains (BGGO9-27, BGGO9-33, and BGGO9-56) showed moderate biofilm formation ability (**Figure 1E**). Two strains, BGGO9-28 and BGGO9-32, belong to the aforementioned group I of strains (among the tested enterococci), which also showed strong auto-aggregation ability and adhesion to components of ECM. This is the first study that indicates the existence of a relationship between biofilm formation and aggregation in non-pathogenic enterococcal strains.

Localization of *aggE* Gene Responsible for Auto-Aggregation Phenotype

The autochthonous plasmids of the selected enterococcal strains were analyzed to confirm the location of genes correlated with auto-aggregation ability (**Figure 2**). To determine the relationship between the presence of plasmids and the auto-aggregation phenotype, which was very similar to that obtained for lactococci and lactobacilli (Kojic et al., 2011; Miljkovic et al., 2015), Southern blot hybridizations with *aggL* and *aggLb* gene probes from *Lc. lactis* BGKP1 and *Lb. paracasei* subsp. *paracasei* BGNJ1-64 were performed (separately) using plasmid DNA isolated from all selected enterococci. The results indicate that the gene(s) similar to *aggL* determining auto-aggregation in all selected enterococcal strains are plasmid located (on the largest common plasmid; **Figure 2**), which allows fast horizontal transfer among bacteria of the same niche and most probably a selective advantage for carriers. It is interesting that in enterococci, like in lacococci and lactobacilli, genes encoding

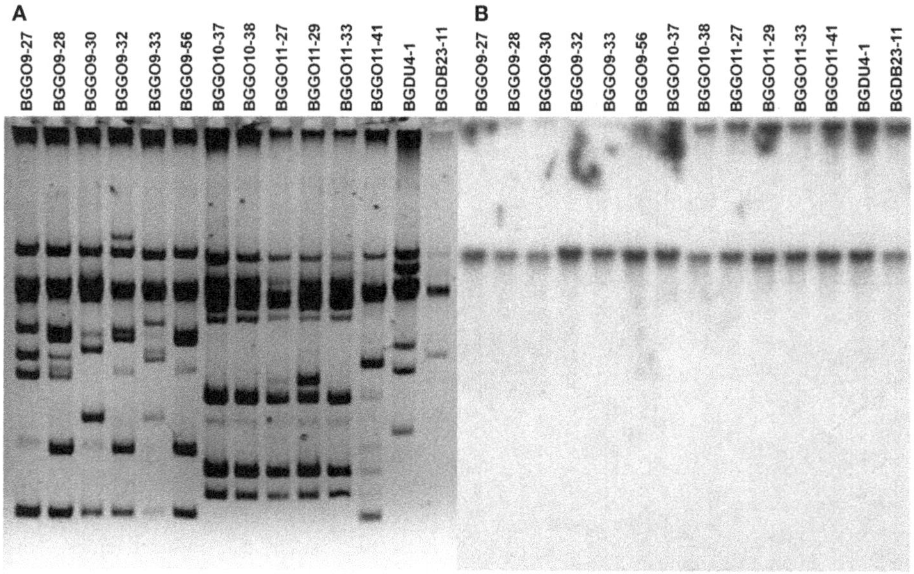

FIGURE 2 | Localization of genes correlated with auto-aggregation ability. **(A)** The electrophoresis of total plasmid DNA of selected enterococcal strains expressing aggregation ability from laboratory collection on 1% agaroze gel; **(B)** Southern blot hybridization with *aggL* gene probe.

for this type of aggregation factor are located on plasmids of different size indicating possible common plasmid origin. In selected enterococci it seems that plasmids carrying *aggE* gene are almost the same size even aggregation positive strains were isolated from different locations. According to plasmid profiles of selected strains it is possible to noted four groups of strains: two big groups (consisted of seven and five strains) with many common plasmids and two groups each consisted of one strain. Unfortunately, it is not possible to give final conclusion regarding plasmids carrying *aggE* gene since all analyzed strains belong to the same collection isolated from narrow distance; additional data from other groups are necessary. During propagation of selected enterococcal strains no loss of aggregation phenotype was noticed, indicating that plasmids are stable (structurally and segregationally) without any selection indicating that it could contributes to the fitness of carrier strains.

Cloning and Heterologous Expression of AggE Aggregation Factor from Strain BGGO9-28

Since the strain BGGO9-28 showed the strongest adhesion capability among selected enterococal strains, it was chosen for the cloning of *aggE* by constructing a plasmid library in pAZIL vector. All plasmid library constructs, carrying different fragments of the total plasmids of strain BGGO9-28, amplified in *E. coli*, were transferred into non-aggregating heterologous plasmid-free lactococcal strain MG7284 and enterococcal strain BGZLS10-27. Only the construct pAggES10 (carrying a *Stu*I fragment of 8,944 bp) provided auto-aggregation ability to strains MG7284 and BGZLS10-27. After the auto-aggregation capacity of construct pAggES10 was confirmed, the cloned fragment was completely sequenced. On the fragment was found an ORF with 70.6% identity with *aggL* from *Lc. lactis* BGKP1 (Kojic et al., 2011), responsible for aggregation in lactococci, and was named *aggE*. In addition, an upstream promoter region of *aggE* showed very high identity (96%) with the promoter region of *aggL* gene from lactococci. The DNA sequence of the region carrying the *aggE* from strain BGGO9-28 was submitted to the European Nucleotide Archive under accession No: LT222050.

Based on the sequence analysis, a shortened *Pvu*I/*Xba*I fragment of 7,115 bp that contained only the *aggE* was subcloned into the pAZIL vector. The resulting construct, named pAggEPX48, successfully restored aggregation phenotype in strains MG7284 and BGZLS10-27, after transformation (**Figure 3**). It was noted that *aggE* is sufficient for the expression of aggregation phenotype in closely related LAB species (lactococci and enterococci). The result supports the conclusion that aggregation ability was stronger in transformants of enterococcal strain BGZLS10-27 compared to that of lactococcal MG7284, in contrast to results obtained with lactococcal *aggL* indicating that there are structural adaptations specific to each group of bacteria. It was found that *aggE* is surrounded by two integrase genes; upstream of *aggE* gene are located genes for RepA protein and for an integrase with high identity with the same genes on an unnamed plasmid from *En. faecium* strain UW8175, and downstream are located genes for integrase, magnesium and cobalt transport protein CorA, and a gene for protein OrfX. A constellation of genes on the sequenced fragment (RepA and OrfX separated by a cassette) and the presence of the genes for integrase on both sides of *aggE* gene indicate a possible horizontal gene transfer.

In Silico Analysis of AggE Protein

Primary structural analysis of AggE protein revealed that it is a 178 kDa (1,637 amino acids) membrane-anchored protein rich

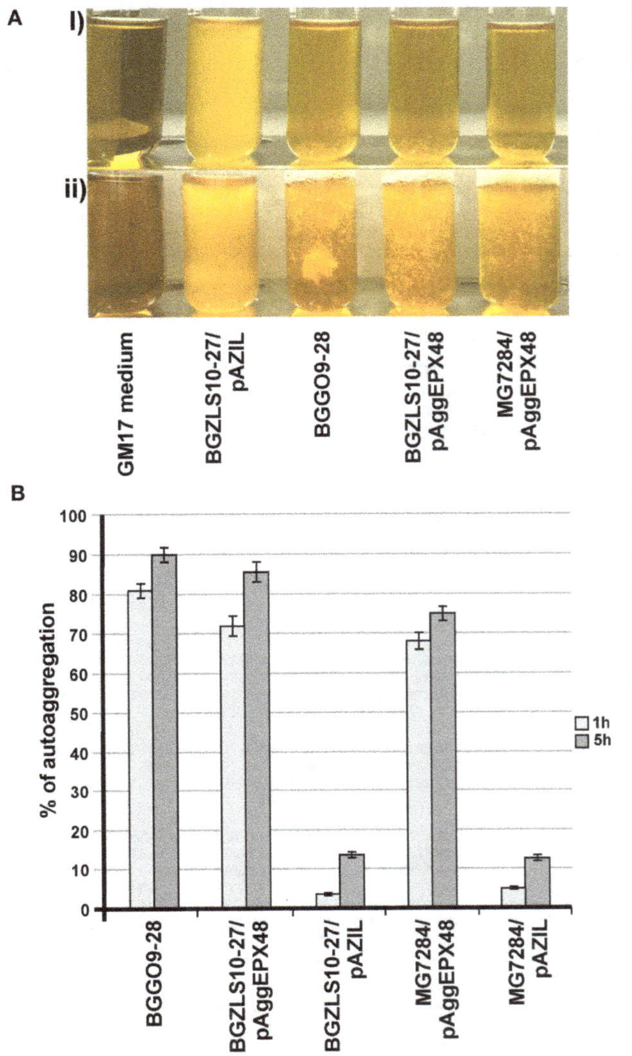

FIGURE 3 | Heterologous expression of AggE aggregation factor from BGGO9-28. Aggregation ability of *En. faecium* BGGO9-28 and transformants (carryng construct pAggEPX48) in growth medium after **(A-i)** overnight cultivation and **(A-ii)** vigorous mixing; **(B)** graphical presentation of results obtained in auto-aggregation assay; auto-aggregation ability is expressed as percentages; the error bars show the standard deviations of three independent observations.

with amino acids threonine (12.6%) and lysine (9.3%). A BLAST search showed that AggE shares the highest identity with AggL from lactococci (81.4%) and a recently discovered hypothetical protein from *En. faecium* (WP_058138517.1) (69.6%), which is shorter by 386 amino acids. It was shown that AggE contains several motifs in relation to cell adhesion, like collagen-binding (three heterologous domains with less than 25% identity at positions 411–534, 829–944, and 964–1,089), collagen-binding B domains (four almost identical domains with consensus sequence TSVSGQKTWSDHDNQDGVRPDEITVNLLADGK KVDSKTVTAKDGWKYEFNDLDKFKGQEIKYTVAEAAVD GYKTTYDGNNIVNTH at positions 1,214–1,299, 1,304–1,389, 1,394–1,479, and 1,484–1,567), a CnaB-like domain (at position 1,132–1,200) as well as a cell wall anchoring domain (LPXTG) at the C-terminus (**Figure 4**).

Aggregation substance (AS) of *En. faecalis*, a sex pheromone plasmid encoded cell surface proteins (Asp1, Asa1 and Asc10; these proteins share more than 90% identity throughout of the protein), mediates the formation of bacterial aggregates, thereby promoting plasmid transfer. The aggregation ability encoded by *asp1* gene was first characterized as a virulence factor of 142 kDa (Galli et al., 1990). It was proposed that amino acid motifs Arg-Gly-Asp-Ser (RGDS) and Arg-Gly-Asp-Val (RGDV) in that aggregation protein play a crucial role in adherence to eukaryotic cells. In this study we have discovered a novel aggregation promoting factor, AggE, responsible for strong aggregation of enterococcal cells. Both types of the enterococcal aggregation proteins (AS and AggE) are high molecular mass proteins rich by amino acids threonine and lysine. The difference between them is that novel aggregation factor AggE from enterococci shows different architecture compared to that characterized as a virulence factor and does not contain RGDS or RGDV amino acid motifs. In addition these two types of aggregation proteins exhibit different binding affinity to ECM proteins: the presence of AS increased enterococcal adherence to fibronectin more than eight-fold and to type I collagen more than two-fold (Rozdzinski et al., 2001) while AggE protein provides an almost identical affinity for both the collagen and the fibronectin, which has been increased more than 10 times. AggE enterococcal aggregation promoting factor showed a structure similar to aggregation factors discovered in other LAB composed of collagen binding and CnaB-like domains (Kojic et al., 2011; Miljkovic et al.,

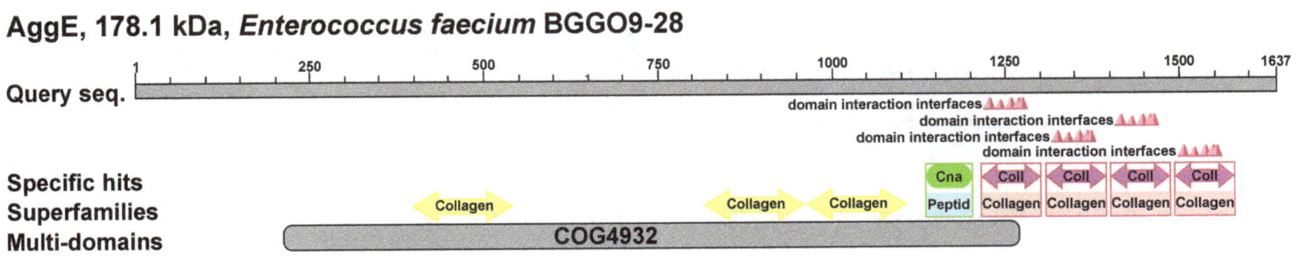

FIGURE 4 | Schematic representation of AggE protein, 178.1 kDa *Enterococcus faecium* BGGO9-28. Prediction of putative conserved domains in AggE protein was analyzed by protein BLASTP search. COG4932-Uncharacterized surface anchored protein, Collagen, Collagen binding domain; Peptid, peptidase associated domain; Coll, repeat unit of collagen binding protein domain B; Cna, Cna protein B-type domain.

2015). The highest level of identity, 81.4%, was detected with an aggregation protein of lactococci (AggL). Comparative analysis of these two proteins indicated their common origin. Differences between these two proteins were seen only in two regions: a region between amino acids 171 and 228 of AggE (that region is deleted in AggL since it is composed of multiple repeated SSTSTT

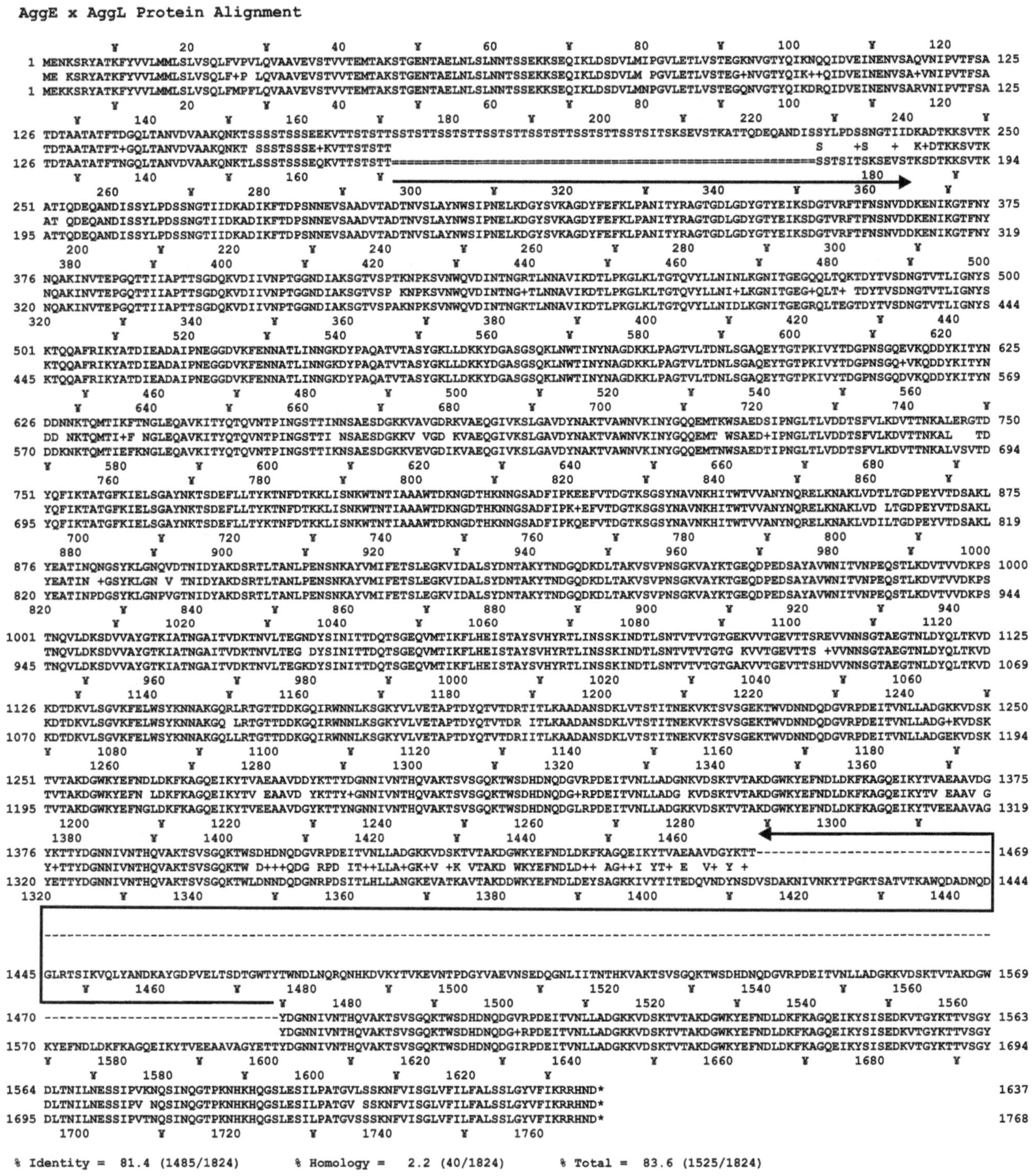

FIGURE 5 | Comparison of the amino acid sequence of AggL and AggE aggregation factors using Strider software. Black arrow oriented to the right indicates the absence of amino acids in AggL protein corresponding to the region between amino acids 171 and 228 of AggE. Black arrow oriented to the left indicates the absence of amino acids in AggE protein corresponding to the region between amino acids 1,413 and 1,600 of AggL. +, − Indicates for amino acids belonging to the same physicochemical group.

sequences), and a second region between amino acids 1,400 and 1,600 of AggL that is not present in AggE and contains two collagen binding B domains (**Figure 5**). These two differences may be the result of an independent selection in each organism and are most likely responsible for the different expression of aggregation proteins in lactococci and enterococci (AggL is better expressed in *Lactococcus* while AggE is better expressed in *Enterococcus*). The hypothesis of a common origin of these two genes is supported by two additional facts; an almost identical promoter region and the presence of the integrase genes close to *agg* gene. In order to determine whether the differences in *aggE* (from BGGO9-28) are a feature of all Agg^+ enterococci, the region (which surrounds the first deletion in *aggL*, positioned between nucleotides 511–680 of *aggE*) was amplified using primers AggE-1DF (positioned in both, *aggL* and *aggE* genes between nucleotides 129–148) and AggE-1DR (positioned in *aggL* between nucleotides 817–835 and in *aggE* between 985 and 1,003), resulting in amplified fragments for *aggL* of 707 bp and for *aggE* of 875 bp (**Figure 5**). For the second deleted region, since it is located in a repeated region composed of sequences completely identical to each other, it was not possible to design primers with a unique position. The results of PCR amplification support the conclusion that this region is variable, not only between lactococci and enterococci, but also among enterococci, or is still under stabilizing selection (**Figure 6**). A comparison of the ability of aggregation and the size of the deleted region in *aggE* gene/protein indicates that there is no corelation between the size of deletion and agregation, collagen, fibronectin and mucin binding ability, and biofilm formation. It seems that the structure and the presence of the respective domains, not the length of the peptide, is responsible for the expression of certain auto-aggregation phenotypes or adhesion ability, as demonstrated previously for AggLb (Miljkovic et al., 2016).

The Role of AggE in Auto-Aggregation, Adhesion to Components of ECM, and Biofilm Formation

The auto-aggregation ability of the wild-type strain BGGO9-28, derivatives of which carry *aggE* gene (BGZLS10-27/pAggEPX48 and MG7284/pAggEPX48) and their non-aggregating derivative carrying an empty plasmid (BGZLS10-27/pAZIL and MG7284/pAZIL) was measured for a period of 5 h and the results are presented in **Figure 3B**.

Earlier it was shown that isolates carrying *aggL* (the aggregation promoting factors from lactococci, AggL) or *aggLb* gene (the aggregation promoting factors from lactobacilli, AggLb) exhibited a direct correlation between auto-aggregation and their collagen binding ability, we tested the binding abilities of derivatives which carry *aggE* gene (BGZLS10-27/pAggEPX48 and MG7284/pAggEPX48) and their non-aggregating derivatives (BGZLS10-27/pAZIL and MG7284/pAZIL) to collagen. The different extents of adhesion to immobilized collagen (**Figure 7A**) and fibronectin (**Figure 7B**) were observed. BGGO9-28 exhibited the highest adhesion ability (absorbance value 3.54 to collagen and 3.48 to fibronectin), while the derivatives MG7284/pAggEPX48 (absorbance value 2.32 to collagen and 2.95 to fibronectin) and BGZLS10-27/pAggEPX48 (absorbance value 2.95 to collagen and 2.47 to fibronectin) possess slightly lower adhesion ability. Significant differences in the adherence to immobilized collagen and fibronectin were apparent between the mentioned aggregation-positive strains (BGGO9-28, MG7284/pAggEPX48, and BGZLS10-27/pAggEPX48) and their aggregation-negative controls, which showed almost no ability to bind to collagen or fibronectin (MG7284/pAZIL and BGZLS10-27/pAZIL). These results indicate a role for AggE in the specific interaction of BGGO9-28 with collagen and fibronectin on the cell surface. The higher adhesion ability of strain BGGO9-28 compared to the

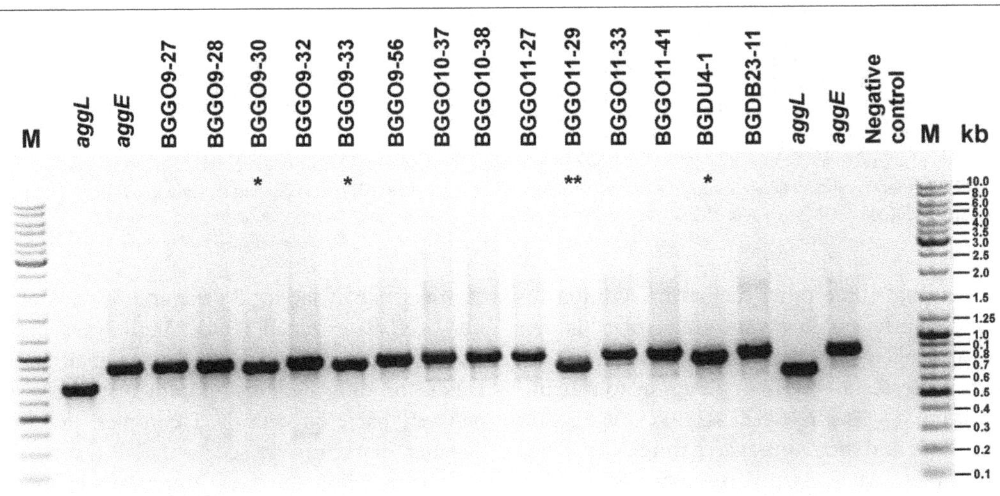

FIGURE 6 | Comparation of *aggE* and *aggL* genes by PCR analyses. The electrophoresis of PCR fragments amplified using primers AggE-1DF and AggE-1DR on plasmid DNA of enterococcal strains and clones (*aggE* and *aggL*) on 1% agarose gel. *Little shorter fragment than obtained for *aggE*; **Fragment thereof according to the size of between *aggE* and *aggL*; M, GeneRuler DNA Ladder Mix (Thermo Scientific); kb, kilobase.

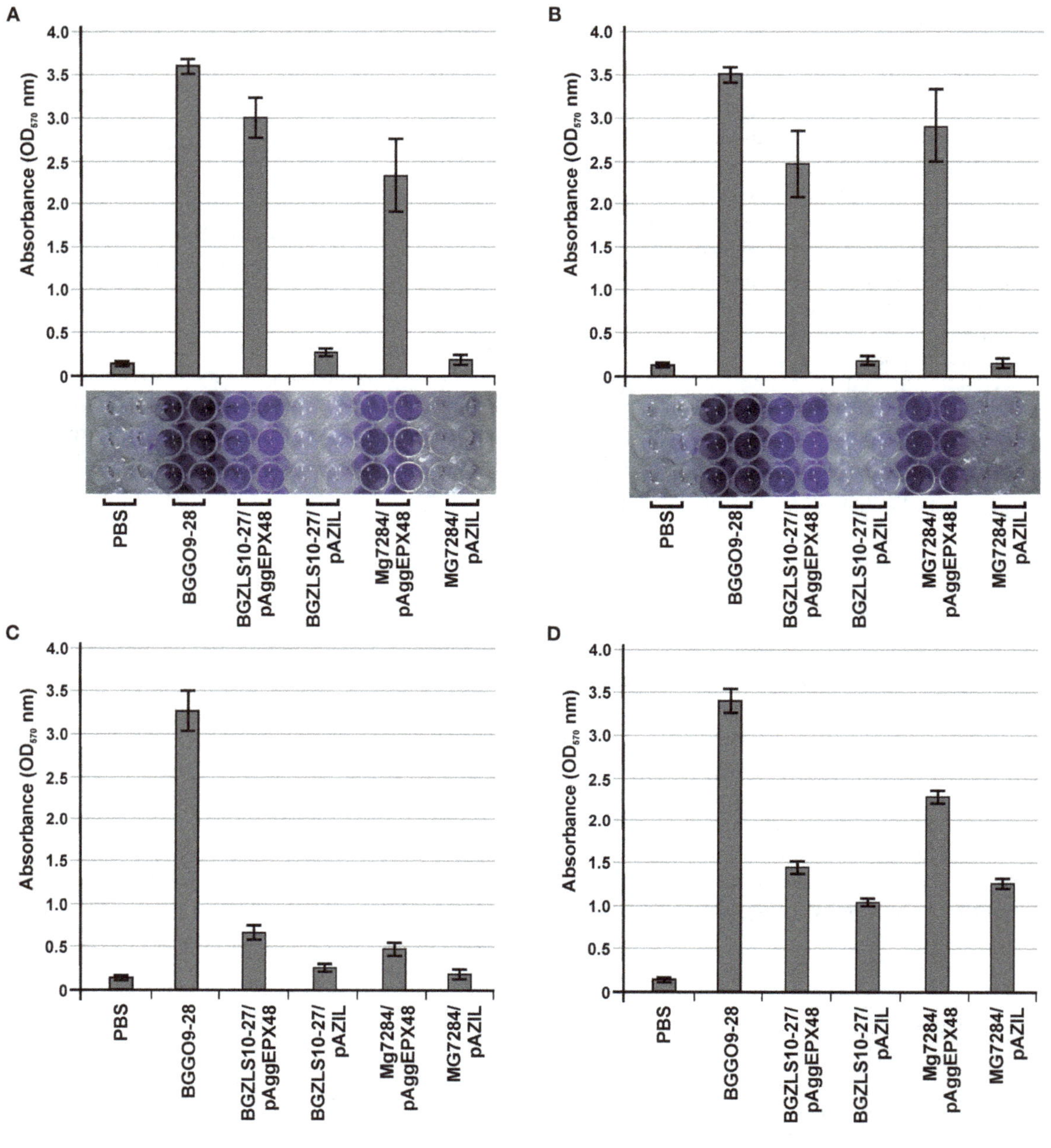

FIGURE 7 | The role of AggE in adhesion to components of ECM and biofilm formation. Graphical presentation and photo of microtiter plates of results obtained in **(A)** collagen-binding assay; **(B)** fibronectin-binding assay; Graphical presentation of results obtained in **(C)** mucin binding assay and **(D)** biofilm formation assay. Results were expressed as average of normalized A_{570} values. The error bars show the standard deviations of three independent observations.

transformants indicates that some other factors in addition to AggE, present on the cell surface of the strain, are involved in the binding interaction to collagen and fibronectin.

Strain BGGO9-28 possesses a very high adhesion to mucin, while derivatives carrying *aggE* gene (BGZLS10-27/pAggEPX48 and MG7284/pAggEPX48) and their non-aggregating derivatives (BGZLS10-27/pAZIL and MG7284/pAZIL) showed lower adhesion abilities to mucin, with a small difference between them (clones showed only about two times higher binding ability) in contrast to binding to collagen and fibronectin (**Figure 7C**). It can be assumed that a direct correlation between the presence of the *aggE* gene and binding ability to mucin has not been determined (since AggE gives little contribution to mucin binding), confirming the specificity of the AggE binding factor for only certain components of the ECM. Interaction between bacterial cells is a complex process that involves a number of factors. It seems that for some processes such as auto-aggregation the most important is *aggE*/AggE, but other cell surface properties or environmental factors can contribute to the modulation of the expression of a given phenotype.

Evaluation of the formation of biofilms and their interaction with the bacterial surface molecules is a complementary approach to better understanding the mechanisms by which bacteria colonize a niche as a consequence of adaptation to environmental stresses (Peter et al., 2013). Aggregation and biofilm formation are multicellular processes that allow a community to be more resistant to stress conditions. Given that these are similar processes, it is not surprising that the same protein could be involved in both functions (Miljkovic et al., 2016). It is considered that the expressed *aggE* gene contributes to the increase of biofilm formation in a heterologous host, but it is not entirely (clones carrying AggE increased only about two times formation of biofim), indicated that additional factors/genes in enterococci are responsible for the full expression of this phenotype (**Figure 7D**).

Probiotic Characteristics of BGGO9-28 Strain

The susceptibility of dairy isolate *En. faecium* BGGO9-28 to antibiotics according to CLSI (2015), and the presence of putative virulence genes, were determined in this study in the interest of safety considerations. Strain BGGO9-28 is sensitive to all of the antibiotics tested, without hemolytic or gelatinase activity, and does not carry any of the tested virulence determinants. Our results are in accordance with data that report the absence of these virulence factors in food-isolated *En. faecium* strains (Zheng et al., 2015); although previously, several starter and food-originated enterococci were shown to harbor some of the virulence factors, suggesting the importance of strain-specific properties for carrying certain virulence factors (Eaton and Gasson, 2001).

The main desirable characteristic required for probiotic bacteria is their ability to survive during GI tract passage, in which low pH, bile salts, and digestion conditions are the main factors affecting this ability (Tan et al., 2013). The cells of strain BGGO9-28 were strongly maintained, with 8.30 log units in artificial gastric juice, 8.39 log units in bile salt juice and 8.22 log units for artificial intestine juice, respectively (**Figure 8**). It has been revealed that *En. faecium* BGGO9-28 was stable in acidic conditions (pH 2.0 for 3 h) and high bile salt, and had a high level of tolerance to pancreatin. BGGO9-28 has a high survival ability in the GI tract, which is similar to previous observations (Nueno-Palop and Narbad, 2011) reporting high levels of survival for enterococci.

Like the ability to survive under harsh conditions, adhesion is also an important functional characteristic of probiotic strains. The adhesion ability of *En. faecium* BGGO9-28 to the epithelial intestinal cell line Caco-2 was determined in order to define a percentage of attachment of the potential probiotic strain. The results obtained in this study clearly indicate that the strain possesses high adhesion abilities, about 80% adhesion to the Caco-2 cell line (data not shown).

The capability of probiotic strains to neutralize the negative effects of pathogens is their important health promoting property (FAO-WHO, 2006). One of the mechanisms of action is antimicrobial activity related to the production of bacteriocins, and colonization competition, or pathogen exclusion (Gareau et al., 2010; Satish-Kumar et al., 2011). Since strain BGGO9-28 does not exhibit antimicrobial activity, it has been proposed that the cell surface components involved in desirable probiotic features could be cell surface associated proteins, S-layer macromolecules built from proteins (Zhang et al., 2010) and auto-aggregation factors (Miljkovic et al., 2015).

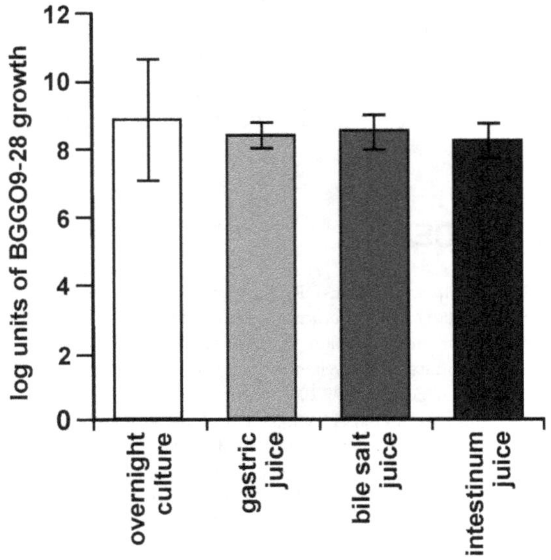

FIGURE 8 | Survival of BGGO9-28 strain in GI tract conditions. Bacterial counts in suspensions made in 10% skimmed-milk of the *En. faecium* BGGO9-28 after chemically simulating the GI tract: in gastric, bile salt and intestinal juices. The error bars show the standard deviations of three independent observations.

It is important to emphasize that *in vitro* tests have many limits, because adhesion properties and mucus production depend on the cell line used in the study (Turpin et al., 2012). Additionally, some *in vitro* studies that estimated the degree of adhesion also indicate the cytotoxicity of tested strains to the target cells (Miquel et al., 2015). This suggests that adhesion and/or long-term colonization of probiotic agents usually is not without consequences.

This paper describes a new aggregation factor in enterococci, AggE, which belongs structurally to those of the other LAB, responsible for auto-aggregation and binding of carrier cells to specific components of the ECM. In conclusion, our findings indicate that there is a relationship between the auto-aggregation and adhesiveness of BGGO9-28 that is mediated by AggE on the cell surface. In particular, it should be noted that despite the fact that the adhesion of enterococci is generally extremely high, specificity of interaction with certain components of ECM is determined by AggE protein. The results of this study emphasize the direct link between AggE protein and auto-aggregation and binding to components of ECM, but also note the importance of other host and environmental factors on the overall adhesion of the bacterial cells.

AUTHOR CONTRIBUTIONS

MK conceived, designed and coordinated this study, interpreted all of results and wrote this paper. KV, NP, and MM designed, performed, analyzed the experiments and wrote this paper. MT and AT provided experimental assistance, contributed to the preparation of the figures, provided technical assistance and contributed to the preparation of this paper. All authors reviewed the results and approved the final version of the manuscript.

FUNDING

This work was supported by the Ministry of Education, Science and Technological Development, Republic of Serbia (Grant number 173019).

REFERENCES

Ahmed, S., Meghji, S., Williams, R. J., Henderson, B., Brock, J. H., and Nair, S. P. (2001). *Staphylococcus aureus* fibronectin binding proteins are essential for internalization by osteoblasts but do not account for differences in intracellular levels of bacteria. *Infect. Immun.* 69, 2872–2877. doi: 10.1128/IAI.69.5.2872-2877.2001

Bhardwaj, A., Kaur, G., Gupta, H., Vij, S., and Malik, R. K. (2011). Interspecies diversity, safety and probiotic potential of bacteriocinogenic *Enterococcus faecium* isolated from dairy food and human faeces. *World J. Microbiol. Biotechnol.* 27, 591–602. doi: 10.1007/s11274-010-0494-4

Clinical and Laboratory Standarsd Institute (CLSI). (2015). *Performance Standarsd for Antimicrobial Susceptibility Testing; 23rd Informational Supplement.* CLSI document M100-S23. Wayne, PA: Clinical Laboratory Standarsd, Institute.

Del Re, B., Sgorbati, B., Miglioli, M., and Palenzona, D. (2000). Adhesion, autoaggregation and hydrophobicity of 13 strains of *Bifidobacterium longum*. *Lett. Appl. Microbiol.* 31, 438–442. doi: 10.1046/j.1365-2672.2000.00845.x

Eaton, T. J., and Gasson, M. J. (2001). Molecular screening of *Enterococcus* virulence determinants and potential for genetic exchange between food and medical isolates. *Appl. Environ. Microbiol.* 67, 1628–1635. doi: 10.1128/A.E.M.67.4.1628-1635.2001

FAO-WHO (2006). *Probiotics in Food: Health and Nutritional Properties and Guidelines for Evaluation.* FAO Food and Nutritional Paper No. 85 (ISBN92-5-105513-105510). Rome: Food and Agriculture Organization of the United Nations, World Health Organization.

Foulquié-Moreno, M. R., Sarantinopoulos, P., Tsakalidou, E., and De Vuyst, L. (2006). The role and application of enterococci in food and health. *Int. J. Food Microbiol.* 106, 1–24. doi: 10.1016/j.ijfoodmicro.2005.06.026

Galli, D., Lottspeich, F., and Wirth, R. (1990). Sequence analysis of *Enterococcus faecalis* aggregation substance encoded by the sex pheromone plasmid pAD1. *Mol. Microbiol.* 4, 895–904. doi: 10.1111/j.1365-2958.1990.tb00662.x

García-Cayuela, T., Korany, A. M., Bustos, I., Gómez de Cadiñanos, L. P., Requena, T., Peláez, C., et al. (2014). Adhesion abilities of dairy *Lactobacillus plantarum* strains showing an aggregation phenotype. *Food Res. Int.* 57, 44–50. doi: 10.1016/j.foodres.2014.01.010

Gareau, M. G., Sherman, P. M., and Walker, W. A. (2010). Probiotics and the gut microbiota in intestinal health and disease. *Nat. Rev. Gastroenterol. Hepatol.* 7, 503–514. doi: 10.1038/nrgastro.2010.117

Gasson, M. J. (1983). Plasmid complements of *Streptococcus lactis* NCDO 712 and other lactic streptococci after protoplast-induced curing. *J. Bacteriol.* 154, 1–9.

Giraffa, G. (2003). Functionality of enterococci in dairy products. *Int. J. Food Microbiol.* 88, 215–222. doi: 10.1016/S0168-1605(03)00183-1

Golić, N., Cadež, N., Terzić-Vidojević, A., Suranská, H., Beganović, J., Lozo, J., et al. (2013). Evaluation of lactic acid bacteria and yeast diversity in traditional white pickled and fresh soft cheeses from the mountain regions of Serbia and lowland regions of Croatia. *Int. J. Food Microbiol.* 166, 294–300. doi: 10.1016/j.ijfoodmicro.2013.05.032

Gomes, B. C., Esteves, C. T., Palazzo, I. C., Darini, A. L., Felis, G. E., Sechi, L. A., et al. (2008). Prevalence and characterization of *Enterococcus* spp. isolated from Brazilian foods. *Food Microbiol.* 25, 668–675. doi: 10.1016/j.fm.2008.03.008

Hanahan, D. (1983). Studies on transformation of *Escherichia coli* with plasmids. *J. Mol. Biol.* 166, 557–580. doi: 10.1016/S0022-2836(83)80284-8

Jovcic, B., Begovic, J., Lozo, J., Topisirovic, L., and Kojic, M. (2009). Dynamic of sodium dodecyl sulfate utilization and antibiotic susceptibility of strain *Pseudomonas* sp. ATCC19151. *Arch. Biol. Sci.* 61, 159–165. doi: 10.2298/ABS0902159J

Kirkman, T. W. (1996). *Statistics to Use.* Available online at: http://www.physics.csbsju.edu/stats/ (Accessed May 01, 2017).

Kojic, M., Jovcic, B., Strahinic, I., Begovic, J., Lozo, J., Veljovic, K., et al. (2011). Cloning and expression of a novel lactococcal aggregation factor from *Lactococcus lactis* subsp. *lactis* BGKP1. *BMC Microbiol.* 11:265. doi: 10.1186/1471-2180-11-265

Kravtsov, E. G., Yermolayev, A. V., Anokhina, I. V., Yashina, N. V., Chesnokova, V. L., and Dalin, M. V. (2008). Adhesion characteristics of lactobacillus is a criterion of the probiotic choice. *Bull. Exp. Biol. Med.* 145, 232–234. doi: 10.1007/s10517-008-0058-x

Lebreton, F., Riboulet-Bisson, E., Serror, P., Sanguinetti, M., Posteraro, B., Torelli, R., et al. (2009). Ace, which encodes an adhesin in *Enterococcus faecalis*, is regulated by Ers and is involved in virulence. *Infect. Immun.* 77, 2832–2839. doi: 10.1128/IAI.01218-08

Lopes, M. F., Simões, A. P., Tenreiro, R., Marques, J. J., and Crespo, M. T. (2006). Activity and expression of a virulence factor, gelatinase, in dairy enterococci. *Int. J. Food Microbiol.* 112, 208–214. doi: 10.1016/j.ijfoodmicro.2006.09.004

Lorca, G., Torino, M. I., Font de Valdez, G., and Ljungh, A. A. (2002). Lactobacilli express cell surface proteins which mediate binding of immobilized collagen and fibronectin. *FEMS Microbiol. Lett.* 206, 31–37. doi: 10.1111/j.1574-6968.2002.tb10982.x

Lozo, J., Jovcic, B., Kojic, M., Dalgalarrondo, M., Chobert, J. M., Haertlé, T., et al. (2007). Molecular characterization of a novel bacteriocin and an unusually large aggregation factor of *Lactobacillus paracasei* subsp. *paracasei* BGSJ2-8, a natural isolate from homemade cheese. *Curr. Microbiol.* 55, 266–271. doi: 10.1007/s00284-007-0159-1

Martín-Platero, A. M., Valdivia, E., Maqueda, M., and Martínez-Bueno, M. (2009). Characterization and safety evaluation of enterococci isolated from Spanish goats' milk cheeses. *Int. J. Food Microbiol.* 132, 24–32. doi: 10.1016/j.ijfoodmicro.2009.03.010

McNaught, C. E., and MacFie, J. (2001). Probiotics in clinical practice: a critical review of the evidence. *Nutr. Res.* 21, 343–353. doi: 10.1016/S0271-5317(00)00286-4

McNulty, N. P., Yatsunenko, T., Hsiao, A., Faith, J. J., Muegge, B. D., Goodman, A. L., et al. (2011). The impact of a consortium of fermented milk strains on the gut microbiome of gnotobiotic mice and monozygotic twins. *Sci. Transl. Med.* 3:106ra106. doi: 10.1126/scitranslmed.3002701

Miljkovic, M., Bertani, I., Fira, D., Jovcic, B., Novovic, K., Venturi, V., et al. (2016). Shortening of the *Lactobacillus paracasei* subsp. *paracasei* BGNJ1-64 AggLb protein switches its activity from auto-aggregation to biofilm formation. *Front. Microbiol.* 7:1422. doi: 10.3389/fmicb.2016.01422

Miljkovic, M., Strahinic, I., Tolinacki, M., Zivkovic, M., Kojic, S., Golic, N., et al. (2015). AggLb is the largest cell-aggregation factor from *Lactobacillus paracasei* subsp. *paracasei* BGNJ1-64, functions in collagen adhesion, and pathogen exclusion *in vitro*. *PLoS ONE* 10:e0126387. doi: 10.1371/journal.pone.0126387

Miquel, S., Beaumont, M., Martín, R., Langella, P., Braesco, V., and Thomas, M. (2015). A proposed framework for an appropriate evaluation scheme for microorganisms as novel foods with a health claim in Europe. *Microb. Cell Fact.* 14:48. doi: 10.1186/s12934-015-0229-1

Mohamed, J. A., and Huang, D. B. (2007). Biofilm formation by enterococci. *J. Med. Microbiol.* 56, 1581–1588. doi: 10.1099/jmm.0.47331-0

Muñoz-Provencio, D., Llopis, M., Antolín, M., de Torres, I., Guarner, F., Pérez-Martínez, G., et al. (2009). Adhesion properties of *Lactobacillus casei* strains to resected intestinal fragments and components of the extracellular matrix. *Arch. Microbiol.* 191, 153–161. doi: 10.1007/s00203-008-0436-9

Nikolic, M., López, P., Strahinic, I., Suárez, A., Kojic, M., Fernández-García, M., et al. (2012). Characterisation of the exopolysaccharide (EPS)-producing *Lactobacillus paraplantarum* BGCG11 and its non-EPS producing derivative strains as potential probiotics. *Int. J. Food Microbiol.* 158, 155–162. doi: 10.1016/j.ijfoodmicro.2012.07.015

Nueno-Palop, C., and Narbad, A. (2011). Probiotic assessment of *Enterococcus faecalis* CP58 isolated from human gut. *Int. J. Food Microbiol.* 145, 390–394. doi: 10.1016/j.ijfoodmicro.2010.12.029

O'Sullivan, D. J., and Klaenhammer, T. R. (1993). Rapid mini-prep isolation of high-quality plasmid DNA from *Lactococcus* and *Lactobacillus* ssp. *Appl. Environ. Microbiol.* 59, 2730–2733.

O'Toole, P. W., and Cooney, J. C. (2008). Probiotic bacteria influence the composition and function of the intestinal microbiota. *Interdiscip. Perspect. Infect. Dis.* 2008:175285. doi: 10.1155/2008/175285

Peter, A., Zacharia, S., and Mathew, J. (2013). Biofilm formation in enterococci from different sources. *Int. J. Biopharm.* 4, 140–144.

Pieniz, S., Andreazza, R., Anghinoni, T., Camargo, F., and Brandelli, A. (2014). Probiotic potential, antimicrobial and antioxidant activities of *Enterococcus durans* strain LAB18s. *Food Control* 37, 251–256. doi: 10.1016/j.foodcont.2013.09.055

Piwat, S., Sophatha, B., and Teanpaisan, R. (2015). An assessment of adhesion, aggregation and surface charges of *Lactobacillus* strains derived from the human oral cavity. *Lett. Appl. Microbiol.* 61, 98–105. doi: 10.1111/lam.12434

Prince, T., McBain, A. J., and O'Neill, C. A. (2012). *Lactobacillus reuteri* protects epidermal keratinocytes from *Staphylococcus aureus*-induced cell death by competitive exclusion. *Appl. Environ. Microbiol.* 78, 5119–5126. doi: 10.1128/AEM.00595-12

Rozdzinski, E., Marre, R., Susa, M., Wirth, R., and Muscholl-Siberhom, A. (2001). Aggregation substance-mediated adherence of *Enterococcus faecalis* to immobilized extracellular matrix proteins. *Microb. Pathog.* 30, 211–220. doi: 10.1006/mpat.2000.0429

Sánchez, B., Fernández-García, M., Margolles, A., de los Reyes-Gavilán, C. G., and Ruas-Madiedo, P. (2010). Technological and probiotic selection criteria of a bile-adapted *Bifidobacterium animalis* subsp. *lactis* strain. *Int. Dairy J.* 20, 800–805. doi: 10.1016/j.idairyj.2010.06.004

Satish-Kumar, R., Kanmani, P., Yuvaraj, N., Paari, K. A., Pattukumar, V., and Arul, V. (2011). *Lactobacillus plantarum* AS1 binds to cultured human intestinal cell line HT-29 and inhibits cell attachment by enterovirulent bacterium *Vibrio parahaemolyticus*. *Lett. Appl. Microbiol.* 53, 481–487. doi: 10.1111/j.1472-765X.2011.03136.x

Shankar, N., Lockatell, C. V., Baghdayan, A. S., Drachenberg, C., Gilmore, M. S., and Johnson, D. E. (2001). Role of *Enterococcus faecalis* surface protein Esp in the pathogenesis of ascending urinary tract infection. *Infect. Immun.* 69, 4366–4372. doi: 10.1128/IAI.69.7.4366-4372.2001

Tan, Q., Xu, H., Aguilar, Z. P., Peng, S., Dong, S., Wang, B., et al. (2013). Safety assessment and probiotic evaluation of *Enterococcus faecium* YF5 isolated from sourdough. *J. Food Sci.* 78, M587–M593. doi: 10.1111/1750-3841.12079

Terzic-Vidojevic, A., Mihajlovic, S., Uzelac, G., Golic, N., Fira, A., Kojic, M., et al. (2014). Identification and characterization of lactic acid bacteria isolated from artisanal white brined Golija cows' milk cheeses. *Arch. Biol. Sci.* 66, 179–192. doi: 10.2298/ABS1401179T

Terzić-Vidojević, A., Veljović, K., Begović, J., Filipić, B., Popović, D., Tolinački, M., et al. (2015). Diversity and antibiotic susceptibility of autochthonous dairy enterococci isolates: are they safe candidates for autochthonous starter cultures? *Front. Microbiol.* 6:954. doi: 10.3389/fmicb.2015.00954

Turpin, W., Humblot, C., Noordine, M. L., Thomas, M., and Guyot, J. P. (2012). *Lactobacillaceae* and cell adhesion: genomic and functional screening. *PLoS ONE* 7:e38034. doi: 10.1371/journal.pone.0038034

Valenzuela, A. S., ben Omar, N., Abriouel, H., López, R. L., Veljovic, K., Cañamero, M. M., et al. (2009). Virulence factors, antibiotic resistance, and bacteriocins in enterococci from artisan foods of animal origin. *Food Control* 20, 381–385. doi: 10.1016/j.foodcont.2008.06.004

Vankerckhoven, V., Van Autgaerden, T., Vael, C., Lammens, C., Chapelle, S., Rossi, R., et al. (2004). Development of a multiplex PCR for the detection of *asa1*, *gel*E, *cyl*A, *esp*, and *hyl* genes in enterococci and survey for virulence determinants among European hospital isolates of *Enterococcus faecium*. *J. Clin. Microbiol.* 42, 4473–4479. doi: 10.1128/JCM.42.10.4473-4479.2004

Xu, Y., Singh, K. V., Qin, X., Murray, B. E., and Weinstock, G. M. (2000). Analysis of a gene cluster of *Enterococcus faecalis* involved in polysaccharide biosynthesis. *Infect. Immun.* 68, 815–823. doi: 10.1128/IAI.68.2.815-823.2000

Yadav, A. K., Tyagi, A., Kaushik, J. K., Saklani, A. C., Grover, S., and Batish, V. K. (2013). Role of surface layer collagen binding protein from indigenous *Lactobacillus plantarum* 91 in adhesion and its anti-adhesion potential against gut pathogen. *Microbiol. Res.* 168, 639–645. doi: 10.1016/j.micres.2013.05.003

Zhang, Y. C., Zhang, L. W., Tuo, Y. F., Guo, C. F., Yi, H. X., Li, J. Y., et al. (2010). Inhibition of *Shigella sonnei* adherence to HT-29 cells by lactobacilli from Chinese fermented food and preliminary characterization of S-layer protein involvement. *Res. Microbiol.* 161, 667–672. doi: 10.1016/j.resmic.2010.06.005

Zheng, W., Zhang, Y., Lu, H. M., Li, D. T., Zhang, Z. L., Tang, Z. X., et al. (2015). Antimicrobial activity and safety evaluation of *Enterococcus faecium* KQ 2.6 isolated from peacock feces. *BMC Biotechnol.* 15:30. doi: 10.1186/s12896-015-0151-y

17

Bile-Salt-Hydrolases from the Probiotic Strain *Lactobacillus johnsonii* La1 Mediate Anti-Giardial Activity *In Vitro* and *In Vivo*

***Thibault Allain*[1,2], *Soraya Chaouch*[2], *Myriam Thomas*[3], *Isabelle Vallée*[3], *André G. Buret*[4], *Philippe Langella*[1], *Philippe Grellier*[2], *Bruno Polack*[5], *Luis G. Bermúdez-Humarán*[1*†] and *Isabelle Florent*[2*†]**

[1] Commensal and Probiotics-Host Interactions Laboratory, Micalis Institute, Institut National de la Recherche Agronomique, AgroParisTech, Jouy-en-Josas, France, [2] UMR7245, Muséum National d'Histoire Naturelle, Centre National de la Recherche Scientifique, Sorbonne-Universités, Paris, France, [3] JRU BIPAR, ANSES, Ecole Nationale Vétérinaire d'Alfort, INRA, Université Paris-Est, Animal Health Laboratory, Maisons-Alfort, France, [4] Department of Biological Sciences, University of Calgary, Calgary, AB, Canada, [5] JRU BIPAR, Ecole Nationale Vétérinaire d'Alfort, ANSES, INRA, Université Paris-Est, Maisons-Alfort, France

***Correspondence:**
Luis G. Bermúdez-Humarán
luis.bermudez@inra.fr
Isabelle Florent
isabelle.florent@mnhn.fr

† These authors have contributed equally to this work.

Giardia duodenalis (syn. *G. lamblia, G. intestinalis*) is the protozoan parasite responsible for giardiasis, the most common and widely spread intestinal parasitic disease worldwide, affecting both humans and animals. After cysts ingestion (through either contaminated food or water), *Giardia* excysts in the upper intestinal tract to release replicating trophozoites that are responsible for the production of symptoms. In the gut, *Giardia* cohabits with the host's microbiota, and several studies have revealed the importance of this gut ecosystem and/or some probiotic bacteria in providing protection against *G. duodenalis* infection through mechanisms that remain incompletely understood. Recent findings suggest that Bile-Salt-Hydrolase (BSH)-like activities from the probiotic strain of *Lactobacillus johnsonii* La1 may contribute to the anti-giardial activity displayed by this strain. Here, we cloned and expressed each of the three *bsh* genes present in the *L. johnsonii* La1 genome to study their enzymatic and biological properties. While BSH47 and BSH56 were expressed as recombinant active enzymes, no significant enzymatic activity was detected with BSH12. *In vitro* assays allowed determining the substrate specificities of both BSH47 and BSH56, which were different. Modeling of these BSHs indicated a strong conservation of their 3-D structures despite low conservation of their primary structures. Both recombinant enzymes were able to mediate anti-giardial biological activity against *Giardia* trophozoites *in vitro*. Moreover, BSH47 exerted significant anti-giardial effects when tested in a murine model of giardiasis. These results shed new light on the mechanism, whereby active BSH derived from the probiotic strain *Lactobacillus johnsonii* La1 may yield anti-giardial effects *in vitro* and *in vivo*. These findings pave the way toward novel approaches for the treatment of this widely spread but neglected infectious disease, both in human and in veterinary medicine.

Keywords: *Giardia duodenalis*, lactobacilli, *Lactobacillus johnsonii*, bile salt hydrolases, BSH, conjugated bile salts, anti-giardial activity

INTRODUCTION

Giardia duodenalis (syn. *Giardia lamblia* and *Giardia intestinalis*) is a flagellated protozoan parasite responsible for giardiasis, an intestinal zoonotic disease infection that may cause acute or chronic diarrhea, weight loss, malabsorption, abdominal pain, and nausea (Ankarklev et al., 2010; Cotton et al., 2011). It is one of the most common intestinal parasites and one of the most frequent causes of diarrhea, with over 280 million human symptomatic cases worldwide (Lane and Lloyd, 2002; Platts-Mills et al., 2015). Infections occur mainly by the ingestion of cysts present in contaminated food and water. After ingestion, infectious cysts differentiate into trophozoite stages, which in turn colonize the upper small intestine. Included in the "Neglected Disease Initiative" of the World Health Organization (WHO) in 2004, giardiasis has a significant public health impact in both developed and developing countries (Savioli et al., 2006; Platts-Mills et al., 2015). Metronidazole is the most frequently used drug for treating *G. duodenalis* infections, whereas albendazole, tinidazole, and nitazoxanide may also be used with efficacy (Gardner and Hill, 2001; Petri, 2005). Although these drugs have different modes of action, there is an increasing incidence of parasite resistance, and treatment failure is relatively common (Ansell et al., 2015). Moreover, these standard treatments are commonly associated with undesirable side effects in both medical and veterinary usages (Barr et al., 1994; Gardner and Hill, 2001). A successful vaccine has proven elusive, and *Giardia* is able to escape host immunity by switching its variant-specific surface proteins (Singer et al., 2001). Together, these observations underscore the need for new therapeutic alternatives for the treatment of giardiasis.

In the last decade, some probiotics (i.e., live microorganisms which, when administered in adequate amounts, confer a health benefit on their hosts, WHO 2001), in particular several species belonging to the genus *Lactobacillus*, have shown anti-giardial efficacy in various murine models (see Travers et al., 2011 for review). The mechanisms remain incompletely understood but may involve host immunomodulation and/or extracellular compounds released by the bacteria (Perez et al., 2001; Humen et al., 2005; Shukla et al., 2008; Shukla and Sidhu, 2011; Goyal et al., 2013). In this context, we have recently shown that unconjugated bile salts, generated by secreted or released enzymes by the probiotic strain of *Lactobacillus johnsonii* La1 (also known as *L. johnsonii* NCC533), may contribute to the inhibition of *Giardia* trophozoite growth *in vitro* (Perez et al., 2001; Travers et al., 2016). BSH (also called cholylglycine hydrolase, EC 3.5.1.2) are enzymes that hydrolyze the amide bond of conjugated bile salts, liberating the amino acid moiety from the steroid core and generating deconjugated bile salts (i.e., cholic acid, deoxycholic acid and chenodeoxycholic acid) (Begley et al., 2006). Conjugated-bile salts are synthesized in the liver where conjugation to either glycine or taurine occurs, and these conjugated-bile salts play an important role in the solubility and absorption of lipids and cholesterol in the intestinal tract (Eyssen, 1973; Kim et al., 2005; Begley et al., 2006). Moreover, glyco- and tauro-conjugated bile salts exert detergent and antimicrobial properties (Ruiz et al., 2013). BSH activities lead to bile salt detoxification and confer a competitive advantage to the microbial communities that express them, such as lactobacilli in the upper part of the small intestine (Ridlon et al., 2006; Ruiz et al., 2013).

In this study, we cloned and expressed each one of the three-*bsh* genes (i.e., *bsh12, bsh47,* and *bsh56*) from *L. johnsonii* La1 (Pridmore et al., 2004) in *Escherichia coli* in order to evaluate their substrate specificities and to assess their anti-*Giardia* activities, both *in vitro* and *in vivo*. A comparative structural analysis of the three BSHs was also performed using *in silico* approaches to explore whether structural differences could explain possible differences in substrate specificities. The three recombinant BSHs, rBSH12, rBSH47, and rBSH56, were tested against two different strains of the human assemblage A of *G. duodenalis* (WB6 and NF) *in vitro*. Then, rBSH47 was selected to be tested *in vivo* on OF1 suckling mice infected with the *G. duodenalis* strain WB6.

MATERIALS AND METHODS

In Silico Analysis of BSHs

Bile salt hydrolases amino acid sequences from different bacterial species were retrieved from databases using BLASTP program from the National Center for Biotechnology Information (NCBI, http://www.ncbi.nlm.nih.gov/) and analyzed *in silico*. Multiple sequence alignments of BSH amino acid sequences were performed using CLUSTALO 1.2.1 (http://www.ebi.ac.uk/Tools/msa/clustalo/) to identify the conserved motifs between the different enzymes. Phylogenetic relationships and phylogenic clustering of BSHs from different species were established by neighbor-joining methods using MEGA5 software (http://www.megasoftware.net/; Tamura et al., 2011). Three-dimensional modeling of *L. johnsonii* La1-BSHs was performed using I-TASSER from University of Michigan (http://zhanglab.ccmb.med.umich.edu/I-TASSER/; Roy et al., 2010). According to C-score results, the BSH from *Bifidobacterium longum* (Kumar et al., 2006) was chosen as template for modeling BSH56, whereas the BSH from *Clostridium perfringens* was used as template for modeling both BSH12 and BSH47 (Rossocha et al., 2005). Models for structure predictions were selected according to the highest values of their C-score (measured for evaluating global and local similarity between query and template protein). Protein structure analysis was performed using Pymol (PyMOL Molecular Graphics System, Version 1.8 Schrödinger, LLC).

Bacteria and Growth Conditions

Lactobacillus johnsonii La1 strain (Pridmore et al., 2004) was cultured in Man Rogosa Sharpe broth (MRS, Difco) and grown at 37°C in an anaerobic jar using BBL GasPak Anaerobic System (BD), incubated overnight (ON). *E. coli* TOP10 chemically competent cells (Invitrogen) were used for the subcloning of PCR fragments. *E. coli* CYS21 and SE1 chemically competent strains (DelphiGenetic, Belgium) were used, respectively, for the cloning and expression of BSHs. *E. coli* strains were grown in Luria-Bertani (LB) medium at 37°C ON with vigorous shaking at 180 rpm. All bacterial strains were stored at −80°C with 15% (v/v) glycerol for cryoprotection.

Cloning of *bsh* Genes from *L. johnsonii* La1

Genomic DNA of *L. johnsonii* La1 was extracted from 2 mL of an ON culture using Wizard Genomic DNA Purification Kit Protocol (Promega) and used as template to amplify the 3 *bsh* genes: *bsh12* (Gene ID: 2743525), *bsh47* (Gene ID: 2743183), and *bsh56* (Gene ID: 2743142) (Pridmore et al., 2004). The coding sequences of *bsh*12, *bsh*47, and *bsh*56 genes (excluding the putative signal sequences) were amplified by PCR (Phusion Taq, Thermo Fisher Scientific) using primers described in **Table 1**. These primers were designed to incorporate two restriction sites: *Nhe*I (forward primer) and *Xho*I (reverse primer). The amplified PCR fragments were purified using SV Gel and PCR Clean-Up System (Wizard) and were subcloned into the vector pCR®2.1-TOPO® (Invitrogen). The resulting constructions (pLB487, pLB488, and pLB489) were validated by sequencing (MWG-Genomic Company, Germany) before recovering the *bsh* genes with *Nhe*I and *Xho*I restriction enzymes and cloning them into pStaby 1.2 vector (DelphiGenetics) previously digested with the same enzymes. The pStaby 1.2 plasmid was used for intermediate cloning to introduce a C-terminal six-Histidine tag (His-tag), allowing subsequent purification of rBSHs using affinity chromatography. The resulting plasmids were transferred into *E. coli* CYS21 strains and transformants were grown at 37°C ON in 10 mL of LB containing ampicillin (Amp, 100 μg/ml) with shaking at 180 rpm. Plasmid DNA were extracted from positive clones, sequenced to confirm identity, and subsequently transformed into *E. coli* SE1 expression strain. Bacterial strains, plasmids, and primer sequences used in this study are described in **Table 1**. Immunoblotting experiments were performed on *E. coli* SE1 (pLB490), *E. coli* SE1 (pLB491), and *E. coli* SE1 (pLB492) strains lysates (see below) using mouse monoclonal 6x-His Epitope Tag Antibody (Thermo Fisher Scientific) to detect recombinant BSHs.

TABLE 1 | Bacterial strains, plasmids, primers used in this study.

Material	Relevant properties	Source/ reference
STRAINS		
L. johnsonii		
La1 (NCC533)	Wild type strain	Nestlé collection center NCC533
E. coli		
TOP10	Cloning strain	Invitrogen
CYS21	Cloning strain	DelphiGenetics
SE1	Expression strain	DelphiGenetics
PLASMIDS		
pCR2.1-TOPO	*Amp^r, subcloning vector	Invitrogen
pLB487	*Amp^r, TOPO harboring *bsh12* gene	This study
pLB488	*Amp^r, TOPO harboring *bsh47* gene	This study
pLB489	*Amp^r, TOPO harboring *bsh56* gene	This study
pStaby express	Amp^r, subcloning vector	DelphiGenetics
pLB490	*Amp^r, pStaby harboring *bsh12* gene	This study
pLB491	*Amp^r, pStaby harboring *bsh47* gene	This study
pLB492	*Amp^r, pStaby harboring *bsh56* gene	This study
Primers	Sequence	
bsh12Fw	5′CCGCTAGCTGTACCTCAATTGTTTATAGTTC 3′	This study
bsh12Rev	3′GGCTCGAGATTTTGATAATTAATTGTTTGC 5′	This study
bsh47Fw	5′CCGCTAGCTGTACTGGTTTAAGATTCAC 3′	This study
bsh47Rev	3′GGCTCGAGGTAAGTCACAAGACTGGTTG 5′	This study
bsh56Fw	5′CCGCTAGCTGTACATCAATTTTATATAGTCC 3′	This study
bsh56Rev	3′GGCTCGAGATTTTCAAATTTAATGGCTTG 5′	This study

Expression and Purification of Recombinant BSH12, BSH47, and BSH56 in *E. coli*

E. coli SE1 strains harboring pLB490 (*bsh12*), pLB491 (*bsh47*), and pLB492 (*bsh56*) were grown at 37°C ON in 10 mL of LB supplemented with ampicillin (100 μg/mL) with vigorous shaking at 180 rpm and subsequently grown in 1.5 L of LB/ampicillin (100 μg/mL) at 37°C. When an optical density ($OD_{600\,nm}$) = 0.6–0.8 was reached, gene expression was induced by the addition of 1 mM of Isopropyl β-D-1-Thiogalactopyranoside (IPTG), and cultures were incubated at 21°C ON with shaking at 180 rpm. Bacteria were harvested by centrifugation and cell pellets were washed with PBS and resuspended in 15 ml of Tris-KCl buffer (Tris 50 mM, KCl 100 mM, $MgCl_2$ 10 mM, pH 7.5) supplemented with Triton-X-100 (Sigma-Aldrich) to a final concentration of 1% and protease inhibitors 1X (Roche). Cells were subsequently sonicated for 4 min with alternated pulses on ice (on: 5 s, off: 30 s). The lysed cells were then placed in ultracentrifuge tubes and spun at 220,000 × g at 4°C for 45 min to separate soluble supernatants from pellets.

The soluble fractions containing the recombinant BSH (rBSH) were then collected and rBSHs were purified using affinity chromatography. Briefly, columns kept in nickel-nitrilotriacetic acid (Ni-NTA; Qiagen) agarose were first washed with milliQ water and equilibrated with 50 mM Tris-KCl buffer pH 7.5 according to the supplier's protocol. Soluble lysates were passed through Ni-NTA columns and washed with 50 mM Tris-KCl buffer pH 7.5 to remove unbound proteins. Finally, rBSHs were eluted by increasing imidazole concentrations (25, 75, and 500 mM) as recommended by the supplier. The eluted proteins were desalted using Sephadex G-25 columns (Amersham Biosciences). All fractions were analyzed on Sodium Dodecyl Sulfate-PolyAcrylamide Gel Electrophoresis (SDS-PAGE) and stained with Coomassie Brilliant Blue.

Bile Salt Hydrolase Activity Assays

The substrate specificity of each rBSHs was assessed on plates using an agar test. *E. coli* strains harboring pLB490, pLB491, and pLB492 were cultured in LB broth in presence of ampicillin (100 μg/ml). Overnight cultures were then spotted on LB agar plates supplemented with either 0.5% taurodeoxycholic acid (TDCA, Sigma-Aldrich) or 0.5% glycodeoxycholic acid (GDCA, Merck Millipore) and incubated at 37°C for 48 h.

The BSH hydrolyzing activities were also monitored using purified recombinant enzymes in presence of conjugated bile salts, in solution, by measuring the liberation of amino acids (glycine or taurine) as previously described (Grill et al., 2000). A volume of 100 μl of rBSH (20 μg) was mixed with 100 μl of 2.4 g/L of each conjugated bile salts (GDCA, TDCA, glycocholic acid, or taurocholic acid) and incubated for 30 min at 37°C. BSH from *C. perfringens* (Sigma-Aldrich, reference C4018) was used as a positive control. A solution without bile salts was used as a negative control. The hydrolysis of bile salts was stopped by adding 200 μl of 15% trichloroacetic acid (TCA) (v/v%) and the mixture was spun at 10,000 g for 15 min to remove precipitated proteins. The supernatant (80 μl) was subsequently collected and added to 680 μl of 0.3 M borate buffer, 1% SDS (pH 9.5), and 80 μl of 0.3% picrylsulfonic acid solution (Sigma-Aldrich). Mixtures were incubated for 30 min in the dark at room temperature and 800 μL of 0.6 mM HCl was added to stop the colorimetric reaction. The amount of glycine or taurine released was measured at 416 nm using a spectrophotometer and standard curves were established with free glycine and taurine.

Giardia duodenalis Cultures

Two different isolates of assemblage A were used in this study: *G. duodenalis* strains WB clone 6 (WB6, ATCC50803), isolated from a patient with chronic giardiasis, and *G. duodenalis* NF (kindly provided by Dr. André Buret, University of Calgary), obtained from an outbreak of human giardiasis. Trophozoites were cultured in axenic conditions grown in Keiser's modified TYI-S-33 medium (KM) adjusted at pH 6.0 and supplemented with heat-inactivated fetal calf serum (10%) (FCS, reference A15-101, PAA laboratories, GE Healthcare) as recently described (Travers et al., 2016). *In vitro* experiments were performed with or without bovine bile (Difco, DB Diagnostic System, reference 212820) supplementation (0.6 g/L).

Anti-giardial Activity Assays

Increasing concentrations of rBSHs were co-incubated with fresh cultures of *G. duodenalis* WB6 trophozoites (2×10^5 parasites/ml) in KM medium supplemented with 10% FCS in a final volume of 480 μl, at 37°C in anaerobic conditions for 22 h. Experiments were performed with or without bovine bile (0.6 g/L) supplementation. BSH from *C. perfringens* (1U, Sigma-Aldrich, reference C4018) was used as a positive control. Trophozoites were detached from tubes by chilling on ice for 10 min and the parasite load was measured by using hemocytometer (flagella mobility was used as viability criteria). The inhibition levels were determined in comparison with values of non-treated trophozoite cultures (percentage of growth). Three biological replicates were performed, each in duplicates. The half maximal inhibitory concentrations (IC_{50}) were calculated using Prism 5 software (GraphPad).

G. duodenalis Viability Assays on Cell Cultures

Caco-2 epithelial cells (human colonic adenocarcinoma, ATTC HTB-37) were grown in Dulbecco's Modified Eagle's Medium (DMEM) containing 200 mM L-glutamine, 100 U/mL penicillin, 100 U/mL streptomycin, and 10% fetal bovine serum (FBS) (Gibco, reference 12484-028) at 37°C and 5% CO_2. Caco-2 cells were cultured (passage 28–32) at 80% confluence with trypsin-EDTA and seeded at 10^5 cells/mL onto 12-wells plates (Caco-2 growth medium). Cells were cultured until the monolayer was confluent (3–4 days) with medium changes every 48 h. 3 days prior to co-incubation, cultures of *G. duodenalis* NF strain trophozoites were axenically cultured in KM medium supplemented with 10% heat-inactivated FBS at 37°C to confluence. Parasites were ice-chilled for 15 min, harvested by centrifugation for 10 min at 1,300 × *g* (4°C), and resuspended in Caco-2 growth medium supplemented with bovine bile (0.6 g/L). For co-culture experiments, trophozoites were seeded at a multiplicity of infection (MOI) of 10:1. Recombinant BSHs were then added to co-cultures at different concentrations and the plates were incubated at 37°C and 5% CO_2. After 20 h of incubation, trophozoites were collected after chilling of plates on ice and the parasite load was determined using hemocytometer (flagella mobility was used as viability criteria).

Scanning Electron Microscopy

For scanning electron microscopy (SEM), fresh cultures of *G. duodenalis* trophozoites WB6 strain were treated with either rBSH47 (0.5 μg/ml), rBSH56 (0.08 μg/ml), or DCA (0.1 g/L and 0.2 g/L) in KM supplemented with 10% heat-inactivated FCS (10%), with or without bovine bile (0.6 g/L) supplementation. Cultures of treated and untreated *Giardia* trophozoites were subsequently seeded in 12 wells plates on poly-lysine glass coverslips placed at the bottom, and parasites were let to settle on the glass coverslips. After 16 h incubation, the supernatants were removed gently and cells were fixed on the glass coverslips with cacodylate 0.1 M and glutaraldehyde 2.5% (pH 7.2) overnight at 4°C. After two washing steps with 0.1 M cacodylate (pH 7.2), cells were dehydrated in a graded ethanol series (50, 70, 90, and 100%) and critical point-dried in liquid CO_2 (Emitech K850, Quorum Technologies). Coverslips were then mounted onto holders and coated with 20 nm of gold (JEOL Fine Coater JFC-1200). The samples were then examined with a Hitachi Scanning Electron SU3500 Premium.

Experimental Infection Model

OF1 mice were obtained from Charles River (Saint-Germain-Nuelles, France). Mice were housed in pathogen-free conditions and all experiments were performed under a laminar flow hood. Neonatal (suckling) mice were challenged with 10^5 *G. duodenalis* WB6 trophozoites at day 10 by intragastric gavage (100 μl). Recombinant BSH47 was diluted in DMEM with $NaHCO_3$ 16.4% (vehicle) and daily administered by intragastric gavage to neonatal mice from days 10 to 15. Control animals received vehicle instead of rBSH47. Animals were sacrificed by cervical dislocation at day 16 (peak of infection, as determined in parallel assays) and assayed for the presence of *G. duodenalis* trophozoites in the small intestine. Small intestines were resuspended in 5 ml of cold PBS, incubated on ice for 10 min, and mixed thoroughly. The parasite load was estimated using hemocytometer chambers. Mice with no detectable trophozoites (threshold: $<10^3$ parasites/5 ml intestine suspension) were considered as parasite-free. All protocols were carried out in accordance with the institutional ethical guidelines of the ethics committee ANSES's Animal Health Laboratory at Maisons-Alfort on the campus of the French National Veterinary School of Alfort (ENVA), which approved this study.

Statistical Analysis

Data analysis was performed with Prism 5 software (GraphPad). One-way ANOVA, Mann-Whitney, and *t*-test were used to evaluate difference between means. Results were presented as means ± standard error of the mean (SEM). Statistical significance was calculated at a P value of 0.05 and 95% confidence interval.

RESULTS

In Silico Analysis of *L. johnsonii* La1-BSHs Protein Sequences

The amino acid sequences of *L. johnsonii*-BSH12, BSH47, and BSH56 enzymes were blasted against reported sequences from several Gram-positive bacteria using Blastp. For the three *L. johnsonii* Lal BSH, results indicated high identity levels with BSH of different *Lactobacillus* species ranging from 54 to 100% but lower levels of identity (less than 54%) with BSH from *Bifidobacterium* and *Clostridium* species. In particular, the *L. johnsonii*-BSH12 shared 54, 57, 60, 79–84, and 60–100% identities with BSHs from *C. perfringens*, *L. acidophilus*, *L. reuteri*, *L. gasseri*, and *L. johnsonii*, respectively. *L. johnsonii*-BSH47 shared 54–55, 56–58, 60–66, 57, 70, and 97–100% identities with BSHs from *L. crispatus*, *L. reuteri*, *L. gasseri*, *L. acidophilus*, *L. amylovorus*, and *L. johnsonii*, respectively. Finally, *L. johnsonii*-BSH56 showed 94 and 99% identity with BSHs from *L. gasseri* and both *L. acidophilus* and *L. johnsonii*, respectively.

The 3D structures of CBAH-1 from *C. perfringens* (Rossocha et al., 2005) and BlBSH from *B. longum* (Kumar et al., 2006) have been determined (PDB: 2BJF and PDB: 2RF8, respectively), revealing the presence of key residues in the enzymatic active site (Cys-2, Arg-18, Asp-21, Asn-82, Asn-172, and Arg-225; numbering referring to CBAH-1). In addition, experimental studies validated the importance of Arg-18 in the catalytic site (Fang et al., 2009; Lin, 2014; Lin et al., 2014). Therefore, multiple amino acid sequence alignments of BSH12, BSH47, and BSH56 with CBAH-1 and BlBSH were performed using ClustalO program (GONNET PAM 250 matrix), thereby indicating that these key residues were indeed highly conserved in all three *L. johnsonii* Lal-BSHs (**Figure 1**). Moreover, motifs surrounding these key amino acid positions were also found to be well conserved such as ^{16}FGRNXD, ^{72}NEXGLXXAGLNF, ^{170}VXXLTNXPXF, and ^{213}GXGXGXXGXPGD, a point that has been also reported in other studies (Elkins et al., 2001; Kim and Lee, 2008). However, residues, which are predicted to be involved in the substrate-binding site based on the 3D structure of *C. perfringens*, did not appear to be conserved in either *L. johnsonii* BSH enzyme (Ridlon et al., 2006).

Predicted tridimensional structures of *L. johnsonii* BSH12, BSH47, and BSH56 were modeled with I-TASSER software, using existing 3D structures (**Figure S1**, BSH47 and BSH56 and **Figure S2**, BSH12). *Clostridium perfringens* CBAH-1 was used as a template for BSH47 modeling (RMSD: 0.64; TM-score: 0.991; Identity, 35.4%) and BSH12 (RMSD: 1.5; TM-score: 0.967; Identity: 37.3%). *Bifidobacterium longum* BlBSH was used as a template for BSH56 modeling (RMSD: 1.16; TM-score: 0.966; Identity: 43.8%). A superimposition of BSH47 and BSH56 models revealed very similar structures. In particular, the distinctive αββα-folding pattern is conserved in both proteins (Patel et al., 2010; Lin et al., 2014). In addition, the residues involved in the catalytic site are superimposed which confirms a conservation of 3D structure despite a high variability of amino acid sequence among BSHs. Similar results were obtained with BSH12 (**Figure S2**).

Heterologous Expression and Purification of BSHs in *E. coli*

To study the biochemical and enzymatic characteristics of *L. johnsonii* Lal-BSHs, *bsh* genes (i.e., *bsh12*, *bsh47*, and *bsh56*) were cloned in *E. coli* CYS21 strain and expressed in *E. coli* SE1 strain. Western blot analysis from *E. coli* SE1 cells expressing His-tagged BSHs showed an efficient production of BSH12, BSH47, and BSH56, respectively (**Figure 2A**). High yields of heterologous proteins were produced from 1.5 L of recombinant *E. coli* cultures upon 1 mM IPTG induction. No cytotoxic effects were observed during bacterial growth. C-terminal His-tagged rBSHs were subsequently purified using Ni-NTA agarose affinity chromatography and desalted. The purity of BSHs was assessed by Coomassie-blue staining of SDS-PAGE (**Figure 2B**). The molecular weights observed on SDS-PAGE corresponded with those expected (based on theoretical predictions) for rBSH 47 (37.1 kDa) and rBSH56 (35.8 kDa). However, the molecular weight for rBSH12 appeared slightly higher than theoretically expected (37.4 kDa). Nanodrop quantifications of desalted proteins showed that 35 mg of rBSH47 and 28 mg of rBSH56 were successfully purified from 1.5 L of culture. However, only 3 mg of rBSH12 could be recovered.

L. johnsonii La1 BSH Activities and Substrate Specificities

The substrate specificities of the *L. johnsonii* BSHs were assayed by two approaches. Enzymatic activities were monitored in solution, using recombinant enzymes, by measuring amino acids released from the hydrolysis of conjugated bile salts as described in materials and methods. These enzymatic activity assays revealed a slight activity toward glycocholic acid, but a much higher level of activity toward taurocholic acid, for both rBSH47 and rBSH56 (**Table 2**). No significant enzymatic activity was detected with the purified rBSH12 with any substrate (**Table 2**). In parallel, the substrate specificities of the three *L. johnsonii* BSHs (produced in *E. coli*) were determined using LB agar supplemented with either taurodeoxycholic (0.3%) or glycodeoxycholic (0.3%) acids. A white and iridescent precipitate around colonies is indicative of BSH hydrolytic activity. *E. coli* SE1 strain expressing rBSH47 efficiently hydrolyzed tauro-conjugated bile salts, whereas no BSH activity was detected for glyco-conjugated bile salts (**Figure 3A**). *E. coli* SE1 strain expressing rBSH56 efficiently hydrolyzed both tauro- and glycol-conjugated bile salts (data not shown). A slight deconjugation

```
BSH12   MCTSIVYSSN-NHHYFGRNLDLEISFGEHPVITPRNYEFQYRKLPS-KKAKYAMVGMAIV 58
BSH47   MCTSILYSPK--DNYFGRNLDYEIAYGQKVVITPRNYQLNYRHLPT-QDTHYAMIGVSVV 57
CBAH-1  MCTGLALETKDGLHLFGRNMDIEYSFNQSIIFIPRNFKCVNKSNKKELTTKYAVLGMGTI 60
BSH56   MCTGLRFTDDQGNLYFGRNLDVGQDYGEGVIITPRNYPLPYKFLDN-TTTKKAVIGMGIV 59
B1BSH   MCTGVRFSDDEGNTYFGRNLDWSFSYGETILVTPRGYHYDTVFGAGGKAKPNAVIGVGVV 60
         **.:    .     ****:*    : :  :. ** :               *::*:. :

BSH12   ENNYPLYFDAANEEGLGIAGLNFDGPCHYFPEN-AEKNNVTPFELIPYLLSQCTTVAEVK 117
BSH47   ANDYPLYCDAINEKGLGIAGLNFTGPGKYFSVD-ESKKNVTSFELIPYLLSNCETIEDVK 116
CBAH-1  FDDYPTFADGMNEKGLGCAGLNFPVYVSYSKEDIEGKTNIPVYNFLLWVLANFSSVEEVK 120
BSH56   VDGYPSYFDCYNEDGLGIAGLNFPHFAKFSDGPIDGKINLASYEIMLWVTQNFTHVSEVK 119
B1BSH   MADRPMYFDCANEHGLAIAGLNFPGYASFVHEPVEGTENVATFEFPLWVARNFDSVDEVE 120
            * : *  **.**. *****     :       . *:  :::  ::  :   : :*:

BSH12   DALKDVSLVNINFSEKLPLSPLHWLMADKTGESIVVESTLSGLHVYDNPVHVLTNNPEFP 177
BSH47   KLLSETNITDESFSKDLPVTTLHWLMGDKSGKSIVIESTETGLHVYDNPVNTLTNNPVFP 176
CBAH-1  EALKNANIVDIPISENIPNTTLHWMISDITGKSIVVEQTKEKLNVFDNNIGVLTNSPTFD 180
BSH56   EALKNVNLVNEAINTSFAVAPLHWIISDSDEAIIVEVSKQYGMKVFDDKVGVLTNSPDFN 179
B1BSH   ETLRNVTLVSQIVP-GQQESLLHWFIGDGKRSIVVEQ-MADGMHVHHDDVDVLTNQPTFD 178
        . * :..:..  .      : ***::.*     :*       :.*..: : .***.* *

BSH12   GQLRNLANYSNIAPAPQKNTLVPGVDLNLYSRGLGTHFLPGGMDSASRFVKIAFVRAHSP 237
BSH47   AQVETLANFASVSPAQPKNTLVPNADINLYSRGLGTHHLPGGTDSNSRFIKASFVLAHSP 236
CBAH-1  WHVANLNQYVGLRYNQVPEFKLGDQSLTALGQGTGLVGLPGDFTPASRFIRVAFLRDAMI 240
BSH56   WHLTNLGNYTGLNPHDATAQSWNGQKVAPWGVGTGSLGLPGDSIPADRFVKAAYLNVNYP 239
B1BSH   FHMENLRNYMCVSNEMAEPTSWGKASLTAWGAGVGMHGIPGDVSSPSRFVRVAYTNAHYP 238
         :: .* ::  :             .:   . * *   :**     .**:: ::

BSH12   QGNNELSSVTNYFHILHSVEQPKGTDEVGPNSYEYTIYSDGTNLETGTFYYTNYENNQIN 297
BSH47   KGNDEVENVTNFFHVLHSVEQAKGTDEVEDNVFEFTMYSDCMNLDKGILYFTTYDNNQIN 296
CBAH-1  KNDKDSIDLIEFFHILNNVAMVRGSTRTVEEKSDLTQYTSCMCLEKGIYYYNTYENNQIN 300
BSH56   TAKGEKANVAKFFNILKSVAMIKGSVVNDQGKDEYTVYTACYSSGSKTYYCNFEDDFELK 299
B1BSH   QQNDEAANVSRLFHTLGSVQMVDGMAKMGDGQFERTLFTSGYSSKTNTYYMNTYDDPAIR 298
          . :  .: . *. * .*    *         : * ::      .   * .  ::  :.

BSH12   AIELNKENLNGDELTDYKLIEKQTINYQN 326
BSH47   AVDMNNEDLGTSDLITYELFKDQAIKFEN 325
CBAH-1  AIDMNKENLDGNEIKTYKYNKTLSINHVN 329
BSH56   TYKLDDHTMNSTSLVTY------------ 316
B1BSH   SYAMADYDMDSSELISVAR---------- 317
        :  : .  :   .:
```

FIGURE 1 | *L. johnsonii* La1 BSH possess conserved key amino acids in their predicted active sites. Multiple sequence alignments of BSH were performed with the ClustalO program (http://www.ebi.ac.uk/Tools/msa/clustalo/) using GONNET 250 matrix. An "*" (asterisk) indicates positions of fully conserved residues in all five sequences; a ":" (colon) indicates conservation of amino acid with strongly similar chemical properties (Gonnet PAM 250 matrix score > 0.5); a "." indicates conservation of amino acid with similar chemical properties (Gonnet PAM 250 matrix score ≤ 0.5). Residues highlighted in light gray correspond to the predicted key active site amino acids, based on the 3D structures of BSHs from both *C. perfringens* (CBAH-1, PDB: 2BJF) (Rossocha et al., 2005) and *B. longum* (BlBSH, PDB: 2RF8) (Kumar et al., 2006). Residues highlighted in dark gray indicate amino acids putatively involved in substrate binding based on CBAH-1 3D structure (Rossocha et al., 2005; Ridlon et al., 2006). Boxes indicate conserved signatures, i.e., ^{16}FGRNXD, ^{72}NEXGLXXAGLNF, ^{170}VXXLTNXPXF, and ^{213}GXGXGXXGXPGD (CBAH-1 numbering).

was observed with *E. coli* strain producing rBSH12 against glyco-conjugated bile salts. However, BSH12 was not further tested in this study.

Phylogenetic relationship among selected BSH sequences and related substrate predictions were represented on a neighbor-joining tree, constructed using amino acid sequences of BSHs whose substrate specificities have been previously characterized, with 500 bootstrap replications using MEGA5 software (http://www.megasoftware.net/). Such a phylogenetic analysis showed that *L. johnsonii* La1-BSH12 is more closely related to *L. johnsonii* 100-100-BSH-α (**Figure 3B**), an enzyme which is able to hydrolyze both tauro- and glyco-conjugated bile salts. The *L. johnsonii* La1-BSH56 is phylogenetically related to a compact cluster including *L. johnsonii* PF01-BSHB (LjBSHB), *L. acidophilus* PF01-BSH (LaBSH), and *L. johnsonii* 100-100-BSH-β (LjBSH-β). Both BSH56 and LjBSH-β display broad substrate specificity, with a slight preference for tauro-conjugated over glyco-conjugated bile salts, whereas LaBSH and LjBSHB exclusively hydrolyze tauro-conjugated bile salts (Chae et al., 2013). Finally, *L. johnsonii* La1-BSH47 was more closely related to *L. johnsonii* PF01-BSHC (LjBSHC) hydrolyzing only glyco-conjugated bile acids, whereas BSH47 displays a preference for tauro-conjugated substrates. These observations suggest that substrate specificities are not systematically conserved among lactobacilli BSHs, despite a good conservation of their 3D-structures and of key amino acids in their active sites, which makes substrate specificity prediction based on phylogenetic analysis not straightforward for the moment.

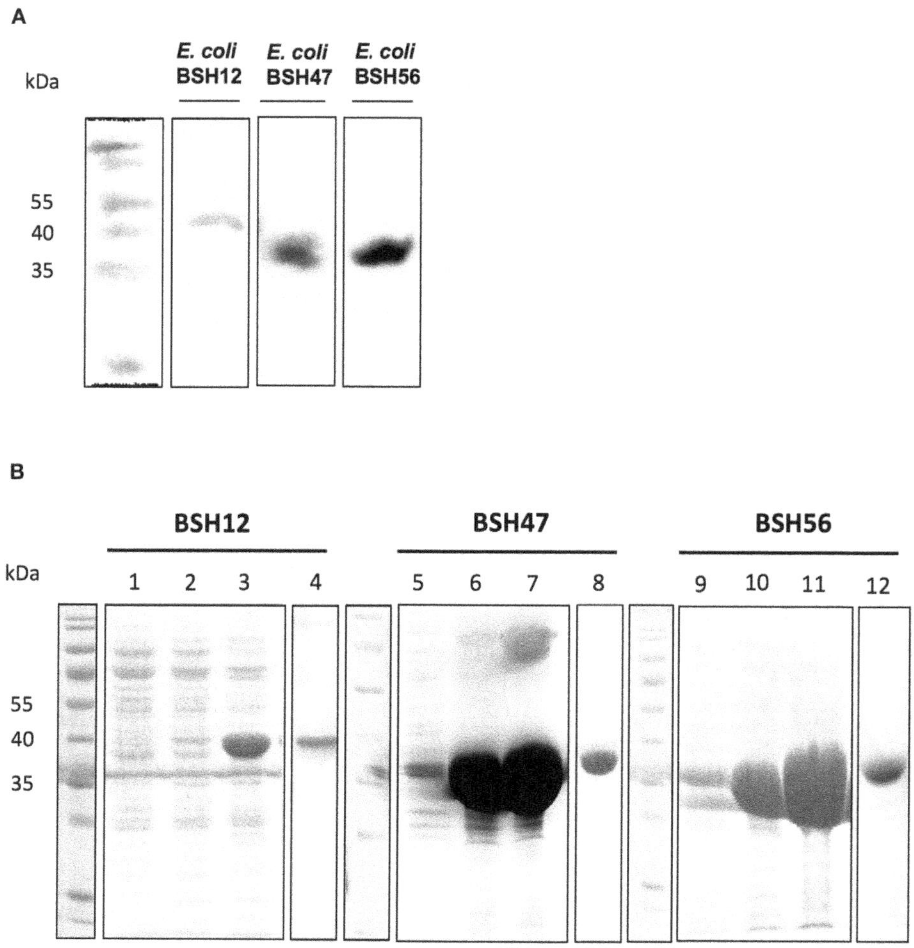

FIGURE 2 | Expression and purification of *L. johnsonii* La1 BSHs. **(A)** Detection of heterologous production of BSH in *E. coli* by Western Blotting using anti-His tag antibody. Production of BSH was done under the control of pStaby system in *E. coli* (induced with 1 mM IPTG). Cytoplasmic fractions were extracted from *E. coli* SE1 harboring pLB490 plasmid (*E. coli* BSH12), pLB491 plasmid (*E. coli* BSH47) or pLB492 plasmid (*E. coli* BSH56). **(B)** SDS–PAGE analysis of purified BSHs. Purification steps of rBSH12, rBSH47, and rBSH56 with Ni-NTA affinity chromatography. Lanes 1–3 correspond to eluted fractions of rBSH12 with imidazole gradient (25, 75, and 500 mM). Lane 4 is rBSH12 after desalting. Lanes 5–7 correspond to eluted fractions of rBSH47 (imidazole gradient: 25, 75, and 500 mM); lane 8 is rBSH47 after desalting step. Lanes 9–11 correspond to eluted fractions of rBSH56 (imidazole gradient: 25, 75, and 500 mM); lane 12 is rBSH56 after desalting step.

TABLE 2 | Activities of *L. johnsonii* BSH against tauro- and glyco-conjugated bile salts.

Enzyme	TDCA hydrolase activity[a]	Relative activity[b]		GDCA hydrolase activity[c]	Relative activity[d]	
		U/g*	%		U/g*	%
BSH12	–	–	Nd	+	–	Nd
BSH47	++	720	100	+	65	9
BSH56	++	2600	100	++	530	21
BSH C. perf	Nd	150	26	Nd	580	100

*μmol/5 min per g of protein.
[a]Based on activity on taurodeoxycholic acid (plate assay).
[b]Based on activity on taurocholic acid (enzymatic assay).
[c]Based on activity on glycodeoxycholic acid (plate assay).
[d]Based on activity on glycocholic acid (enzymatic assay).
Nd, Non-detected. One unit of BSH activity was defined as the amount of enzyme that can liberate 1 μmol of amino acid from a given substrate in 5 minutes.

Besides, enzymatically active BSHs from *L. johnsonii* La1 that could be measured here showed a higher activity for tauro-conjugated than glyco-conjugated substrates, whereas a clear preference has been observed for glyco-conjugated bile salts among other lactobacilli-BSHs characterized so far (Tanaka et al., 1999).

Enzymatic Activities of *L. johnsonii* La1 BSH47 and BSH56 Display Anti-giardial Effects

To evaluate the anti-giardial potential of purified *L. johnsonii* La1-BSHs, *G. duodenalis* WB6 trophozoites were incubated for 22 h in the presence of increasing concentrations of rBSH47 and rBSH56 from 2×10^{-5} to 17.4 μg/ml (rBSH12 was not tested for anti-giardial activity due to weak BSH-activity). Positive controls with *C. perfringens* BSH (Sigma-Aldrich) and negative experimental controls were set up in each independent inhibition

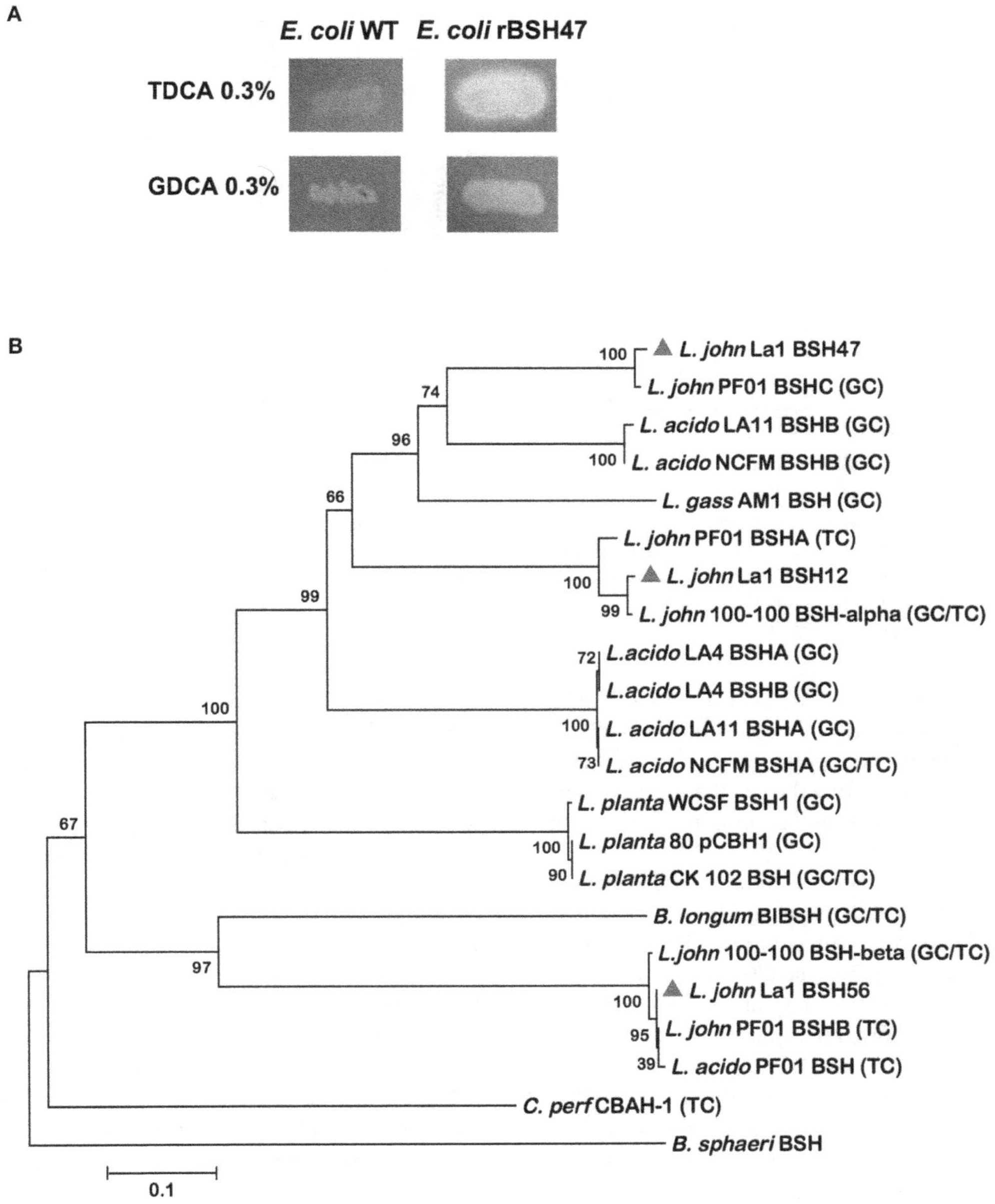

FIGURE 3 | Substrate specificities of *L. johnsonii* La1 BSHs. **(A)** Hydrolase activity of rBSH47 produced in *E. coli* tested on LB plates. *E. coli* SE1 wild type or *E. coli* SE1 expressing rBSH47 were plated in the presence of taurodeoxycholic acid 0.3% (TDCA) or glycodeoxycholic acid 0.3% (GDCA) and incubated for 48–72 h. Activity is detected when a whitish halo forms around colonies. Data with *E. coli* SE1 expressing rBSH12 and rBSH56, respectively, are not shown. **(B)** Phylogenetic relationship among selected BSH sequences and substrate prediction. Programme MEGA5 was used for the phylogenetic tree and for the 500-replication bootstrap analysis. The following predicted amino acid sequences were obtained from UniProtKB/Swiss-Prot databases: BSH12, *L. johnsonii* La1 (Q74IV4_LACJO); BSH47, *L. johnsonii* La1 (Q74JG0_LACJO); BSH12, *L. johnsonii* La1 (Q74LX7_LACJO); CBAH-1, *C. perfringens* strain 13 (P54965.3); BSHA, *L. acidophilus* LA4 (ACL98173.1); BSHB, *L. acidophilus* LA4 (ACL98173.1); BSHA, *L. acidophilus* LA11 (ACL98175.1); BSHB, *L. acidophilus* LA11 (ACL98176.1); BSHA, *L. acidophilus* NCFM (YP_193782.1); BSHB, *L. acidophilus* NCFM (AAV42923.1); BSH, *L. gasseri* AM1 (ACL98172.1); BSH-α, *L. johnsonii* 100-100 (AAG22541.1); BSH-β, *L. johnsonii* 100-100 (AAC34381.1); BSHA, *L. johnsonii* pf01 (EGP12224.1); BSHB, *L. johnsonii* pf01 (EGP13287.1); BSHC, *L. johnsonii* pf01 (EGP12391.1); pCBH1, *L. plantarum* 80 (AAB24746.1); BSH1, *L. plantarum* WCSF (CCC80500.1); BIBSH, *B. longum* subsp. *longum* (2HF0); BSH, *L. acidophilus* PF01 (ABQ01980.1); BSH, *L. plantarum* CK 102 (Ha et al., 2006); Penicillin V Acylase (PVA), *Bacillus sphaericus* (3PVA). Substrate specificity, when known (see text for referenced literature) is indicated for each BSH enzyme (in brackets): (TC), specificity for tauro-conjugated bile salts; (GC), specificity for glyco-conjugated bile salts; (TC/GC), specificity for both tauro and glyco-conjugated bile salts.

assay. Treatments of *Giardia* trophozoites with BSHs showed a dose-dependent inhibition of the parasite growth in presence of bile, when compared to the controls without bile (**Figures 4A,B**). The IC_{50} of rBSH56 ($IC_{50BSH56} = 0.018 \pm 0.002\,\mu g/ml$) was slightly lower than that of rBSH47 ($IC_{50BSH47} = 0.030 \pm 0.003\,\mu g/ml$). Concentrations higher than $1\,\mu g/ml$ of either

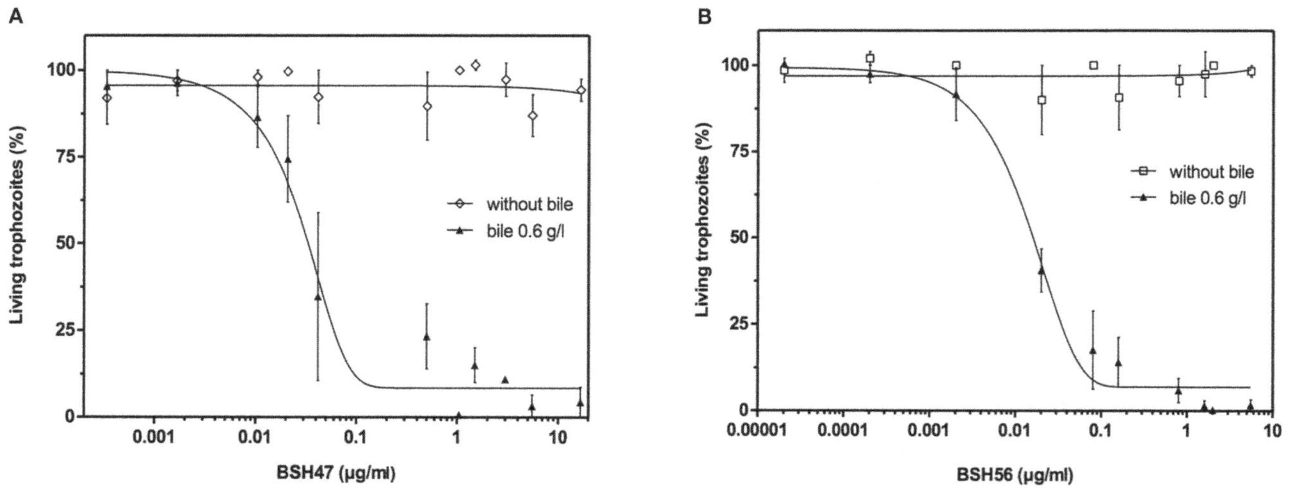

FIGURE 4 | Anti-giardial activity of *L. johnsonii* La1 BSHs *in vitro*. Inhibition of *G. duodenalis* WB6 strain growth by enzymatically active rBSH47 **(A)** and rBSH56 **(B)** from *L. johnsonii* La1 with and without bovine bile supplementation (0.6 g/L) after 22 h of incubation. Increasing doses of BSH were tested ranging from 2×10^{-5} to 17.4 µg/ml. Values are in percentage ± SEM (standard error of the mean). Growth inhibition curves of *G. duodenalis* were calculated using Prism 5 software (GraphPad). $IC50_{BSH56} = 0.018 \pm 0.002$ µg/ml; $IC50_{BSH47} = 0.030 \pm 0.003$ µg/ml.

rBSH47 or rBSH56, respectively, were sufficient to kill 100% of trophozoites in 22 h. Co-cultures of trophozoites and rBSHs in a growth medium without bile supplementation did not exhibit any toxic effects, further supporting the fact that the anti-giardial effect is mediated by BSH activity and requires the presence of an appropriate substrate (bile).

To better characterize the damages induced by BSHs activity, the morphology of *G. duodenalis* trophozoites WB6 was analyzed by SEM after 16 h of treatment with either rBSH56 (0.08 µg/ml), rBSH47 (0.5 µg/ml), or deoxycholic acid (DCA, 0.1 and 0.2 g/L), which is a major product of bile hydrolysis. SEM analysis of non-treated trophozoites showed the characteristic giardial tear-drop shape with no apparent sign of morphological alteration (**Figures 5a,b**). Trophozoites treated with either DCA, or rBSH56 or rBSH47 in presence of bile revealed significant structural damage when compared to controls (**Figures 5c–h**). BSH-treated parasites displayed several alterations such as protrusions and perforations at the surface of their plasma membrane (**Figures 5d,f–h**). In DCA-treated trophozoites, membrane and median body were dramatically disrupted (**Figures 5g,h**). In contrast, with both treatments, the ventral disk microtubule array was still observable.

Assessment of *in Vivo* Anti-giardial Activities of *L. johnsonii* La1 BSH47

Numerous studies have reported that bile acids conjugated to taurine are predominant in mice (Claus et al., 2011). Recombinant BSH47 efficiently hydrolyzed tauro-conjugated bile acids, and its efficacy against *Giardia* has been demonstrated *in vitro*. Since this enzyme was available in larger quantities compared to rBSH56 and rBSH12, rBSH47 was selected to evaluate the potential of rBSH to treat giardiasis in a murine model (**Figure 6A**). OF1 suckling mice were divided into four groups ($n = 7$–12). Mice were challenged with *G. duodenalis* WB6 trophozoites (1×10^5) at day 10 by intragastric gavage. Increasing doses of rBSH47 corresponding to 0.5, 5, and 50 µg (50 µl, diluted in $NaHCO_3$ 16.4%) were thawed and daily administered by intragastric gavage to neonatal mice from day 10 to 15. The control group received vehicle (PBS + $NaHCO_3$ 16.4%). Animals were sacrificed at day 16, corresponding to the peak of trophozoite colonization, and small intestinal contents were sampled and analyzed. Six days after inoculation, trophozoites were able to efficiently colonize and persist in the small intestine with a parasite load 20-fold higher than the inoculum (**Figure 6B**). In groups treated with rBSH47, the parasite burden decreased in a dose-dependent manner (**Figure 6B**). Interestingly, the highest dose of rBSH47 (50 µg daily for 5 days) induced a significant reduction of 68.8% of *G. duodenalis* trophozoites compared to the control group.

DISCUSSION

L. johnsonii La1 is a probiotic strain with pathogen inhibition and host immunomodulation properties (Vidal et al., 2002; Cruchet et al., 2003; Pridmore et al., 2008). The activity of BSH and lactobacilli's bile resistance have been widely accepted as key factors for gut persistence and colonization by these bacteria (Tannock et al., 1994; Tanaka et al., 2000; Begley et al., 2006). Three *bsh* and two bile acid transporters genes were identified in the genome of *L. johnsonii* La1 (Pridmore et al., 2004). In this study, we cloned, purified, and characterized these 3 BSH enzymes in order to assess their antiprotozoal effect on *Giardia*. Nucleotide homology comparisons previously highlighted the similarities between *L. johnsonii* La1 *bsh*12 and *bsh*56 with *cbsHα* and *cbsHβ* from *L. johnsonii* 100-100, respectively (Elkins and Savage, 1998; Elkins et al., 2001; Pridmore et al., 2004). A

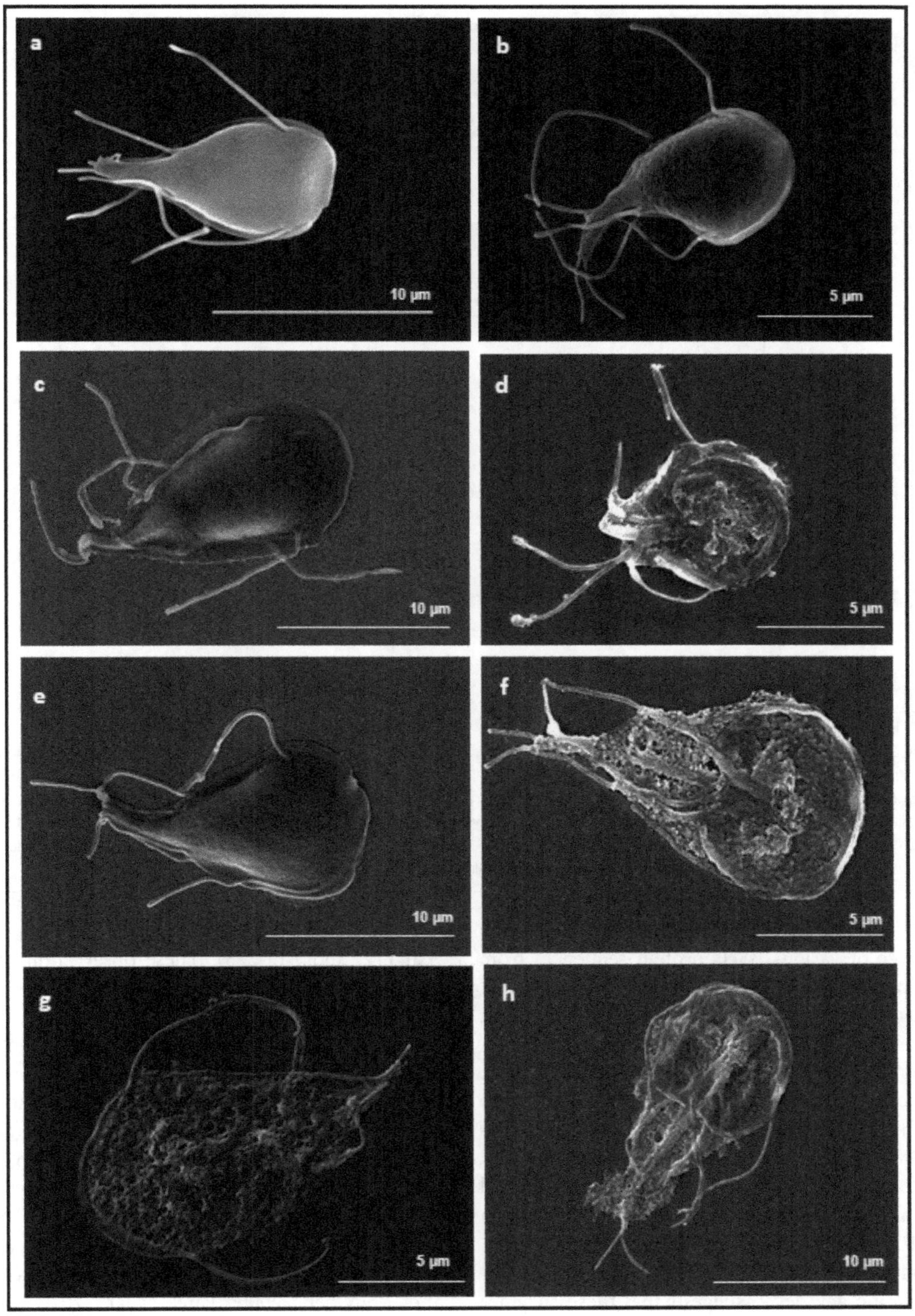

FIGURE 5 | Morphological alterations following *in vitro* treatments of *G. duodenalis* by BSH or deoxycholic acid (DCA). Scanning electron microscopy of *G. duodenalis* trophozoites WB6 strain treated with either BSH47 (0.5 µg/ml), BSH56 (0.08 µg/ml) or DCA (0.1 and 0.2 g/L). **(a)** KM control (KM+ 10% FCS) and **(b)** KM control with bile (bovine bile 0.6 g/l) show the characteristic pear-shaped of trophozoites. **(c)** *G. duodenalis* treated with rBSH47and **(d)** *G. duodenalis* treated with rBSH47 with bile reveal altered morphology and plasma membrane disruption in presence of bile. **(e)** *G. duodenalis* treated with rBSH56 and **(f)** *G. duodenalis* treated with rBSH56 with bile showed similar cell lysis. **(g,h)** DCA-treated (0.1 and 0.2 g/l, respectively) *Giardia* present similar alterations and a disruption of plasma membrane exposing cell interior. Scale bar = 5 µm **(b,d,f,g)** or 10 µm **(a,c,e,h)**.

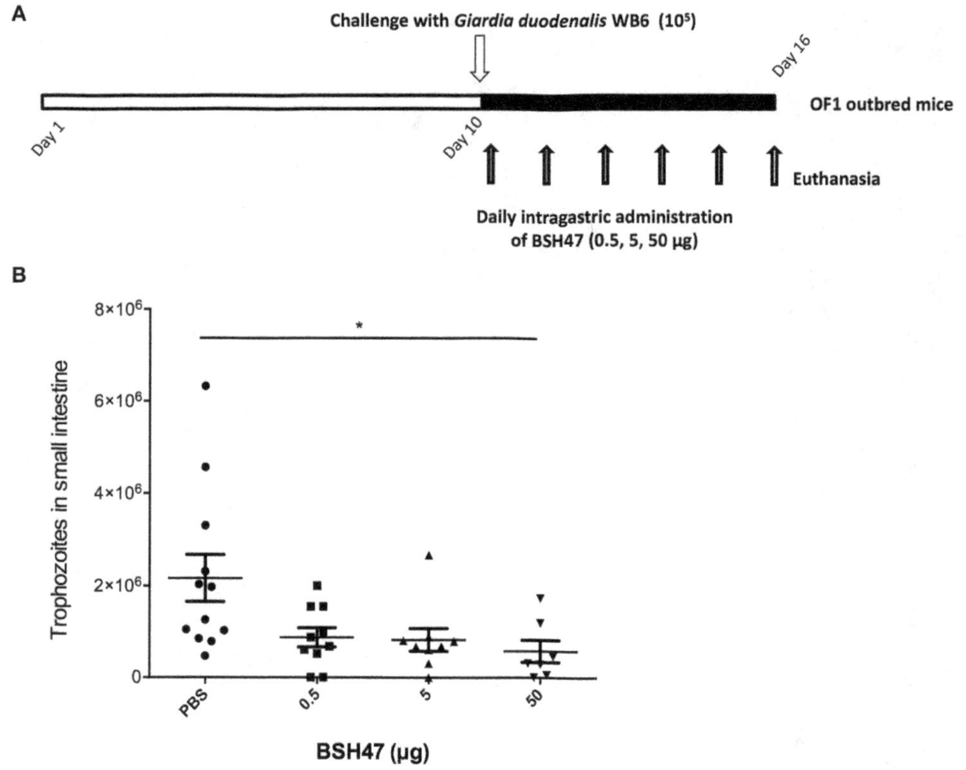

FIGURE 6 | Anti-giardial activity of rBSH47 *in vivo*. **(A)** Experimental design of *G. duodenalis* infection in OF1 suckling mice model. Increasing doses of rBSH47 were daily administered by intragastric gavage (0.5, 5, 50 µg) to OF1 suckling mice from day 10 to 15. Control animals received PBS+ $NaHCO_3$ 16.4% (vehicle). Mice were challenged with *G. duodenalis* WB6 trophozoites (10^5) at day 10 by intragastric gavage. Animals were euthanized by cervical dislocation at day 16. **(B)** *G. duodenalis* trophozoites enumeration in small intestine after rBSH47-treatement. Group I (control): mice received vehicle ($n = 12$); Group II: mice received 0.5 µg of BSH47 daily for 5 days ($n = 10$); Group III: mice received 5 µg of BSH47 daily for 5 days ($n = 9$); mice received 50 µg of BSH47 daily for 5 days ($n = 7$). Small intestines were resuspended in PBS and trophozoites were counted using a hemocytometer. Values are mean ± SEM; $p < 0.0001$.

neighbor-joining tree of various BSHs protein sequences from several lactic acid bacteria confirmed that *L. johnsonii* La1-BSH enzymes are phylogenetically related to BSHs from other species. In addition, they share a high degree of similarity to various subgroups of BSHs; for instance, BSH12 shares 99% identity with *L. johnsonii* 100-100 cbsHα and *L. johnsonii* PF01 BSHA at amino acid level, and BSH56 shares 99% identity with *L. johnsonii* 100-100 cbsHβ and 98% with *L. johnsonii* PF01 BSHB at amino acid level. *L. johnsonii* La1 and *L. johnsonii* PF01 both possess a third BSH gene, *bsh*47 and *bsh*C, respectively, which is absent from *L. johnsonii* 100-100. Besides, the close relationship among *L. johnsonii* La1 BSH47, *L. johnsonii* PF01 BSHC, and *L. acidophilus* NCFM BSHB, at amino acid level, suggests that these enzymes likely share a common ancestor. These observations contribute to the idea that BSH might have been acquired through horizontal gene transfer from microorganisms sharing the same intestinal environment (Corzo and Gilliland, 1999; Franz et al., 2001; McAuliffe et al., 2005; Begley et al., 2006), although this latter hypothesis remains to be tested.

Multiple amino acid sequence alignment of *L. johnsonii* La1 BSHs indicated a high variability among characterized BSHs; however, well-conserved motifs were observed around residues involved in the active site (Cys-2, Arg-18, Asp-21, Tyr-82, Asn-172, and Arg-225). These observations are in agreement with previous studies (Rossocha et al., 2005; Fang et al., 2009; Lin et al., 2014) and highlight that the biological functions of BSHs are strictly conserved despite sequence/phenotypic variabilities. BSHs (EC 3.5.1.24) belong to N-terminal nucleophilic (Ntn) hydrolases, a superfamily of enzymes containing N-terminal cysteine residue involved in the catalytic site (Suresh et al., 1999; Kim et al., 2004). Penicillin V acylases (EC 3.5.1.11), which are closely related to BSH, also belong to Ntn hydrolases and share similar structures. *In silico* modeling, BSH47, BSH56, and BSH12 showed that the typical αββα tertiary structure arrangement, which is characteristic of Ntn superfamily, is conserved (Oinonen and Rouvinen, 2000; Patel et al., 2010; Lin et al., 2014). Taken together, these structural observations indicate that the folding of BSHs remained stable during evolution despite low sequence identity, which suggest a high evolutionary pressure to maintain their functionality (Chothia and Lesk, 1986; Sander and Schneider, 1991; Krieger et al., 2003).

Experimental determination of BSH activities showed that at least 2 of the 3 BSHs from *L. johnsonii* La1 have broad substrate specificities. The enzyme BSH56 exhibited high hydrolysis activities toward tauro- and glyco-conjugated bile salts, with a preference toward tauro-conjugated substrates.

Interestingly, BSH56 belongs to a phylogenetic cluster of BSH enzymes exhibiting activity exclusively directed toward tauro-conjugated bile acids. Similarly, BSH47 was more efficient at hydrolyzing tauro-conjugated bile salts and exhibited a very low relative activity toward glyco-conjugated bile salts. Surprisingly, the amino acid sequence of BSH47 is more closely related to that of *L. johnsonii* BSHC that has been reported to hydrolyze glyco-conjugated bile salts (Chae et al., 2013). Our results, therefore, contrast with previous studies reporting that most BSH enzymes isolated from lactobacilli are very efficient at hydrolyzing glyco-conjugated bile salts (Coleman and Hudson, 1995; Liong and Shah, 2005). In addition, these observations point out the limits of substrate predictions based on phylogenetic relationships considering whole enzyme sequences. The mechanisms responsible for substrate specificity of BSH enzymes are still unclear. Putative amino acids have been associated with substrate binding pockets in *C. perfringens* (Rossocha et al., 2005; Ridlon et al., 2006), but these residues are different in all 3 BSHs from *L. johnsonii*. Several studies emphasized that BSH preferably recognize conjugated substrates at amino acid moieties (Coleman and Hudson, 1995; Tanaka et al., 2000; Kim et al., 2004; Rossocha et al., 2005), whereas others still suggest that steroid moieties are recognized in priority (Moser and Savage, 2001; Begley et al., 2006; Patel et al., 2010) which could explain broad substrate specificities. Experimentally solving the 3D structures of rBSH47 and rBSH56 harboring appropriate substrates would certainly provide invaluable information regarding this important question.

The third BSH isolated from *L. johnsonii* La1, BSH12, was successfully expressed in *E. coli* and clearly observed in SDS-PAGE and by Western blotting, but no specific activity could be detected toward either substrate in liquid tests. However, a slight positive signal was observed with *E. coli* strain-expressing rBHS12 on agar plates supplemented with glyco-specific bile salts, suggesting a weak glyco-specific activity. Similar difficulties to express recombinant BSHs have been observed with BSHs from *L. plantarum* JPP2 (Ren et al., 2011) and BSH2 from *L. plantarum* WCFS1 (Lambert et al., 2008). Proteolytic degradation and misfolding of the recombinant protein produced in *E. coli* may have affected the enzyme's function (Baneyx and Mujacic, 2004). The functionality of BSH12 is, therefore, still under investigation.

As mentioned previously, the putative natural role of BSHs is to decrease the toxicity of conjugated bile salts for bacterial cells (De Smet et al., 1995). In this work, we assessed the anti-parasitic activity of recombinant BSHs and we demonstrated that rBSH47 and rBSH56 were highly active against viable trophozoites of *G. duodenalis* strains WB6 and NF. The minimum concentration found to kill 100% of *G. duodenalis* WB6 trophozoites *in vitro* was 1 μg/mL for both rBSH47 and rBSH56. When tested on human enterocyte Caco-2 cells, both rBSH47 and rBSH56 inhibited the growth of *G. duodenalis* NF in the presence of bile (0.6 g/L) in a dose-dependent fashion and prevented the attachment of the parasites to the cell monolayers (**Figure S3**). The rBSH56 was more effective than rBSH47 in killing both *G. duodenalis* WB6 and NF strains, although it induced more cell damages to Caco-2 cells at high concentrations (**Figure S3**). Recombinant BSH47 was, therefore, chosen to assess the *in vivo* effectiveness of BSH to treat *Giardia* infection in a suckling murine model. Moreover, given that bile acids are predominantly conjugated to taurine in mice (Claus et al., 2011), the ability of BSH47 to preferentially hydrolyze tauro-conjugated bile salts seemed more appropriate. We observed that rBSH47 inhibited *Giardia* growth in a dose-dependent manner *in vivo*, in keeping with the data obtained *in vitro*. At the highest dose (50 μg/mice/day) administered daily for 5 days, the parasite (trophozoite) burden was significantly reduced by 68.8% in the small intestine of the mice. Despite this important decrease of the parasite load, none of the treated mice were free of parasites at 16 days post-inoculation. The anti-giardial effects mediated by rBSH47 *in vivo* were, therefore, modest compared to their efficacy in the *in vitro* assays. This can be explained by a partial degradation of BSHs by acidic proteases and peptidases in the stomach. The activity of BSHs correlates with the amount of conjugated bile salts released in the duodenum, which is highly variable in neonates (Heubi et al., 2007). The production of deconjugated bile salts at inhibiting levels is, therefore, dependent to the bioavailability of BSH in the small intestine.

It has been reported that bile salts, and more specifically conjugated bile salts, have growth promoting effects on *G. duodenalis in vivo* (Halliday et al., 1988). Indeed, bile uptake contributes to cholesterol and exogenous phospholipids needs, which are essentials for parasite growth (Yichoy et al., 2011). So far, to our knowledge, there is no evidence showing that *Giardia* is able to deconjugate bile salts. Conjugated bile salts are, thus, directly consumed by *Giardia* without being detoxified (Farthing et al., 1985). In contrast, bacterial deconjugation aims at reducing the detergent properties of conjugated bile salts, which are more toxic for bacterial cells than secondary bile salts, i.e., cholic acid (CA), deoxycholic acid (DCA), and chenodeoxycholic acid (CDCA) (De Boever and Verstraete, 1999). It is likely that detoxification of bile salts by the duodenal microbiota has a collateral effect on parasite survival. Earlier work carried out in our lab showed that DCA and CDCA exerted cytotoxic effects on *G. duodenalis* trophozoites *in vitro* at non-micellar concentrations (Travers et al., 2016). Therefore, we investigated the morphological perturbations induced by DCA and BSHs on trophozoite cultures and we noticed both induced degenerations and perforations of the parasite plasma membrane. It has been established that DCA perturbs eukaryotic membranes structure by altering the membrane lipid microdomains (Jean-Louis et al., 2006). Furthermore, secondary bile salts induced a redistribution of cholesterol and decrease membrane fluidity. Hence, we hypothesized that secondary bile salt, and more specifically DCA, would kill *Giardia* trophozoites by damaging the cell structure. In the upper parts of the small intestine, where bile salt deconjugation occurs at high rate, the Gram-positive bacteria might be protected against secondary deconjugated bile salts by cell wall peptidoglycan.

A major side effect of BSH-based treatment would be a shift of bile salt balance in the gut. It has been reported in previous studies that an enhancement of BSH activity might impact host physiology by disturbing fat digestion and lipid metabolism (Begley et al., 2006; Lin et al., 2014). Moreover, secondary bile acids resulting from the deconjugation of bile salts have also been linked to DNA damage in bacterial and host cells, colon cancer, and inflammation (Cheah and Bernstein, 1990; Moser and Savage, 2001; Bernstein et al., 2005). On the other hand, BSH activity is a natural process that plays a central role in the reduction of cholesterol (Jones et al., 2013).

The aim of this study was to evaluate the anti-giardial potential of BSHs against *G. duodenalis*. We expressed for the first time the BSHs isolated from the probiotic strain *L. johnsonii* La1 and showed that rBSH47 and rBSH56 exhibited high specific activity and broad substrate specificities. Antiprotozoal assays demonstrated that BSHs were highly effective against *G. duodenalis in vitro* and *in vivo* and represent a promising therapeutic strategy based on their natural catalytic activity. Future studies will determine whether such treatment approaches should be of short duration in order to avoid putative side effects related to the enhancement of bile salt deconjugation. Besides, this anti-giardial effect can be extended to any BSH activity as long as it efficiently converts conjugated bile salts into their deconjugated counterparts. However, further works are still needed to investigate the positive impact of such treatment on the pathophysiology of giardiasis, including protective effects on epithelial permeability, mucosal injury, and malfunction. Moreover, newer galenic formulations are needed in order to provide a better persistence of rBSHs *in vivo*, which can improve health outcomes in routine clinical and veterinary usages.

AUTHOR CONTRIBUTIONS

IF, PG, BP, TA, and LB-H conceived and designed the study. TA, IF, and LB-H produced and isolated the recombinant BSH, performed the biochemical characterizations with SC and the *in silico* analyses. TA, SC, AB, and IF performed the *Giardia* assays *in vitro* and SEM. TA, MT, and BP performed the *Giardia* assays in the suckling mice model. IV, PL, and PG discussed the experiments and results. TA, IF, and LB-H wrote the manuscript with contributions from all authors.

FUNDING

This work was partially funded by Region Ile de France-DIM (Maladies Infectieuses Parasitaires et Nosocomiales Emergentes, programm n° 120092).

ACKNOWLEDGMENTS

We deeply thank Geraldine Toutirais (PTME, Plateau Technique de Microscopie Électronique et de Microanalyses du Museum National d'Histoire Naturelle, Paris) for assistance with SEM imaging. We thank Jasmine Kirati (UMR BIPAR, Anses, ENVA, INRA) for help with *in vivo* assays and Olivier Berteau (Micalis Institute, INRA) for assistance in protein purifications.

SUPPLEMENTARY MATERIAL

Figure S1 | Protein structure prediction of *L. johnsonii* La1 BSHs. Protein structures were modeled for *L. johnsonii* BSH56 **(a)** and BSH47 **(b)** using I-TASSER software (http://zhanglab.ccmb.med.umich.edu/I-TASSER/). CBAH-1 (PDB: 2BJF) from *C. perfringens* (Rossocha et al., 2005) and BlBSH from *B. longum* (Kumar et al., 2006) (PDB: 2HF0) were used as templates for modeling BSH47 and BSH56, respectively. Best values of the C-score were chosen for model structure prediction. Visualization of predicted structures for BSH47 (red, **a**) and BSH56 (blue, **b**) and superimposition **(c,d)** were performed using Pymol software (https://www.pymol.org/).

Figure S2 | Protein structure prediction of *L. johnsonii* La1 BSH12**.** Protein structure was modeled for *L. johnsonii* BSH12 using I-TASSER software (http://zhanglab.ccmb.med.umich.edu/I-TASSER/). Bile salt hydrolase (PDB: 2RF8) from *C. perfringens* was used as a template for modeling. Best value of the C-score was chosen for model structure prediction. Visualization of predicted structure was performed using Pymol software (https://www.pymol.org/).

Figure S3 | Anti-giardial effect of BSH in co-culture with Caco2 cells. To further investigate the effect of *L. johnsonii* La1-BSHs on the adherence of *Giardia* enterocytes, differentiated Caco-2 cells were co-incubated with fresh trophozoites cultures of *G. duodenalis* NF strain and treated with either rBSH47 or rBSH56, over a range of concentrations from 0.005 to 1 μg/ml. *G. duodenalis* NF strain trophozoites were inoculated to Caco2 cells at a multiplicity of infection (MOI) of 10:1 in the presence of increasing doses of rBSH47, rBSH56 or DMEM. Anti-giardial activity assays were performed with bovine bile (0.6 g/l) added to the medium. The results are expressed as relative percentage of growth compared to untreated trophozoites as negative control. Data are presented as mean ± SEM and correspond to triplicates. As expected from previous experiments done with the *G. duodenalis* WB6 strain, both BSHs triggered a growth inhibition of *G. duodenalis* NF trophozoites, in a dose-dependent fashion, after 20 h of exposure (this figure). In contrast, high concentrations of rBSH in assays induced cell damages on Caco-2 monolayer (data not shown). This phenomenon might be due to a putative cytotoxicity of deconjugated bile salt. Interestingly, neither rBSH47 nor rBSH56 displayed cytotoxic effects when tested in absence of bile (data not shown).

REFERENCES

Ankarklev, J., Jerlstrom-Hultqvist, J., Ringqvist, E., Troell, K., and Svard, S. G. (2010). Behind the smile: cell biology and disease mechanisms of Giardia species. *Nat. Rev. Microbiol.* 8, 413–422. doi: 10.1038/nrmicro2317

Ansell, B. R., McConville, M. J., Ma'ayeh, S. Y., Dagley, M. J., Gasser, R. B., Svard, S. G., et al. (2015). Drug resistance in *Giardia duodenalis. Biotechnol. Adv.* 33, 888–901. doi: 10.1016/j.biotechadv.2015.04.009

Baneyx, F., and Mujacic, M. (2004). Recombinant protein folding and misfolding in *Escherichia coli. Nat. Biotechnol.* 22, 1399–1408. doi: 10.1038/nbt1029

Barr, S. C., Bowman, D. D., and Heller, R. L. (1994). Efficacy of fenbendazole against giardiasis in dogs. *Am. J. Vet. Res.* 55, 988–990.

Begley, M., Hill, C., and Gahan, C. G. (2006). Bile salt hydrolase activity in probiotics. *Appl. Environ. Microbiol.* 72, 1729–1738. doi: 10.1128/AEM.72.3.1729-1738.2006

Bernstein, H., Bernstein, C., Payne, C. M., Dvorakova, K., and Garewal, H. (2005). Bile acids as carcinogens in human gastrointestinal cancers. *Mutat. Res.* 589, 47–65. doi: 10.1016/j.mrrev.2004.08.001

Chae, J. P., Valeriano, V. D., Kim, G. B., and Kang, D. K. (2013). Molecular cloning, characterization and comparison of bile salt hydrolases from *Lactobacillus johnsonii* PF01. *J. Appl. Microbiol.* 114, 121–133. doi: 10.1111/jam.12027

Cheah, P. Y., and Bernstein, H. (1990). Modification of DNA by bile acids: a possible factor in the etiology of colon cancer. *Cancer Lett.* 49, 207–210. doi: 10.1016/0304-3835(90)90160-Y

Chothia, C., and Lesk, A. M. (1986). The relation between the divergence of sequence and structure in proteins. *EMBO J.* 5, 823–826.

Claus, S. P., Ellero, S. L., Berger, B., Krause, L., Bruttin, A., Molina, J., et al. (2011). Colonization-induced host-gut microbial metabolic interaction. *MBio* 2, e00271–00210. doi: 10.1128/mBio.00271-10

Coleman, J. P., and Hudson, L. L. (1995). Cloning and characterization of a conjugated bile acid hydrolase gene from *Clostridium perfringens*. *Appl. Environ. Microbiol.* 61, 2514–2520.

Corzo, G., and Gilliland, S. E. (1999). Bile salt hydrolase activity of three strains of *Lactobacillus acidophilus*. *J. Dairy Sci.* 82, 472–480. doi: 10.3168/jds.S0022-0302(99)75256-2

Cotton, J. A., Beatty, J. K., and Buret, A. G. (2011). Host parasite interactions and pathophysiology in giardia infections. *Int. J. Parasitol.* 41, 925–933. doi: 10.1016/j.ijpara.2011.05.002

Cruchet, S., Obregon, M. C., Salazar, G., Diaz, E., and Gotteland, M. (2003). Effect of the ingestion of a dietary product containing *Lactobacillus johnsonii* La1 on Helicobacter pylori colonization in children. *Nutrition* 19, 716–721. doi: 10.1016/S0899-9007(03)00109-6

De Boever, P., and Verstraete, W. (1999). Bile salt deconjugation by *Lactobacillus plantarum* 80 and its implication for bacterial toxicity. *J. Appl. Microbiol.* 87, 345–352. doi: 10.1046/j.1365-2672.1999.00019.x

De Smet, I., Van Hoorde, L., Vande Woestyne, M., Christiaens, H., and Verstraete, W. (1995). Significance of bile salt hydrolytic activities of lactobacilli. *J. Appl. Bacteriol.* 79, 292–301. doi: 10.1111/j.1365-2672.1995.tb03140.x

Elkins, C. A., and Savage, D. C. (1998). Identification of genes encoding conjugated bile salt hydrolase and transport in *Lactobacillus johnsonii* 100-100. *J. Bacteriol.* 180, 4344–4349.

Elkins, C. A., Moser, S. A., and Savage, D. C. (2001). Genes encoding bile salt hydrolases and conjugated bile salt transporters in *Lactobacillus johnsonii* 100-100 and other *Lactobacillus* species. *Microbiology* 147, 3403–3412. doi: 10.1099/00221287-147-12-3403

Eyssen, H. (1973). Role of the gut microflora in metabolism of lipids and sterols. *Proc. Nutr. Soc.* 32, 59–63. doi: 10.1079/PNS19730016

Fang, F., Li, Y., Bumann, M., Raftis, E. J., Casey, P. G., Cooney, J. C., et al. (2009). Allelic variation of bile salt hydrolase genes in *Lactobacillus salivarius* does not determine bile resistance levels. *J. Bacteriol.* 191, 5743–5757. doi: 10.1128/JB.00506-09

Farthing, M. J., Keusch, G. T., and Carey, M. C. (1985). Effects of bile and bile salts on growth and membrane lipid uptake by *Giardia lamblia*. Possible implications for pathogenesis of intestinal disease. *J. Clin. Invest.* 76, 1727–1732. doi: 10.1172/JCI112162

Franz, C. M., Specht, I., Haberer, P., and Holzapfel, W. H. (2001). Bile salt hydrolase activity of Enterococci isolated from food: screening and quantitative determination. *J. Food Prot.* 64, 725–729. doi: 10.4315/0362-028X-64.5.725

Gardner, T. B., and Hill, D. R. (2001). Treatment of giardiasis. *Clin. Microbiol. Rev.* 14, 114–128. doi: 10.1128/CMR.14.1.114-128.2001

Goyal, N., Rishi, P., and Shukla, G. (2013). *Lactobacillus rhamnosus* GG antagonizes Giardia intestinalis induced oxidative stress and intestinal disaccharidases: an experimental study. *World J. Microbiol. Biotechnol.* 29, 1049–1057. doi: 10.1007/s11274-013-1268-6

Grill, J. P., Cayuela, C., Antoine, J. M., and Schneider, F. (2000). Isolation and characterization of a *Lactobacillus amylovorus* mutant depleted in conjugated bile salt hydrolase activity: relation between activity and bile salt resistance. *J. Appl. Microbiol.* 89, 553–563. doi: 10.1046/j.1365-2672.2000.01147.x

Ha, C.-G., Cho, J.-K., Chai, Y.-G., Ha, Y.-A., and Shin, S.-H. (2006). Purification and characterization of bile salt hydrolase from Lactobacillus plantarum CK 102. *J. Microbiol. Biotechnol.* 16, 1047–1052.

Halliday, C. E., Clark, C., and Farthing, M. J. (1988). Giardia-bile salt interactions *in vitro* and *in vivo*. *Trans. R. Soc. Trop. Med. Hyg.* 82, 428–432. doi: 10.1016/0035-9203(88)90153-8

Heubi, J. E., Setchell, K. D., and Bove, K. E. (2007). Inborn errors of bile acid metabolism. *Semin. Liver Dis.* 27, 282–294. doi: 10.1055/s-2007-985073

Humen, M. A., De Antoni, G. L., Benyacoub, J., Costas, M. E., Cardozo, M. I., Kozubsky, L., et al. (2005). *Lactobacillus johnsonii* La1 antagonizes giardia intestinalis *in vivo*. *Infect. Immun.* 73, 1265–1269. doi: 10.1128/IAI.73.2.1265-1269.2005

Jean-Louis, S., Akare, S., Ali, M. A., Mash, E. A. Jr., and Meuillet, E. (2006). Deoxycholic acid induces intracellular signaling through membrane perturbations. *J. Biol. Chem.* 281, 14948–14960. doi: 10.1074/jbc.M506710200

Jones, M. L., Tomaro-Duchesneau, C., Martoni, C. J., and Prakash, S. (2013). Cholesterol lowering with bile salt hydrolase-active probiotic bacteria, mechanism of action, clinical evidence, and future direction for heart health applications. *Expert Opin. Biol. Ther.* 13, 631–642. doi: 10.1517/14712598.2013.758706

Kim, G. B., and Lee, B. H. (2008). Genetic analysis of a bile salt hydrolase in *Bifidobacterium animalis* subsp. lactis KL612. *J. Appl. Microbiol.* 105, 778–790. doi: 10.1111/j.1365-2672.2008.03825.x

Kim, G. B., Brochet, M., and Lee, B. H. (2005). Cloning and characterization of a bile salt hydrolase (bsh) from *Bifidobacterium adolescentis*. *Biotechnol. Lett.* 27, 817–822. doi: 10.1007/s10529-005-6717-3

Kim, G. B., Yi, S. H., and Lee, B. H. (2004). Purification and characterization of three different types of bile salt hydrolases from Bifidobacterium strains. *J. Dairy Sci.* 87, 258-266. doi: 10.3168/jds.S0022-0302(04)73164-1

Krieger, F., Fierz, B., Bieri, O., Drewello, M., and Kiefhaber, T. (2003). Dynamics of unfolded polypeptide chains as model for the earliest steps in protein folding. *J. Mol. Biol.* 332, 265–274. doi: 10.1016/S0022-2836(03)00892-1

Kumar, R. S., Brannigan, J. A., Prabhune, A. A., Pundle, A. V., Dodson, G. G., Dodson, E. J., et al. (2006). Structural and functional analysis of a conjugated bile salt hydrolase from *Bifidobacterium longum* reveals an evolutionary relationship with penicillin V acylase. *J. Biol. Chem.* 281, 32516–32525. doi: 10.1074/jbc.M604172200

Lambert, J. M., Bongers, R. S., De Vos, W. M., and Kleerebezem, M. (2008). Functional analysis of four bile salt hydrolase and penicillin acylase family members in *Lactobacillus plantarum* WCFS1. *Appl. Environ. Microbiol.* 74, 4719–4726. doi: 10.1128/AEM.00137-08

Lane, S., and Lloyd, D. (2002). Current trends in research into the waterborne parasite giardia. *Crit. Rev. Microbiol.* 28, 123–147. doi: 10.1080/1040-840291046713

Lin, J. (2014). Antibiotic growth promoters enhance animal production by targeting intestinal bile salt hydrolase and its producers. *Front. Microbiol.* 5:33. doi: 10.3389/fmicb.2014.00033

Lin, J., Negga, R., Zeng, X., and Smith, K. (2014). Effect of bile salt hydrolase inhibitors on a bile salt hydrolase from *Lactobacillus acidophilus*. *Pathogens* 3, 947–956. doi: 10.3390/pathogens3040947

Liong, M. T., and Shah, N. P. (2005). Acid and bile tolerance and cholesterol removal ability of lactobacilli strains. *J. Dairy Sci.* 88, 55–66. doi: 10.3168/jds.S0022-0302(05)72662-X

McAuliffe, O., Cano, R. J., and Klaenhammer, T. R. (2005). Genetic analysis of two bile salt hydrolase activities in *Lactobacillus acidophilus* NCFM. *Appl. Environ. Microbiol.* 71, 4925–4929. doi: 10.1128/AEM.71.8.4925-4929.2005

Moser, S. A., and Savage, D. C. (2001). Bile salt hydrolase activity and resistance to toxicity of conjugated bile salts are unrelated properties in lactobacilli. *Appl. Environ. Microbiol.* 67, 3476–3480. doi: 10.1128/AEM.67.8.3476-3480.2001

Oinonen, C., and Rouvinen, J. (2000). Structural comparison of Ntn-hydrolases. *Protein Sci.* 9, 2329–2337. doi: 10.1110/ps.9.12.2329

Patel, A. K., Singhania, R. R., Pandey, A., and Chincholkar, S. B. (2010). Probiotic bile salt hydrolase: current developments and perspectives. *Appl. Biochem. Biotechnol.* 162, 166–180. doi: 10.1007/s12010-009-8738-1

Perez, P. F., Minnaard, J., Rouvet, M., Knabenhans, C., Brassart, D., De Antoni, G. L., et al. (2001). Inhibition of giardia intestinalis by extracellular factors from lactobacilli: an *in vitro* study. *Appl. Environ. Microbiol.* 67, 5037–5042. doi: 10.1128/AEM.67.11.5037-5042.2001

Petri, W. A. (2005). Treatment of giardiasis. *Curr. Treat. Options Gastroenterol.* 8, 13–17. doi: 10.1007/s11938-005-0047-3

Platts-Mills, J. A., Babji, S., Bodhidatta, L., Gratz, J., Haque, R., Havt, A., et al. (2015). Pathogen-specific burdens of community diarrhoea in developing countries: a multisite birth cohort study (MAL-ED). *Lancet Glob. Health* 3, e564–e575. doi: 10.1016/S2214-109X(15)00151-5

Pridmore, R. D., Berger, B., Desiere, F., Vilanova, D., Barretto, C., Pittet, A. C., et al. (2004). The genome sequence of the probiotic intestinal bacterium *Lactobacillus johnsonii* NCC 533. *Proc. Natl. Acad. Sci. U.S.A.* 101, 2512–2517. doi: 10.1073/pnas.0307327101

Pridmore, R. D., Pittet, A. C., Praplan, F., and Cavadini, C. (2008). Hydrogen peroxide production by *Lactobacillus johnsonii* NCC 533 and its role in anti-Salmonella activity. *FEMS Microbiol. Lett.* 283, 210–215. doi: 10.1111/j.1574-6968.2008.01176.x

Ren, J., Sun, K., Wu, Z., Yao, J., and Guo, B. (2011). All 4 bile salt hydrolase proteins are responsible for the hydrolysis activity in *Lactobacillus plantarum* ST-III. *J. Food Sci.* 76, M622–M628. doi: 10.1111/j.1750-3841.2011.02431.x

Ridlon, J. M., Kang, D. J., and Hylemon, P. B. (2006). Bile salt biotransformations by human intestinal bacteria. *J. Lipid Res.* 47, 241–259. doi: 10.1194/jlr.R500013-JLR200

Rossocha, M., Schultz-Heienbrok, R., Von Moeller, H., Coleman, J. P., and Saenger, W. (2005). Conjugated bile acid hydrolase is a tetrameric N-terminal thiol hydrolase with specific recognition of its cholyl but not of its tauryl product. *Biochemistry* 44, 5739–5748. doi: 10.1021/bi0473206

Roy, A., Kucukural, A., and Zhang, Y. (2010). I-TASSER: a unified platform for automated protein structure and function prediction. *Nat. Protoc.* 5, 725–738. doi: 10.1038/nprot.2010.5

Ruiz, L., Margolles, A., and Sanchez, B. (2013). Bile resistance mechanisms in *Lactobacillus* and *Bifidobacterium*. *Front. Microbiol.* 4:396. doi: 10.3389/fmicb.2013.00396

Sander, C., and Schneider, R. (1991). Database of homology-derived protein structures and the structural meaning of sequence alignment. *Proteins* 9, 56-68. doi: 10.1002/prot.340090107

Savioli, L., Smith, H., and Thompson, A. (2006). Giardia and Cryptosporidium join the 'neglected diseases initiative'. *Trends Parasitol.* 22, 203–208. doi: 10.1016/j.pt.2006.02.015

Shukla, G., and Sidhu, R. K. (2011). Lactobacillus casei as a probiotic in malnourished *Giardia lamblia*-infected mice: a biochemical and histopathological study. *Can. J. Microbiol.* 57, 127–135. doi: 10.1139/W10-110

Shukla, G., Devi, P., and Sehgal, R. (2008). Effect of *Lactobacillus casei* as a probiotic on modulation of giardiasis. *Dig. Dis. Sci.* 53, 2671–2679. doi: 10.1007/s10620-007-0197-3

Singer, S. M., Elmendorf, H. G., Conrad, J. T., and Nash, T. E. (2001). Biological selection of variant-specific surface proteins in *Giardia lamblia*. *J. Infect. Dis.* 183, 119–124. doi: 10.1086/317659

Suresh, C. G., Pundle, A. V., Sivaraman, H., Rao, K. N., Brannigan, J. A., McVey, C. E., et al. (1999). Penicillin V acylase crystal structure reveals new Ntn-hydrolase family members. *Nat. Struct. Biol.* 6, 414–416. doi: 10.1038/8213

Tamura, K., Peterson, D., Peterson, N., Stecher, G., Nei, M., and Kumar, S. (2011). MEGA5: molecular evolutionary genetics analysis using maximum likelihood, evolutionary distance, and maximum parsimony methods. *Mol. Biol. Evol.* 28, 2731–2739. doi: 10.1093/molbev/msr121

Tanaka, H., Doesburg, K., Iwasaki, T., and Mierau, I. (1999). Screening of lactic acid bacteria for bile salt hydrolase activity. *J. Dairy Sci.* 82, 2530–2535. doi: 10.3168/jds.S0022-0302(99)75506-2

Tanaka, H., Hashiba, H., Kok, J., and Mierau, I. (2000). Bile salt hydrolase of *Bifidobacterium longum*-biochemical and genetic characterization. *Appl. Environ. Microbiol.* 66, 2502–2512. doi: 10.1128/AEM.66.6.2502-25 12.2000

Tannock, G. W., Luchansky, J. B., Miller, L., Connell, H., Thode-Andersen, S., Mercer, A. A., et al. (1994). Molecular characterization of a plasmid-borne (pGT633) erythromycin resistance determinant (ermGT) from *Lactobacillus reuteri* 100-63. *Plasmid* 31, 60–71. doi: 10.1006/plas.19 94.1007

Travers, M. A., Florent, I., Kohl, L., and Grellier, P. (2011). Probiotics for the control of parasites: an overview. *J. Parasitol. Res.* 2011:610769. doi: 10.1155/2011/610769

Travers, M. A., Sow, C., Zirah, S., Deregnaucourt, C., Chaouch, S., Queiroz, R. M., et al. (2016). Deconjugated bile salts produced by extracellular bile-salt hydrolase-like activities from the probiotic *lactobacillus johnsonii* La1 inhibit *Giardia duodenalis in vitro* growth. *Front. Microbiol.* 7:1453. doi: 10.3389/fmicb.2016.01453

Vidal, K., Donnet-Hughes, A., and Granato, D. (2002). Lipoteichoic acids from *Lactobacillus johnsonii* strain La1 and *Lactobacillus acidophilus* strain La10 antagonize the responsiveness of human intestinal epithelial HT29 cells to lipopolysaccharide and gram-negative bacteria. *Infect. Immun.* 70, 2057–2064. doi: 10.1128/IAI.70.4.2057-2064.2002

Yichoy, M., Duarte, T. T., De Chatterjee, A., Mendez, T. L., Aguilera, K. Y., Roy, D., et al. (2011). Lipid metabolism in giardia: a post-genomic perspective. *Parasitology* 138, 267–278. doi: 10.1017/S0031182010001277

18

Functional Characterization of Novel *Faecalibacterium prausnitzii* Strains Isolated from Healthy Volunteers: A Step Forward in the Use of *F. prausnitzii* as a Next-Generation Probiotic

***Rebeca Martín*[1†]*, Sylvie Miquel*[1,2†]*, Leandro Benevides*[1,3]*, Chantal Bridonneau*[1]*, Véronique Robert*[1]*, Sylvie Hudault*[1]*, Florian Chain*[1]*, Olivier Berteau*[1]*, Vasco Azevedo*[3]*, Jean M. Chatel*[1]*, Harry Sokol*[1,4,5]*, Luis G. Bermúdez-Humarán*[1]*, Muriel Thomas*[1] *and Philippe Langella*[1*]**

[1] Commensals and Probiotics-Host Interactions Laboratory, Micalis Institute, Institut National de la Recherche Agronomique, AgroParisTech, Université Paris-Saclay, Jouy-en-Josas, France, [2] Université Clermont Auvergne, Centre National de la Recherche Scientifique UMR 6023 Laboratoire Microorganismes: Génome et Environnement, Clermont-Ferrand, France, [3] Department of General Biology, Federal University of Minas Gerais, Belo Horizonte, Brazil, [4] AVENIR Team Gut Microbiota and Immunity Equipe de Recherche Labélisée (ERL), Institut National de la Santé et de la Recherche Médicale U1157/UMR7203, Faculté de Médecine Saint-Antoine, Université Pierre et Marie Curie, Paris, France, [5] Service de Gastroentérologie, Hôpital Saint-Antoine, Assistance Publique—Hôpitaux de Paris, Paris, France

***Correspondence:**
Philippe Langella
philippe.langella@infra.fr

[†]These authors have contributed equally to this work.

Faecalibacterium prausnitzii is a major member of the Firmicutes phylum and one of the most abundant bacteria in the healthy human microbiota. *F. prausnitzii* depletion has been reported in several intestinal disorders, and more consistently in Crohn's disease (CD) patients. Despite its importance in human health, only few microbiological studies have been performed to isolate novel *F. prausnitzii* strains in order to better understand the biodiversity and physiological diversity of this beneficial commensal species. In this study, we described a protocol to isolate novel *F. prausnitzii* strains from feces of healthy volunteers as well as a deep molecular and metabolic characterization of these isolated strains. These *F. prausnitzii* strains were classified in two phylogroups and three clusters according to 16S rRNA sequences and results support that they would belong to two different genomospecies or genomovars as no genome sequencing has been performed in this work. Differences in enzymes production, antibiotic resistance and immunomodulatory properties were found to be strain-dependent. So far, all *F. prausnitzii* isolates share some characteristic such as (i) the lack of epithelial cells adhesion, plasmids, anti-microbial, and hemolytic activity and (ii) the presence of DNAse activity. Furthermore, Short Chain Fatty Acids (SCFA) production was assessed for the novel isolates as these products influence intestinal homeostasis. Indeed, the butyrate production has been correlated to the capacity to induce IL-10, an anti-inflammatory cytokine, in peripheral blood mononuclear cells (PBMC) but not to the ability to block IL-8 secretion in TNF-α-stimulated HT-29 cells, reinforcing the hypothesis of a complex anti-inflammatory pathway driven by *F. prausnitzii*. Altogether, our results suggest that some *F. prausnitzii* strains could represent good candidates as next-generation probiotic.

Keywords: probiotic, commensal, *Faecalibacterium*, molecular and metabolic characterization, immune-modulatory properties

INTRODUCTION

Despite a large number of bacteria, archaea, viruses, and unicellular eukaryotes inhabit the human body, only a few bacterial genera (*Bacteroides, Clostridium, Bifidobacterium,* and *Faecalibacterium*) predominate in the human gut microbiome (Schmidt, 2013). Nowadays it is recognized that *Faecalibacterium prausnitzii* represents around 5% from the total fecal microbiota in healthy adults (Hold et al., 2003). Furthermore, this bacterium has been proposed to be a sensor and an actor of the human intestinal health. Indeed, the levels of *F. prausnitzii* have been found to be decreased in patients suffering from intestinal and metabolic disorders such as inflammatory bowel diseases (IBD), irritable bowel syndrome (IBS), colorectal cancer (CRC), obesity, and celiac disease among others (Balamurugan et al., 2008; Sokol et al., 2008; Neish, 2009; De Palma et al., 2010; Furet et al., 2010; Rajilic-Stojanovic et al., 2011) as well as in frail elderly (van Tongeren et al., 2005). Moreover, this species may be a biomarker of choice to assist in Ulcerative colitis (UC) and Crohn's disease (CD) discrimination (Lopez-Siles et al., 2017).

F. prausnitzii has been only described in detail recently probably because it is very difficult to grow as it is an Extremely Oxygen Sensitive (EOS) bacterium (Duncan et al., 2002). Similar to other EOS bacteria, little is known about the biology of *F. prausnitzii* despite its relevance in the human gut ecosystem (Miquel et al., 2014). Most of the data referring *F. prausnitzii* are based on metagenomic studies (Miquel et al., 2013), with only few studies with isolated strains and functional approach (Duncan et al., 2002; Ramirez-Farias et al., 2009; Lopez-Siles et al., 2012; Foditsch et al., 2014). This gap between metagenomic and microbiological data is striking for microbiota-derived EOS bacteria. To reduce this gap, it is now essential to increase the knowledge of several commensal bacterial strains in order to better understand the beneficial effect of this species.

Most of the commercial probiotics do not include dominant commensal human isolates. This is a reason why these probiotic strains do not colonize the human gut and their effects persist only during a short period of time (Schmidt, 2013). Nowadays, there is an increasing interest in the use of commensal bacteria as potential probiotic agents. The reasons are multiple and the most evident is that the role of commensal bacteria in homeostatic crosstalk has started to be unraveled in the last decade (Wrzosek et al., 2013). The domestic probiotic market, with a turnover approaching \$7 billion in Europe and \$1.7 billion in the US in 2013 (Schmidt, 2013), is expected to grow in the next years. However, these next-generation probiotic-commensal candidates must meet the same criteria than the conventional ones. It means that they should (i) be isolated and well-characterized, (ii) achieve safety requirements, such as the acceptable resistance to antibiotics or the lack of lytic and adhesion capacities, and (iii) show beneficial effects on the host before being considerate as a probiotic. In this sense, the Food and Agriculture Organization of the United Nations (FAO) and the European Food Safe Administration (EFSA) have established several guidelines for the correct definition and evaluation of probiotics on food (FAO/WHO, 2002; Pineiro and Stanton, 2007; Binnendijk and Rijkers, 2013). Regarding *F. prausnitzii*, although little is known about its safety, there is a clear potential of this species as a next-generation probiotic. This was already proposed for livestock animals with the isolation and characterization of *F. prausnitzii* strains from stool of calves and piglets (Foditsch et al., 2014) but also for patients with intestinal dysbiosis-associated illness with the development of specific formulation keeping this EOS bacteria alive at ambient air (Khan et al., 2014). Besides, its beneficial anti-inflammatory effect has been only analyzed *in vitro* and *in vivo* with the reference strain *F. prausnitzii* A2-165 (Sokol et al., 2008) and the biofilm forming strain HTF-F (Rossi et al., 2015). As the probiotic properties are usually strain-specific ones (Pineiro and Stanton, 2007), individual studies are required to assess the anti-inflammatory properties of other *F. prausnitzii* isolated strains.

The aim of this work is to isolate a collection of novel *F. prausnitzii* strains from healthy volunteers in order to characterize them as potential probiotic bacteria in accordance with Novel Food regulatory (Miquel et al., 2015a). We have also validated the collection of viable isolated strains by metabolic and safety tests in order to better understand their biology especially in the gastrointestinal tract. Furthermore, the anti-inflammatory properties of all these strains were validated *in vitro* in order to identify the best potential *F. prausnitzii* strain to be used as a next-generation probiotic.

MATERIALS AND METHODS

Isolation of Novel Extremely Oxygen Sensitive (EOS) Strains

A cohort of healthy volunteers was first established (**Table 1**) to collect freshly emitted fecal samples used as inocula. All volunteers signed informed consent to provide the samples and an agreement of confidentiality. The complete isolation of EOS strain procedure was performed in an anaerobic chamber (N_2 = 90%, CO_2 = 5% and H_2 = 5%). Briefly, fecal samples were homogenized and serial dilutions performed in order to plate dilutions 10^{-8} and 10^{-9} on YBHI [Brain–heart infusion medium supplemented with 0.5% yeast extract (Difco)] agar

TABLE 1 | Studied cohort of healthy humans' volunteers and new *F. prausnitzii* strain identified.

Subject	Sex	Age (years)	Fecal SCFA (mM)			CFU/g	% EOS	Identified *F. prausnitzii* strains	Cultivability of the strain
			Butyrate	Propionate	Acetate				
A	M	81	nd	nd	nd	4.4×10^9	51	CNCM-I4540	Yes
B	F	59	nd	nd	nd	8.7×10^9	30.7	X	
C	M	54	nd	nd	nd	8.0×10^9	67.7	CNCM-I4541	Yes
								CNCM-I4542	Yes
								S3C12	No
								S3G1	No
D	M	54	21.7	14.8	65.4	8.0×10^9	69	X	
E	F	60	nd	nd	nd	3.5×10^{10}	40	X	
F	M	53	3.7	4.4	11.6	3.0×10^9	35.4	X	
G	F	26	3	3.9	14	2.0×10^9	37.5	X	
H	F	56	15.8	10.2	27.6	4.8×10^9	56.2	CNCM-I4574	Yes
								CNCM-I4543	Yes
I	M	59	10.1	9.5	27.3	7.8×10^9	33	S9G3	No
								S9D8	No
J	M	34	9.9	12.3	26.8	7.7×10^9	30.7	CNCM-I4644	Yes
								CNCM-I4544	Yes
								S10H3	No
K	F	60	1.1	2	5.3	2.0×10^9	28.1	X	
L	M	40	1.7	2	6.9	7.4×10^9	29.6	CNCM-I4575	Yes
								CNCM-I4573	Yes
								S13A12	No
								S13E3	No
M	F	51	2.5	3.1	10.8	4.6×10^9	53.1	CNCM-I4546	Yes

All the isolates were obtained from human fecal samples of healthy volunteers consuming omnivorous diets. F, female; M, male; nd, not determined, X, no identified F. prausnitzii strain.

supplemented with rumen fluid 20%. After 4 days of incubation at 37°C, single colonies were obtained on plates and 96 varied colonies were selected and isolated in duplicate on YHBHI supplemented with rumen fluid 20% agar plate. A group of plates was placed brought out of the anaerobic chamber for 1 h to eliminate EOS strains and after a long period of incubation (usually between 48 h and 4 days), we performed a negative screening. The EOS colonies were further re-isolated and a specific *F. prausnitzii* PCR (primers Fprau07/Fprau02) was done to identify strains of this specie (**Table 2**). Finally, a 16S rRNA gene sequencing was performed after complete 16S rRNA amplification using primer FP1 to FP5 (**Table 2**; MWG France). The viable isolates were stocked at −80°C with 16% of glycerol.

Bacterial Strains, Cell Culture, and Growth Conditions

The reference strains A2-165 (DSM 17677; Duncan et al., 2002), L2/6 (Barcenilla et al., 2000) and M21/2 (Louis et al., 2004) and the *F. prausnitzii* isolated strains (**Table 1**) were grown at 37°C in YBHI medium supplemented with cellobiose (1 mg/ml; Sigma), maltose (1 mg/ml; Sigma), and cysteine (0.5 mg/ml; Sigma) in an anaerobic chamber filled with $N_2 = 90\%$, $CO_2 = 5\%$ and $H_2 = 5\%$.

HT-29 (ATCC HTB-38) (LGC-Standars) cell line was grown in Dulbecco's Modified Eagle's minimal essential medium (DMEM) (Sigma-Aldrich) supplemented with 10% (w/v) heat-inactivated fetal bovine serum (FBS) (GibcoBRL, Eragny, France) and with penicillin G/ streptomycin (5,000 IU/mL, 5,000 μg/mL) (Sigma-Aldrich). Cultures were incubated in 25 cm^2 tissue culture flasks (Nunc, Roskilde, Denmark) at 37°C in a 5% (v/v) CO_2 atmosphere until confluence.

16S rRNA Gene Analysis

DNA was extracted from isolated colonies of the different *F. prausnitzii* strains by alkaline lysis in 50 μL of NaOH 0.5 M during 30 min and 50 μL of Tris 1M pH7 and 100 μL H_2O were added. 16S rRNA sequences were amplified using FP1 and FP2 primers (**Table 2**) and PCR products purified with the Wizard SV Gel. PCR Clean-Up system (Promega) was used to obtain bidirectional partial 16S rRNA gene sequences by using primers FP1, FP2, FP3, FP4, and FP5 (**Table 2**). All DNA sequences were confirmed by sequencing (Eurofins MWG Operon, Ebersberg, Germany). Sequences for the novel isolates were deposited in the NCBI database under the accession numbers MF185398 to MF186168.

Phylogenetic analysis based on 16S rRNA were performed using the multiple sequence alignment—CLUSTALW (Thompson et al., 1994) integrated in MEGA6 software (Tamura et al., 2013). After that, the most appropriate evolutionary model was defined and the evolutionary history was inferred

TABLE 2 | Oligonucleotides used in this study and PCR product sizes.

Primer	Oligonucleotide sequence (5′–3′)	PCR product size (bp)	Use	References
Fprau07	CCATGAATTGCCTTCAAAACTGTT	141	PCR *F. prausnitzii* specific	Sokol et al., 2008
Fprau02	GAGCCTCAGCGTCAGTTGGT			
FP1	AGAGTTTGATCCTGGCTCAG	1,474	16S rRNA complete sequence amplification and sequencing	This study
FP2	ACGGCTACCTTGTTACGACTT			
FP3	GTTGCGGGACTTAACCCAACATC		16S rRNA sequencing	This study
FP4	GTTTTTCTTGAGTAGTGCAGAGG		16S rRNA sequencing	This study
FP5	GATGTTGGGTTAAGTCCCGCAAC		16S rRNA sequencing	This study

using the Maximum likelihood (ML) criterion, based on the Kimura 2-parameter model (Kimura, 1980), with 1,000 bootstrap replicates. A discrete Gamma distribution was used to model evolutionary rate differences among sites [five categories (+G, parameter = 0.1846)]. The rate variation model allowed for some sites to be evolutionarily invariable ([+I], 64.70% sites). Initial tree(s) for the heuristic search were obtained by applying the Neighbor-Joining method to a matrix of pairwise distances estimated using the Maximum Composite Likelihood (MCL) approach and all positions containing gaps and missing data were eliminated. The tree with the highest log likelihood (−3073.67) is shown (**Figure 3**). The tree is drawn to scale, with branch lengths measured in the number of substitutions per site. The analysis involved 36 nucleotide sequences. There were a total of 1090 positions in the final dataset. In this analysis, sequences used by Lopez-Siles et al. (Duncan et al., 2002; Ramirez-Farias et al., 2009; Lopez-Siles et al., 2012) were included with the objective of compare the new strains to the two phylogroups proposed by that study. *Eubacterium desmolans* was used to root the tree.

Plasmid Presence

The presence of plasmids in the isolated strains were determined following Wizard® Plus SV Minipreps DNA Purification System (Promega) with modifications to adapt it for use with Gram positive bacteria. Briefly, an extra lysis step was performed after centrifugation of liquid overnight (ON) cultures by incubation for 1 h at 37°C with lysozyme (Sigma; 10 mg/ml) in the cell resuspension solution.

Scanning Electron Microscopy

Scanning electron microscopy analyses were performed on the MIMA2 platform (INRA, France) with pure pellet of bacterial culture suspended and fixed in 200 μL of glutaraldehyde and 3% ruthenium red during 2 h in an anaerobic chamber and stored at 4°C. Scanning electron microscopy was performed as previously reported (Joly et al., 2010).

Determination of Antibiotics Resistance

The minimum inhibitory concentrations (MIC) for 13 antibiotics (including tetracycline, kanamycin, chloranphenicol, linezolid, nupri/dalfopri, trimethoprim, gentamicin, erythromycin, cefpirome, clindamycin, streptomycin, vanomycin, and ampicillin) were determined on Wilkins-Chalgren agar (Difco) according to the E-test procedure, in accordance with the conditions recommended by the supplier (Biomerieux, France). The results were recorded after 48 h of incubation.

Anti-bacterial Assays

The anti-bacterial effect of *F. prausnitzii* supernatants were investigated *in vitro* using the bacteriocin activity assay as previously described (Ramirez-Farias et al., 2009). This anti-bacterial effect was tested on six different bacterial species: three aerobic bacteria (*E. coli* Nissle 1917, *E. coli* DH10B, and *Listeria monocytogenes* 11765), one facultative anaerobic bacterium (*Lactococcus* subsp *cremoris* MG1363), and two obligate anaerobic bacteria (*Clostridium perfringens* ATCC13124 and *Bifidobacterium infantis* DSM20088/ATCC15697). YBHI liquid medium alone was used as negative control.

Metabolic Activities

To determine the metabolic activities of the cultivable strains, API-20A galleries and the gelatin degradation test of API-20E galleries were used according to manufacturer's instructions. For detection of DNase and hemolytic activity, the strains were grown ON and then plated into Methyl green-DNA agar plates (Difco) or blood agar plates (Biomérieux) respectively. The results were recorded after 48 h of incubation. The capacity to grow in presence of mucin was assayed using a defined medium (KH_2PO_4: 5.236 g/L, $(NH_4)_2SO_4$: 4 g/L, NaCl: 4 g/L, $CaCl_2$: 30 mg/L, $MgCl_2$: 300 mg/L, $MnCl_2$: 30 mg/L, $FeCl_2$: 8 mg/L, Vitamin B12: 5 mg/L, Vitamin B1: 1 mg/L, Biotin: 1 mg/L, PABA: 1 mg/L, Folic acid: 1 mg/L, Vitamin K: 2 mg/L, cystein 0.5 mg/mL) supplemented with 1.5% mucin (Type II, Sigma-Aldrich).

Short Chain Fatty Acid (SCFA) Analysis

Supernatant concentrations of propionate, acetate, and butyrate were analyzed using gas liquid chromatography (Nelson 1020, Perkin-Elmer, St Quentin en Yvelines, France) as previously described (Lan et al., 2008). Overnight culture (20 h) of *F. prausnitzii* strains were used and culture media as negative control; each measurement for performed at least in triplicate except for fecal samples. SCFA concentrations are expressed in mM.

Dosage of D- and L-Lactate

D- and L-lactate was measured in supernatant of bacterial cultures. This supernatant was precipitated with trichloroacetic acid (10%) and centrifuged at 4,500 g for 20 min at 4°C. Lactate was then measured in the supernatants with the Biosentec D/L lactic acid enzymatic kits according to the manufacturer instructions (Biosentec, Toulouse, France). Overnight culture (20 h) of *F. prausnitzii* strains were used and culture media as negative control; each measurement was performed at least in triplicate.

Adhesion Assays

Monolayers of HT-29 cells were seeded in 24-well tissue culture plates (Nunc) with 1.83 × 10^5 HT-29 cells/well and cultivated until confluence, culture medium was changed daily. Monolayers were then infected in 1 ml of the cell culture medium without antibiotics and with heat-inactivated FBS at a multiplicity of infection (MOI) of 100 bacteria per epithelial cell. After, 3 h of incubation at 37°C in anaerobic conditions (as describe above), monolayers were washed three times in phosphate-buffered saline (PBS; pH 7.2). The epithelial cells were then lysed with 1% Triton X-100 (Sigma Chemical Company, St Louis, Mo.) in water. Samples were plated onto YHBHI supplemented agar plates to determine the number of CFU corresponding to the total number of cell-associated bacteria. Adhesion to mucin has been performed as previously described by Radziwill-Bienkowska et al. (2014, 2016) Briefly, after an overnight coating of 96 plates (Nunc) with a solution of 10 mg/ml of mucin [Type III mucin from porcine stomach (lyophilized powder, Sigma-Aldrich)] a bacterial suspension (OD_{600nm} = 1) in PBS of each strain was incubated 3-h at 37°C in the anaerobic chamber. Bound cells were stained with crystal violet. Stained bacteria were suspended in 96% ethanol and optical density was determined at 583 nm. All the experiments were performed in triplicate. The adhesion values have been normalized using *Lactobacillus rhamnosus* GG (LGG) a positive control know by their good adhesion properties to mucin (Martin et al., 2015). Results are presented by the mean and the standard deviation.

Immuno-Modulatory Properties Using HT-29 Cells

Anti-inflammatory assays were done following the procedure described by Kechaou et al. (2012). Briefly, 50,000 HT-29 cells per well were seeded in 24-well culture plates (Nunc). Twenty-four h before bacterial co-culture (day 6), the culture medium was changed for a medium with 5% heat-inactivated FBS and 1% glutamine. On the day of co-culture, 10% of bacterial supernatant or bacterial medium (YBHI) were added in DMEM in a total volume of 500 μL. Cells were stimulated simultaneously with human TNF-α (5 ng/ml; Peprotech, NJ) for 6 h at 37°C in 10% CO_2. All samples were analyzed in triplicate. After co-incubation, cell supernatants were collected and stocked at −80°C until further analysis of interleukin-8 (IL-8) concentrations by ELISA (Biolegend, San Diego, CA). Total protein was determined by Bradford Reagent test (Sigma-Aldrich). Experiments have been done at least in triplicate. Results are expressed as IL-8/protein (pg/mg) and have been normalized using as reference value the IL-8 produced after the co-incubation with PBS as a negative control.

Experiments on Peripheral Blood Mononuclear Cells (PBMCs)

The protocol used in this study was adapted from Kechaou et al. (2012). Commercial PBMCs (StemCell Technologies, France) from five healthy donors were used in this assay. Donors presented the following characteristics: men, age under 65, body mass index <30, non-smoking, no drugs with anti-inflammatory known effects taken during the 15 days prior to sampling, and tested negative for HIV, hepatitis A and B viruses. After reception, cells were stored in liquid nitrogen until use. To prepare PBMCs for co-culture experiments with bacteria, the vial were thawed at 37°C in a water bath and then transferred into a medium containing RPMI-1640 medium supplemented with 10% heat-inactivated FCS, 1% L-glutamine and 0.1% Penicillin/Streptavidin (medium components were bought from Lonza, Switzerland). DNase (100 μg/mL, Roche Applied Science, France) was added to this mix to avoid cell clumping. Cells were then centrifuged at 200 g for 15 min, counted using trypan blue and spread on 24-well plates at 1 × 10^6 cells/well. Supernatants were added in triplicates (three wells per donor) at 10% in a total volume of 1 ml. Plates were incubated for 24 h at 37°C with 10% CO_2. Culture supernatant were collected, mixed with an antiprotease cocktail according to manufacturer's instructions (Complete EDTA-Free protease inhibitor, Roche Applied Bioscience) and stored at −80°C until further analysis of IL-10 concentrations by ELISA (Mabtech, Sweden).

Statistical Analysis

GraphPad software (GraphPad Sofware, La Jolla, CA, USA) was used for statistical analysis. Results are presented as bar graphs ±SEM. Comparisons were realized with the non-parametric Kruskal–Wallis test followed by a Dunn's Multiple Comparison test. Correlation test were performed using spearman test. A $p < 0.05$ was considered significant.

RESULTS AND DISCUSSION

Construction of EOS and *F. prausnitzii* Libraries

The vast majority of intestinal bacteria are EOS and thus mostly very difficult to culture (Qin et al., 2010). Although metagenomic approaches recently allow identifying some uncultivable organisms, the use of cultivable strains is requested to determine their biological activities. In this study, we report a method for isolation of novel EOS strains from human fecal samples on a complete medium (**Figure 1**). For this, a negative screening was performed through the exposition of bacterial isolates to oxygen and in parallel, these same strains were cultivated in an anaerobic chamber, which maintains a consistent anaerobic environment to ensure proper conditions for optimal EOS growth. We identified between 28.1 and 67.7% of EOS strains in the microbiota of healthy volunteers (**Table 1**). Interestingly, the proportion of EOS strains in the human microbiota was positively and significantly correlated to the amount of fecal acetate ($r = 0.7$; $p = 0.0433$) and tend to be correlated to the amount of fecal butyrate ($r =$

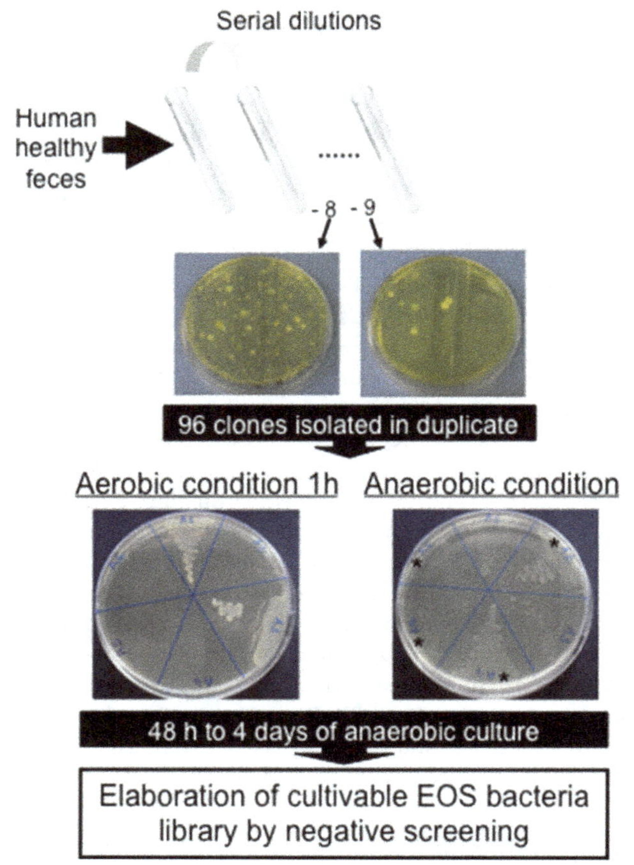

FIGURE 1 | Negative screening for isolation of new Extremely Oxygen Sensitive (EOS) strains from human healthy feces.

0.6833; $p = 0.0503$). These observations suggest that EOS population has an important metabolic impact that could participate to intestinal homeostasis (Wrzosek et al., 2013). The EOS isolates were identified by 16S rRNA gene sequencing and among them *F. prausnitzii* candidate strains were selected for further characterization. These isolation and screening set up can have a small inspecificity rate and no-*F. prausnitzii* strains can be recovered as well as the strain S13E3. After three subcultures, cultivable strains were stored at −80°C in 16% glycerol. Among 17 identified *F. prausnitzii* strains, only 10 were cultivable in the tested conditions (**Table 1**) with an $OD_{600\ nm}$ lower than 2 corresponding to $>1 \times 10^8$ CFU/mL (**Figure 2**). There was no direct correlation between CFU counts and OD_{600nm} due to difference of viability between strains. We substantially increased the number of cultured *F. prausnitzii* isolates from human origin and provided new tools for a better understanding of the diversity and microbial ecology of the colon.

Phylogenetic Diversity of *Faecalibacterium prausnitzii*

Full-length 16S rRNA gene sequences were determined for the 17 isolates of *F. prausnitzii* from healthy individuals (**Table 1**). The sequences from the literature (Barcenilla et al., 2000; Duncan et al., 2002; FEEDAP, 2012; Lopez-Siles et al., 2012) were included in order to classify the new isolates in the two phylogroups proposed by Lopez-Siles et al. (Barcenilla et al., 2000; Duncan et al., 2002; FEEDAP, 2012; Lopez-Siles et al., 2012; **Figure 3**). Each of these 16S rRNA sequences were unique, came from a different colony, and share >97% 16S rRNA sequences similarity. Cultivability of strains was not linked to phylogroups affiliation (**Figure 3**). Of note, all strains have a similar morphotype with cell wall extensions, like "swellings" (**Figure 4**) already described but with yet unknown function (Miquel et al., 2013). The average nucleotide identity between strains of the two phylogroups (S3L/3 and L2/6 = 94%) supports the hypothesis of the existence of two genomospecies without phenotypic properties defined yet (Lopez-Siles et al., 2017). Although, as was previously described for another library, there was a tendency for some sequences to group by isolation and individual with a clustering of strains (subgroup B of the phylogroup II; Lopez-Siles et al., 2012). For example, CNCM I-4574 and CNCM I-4543 strains were isolated from the same volunteer and present 99.8% of homology at 16S rRNA level.

Interestingly, the existence of strains that do not fit in any phylogroup (as CNCM I-4541) suggest that biodiversity of *F. prausnitzii* remains poorly known, maybe since only few strains have been isolated. Moreover, the strain S13E3, could be not an *F. prausnitzii* stain.

Resistance to Antibiotics

The MIC for the different antibiotics tested are represented in the **Table 3**. Concerning the breakpoints for Gram positive bacteria from EFSA (Duncan et al., 2004) which classify bacteria as resistant or not to a specific antibiotic, all *F. prausnitzii* isolates were susceptible to clindamycin, vancomycin, ampicillin, quinupristin+dalfopristin, and chloramphenicol (MICs lower than 0.25, 2, 1, 0.5, and 2 mg/L respectively). Only one isolate, the CNCM I-4541 strain was resistant to erythromycin (MICs > 0.5mg/L). Surprisingly, all tested strains were resistant to streptomycin (MICs ranging from 14 to 50 mg/L) excepted for the CNCM I-4575 isolate. Regarding gentamicin, kanamycin, and tetracycline, different results were obtained for the different isolates: with up to 5 isolates displaying resistance to higher concentrations of the tested antibiotics than the determined breakpoint. Finally, three antibiotics (not included in the EFSA guidance) were also analyzed due to their importance in the clinical treatments: trimetroprim, linezolid, and cefpirome. All strains were resistant to trimethoprim, as expected for an anaerobic bacteria (MICs >32 mg/L; data not shown), while they tended to be susceptible to linezolid (MICs ranging from 0.032 to 3.3 mg/L) and resistant to cefpirome (from 4.66 to >256 mg/L) which, when linked to the general susceptibility to ampicillin, might indicate that the penicillin binding proteins of *Faecalibacterium* are poorly recognized by cephalosporins. Remarkably, CNCM I-4543 and CNCM I-4574 isolates were resistant to cefpirome, a fourth-generation cephalosporin

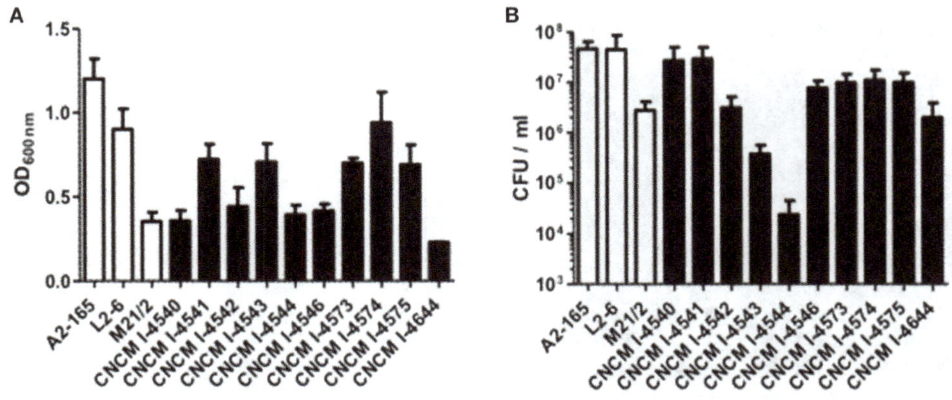

FIGURE 2 | Growth profile of *F. prausnitzii* strains. **(A)** $OD_{600\,nm}$ determination after 20 h growth in YBHI supplemented medium and **(B)** determination of viable bacteria: the CFU/mL numeration in the same cultures. Each measurement have been done at least in triplicate.

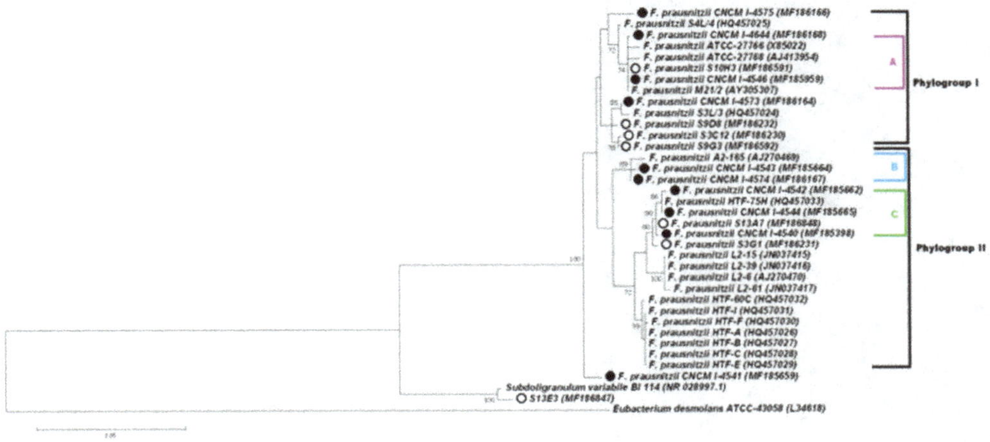

FIGURE 3 | Phylogenetic tree of *F. prausnitzii* strains based on 16S rRNA gene sequences. The tree was constructed with the MEGA6 software package using the Maximum Likelihood method. The bootstrap values above 70% are shown next to the branches. The *F. prausnitzii* isolates incorporated in this study have circles besides. The black circles represent the cultured strains and white circles represent uncultured isolates. Colors (purple, blue, and green) and letters (A, B, and C) indicate the tree groups with high bootstrap values, formed by our cultured strains.

stable against most plasmid- and chromosome-mediated beta-lactamases (Wiseman et al., 1997), with a MIC higher than 256 mg/L.

The analysis of antimicrobial resistance is of major importance due to the fast evolution of antibiotic resistance in response to the extensive use of antimicrobials. However, the microbiological breakpoints marked by the EFSA for most of Gram positive bacteria is probably not the most correct for the analysis of *F. prausnitzii* isolates as no so many information about their natural or acquired resistance patters is reported, to our knowledge, up to day in the literature. Foditsch et al. (2014) have identify that more of the 50% of the *F. prausnitzii* strains that they isolated from fecal samples of healthy calves and piglets were resistant to tetracycline, amikacin, cefepime, and cefoxitin comparing the MIC values with the standard values determined by CLSI for *Bacteroides fragilis* ATCC 25285. This fact highlights the need of more microbiological studies of antibiotic resistance in this species in order to determine a correct standard values for *Faecalibacterium* as well as the search for genes codifying for the most important resistance mechanisms for, at least, some of the antibiotics tested in this study.

Metabolic Activities

Enzymatic activities detected by API-20A gallery system are reported in **Table 4**. Interestingly, only one enzyme was detected and active in all the tested strains: the beta-galactosidase. Otherwise, all the strains were not able to ferment mannose or raffinose, to reduce nitrate and to produce indole (data not shown). Furthermore, all the isolates were negative for the presence of urease, arginine dihydrolase, beta-glucosidase, alpha-arabinosidase, N-acetyl-beta-glucosaminidase, glutamic acid decarboxylase, alkaline phosphatase, phenylalanine arylamidase, leucine arylamidase, pyroglutamic acid arylamidase, tyrosin arylamidase, alanine arylamidase, glutamyl glutamic acid arylamidase, and serin arylamidase (data not shown). These results confirm previous observations where no strain was able

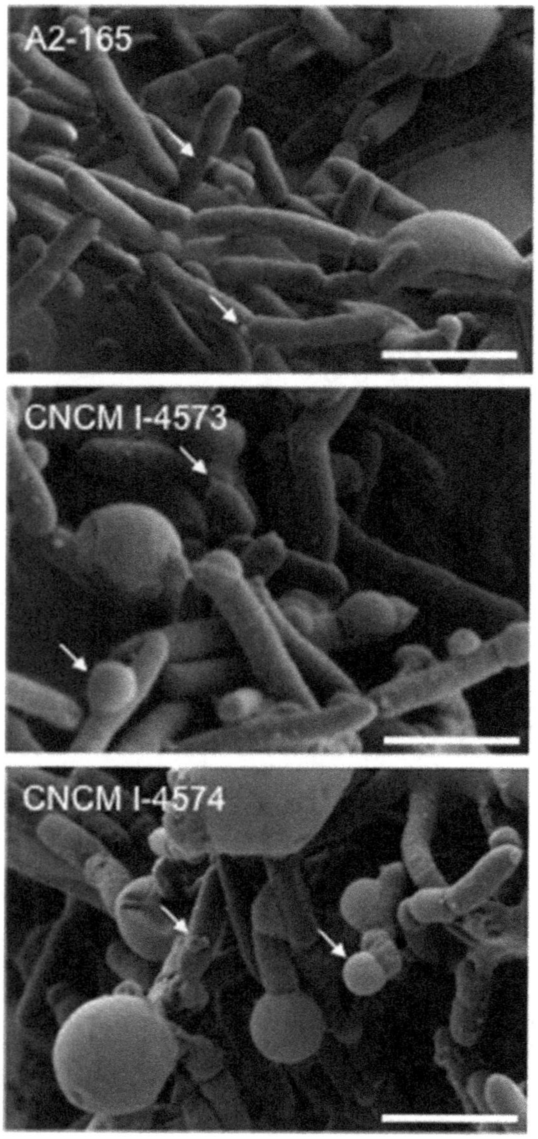

FIGURE 4 | Scanning electron microscopy images of *F. prausnitzii* strains phylogroup II. Strains were grown in YBHI liquid medium 20 h. Scale bars indicate 2 μm. Arrows indicates "swelling."

to metabolize arabinose and raffinose among others as the sole energy source (Duncan et al., 2002; Lopez-Siles et al., 2012).

For all the other enzymes (6 phospho-beta galactosidase, alpha-glucosidase, beta-glucuronidase, arginine arylamiase, leucyl glycerine-arylamidase, glycine-arylamidaseycine, and histidine-arylamidase), differences inter-strains were detected (**Table 4**). Beta-glucuronidase activity has been previously reported in some *F. prausnitzii* isolates (Lopez-Siles et al., 2012). While six strains showed individual profiles, the other seven are included in three different profiles. Two of them corresponds to the group A from phylogroup I (CNCM I-4546 and M21/2). The strains CNCM I-4543 and CNCM I-4574 (group B, phylogroup II), which are the only ones resistant to cefpirome, share also the same metabolic profile and donor. And the third metabolic

TABLE 3 | Minimum inhibitory concentrations (MIC) (mg/L) for the different antibiotics tested.

EFSA Breakpoint (other Gram +)	GEN	STR	KM	ERY	CLI	VAN	TET	QD	CM	AMP	CPO	LZD
	4	8	16	0.5	0.25	2	2	0.5	2	1	nd	nd
A2-165	1.37 ± 0.12	**96 ± 18.47**	**8.67 ± 1.76**	0.20 ± 0.08	0.016 ± 0	0.27 ± 0.05	0.016 ± 0	0.03 ± 0.01	0.08 ± 0.02	0.11 ± 0.02	9 ± 1	1.25 ± 0.25
L2-6	**4.33 ± 0.88**	**32 ± 7.15**	0.42 ± 0.08	0.10 ± 0.02	0.023 ± 0	0.47 ± 0.12	**4.21 ± 0.62**	0.58 ± 0.46	**20 ± 5.66**	0.06 ± 0.03	24 ± 4.62	0.62 ± 0.12
M21/2	**4.75 ± 1.49**	**21 ± 4.43**	**51 ± 45**	0.05 ± 0.01	0.016 ± 0	0.25 ± 0	1.09 ± 0.63	0.016 ± 0	0.15 ± 0.03	0.04 ± 0.03	16.67 ± 7.86	0.75 ± 0
CNCM I-4540	1.25 ± 0.25	**21.33 ± 2.67**	**122.67 ± 66.83**	0.11 ± 0.02	0.016 ± 0	0.71 ± 0.18	0.016 ± 0	0.011 ± 0.004	0.05 ± 0.04	0.11 ± 0.02	24 ± 4.62	0.04 ± 0.06
CNCM I-4541	1.62 ± 0.47	**24 ± 0**	**14 ± 2**	**20 ± 4**	0.016 ± 0	0.125 ± 0	**8 ± 0**	0.27 ± 0.24	0.17 ± 0.07	0.06 ± 0	40 ± 8	1.25 ± 0.25
CNCM I-4542	2.87 ± 1.12	**23.67 ± 3.26**	**20 ± 4**	0.11 ± 0.07	0.016 ± 0	0.67 ± 0.17	0.016 ± 0	0.016 ± 0	0.29 ± 0.40	0.08 ± 0.03	20.67 ± 7.69	3.17 ± 1.42
CNCM I-4543	2 ± 0.40	**16 ± 0**	**20 ± 4**	0.08 ± 0.02	0.016 ± 0	0.29 ± 0.04	0.2 ± 0.002	0.07 ± 0.03	0.31 ± 0.09	0.12 ± 0	**≥256 ± 0**	1.25 ± 0.38
CNCM I-4544	**6 ± 1.15**	**21.2 ± 7.31**	**100 ± 52.41**	0.12 ± 0	0.016 ± 0	0.92 ± 0.08	0.016 ± 0	0.023 ± 0	0.11 ± 0.02	0.09 ± 0.02	53.33 ± 5.33	0.5 ± 0
CNCM I-4546	**10 ± 66**	**50.67 ± 13.33**	**256 ± 0**	0.22 ± 0.61	0.018 ± 0.002	0.56 ± 0.31	**2.6 ± 0.6**	0.16+0.07	1.25 ± 1.51	0.07 ± 0.02	24.8 ± 6.24	3 ± 1
CNCM I-4573	**7 ± 1**	**32 ± 0**	**234 ± 21.33**	0.01 ± 0.03	0.024 ± 0.007	0.28 ± 0.05	0.028 ± 0.003	0.04 ± 0.005	0.38 ± 0	0.25 ± 0	22 ± 3.83	3.3 ± 0.8
CNCM I-4574	1.75 ± 0.25	**14 ± 0**	6 ± 2	0.07 ± 0.02	0.016 ± 0	0.25 ± 0	0.016 ± 0	0.03 ± 0.01	0.09 ± 0.02	0.22 ± 0.03	**≥256 ± 0**	0.5 ± 0.14
CNCM I-4575	1.25 ± 0.25	5 ± 1	4 ± 1	0.07 ± 0.01	0.016 ± 0	0.5 ± 0	0.032 ± 0	0.03 ± 0.03	0.016 ± 0	0.084 ± 0.02	4.67 ± 1.67	0.03 ± 0.01
CNCM I-4644	0.91 ± 0.08	**9.33 ± 1.33**	**135 ± 69.84**	0.10 ± 0.05	0.026 ± 0.01	0.23 ± 0.02	0.83 ± 0.32	0.04 ± 0.01	0.079 ± 0.04	0.026 ± 0.01	9.333 ± 1.33	0.58 ± 0.08

Gentamicin (GEN), streptomycin (STR), kanamycin (KM), erythromycin (ERY), clindamycin (CLI), vancomycin (VAN), tetracycline (TET), quinupristin/dalfopristin (QD), chloramphenicol (CM), ampicillin (AMP), cefpirome (CPO), and linezolid (LZD). Experiments have been done in triplicate and the results are expressed as the media ± SEM. nd, Not defined. In bold, Resistances.

TABLE 4 | Metabolic capacities of *F. prausnitzii* strains detected by API 32A galleries.

	bGal	bGP	αGLU	bGUR	ArgA	Lga	GlyA	HisA
	beta–galactosidase	beta Galactosidase 6 phosphate	Alpha glucosidase	beta glucuronidase	Arginine Arylamidase	Leucyl Glycine Arylamidase	Glycine Arylamidaseycine	Histidine Arylamidase
A2–165	+	+	+	+	+	+	+	+
L2–6	+	−	+	+	+	+	+	+
M21/2	+	−	−	−	+	−	+	+
CNCM I–4540	+	+	−	−	−	−	−	−
CNCM I–4541	+	+	−	−	+	−	−	−
CNCM I–4542	+	+	−	−	−	−	−	−
CNCM I–4543	+	+	−	+	+	+	+	−
CNCM I–4544	+	−	−	−	−	−	−	−
CNCM I–4546	+	−	−	−	+	−	+	+
CNCM I–4573	+	−	−	−	+	−	+	+
CNCM I–4574	+	+	−	+	+	+	+	−
CNCM I–4575	+	+	−	+	+	−	+	+
CNCM I–4644	+	−	−	−	+	+	+	+

+, Presence; −, absence. Experiments have been done in triplicate.

profile is shared by strains CNCM I-4540 and CNCM I-4542 that belong to the group C of phylogroup II.

It is now well-establish that *F. prausnitzii* is an acetate-consumer and butyrate-producer species (Duncan et al., 2002; Lopez-Siles et al., 2012). Here, we report that in pure cultures, our new isolated strains are also able to produce butyrate and this production is significantly and positively correlated to their growth (OD_{600nm}; $r = 0.8462$; $p = 0.003$; **Figures 5A,B**). It is interesting to highlight that the production level of butyrate was not linked to a particular phylogroup (Phylogroup I 3.91 mM ± 0.43 and Phylogroup II 4.89 mM ± 0.62). Moreover, all strains could metabolize acetate present in the culture medium at around the same level (**Figure 5A**). This consumption was not directly correlated to bacterial growth ($r = -0.3132$, $p = 0.2975$) and tended to be more correlated to butyrate production ($r = -0.544$, $p = 0.0546$). This observation is in agreement with the literature which describes that most of the carbon present in the butyrate produced (around 85%) is derived from external acetate, with only 15% provided directly from glucose (FEEDAP, 2012).

F. prausnitzii can also produce a few amount of D-lactate (FEEDAP, 2012). Indeed, among our strain collection, no L-lactate was detected and only few amounts of D-lactate were detected (1.09 mM ± 0.15 and 1.07 mM ± 0.39 phylogroup I and II respectively; data not shown). This production, not correlated with phylogroup affiliation, was correlated to the OD_{600nm}($r = 0.6209$, $p = 0.0235$). Bacterial D-Lactate production can be viewed as harmful since accumulation of this metabolite into the blood may be neurotoxic and leads to acidosis (Mack, 2004). In particular, humans with short bowel syndrome (in which small intestine has been surgically removed), the D/L fecal lactate ratio seems to be the most relevant index with a higher D-encephalopathy risk (Mayeur et al., 2013). However, in healthy adults, there is no lactate detectable in fecal samples, because lactobacilli (main producer of D-lactate) are minor groups in microbiota and lactate is degraded by other major bacterial groups (36, He, 2008 #41). This observation also suggested that the weak production of D-lactate by *F. prausnitzii* strains, major component of the microbiota, could not have metabolic deleterious impact on the host.

All strains were unable to growth in the presence of mucin as the only carbon source in a defined medium (data not shown). This data agrees with previous results where no evidence of fermentation of porcine gastric mucin by *F. prausnitzii* was detected (Lopez-Siles et al., 2012). Nevertheless, SCFA concentrations and OD_{600nm} measures taken after 2 days of incubation showed the ability of the different strains to survive but metabolically inactive as it could be deduced by the absence of butyrate in the supernatants of the cultures and the almost minimal OD_{600nm} recorded (data no shown). A decrease in butyrate production due to non-optimal growth conditions have been already reported for *F. prausnitzii* A2-165 strain (Lopez-Siles et al., 2012). This characteristic pointed out the intrinsic growth requirements of this species which, in addition to be an EOS, needs strain specific nutritional environment and has the ability to switch between substrates derived from the diet or the host (Lopez-Siles et al., 2017).

Lytic Activities

Gelatin is a heterogeneous mixture of water-soluble protein that is usually used in microbiological procedures to detect the presence of proteolytic activities. None of the strains were able to degrade gelatin in the conditions recommended by the API gallery supplier (data not shown). However, when the strains were inoculated in the gallery in a defined medium instead of API suspension medium, they were able to degrade partially this compound after 3 days of incubation. This fact suggests that the strains are able to hydrolyze gelatin although, maybe due to the growth limitations present in this culture media, the existence of this compound is not enough to allow the metabolic development of this activity in the strains.

The presence of hemolytic activity was tested using blood agar plates. None of the strains showed hemolytic activity under the conditions tested. In contrast, all the strains reveal a DNAse activity in green methyl-DNA medium (data not

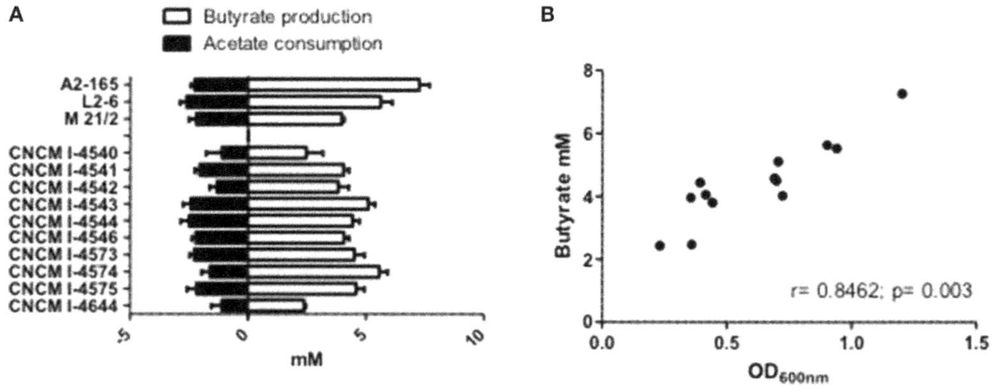

FIGURE 5 | SCFA metabolism of *F. prausnitzii* strains *in vitro*. **(A)** Acetate and butyrate concentrations after 20 h growth of strain in YBHI supplemented medium. The concentration of control media was subtracted for each measurement have been done at least in triplicate. **(B)** Correlation between $OD_{600\,nm}$ and butyrate production.

shown). Furthermore, the presence of a magnesium dependent DNase activity has been previously reported in at least three of five strains already sequenced [A2-165 (gi:257439194), SL3/3 (gi:295105207), and L2/6 (gi:295102777)].

The presence of these extracellular activities is often linked to a virulence status in some bacterial species such as *Enterococcus* spp. (Eaton and Gasson, 2001). However, these factors also contribute to the survival of microorganisms in the mammalian gut being characteristic of several members of the natural microbiota (Sanders et al., 2010). This can be the case of *Faecalibacterium* isolates, which are extremely well-adapted to the gut environment (Lopez-Siles et al., 2012).

Antibacterial Activities

We investigated antibacterial properties of *F. prausnitzii* supernatants, using the bacteriocin activity assay. We did not reveal any antibacterial effect on several anaerobic and aerobic bacterial species under the conditions tested. This fact is a desirable characteristic of a strain to be considered as a probiotic candidate.

Ability to Stimulate the Immune Response

The reference strain *F. prausnitzii* A2-165 is well-known for its immuno-modulatory properties and more specifically for its anti-inflammatory effects both *in vitro* and *in vivo* in different murine models of colitis (Sokol et al., 2008; Martin et al., 2014). To determine whether the newly isolated *F. prausnitzii* strains are able to modulate the immune response, we tested *in vitro* the immuno-modulatory properties of the supernatants from all the isolates in two different cellular models: HT-29 and PBMC. The first one is based on the capacity to block IL-8 production (a pro-inflammatory cytokine) induced by TNF-α stimulation in HT-29 epithelial cells and the second is based on the stimulation of PBMC cells and the measure of the anti-inflammatory cytokine IL-10. As shown in **Figure 6A**, all the strains tend to decrease IL-8 concentrations. However, this decrease was not equivalent in all the strains and does not correlate either with growth ratio ($r = -0.2857$, $p = 0.344$) or butyrate production ($r = -0.3357$, $p = 0.2869$).

For the PBMC assay, although all the strains tend to increase the production of IL-10 cytokine, only four strains (two controls and two new isolates from this study) were able to induce statistically significant increase production of this cytokine (**Figure 6B**) The two most performing strains (A2-165 and 4543) belong to the phylogroup II, group B. Notably, the IL-10 production was correlated with both growth ratio ($r = 0.6813$, $p = 0.0103$) and butyrate production ($r = -0.6923$, $p = 0.0126$). This different phenotype may suggest the presence of different molecule(s) responsible of the anti-inflammatory effects *in vitro*. The anti-inflammatory properties of butyrate have been already reported in the literature (Fusunyan et al., 1999; Kamitani et al., 1999) and its ability to block IL-8 production under the conditions tested in this study were confirmed *in vitro* in similar concentrations to those founds in *F. prausnitzii* supernatants (data not shown). However, its role remains controversial as its effects seems to be dose- and time-dependent as well as depended on the cellular model used (Martin et al., 2013). For instance, regarding cells from intestinal origin, butyrate has been found to decrease the secretion of IL-8 in Caco-2 and HIPEC cells and, in contrast to this study, to enhance IL-8 production in HT-29 and HT-29 MTX cells (Bocker et al., 2003).

However, several authors have found different candidate molecules/structures responsible for *F. prausnitzii* anti-inflammatory effects. MAM protein, found in *F. prausnitzii* supernatant, has been found to block NF-κB activation and the production of the pro-inflammatory cytokine IL-8 (Quevrain et al., 2016). *F. prausnitzii* is also able to produce bioactive anti-inflammatory molecules such as shikimic and salicylic acids (Miquel et al., 2015b). Besides, Rossi and co-workers showed the ability of *F. prausnitzii* strain HTF-F and its extracellular polymeric matrix to develop immunomodulatory effects through the TLR2 dependent modulation of IL-12 and IL-10 cytokine production in human monocyte-derived dendritic cells (Rossi et al., 2015) and *F. prausnitzii* has been found to be a strong inducer of regulatory T cells secreting IL-10 (Sarrabayrouse et al., 2014). All these results point out the complex anti-inflammatory mechanisms underlying this species.

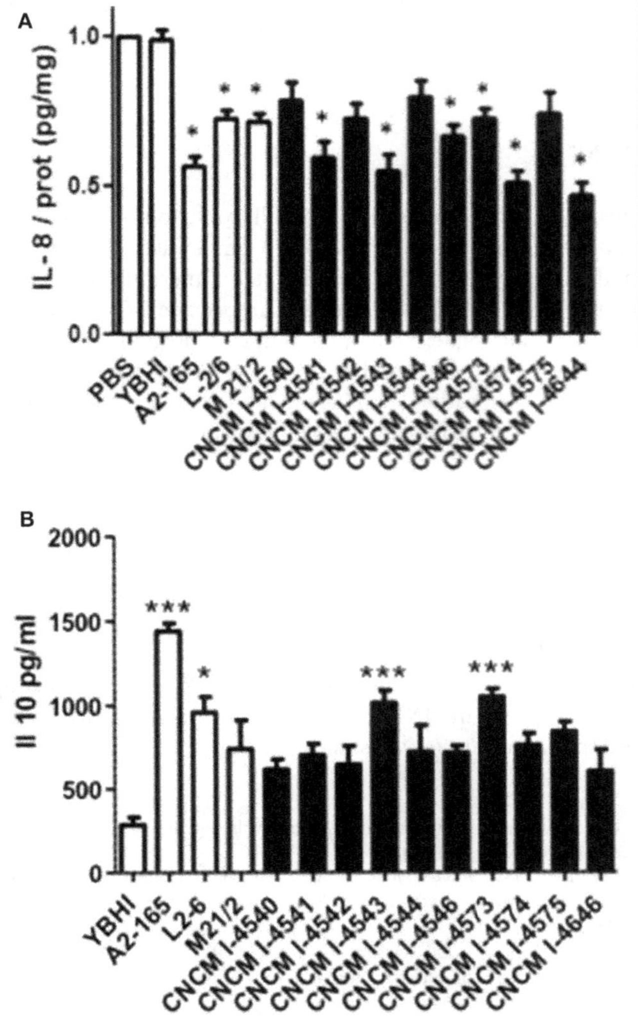

FIGURE 6 | Immuno-modulation capacities of *F. prausnitzii* strains *in vitro*. **(A)** IL-8 production in HT-29 TNF-α stimulated cells. Experiments have been done at least in triplicate. Results are expressed as IL-8/ protein (pg/mg) and have been normalized using as reference value the IL-8 produced after the co-incubation with PBS as a negative control. **(B)** IL-10 production in peripheral blood mononuclear cells. Experiments have been done at least in triplicate. Results are expressed as IL-10 concentration (pg/mL). Significant differences from the control (YBHI) was specified as: $^*p < 0.05$ and $^{***}p < 0.001$.

Adhesion to Epithelial Cells *In vitro*

In parallel, we also sought for the adhesion capacities of the new *F. prausnitzii* isolates to the intestinal epithelial cells HT-29 and mucin. All the tested strains were not able to adhere to HT-29 cells *in vitro* (data not shown) in anaerobic conditions. Regarding mucin, some of the strains were able to adhere to this compound after 3 h of incubation in the anaerobic chamber (**Figure 7**), Even if our conditions were not representative of physiological conditions (death of our eukaryotic cells), this result gives ecological clues about the processes of colonization of the gastro-intestinal tract by *F. prausnitzii*. In fact, this species is a late but major commensal colonizer of the gut which

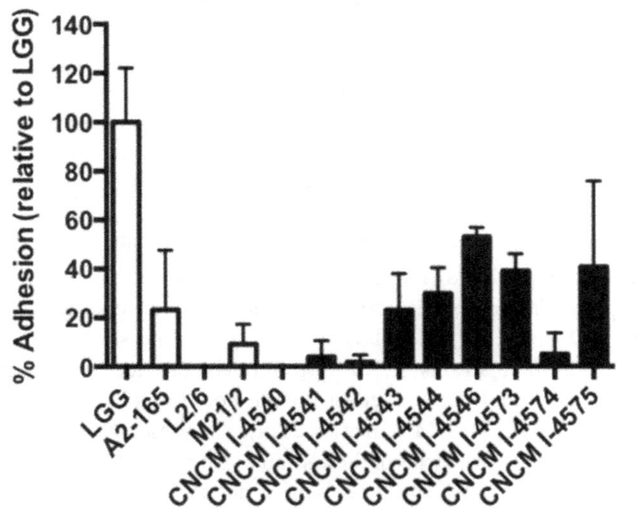

FIGURE 7 | Adhesion to mucin of *F. prausnitzii* strains. Experiments have been done in triplicate. The adhesion values have been normalized using *Lactobacillus rhamnosus* GG (LGG) a positive control know by their good adhesion properties to mucin (50). Results are presented by the mean and the standard deviation.

implantation requires a likely copro-cooperation maybe for the establishment of a trophic chain (Wrzosek et al., 2013).

CONCLUDING REMARKS

The development of new probiotic products containing human isolated strains with beneficial properties for the host requires the development of new techniques in order to: (i) isolate strains belonging to the major groups of the intestinal microbiota, (ii) determinate their safe status and (iii) infer in their potential beneficial effects. This study meets these entire three requests. Work with anaerobic and more precisely EOS bacteria are a prerequisite to succeed in the isolation of representative strains that can impact on intestinal homeostasis. For this reason, in this study, we have used a new procedure to isolate EOS strains from feces that has enabled us to build a collection of *F. prausnitzii* strains. The lack of knowledge about this species prompts us to further analyze their genetic diversity by comparing the new isolates with those already available in the databases. This has allowed us to point out the high diversity of our collection ranged on two different phylogroups with different clusters. *F. prausnitzii* strain genomes should be established or/and a metabolic comparison of several strains in the same culture conditions whether the phylogroups belong to genomovars or genomospecies.

Regarding safety concerns, this study is the first step toward a better understanding of *F. prausnitzii* properties. Up to date, little was known about *F. prausnitzii* resistance to antibiotics, lytic activities or adhesion properties. Here, we have shown for the first time the profile of all these characteristics in a collection of human *Faecalibacterium* strains. A positive remark is that all the strains were not antibacterial producers, not hemolytic and weak producer of D-lactate. Furthermore, although some of the strains were able to adhere to mucin, this trait can be considered as factor favoring durable implantation and a highly effective probiotic (Miquel et al., 2015a). However, further analyses are required to better determine the presence of acquired or natural resistances as well as to distinguish between the pathogenic or adaptative nature of some of the properties detected such as the presence of DNase activity.

Finally, the anti-inflammatory properties of all the strains have been analyzed. There is a well-known correlation between *F. prausnitzii* dysbiosis and a large set of human diseases such as IBD and IBS (Miquel et al., 2013). Recent studies using *F. prausnitzii* strains in *in vivo* models provide arguments concerning its beneficial effect on the host (Sokol et al., 2008; Wrzosek et al., 2013; Martin et al., 2014). The presence of the anti-inflammatory properties of these strains also opens the possibility to test them in murine models in order to further determine their beneficial effects before testing them in human clinical trials.

AUTHOR CONTRIBUTIONS

RM, SM, JC, HS, LGBH, MT, and PL participate in the design of the project. RM, SM, JC, HS, OB, VA, LGBH, MT, and PL designed the experiments. RM, SM, LB, CB, VR, SH, and FC performed the experiments and analysis. RM and SM draft the manuscript. VR, CB, FC, JC, HS, LGBH, MT, and PL revised the manuscript critically. All the authors have read and approved the last version of the manuscript.

FUNDING

This paper was a part of FPARIS collaborative project selected and supported by the Vitagora Competitive Cluster and funded by the French FUI (Fond Unique Interministériel; FUI: n°F1010012D), the FEDER (Fonds Européen de Développement Régional; Bourgogne: 34606), the Burgundy Region, the Conseil Général 21 and the Grand Dijon. This work was also supported by Merck Médication Familiale (Dijon, France) and Biovitis (Saint Etienne de Chomeil, France). RM and SM receive a salary from the same grants.

ACKNOWLEDGMENTS

Authors thank Prof. Juan Evaristo Suárez for the critical reading of the manuscript and Stéphanie Courau and Pascal Molimard for fruitful discussions during the project. We gratefully acknowledge T. Meylheuc for scanning electron microscopy (MIMA2 platform, INRA, France) and Harry Flint for the reference *Faecalibacterium* strains.

REFERENCES

Balamurugan, R., Rajendiran, E., George, S., Samuel, G. V., and Ramakrishna, B. S. (2008). Real-time polymerase chain reaction quantification of specific butyrate-producing bacteria, Desulfovibrio and *Enterococcus faecalis* in the feces of patients with colorectal cancer. *J. Gastroenterol. Hepatol.* 23(8 Pt 1), 1298–1303. doi: 10.1111/j.1440-1746.2008.05490.x

Barcenilla, A., Pryde, S. E., Martin, J. C., Duncan, S. H., Stewart, C. S., Henderson, C., et al. (2000). Phylogenetic relationships of butyrate-producing bacteria from the human gut. *Appl. Environ. Microbiol.* 66, 1654–1661. doi: 10.1128/AEM.66.4.1654-1661.2000

Binnendijk, K. H., and Rijkers, G. T. (2013). What is a health benefit? An evaluation of EFSA opinions on health benefits with reference to probiotics. *Benef. Microbes* 4, 223–230. doi: 10.3920/BM2013.0019

Bocker, U., Nebe, T., Herweck, F., Holt, L., Panja, A., Jobin, C., et al. (2003). Butyrate modulates intestinal epithelial cell-mediated neutrophil migration. *Clin. Exp. Immunol.* 131, 53–60. doi: 10.1046/j.1365-2249.2003.02056.x

De Palma, G., Nadal, I., Medina, M., Donat, E., Ribes-Koninckx, C., Calabuig, M., et al. (2010). Intestinal dysbiosis and reduced immunoglobulin-coated bacteria associated with coeliac disease in children. *BMC Microbiol.* 10:63. doi: 10.1186/1471-2180-10-63

Duncan, S. H., Hold, G. L., Harmsen, H. J., Stewart, C. S., and Flint, H. J. (2002). Growth requirements and fermentation products of Fusobacterium prausnitzii, and a proposal to reclassify it as *Faecalibacterium prausnitzii* gen. nov., comb. nov. *Int. J. Syst. Evol. Microbiol.* 52(Pt 6), 2141–2146. doi: 10.1099/00207713-52-6-2141

Duncan, S. H., Holtrop, G., Lobley, G. E., Calder, A. G., Stewart, C. S., and Flint, H. J. (2004). Contribution of acetate to butyrate formation by human faecal bacteria. *Br. J. Nutr.* 91, 915–923. doi: 10.1079/BJN20041150

Eaton, T. J., and Gasson, M. J. (2001). Molecular screening of Enterococcus virulence determinants and potential for genetic exchange between food and medical isolates. *Appl. Environ. Microbiol.* 67, 1628–1635. doi: 10.1128/AEM.67.4.1628-1635.2001

EFSA Panel on Additives and Products or Substances used in Animal Feed (FEEDAP) (2012). Guidance on the assessment of bacterial susceptibility to antimicrobials of human and veterinary importance. *EFSA J.* 10:2740. doi: 10.2903/j.efsa.2012.2740

FAO/WHO (2002). *FAO/WHO and Agriculture Organization Guidelines for the Evaluation of Probiotics in Food.* London: Food and Agriculture Organization, 11.

Foditsch, C., Santos, T. M., Teixeira, A. G., Pereira, R. V., Dias, J. M., Gaeta, N., et al. (2014). Isolation and characterization of *Faecalibacterium prausnitzii* from calves and piglets. *PLoS ONE* 9:e116465. doi: 10.1371/journal.pone.0116465

Furet, J. P., Kong, L. C., Tap, J., Poitou, C., Basdevant, A., Bouillot, J. L., et al. (2010). Differential adaptation of human gut microbiota to bariatric surgery-induced weight loss: links with metabolic and low-grade inflammation markers. *Diabetes* 59, 3049–3057. doi: 10.2337/db10-0253

Fusunyan, R. D., Quinn, J. J., Fujimoto, M., MacDermott, R. P., and Sanderson, I. R. (1999). Butyrate switches the pattern of chemokine secretion by intestinal epithelial cells through histone acetylation. *Mol. Med.* 5, 631–640.

Hold, G. L., Schwiertz, A., Aminov, R. I., Blaut, M., and Flint, H. J. (2003). Oligonucleotide probes that detect quantitatively significant groups of butyrate-producing bacteria in human feces. *Appl. Environ. Microbiol.* 69, 4320–4324. doi: 10.1128/AEM.69.7.4320-4324.2003

Joly, F., Mayeur, C., Bruneau, A., Noordine, M. L., Meylheuc, T., Langella, P., et al. (2010). Drastic changes in fecal and mucosa-associated microbiota in adult patients with short bowel syndrome. *Biochimie* 92, 753–761. doi: 10.1016/j.biochi.2010.02.015

Kamitani, H., Ikawa, H., Hsi, L. C., Watanabe, T., DuBois, R. N., and Eling, T. E. (1999). Regulation of 12-lipoxygenase in rat intestinal epithelial cells during differentiation and apoptosis induced by sodium butyrate. *Arch. Biochem. Biophys.* 368, 45–55. doi: 10.1006/abbi.1999.1284

Kechaou, N., Chain, F., Gratadoux, J. J., Blugeon, S., Bertho, N., Chevalier, C., et al. (2012). Identification of one novel candidate probiotic *Lactobacillus plantarum* strain active against influenza virus infection in mice by a large-scale screening. *Appl. Environ. Microbiol.* 79, 1491–1499. doi: 10.1128/AEM.03075-12

Khan, M. T., van Dijl, J. M., and Harmsen, H. J. (2014). Antioxidants keep the potentially probiotic but highly oxygen-sensitive human gut bacterium *Faecalibacterium prausnitzii* alive at ambient air. *PLoS ONE* 9:e96097. doi: 10.1371/journal.pone.0096097

Kimura, M. (1980). A simple method for estimating evolutionary rates of base substitutions through comparative studies of nucleotide sequences. *J. Mol. Evol.* 16, 111–120. doi: 10.1007/BF01731581

Lan, A., Bruneau, A., Bensaada, M., Philippe, C., Bellaud, P., Rabot, S., et al. (2008). Increased induction of apoptosis by *Propionibacterium freudenreichii* TL133 in colonic mucosal crypts of human microbiota-associated rats treated with 1,2-dimethylhydrazine. *Br. J. Nutr.* 100, 1251–1259. doi: 10.1017/S0007114508978284

Lopez-Siles, M., Duncan, S. H., Garcia-Gil, L. J., and Martinez-Medina, M. (2017). *Faecalibacterium prausnitzii*: from microbiology to diagnostics and prognostics. *ISME J.* 11, 841–852. doi: 10.1038/ismej.2016.176

Lopez-Siles, M., Khan, T. M., Duncan, S. H., Harmsen, H. J., Garcia-Gil, L. J., and Flint, H. J. (2012). Cultured representatives of two major phylogroups of human colonic *Faecalibacterium prausnitzii* can utilize pectin, uronic acids, and host-derived substrates for growth. *Appl. Environ. Microbiol.* 78, 420–428. doi: 10.1128/AEM.06858-11

Louis, P., Duncan, S. H., McCrae, S. I., Millar, J., Jackson, M. S., and Flint, H. J. (2004). Restricted distribution of the butyrate kinase pathway among butyrate-producing bacteria from the human colon. *J. Bacteriol.* 186, 2099–2106. doi: 10.1128/JB.186.7.2099-2106.2004

Mack, D. R. (2004). D(-)-lactic acid-producing probiotics, D(-)-lactic acidosis and infants. *Can. J. Gastroenterol.* 18, 671–675. doi: 10.1155/2004/342583

Martin, R., Chain, F., Miquel, S., Lu, J., Gratadoux, J. J., Sokol, H., et al. (2014). The commensal bacterium *Faecalibacterium prausnitzii* is protective in DNBS-induced chronic moderate and severe colitis models. *Inflamm. Bowel Dis.* 20, 417–430. doi: 10.1097/01.MIB.0000440815.76627.64

Martin, R., Miquel, S., Ulmer, J., Kechaou, N., Langella, P., and Bermudez-Humaran, L. G. (2013). Role of commensal and probiotic bacteria in human health: a focus on inflammatory bowel disease. *Microb. Cell Fact.* 12:71. doi: 10.1186/1475-2859-12-71

Martin, R., Sanchez, B., Urdaci, M. C., Langella, P., Suarez, J. E., and Bermudez-Humaran, L. G. (2015). Effect of iron on the probiotic properties of the vaginal isolate *Lactobacillus jensenii* CECT 4306. *Microbiology* 161(Pt 4), 708–718. doi: 10.1099/mic.0.000044

Mayeur, C., Gratadoux, J. J., Bridonneau, C., Chegdani, F., Larroque, B., Kapel, N., et al. (2013). Faecal D/L lactate ratio is a metabolic signature of microbiota imbalance in patients with short bowel syndrome. *PLoS ONE* 8:e54335. doi: 10.1371/journal.pone.0054335

Miquel, S. R., Martìn, Bridonneau, C., Robert, V., Sokol, H., Bermúdez-Humarán, L., Thomas, M., et al. (2014). Ecology and metabolism of the beneficial intestinal commensal bacterium *Faecalibacterium prausnitzii*. *Gut Microbes* 5, 146–151. doi: 10.4161/gmic.27651

Miquel, S., Beaumont, M., Martin, R., Langella, P., Braesco, V., and Thomas, M. (2015a). A proposed framework for an appropriate evaluation scheme for microorganisms as novel foods with a health claim in Europe. *Microb. Cell Fact.* 14, 48. doi: 10.1186/s12934-015-0229-1

Miquel, S., Leclerc, M., Martin, R., Chain, F., Lenoir, M., Raguideau, S., et al. (2015b). Identification of metabolic signatures linked to anti-inflammatory effects of *Faecalibacterium prausnitzii*. *Mbio* 6:e00300-15. doi: 10.1128/mBio.00300-15

Miquel, S., Martin, R., Rossi, O., Bermudez-Humaran, L., Chatel, J., Sokol, H., et al. (2013). *Faecalibacterium prausnitzii* and human intestinal health. *Curr. Opin. Microbiol.* 16, 255–261. doi: 10.1016/j.mib.2013.06.003

Neish, A. S. (2009). Microbes in gastrointestinal health and disease. *Gastroenterology* 136, 65–80. doi: 10.1053/j.gastro.2008.10.080

Pineiro, M., and Stanton, C. (2007). Probiotic bacteria: legislative framework–requirements to evidence basis. *J. Nutr.* 137(3 Suppl. 2), 850S–853S.

Qin, J., Li, R., Raes, J., Arumugam, M., Burgdorf, K. S., Manichanh, C., et al. (2010). A human gut microbial gene catalogue established by metagenomic sequencing. *Nature*, 464, 59–65. doi: 10.1038/nature08821

Quevrain, E., Maubert, M. A., Michon, C., Chain, F., Marquant, R., Tailhades, J., et al. (2016). Identification of an anti-inflammatory protein from *Faecalibacterium prausnitzii*, a commensal bacterium deficient in Crohn's disease. *Gut* 65, 415–425. doi: 10.1136/gutjnl-2014-307649

Radziwill-Bienkowska, J. M., Le, D. T., Szczesny, P., Duviau, M. P., Aleksandrzak-Piekarczyk, T., Loubiere, P., et al. (2016). Adhesion of the genome-sequenced *Lactococcus lactis* subsp. *cremoris* IBB477 strain is mediated by specific molecular determinants. *Appl. Microbiol. Biotechnol.* 100, 9605–9617. doi: 10.1007/s00253-016-7813-0

Radziwill-Bienkowska, J. M., Zochowska, D., Bardowski, J., Mercier-Bonin, M., and Kowalczyk, M. (2014). *Lactococcus lactis* IBB477 presenting adhesive and muco-adhesive properties as a candidate carrier strain for oral vaccination against influenza virus. *Acta Biochim. Pol.* 61, 603–607.

Rajilic-Stojanovic, M., Biagi, E., Heilig, H. G., Kajander, K., Kekkonen, R. A., Tims, S., and de Vos, W. M. (2011). Global and deep molecular analysis of microbiota signatures in fecal samples from patients with irritable bowel syndrome. *Gastroenterology* 141, 1792–1801. doi: 10.1053/j.gastro.2011.07.043

Ramirez-Farias, C., Slezak, K., Fuller, Z., Duncan, A., Holtrop, G., and Louis, P. (2009). Effect of inulin on the human gut microbiota: stimulation of Bifidobacterium adolescentis and *Faecalibacterium prausnitzii*. *Br. J. Nutr.* 101, 541–550. doi: 10.1017/S0007114508019880

Rossi, O., Khan, M. T., Schwarzer, M., Hudcovic, T., Srutkova, D., Duncan, S. H., et al. (2015). *Faecalibacterium prausnitzii* strain HTF-F and its extracellular polymeric matrix attenuate clinical parameters in DSS-induced colitis. *PLoS ONE* 10:e0123013. doi: 10.1371/journal.pone.0123013

Sanders, M. E., Akkermans, L. M., Haller, D., Hammerman, C., Heimbach, J., Hormannsperger, G., et al. (2010). Safety assessment of probiotics for human use. *Gut Microbes* 1, 164–185. doi: 10.4161/gmic.1.3.12127

Sarrabayrouse, G., Bossard, C., Chauvin, J. M., Jarry, A., Meurette, G., Quevrain, E., et al. (2014). CD4CD8αα lymphocytes, a novel human regulatory T cell subset induced by colonic bacteria and deficient in patients with inflammatory bowel disease. *PLoS Biol.* 12:e1001833. doi: 10.1371/journal.pbio.1001833

Schmidt, C. (2013). The startup bugs. *Nat. Biotechnol.* 31, 279–281. doi: 10.1038/nbt.2544

Sokol, H., Pigneur, B., Watterlot, L., Lakhdari, O., Bermudez-Humaran, L. G., Gratadoux, J. J., et al. (2008). *Faecalibacterium prausnitzii* is an anti-inflammatory commensal bacterium identified by gut microbiota analysis of Crohn disease patients. *Proc. Natl. Acad. Sci. U.S.A.* 105, 16731–16736. doi: 10.1073/pnas.0804812105

Tamura, K., Stecher, G., Peterson, D., Filipski, A., and Kumar, S. (2013). MEGA6: molecular evolutionary genetics analysis version 6.0. *Mol. Biol. Evol.* 30, 2725–2729. doi: 10.1093/molbev/mst197

Thompson, J. D., Higgins, D. G., and Gibson, T. J. (1994). CLUSTAL W: improving the sensitivity of progressive multiple sequence alignment through sequence weighting, position-specific gap penalties and weight matrix choice. *Nucleic Acids Res.* 22, 4673–4680. doi: 10.1093/nar/22.22.4673

van Tongeren, S. P., Slaets, J. P., Harmsen, H. J., and Welling, G. W. (2005). Fecal microbiota composition and frailty. *Appl. Environ. Microbiol.* 71, 6438–6442. doi: 10.1128/AEM.71.10.6438-6442.2005

Wiseman, L. R., Lamb, H., and Cefpirome, M. (1997). A review of its antibacterial activity, pharmacokinetic properties and clinical efficacy in the treatment of severe nosocomial infections and febrile neutropenia. *Drugs* 54, 117–140. doi: 10.2165/00003495-199754010-00013

Wrzosek, L., Miquel, S., Noordine, M. L., Bouet, S., Chevalier-Curt, M. J., Robert, V., et al. (2013). Bacteroides thetaiotaomicron and *Faecalibacterium prausnitzii* influence the production of mucus glycans and the development of goblet cells in the colonic epithelium of a gnotobiotic model rodent. *BMC Biol.* 11:61. doi: 10.1186/1741-7007-11-61

19

Lactobacillus plantarum MYS6 Ameliorates Fumonisin B1-Induced Hepatorenal Damage in Broilers

B. V. Deepthi[1], Rakesh Somashekaraiah[1], K. Poornachandra Rao[1], N. Deepa[1], N. K. Dharanesha[2], K. S. Girish[3] and M. Y. Sreenivasa[1]*

[1] Department of Studies in Microbiology, University of Mysore, Mysuru, India, [2] Animal Disease Diagnostic Laboratory and Information Centre, Institute of Animal Health and Veterinary Biologicals, Karnataka Veterinary, Animal and Fisheries Sciences University (KVAFSU), Mysuru, India, [3] Department of Studies and Research in Biochemistry, Tumkur Universty, Tumkur, India

***Correspondence:**
M. Y. Sreenivasa
sreenivasamy@gmail.com;
mys@microbiology.uni-mysore.ac.in

Fumonisin B1 (FB1), a mycotoxin produced by *Fusarium* species is a predominant Group 2B carcinogen occurring in maize and maize-based poultry feeds. It is shown to be nephrotoxic, hepatotoxic, neurotoxic, and immunosuppressing in animals. In this study, we report the ameliorating effects of a probiotic strain, *Lactobacillus plantarum* MYS6 on FB1-induced toxicity and oxidative damage in broilers. A 6-week dietary experiment consisting of 48 broilers was performed in six treatment groups. Probiotic treatment (10^9 cells/mL) involved pre-colonization of broilers with *L. plantarum* MYS6 while co-administration treatment involved supplementation of probiotic and FB1-contaminated diet (200 mg/Kg feed) simultaneously. At the end of the treatment period, growth performance, hematology, serum biochemistry, and markers of oxidative stress in serum and tissue homogenates were evaluated in all the broilers. The histopathological changes in hepatic and renal tissues were further studied. The results demonstrated that administration of *L. plantarum* MYS6 efficiently improved the feed intake, body weight and feed conversion ratio in broilers. It mitigated the altered levels of hematological indices such as complete blood count, hemoglobin, and hematocrit. Serum parameters such as serum glutamic oxaloacetic transaminase, serum glutamic pyruvic transaminase, creatinine, cholesterol, triglycerides, and albumin were significantly restored after administering the probiotic in FB1-intoxicated broilers. Additionally, *L. plantarum* MYS6 alleviated the levels of oxidative stress markers in serum and tissue homogenate of liver. The histopathological data of liver and kidney further substantiated the overall protection offered by *L. plantarum* MYS6 against FB1-induced cellular toxicity and organ damage in broilers. Our results indicated that co-administration of probiotic along with the toxin had better effect in detoxification compared to its pre-colonization in broilers. Collectively, our study signifies the protective role of *L. plantarum* MYS6 in ameliorating the FB1-induced toxicity in the vital organs and subsequent oxidative stress in broilers. The probiotic *L. plantarum* MYS6 can further be formulated into a functional feed owing to its anti-fumonisin attributes and role in mitigating FB1-induced hepatorenal damage.

Keywords: Fumonisin B1, *Lactobacillus plantarum*, poultry, oxidative stress, hepatotoxicity, nephrotoxicity

INTRODUCTION

Fumonisin B1 (FB1), a potentially hazardous mycotoxin, produced mainly by *Fusarium verticillioides* and *F. proliferatum*, is a common contaminant of maize-based poultry feeds contributing to the unpalatability of feed and reduction in nutrient quality. It affects the alimentary value and organoleptic characteristics of feeds resulting in decreased feed intake and animal performance. FB1 entails the risk of mycotoxicoses and other major diseases in farm animals such as poultry (nephrotoxic and immunosuppressing effects), horses (leukoencephalomalacia), swine (pulmonary edema), cattle etc (Fandohan et al., 2005). High exposure to FB1 is hepatotoxic, and also causes lesions in gastrointestinal tract (Escriva et al., 2015). FB1 has been epidemiologically associated with cancer in humans and classified as Group 2B carcinogen by the International Agency for Research on Cancer (International Agency for Research on Cancer [IARC], 2002). The molecular aspects of FB1-induced toxicity are poorly understood, however, the downstream toxic cellular mechanisms of FB1 have been deduced to be complex involving many molecular sites. Studies have ascribed FB1-induced toxicity to the structural similarity between fumonisins and the sphingoid bases (sphinganine and sphingosine) of sphingolipid layer in cell membrane. FB1 inhibits the synthesis of ceramide by specifically binding to the sphinganine and sphingosine *N*-acetyltransferase enzymes thus deregulating the sphingolipid complex formation (Merrill et al., 2001; Riley et al., 2001; Enongene et al., 2002). This leads to the intracellular accumulation of sphingoid bases which further mediate cytotoxicity, apoptosis, cell proliferation, carcinogenicity, DNA damage (Riley et al., 2001; Voss et al., 2007), and oxidative stress (Poersch et al., 2014; Abdellatef and Khalil, 2016). In addition, Domijan and Abramov (2011) demonstrated that FB1 inhibited the complex 1 of mitochondrial electron transport chain in the cell cultures of rat primary astrocytes and human neuroblastoma (SH-SY5Y). This led to a reduction in the rate of mitochondrial and cellular respiration, depolarization of mitochondrial membrane, over production of reactive oxygen species (ROS) in mitochondria, and deregulation of calcium signaling.

Safe elimination of fumonisins from feeds and/or poultry is of paramount importance as the poultry sector suffers great economic losses due to fumonisins compared to other livestock industries. The most commonly employed detoxification method in poultry industry is the use of mycotoxin binders in feed. Nevertheless, a much promising alternative strategy would be the use of microorganisms such as lactic acid bacteria (LAB) having the potential to detoxify fumonisins. LAB constitutes an important group of probiotic organisms used as dietary supplements for humans and animals. Probiotic strains of LAB should be capable of adhering to the host intestinal epithelial cells and surviving in the gastrointestinal conditions. Beneficial aspects of probiotic LAB include increased feed conversion (Cenesiz et al., 2008), enhancement of host immune system, competitive exclusion of pathogens (Chiu et al., 2007), binding of toxic compounds (Niderkorn et al., 2007), synthesis of pathogen inhibitory metabolites (Todorov et al., 2008; Gerez et al., 2013), and mitigation of stress conditions (Poersch et al., 2014; Abdellatef and Khalil, 2016).

TABLE 1 | Feed composition of the basal diet during pre-starter, starter, and finisher adopted in the experiment.

Ingredients	Pre-starter (%)	Starter (%)	Finisher (%)
Maize	55.35	59.08	63.44
Soya meal	35	32.5	27.5
Rice polish	4.8	3	3
Rice bran oil	1	2	3
Limestone powder	1.3	1.14	1.1
Digestible crude protein	0.8	0.64	0.4
Salt	0.42	0.37	0.28
Amino acids	0.51	0.48	0.45
Other supplements	0.82	0.79	0.84

Poultry farming is one of the major agricultural sectors in India contributing greatly to the economy. The majority of studies on mycotoxins from India are aflatoxin-oriented, with less attention being paid to fumonisin B1 contamination in poultry feeds and their toxicity in broilers. A few studies from India demonstrated FB1 toxicity in Japanese quail (Asrani et al., 2006; Sharma et al., 2008). In the present study, we evaluated the *in vivo* potential of a probiotic LAB strain (previously characterized in our laboratory) in ameliorating the FB1-induced toxicity and oxidative stress in broilers.

MATERIALS AND METHODS

Chemicals

All the chemicals used in this study were of the highest purity grade available commercially. Dihydrodichlorofluorescein diacetate (DCFDA) and 4-(2-hydroxyethyl) 1-piperazine ethane sulfonic acid (HEPES) were obtained from Sigma (St. Louis, United States). 2, 4-dinitrophenylhydrazine (DNPH), homovanillic acid (HVA), thiobarbituric acid (TBA), and all other chemicals and solvents were purchased from Sisco Research Laboratories (Mumbai, India). Serum glutamic oxaloacetic transaminase (SGOT), serum glutamic pyruvic transaminase (SGPT), albumin, triglycerides, creatinine, and cholesterol commercial kits were purchased from Swemed Diagnostics (Bengaluru, India).

Diet Preparation and Probiotic Strain

FB1 test diets were prepared using commercially available broiler feed (basal diet; Shresta feeds, Bengaluru). The basal diet composition is given in **Table 1**. Culture jars containing 1 kg of broiler feed ($a_w = 1$, autoclaved at 121°C for 20 min) were inoculated with 20 mL of toxigenic *Fusarium verticillioides* MTCC 1848 (10^6 spores/mL). The jars were shaken thoroughly to ensure complete dispersal of the fungal spores and incubated in dark for 45 days at 28°C ± 2°C. After incubation, jars were dried in hot air oven at 60°C for 8–10 h. The dried feed mixture was ground in a blender to a fine meal. The finely ground feed

TABLE 2 | Treatment groups of *in vivo* study.

Experimental groups	Treatment
Control (C)	Basal diet + PBS control
Positive Control (TOXB)	200 mg FB1/kg feed + 1.0 g/kg feed toxin binder
Group TOX	200 mg FB1/kg feed
Pre-colonization study	
Group LP	10^9 cells/mL *Lactobacillus plantarum* MYS6
Group LP+TOX	200 mg FB1/kg feed + 10^9 cells/mL *L. plantarum* MYS6
Challenge study	
Group TOX_LP	200 mg FB1/kg feed + 10^9 cells/mL *L. plantarum* MYS6

mixture (0.4 g) was taken in a sterile amber vial and suspended in 2.0 mL acetonitrile:water (1:1) and allowed for equilibration overnight in a gel rocker at 28°C ± 2°C. The extracts were syringe filtered using 0.45 μm nylon membrane filters and subjected to liquid chromatography/mass spectrometry (LC/MS) (Waters Acquity/ Synapt G2, United States). Chromatographic separation was achieved on a C18 column maintained at 50°C. Mobile phase A was 0.3% formic acid in water (v/v) and acetonitrile being mobile phase B. The mass spectrometer was operated in the positive electrospray ionization mode (ESI+). The limit of detection (LOD) for FB1 was 10 ng/mL and retention time was found to be 1.77 min. (Deepthi et al., 2016). The cultured broiler feed was mixed with the basal feed to obtain FB1 treatment equivalent to the ingestion of diet containing toxin concentration of 200 mg/kg feed.

The bacterial strain, *Lactobacillus plantarum* MYS6 (LpMYS6) which was previously characterized in our laboratory with respect to its probiotic and antifungal attributes (Deepthi et al., 2016) was used in this study. The bacterium was cultured in de Man Rogosa Sharpe (MRS) broth anaerobically at 37°C for 48 h. Cells were harvested by centrifugation at 8000 rpm for 10 min, washed thrice and re-suspended in phosphate buffered saline (PBS, 100 mM, pH 7.4) to a final concentration of 10^9 cells/mL.

Experimental Design and Treatment

The poultry trial was approved (UOM/IAEC/02/2013) by the Animal Ethical Committee, Department of Zoology, University of Mysore, Mysuru.

One-day old, 48 Cobb variety broiler chicks (male 27, female-21) were used in this study. The 1-day old chicks weighed in a range from 42 to 46 g and were reared in an environmentally controlled room for 42 days. Chicks were randomly distributed into six treatment groups with each treatment having eight chicks. The experimental design involving six treatment groups is described in **Table 2**. The basal diet types included pre-starter feed (0–7 days), starter feed (8–21 days), and finisher feed (22–42 days). Initial 1-week of acclimatization period at high temperature (90°C) was provided to one-day old chicks followed by vaccination on day 7. The experiment was performed in two ways: (a) pre-colonization study which started with the pre-incubation of LpMYS6 from day 8 followed by supplementation of FB1-contaminated feed mixture from day 12 and (b) challenge study involved the co-administration of chicks with LpMYS6 and FB1-contaminated feed simultaneously from day 12. One mL (10^9 cells/mL) of LpMYS6 preparation was administered daily by oral gavage. The positive control consisted of a commercially available multi-spectrum mycotoxin binder (Varishta, Bengaluru, India) that was administered to the chicks from day 12. The toxin binder (TOXB) was a combination of *Picrorhiza kurroa*, activated charcoal, hydrated sodium calcium aluminosilicate (HSCAS), mannan oligosaccharide (MOS), buffered organic acids, and antioxidants. The control (C) group was also a negative control where the chicks were provided with basal diet and PBS. All the chicks were vaccinated for Newcastle disease and Infectious Bursal Disease (IBD) on day 7 and day 14, respectively. Antibiotics and liver stimulants were not supplemented in the basal diet and the basal feed was free from aflatoxins and other major mycotoxins. All the treatment groups were provided with water and basal diet *ad libitum*.

Broiler Performance and Sampling

To evaluate the influence of FB1 and LpMYS6 on broiler performance, body weight of each bird was measured at weekly interval and feed consumption of every pen was monitored throughout the experimental period. The feed conversion ratio (FCR) was calculated for each treatment on the basis of unit feed consumption to unit body weight gain. Treatment groups were observed daily to record the morbidity/mortality. On the conclusion of experiment (day 42), broilers were submitted to pre-slaughter fasting for 18 h. Five birds from each treatment group were randomly selected, weighed, euthanized by cervical dislocation and necropsied for the excision of liver and kidney. Prior to sacrifice, blood samples were collected from the jugular vein in two sets. One set for hematological study was collected in the sterile vials containing the anticoagulant citrate dextrose (ACD) maintained in ice bath. The other set of blood samples was collected in dry sterile tubes, centrifuged at 5000 rpm for 10 min and the serum was separated and stored at −20°C until further use. The excised liver and kidney tissues were blotted free of blood, rinsed with PBS, weighed and stored at −20°C for histopathological studies. The excised liver tissues were homogenized (10% w/v) in ice-cold potassium phosphate buffer (100 mM, pH 7.4) and centrifuged at 5000 rpm for 15 min at 4°C. The resulting supernatant (total liver homogenate) was stored at −20°C for the analysis of different parameters to evaluate oxidative stress.

Determination of Hematological Parameters

Citrated blood samples of five birds from each treatment group were checked for hematological indices using a blood cell counter (ERMA PCE210, Tokyo, Japan). The following parameters were examined: hemoglobin (HGB), red blood corpuscles (RBC), white blood corpuscles (WBC), platelets (PLT), and hematocrit (HCT).

Determination of Serum Biochemical Parameters

Serum samples were screened for routine biochemical parameters such as albumin, triglycerides, creatinine, and cholesterol. Liver function was assessed by the activities of serum glutamic oxaloacetic transaminase (SGOT) and serum glutamic pyruvic transaminase (SGPT). All the above parameters were estimated according to the instructions of assay kits (Swemed Diagnostics, Bengaluru, India) using a versatile biochemistry analyzer ARTOS-SBPL/418 (Swemed Diagnostics, Bengaluru, India).

Analysis of Oxidative Stress Markers

Estimation of Reactive Oxygen Species (ROS)

The levels of endogenously generated ROS were measured in liver homogenate and serum as per the protocol described by Driver et al. (2000). In this assay, an aliquot of liver homogenate (20 μL, 0.5 mg protein) was dispensed into a 96 well microtitre plate containing 170 μL of Locke's buffer (154 mM NaCl, 5.6 mM KCl, 3.6 mM $NaHCO_3$, 5 mM HEPES, 10 mM glucose, 2 mM $CaCl_2$, pH 7.4). To this mixture, 10 μL of DCFDA (10 μM) was added and incubated at room temperature for 30 min. After incubation, fluorescence was measured using a multimode plate reader (Thermo Scientific, United States) with excitation and emission at 480 nm and 530 nm, respectively. To measure the ROS levels in serum, the same assay was followed but the liver homogenate was replaced with 10 μL of serum. Background fluorescence was corrected by the inclusion of parallel blanks. A dichlorofluorescein standard curve was used to quantify ROS levels and the data were expressed as pmol DCF formed per mg protein.

Estimation of Hydrogen Peroxide Level

Another well-known oxidative stress marker, hydrogen peroxide (H_2O_2) was quantified in liver homogenate and serum as per the method followed by Botsoglou et al. (2010) with minor modifications. Here, 20 μL (0.5 mg protein) of liver homogenate was dispensed into 96 well microtitre plate containing HEPES buffered saline (HBS, 145 mM NaCl, 10 mM HEPES, 10 mM glucose, 5 mM KCl, 1 mM $MgSO_4$, pH 7.4) and incubated with 100 μM HVA at room temperature for 45 min. After incubation, reaction mixture was excited at 312 nm and fluorescence was measured at 420 nm. The H_2O_2 levels in serum samples were measured by using 10 μL serum as incubation mixture instead of liver homogenate. The H_2O_2 levels were expressed as nmol H_2O_2 per mg protein.

Assessment of Lipid Peroxidation (LPO)

Lipid peroxidation (LPO) status was assessed in liver homogenate and serum samples by measuring thiobarbituric acid reactive substances (TBARS) and was expressed in terms of malondialdehyde (MDA) content, as described by Ohkawa et al. (1979). In this assay, tubes containing 1.5 mL acetic acid (20% v/v, pH 3.5), 0.2 mL SDS (8% w/v), 1.5 mL TBA (0.8% w/v) were added with 200 μL of test sample (liver homogenate/serum). The reaction mixture was incubated in a boiling water bath for 45 min. After cooling to room temperature, 3 mL of butanol was added to extract adducts formed and were centrifuged at 2000 rpm for 10 min. The absorbance was measured in the supernatant at 532 nm and results were expressed in terms of malondialdehyde equivalents as nmol MDA formed per mg protein.

Measurement of Protein Carbonyl Content (PCC)

Protein carbonyl content (PCC) was estimated in the liver homogenate and serum samples using DNPH following the method described by Levine et al. (1990). Two hundred microliter of sample (liver homogenate/serum; 0.5–1 mg protein) was added into eppendorf tube containing 500 μL of 10 mM DNPH in 2 N HCl and incubated at room temperature for 1 h with intermittent shaking. Corresponding blank was maintained by adding only 2 N HCl to the sample. After incubation, 500 μL 20% TCA was added to the mixture to precipitate proteins followed by centrifugation at 5000 rpm for 10 min. The precipitate was washed twice with acetone and finally suspended in 1 mL of Tris buffer (20 mM, pH 7.4 containing 140 mM NaCl and 2% SDS w/v), vortexed and incubated overnight at 4°C. The absorbance of the mixture was read at 360 nm and expressed as nmol of carbonyl groups per mg protein.

Histopathology

The formalin-fixed tissue samples of liver and kidney were processed routinely, sectioned at 4–5 μm thickness, stained with hematoxylin-eosin dye and observed and photographed using Olympus Bx41 microscope equipped with ProgRes CT3 camera (Tokyo, Japan).

Protein Estimation

The protein concentration of liver homogenate was estimated by the protocol of Lowry et al. (1951) using bovine serum albumin (BSA) as the standard.

Statistical Analysis

The data obtained in this study are the mean of five determinations expressed as mean ± SEM and analyzed by one-way analysis of variance (ANOVA) followed by Bonferroni's *post hoc* test for multiple comparison, with following probability $^{*}P < 0.05$, $^{**}P < 0.01$, and $^{***}P < 0.001$ to be considered statistically significant. The graphs were drawn using GraphPad Prism version 5.03 software (GraphPad Software Inc.).

RESULTS

Growth Performance

On completion of 42 days of feeding experiment, broilers treated with only FB1-contaminated diet (TOX) showed a feed intake 2.725 Kg when compared to the control group (2.948 Kg). Also, FCR was found to be 1.741 ± 0.06 when compared to the control treatment (1.965 ± 0.07). There was no significant difference in the body weight of FB1-intoxicated broilers (TOX) when compared to control. Broilers of pre-colonization treatment (LP and LP+TOX) showed a feed intake of 2.787 and 2.855 Kg, respectively, when compared to the TOXB group (2.933 Kg) and showed a FCR ranging from 1.845 ± 0.27 and 1.860 ± 0.07 when compared to

TABLE 3 | Effect of *L. plantarum* MYS6 and fumonisin B1-supplemented feed on growth performance of broilers after 42 days of feeding experiment.

Groups	Body weight (Kg)	Feed intake (Kg)	FCR	Mortality
C	1.509 ± 0.05	2.948	1.965 ± 0.07	0
LP	1.614 ± 0.17	2.787	1.845 ± 0.27	0
TOX	1.575 ± 0.05	2.726	1.741 ± 0.06	0
LP+TOX	1.545 ± 0.06	2.855	1.860 ± 0.07	0
TOX_LP	1.918 ± 0.01[a]*	2.902	1.507 ± 0.00[b]*	0
TOXB	1.659 ± 0.05	2.933	1.777 ± 0.06	0

*Data are the mean ± SEM of five broiler birds per treatment group. *$P < 0.05$; [a]Significant when compared to 200 mg toxin control, [b]Significant when compared to TOXB group.*

that of TOXB group (1.777 ± 0.06). Our study showed no significant changes of body weight in the broilers of treatment groups. The body weight, feed consumption and FCR of each treatment are tabulated in **Table 3**. No mortality was recorded in any of the treatment groups during the experiment. Broilers fed with FB1 concentration alone, suffered from dysentery 5 days post toxin treatment (TOX) until the end of experiment. While the broilers of TOXB group and challenge study witnessed recurrent episodes of diarrhea during the experiment. It is important to note that, groups of pre-colonization study administered with LpMYS6 alone and along with toxin did not show any signs of illness throughout the experiment.

Postmortem examination of organs revealed yellowish discoloration of liver in broilers fed with 200 mg FB1-contaminated diet, and also witnessed atrophy of liver (**Figure 3i**). Further, broilers of other experimental groups showed dark brown-enlarged liver when compared to normal sized liver of control group (**Figures 3a,e,m,q**). The effects of TOX on relative organs weight are presented in **Table 4**. Increase in the mean weight of liver of 3.86 ± 0.16 g/100g body weight was observed in broilers fed with 200 mg FB1-contaminated diet (TOX) compared to that of the control (2.84 ± 0.13 g/100g body weight). With respect to mean weight of kidney, substantial differences were not observed in the treatment groups in comparison to the control.

TABLE 4 | Relative organ weights of control and treatment broilers after 42 days of feeding experiment.

	Relative organ weights (g/100g body weight)	
Groups	Liver	Kidney
C	2.84 ± 0.13	0.08 ± 0.01
LP	3.04 ± 0.35[a]*	0.10 ± 0.00
TOX	3.86 ± 0.16[b]**	0.13 ± 0.01
LP+TOX	3.69 ± 0.11	0.11 ± 0.00
TOX_LP	3.20 ± 0.09	0.11 ± 0.00
TOXB	3.61 ± 0.15	0.09 ± 0.03

*Data are the mean ± SEM of 5 broiler birds per treatment group. *$P < 0.05$; [a]Significant when compared to toxin control. **$P < 0.01$; [b]Significant when compared to control.*

Hematological Indices

FB1 toxicity in broilers fed with 200 mg toxin damaged the hematological parameters. **Table 5** summarizes the effects of FB1 concentration and LpMYS6 on the hematological indices of broilers. The WBC and PLT count in the control group were 35420 ± 3860 cells/μL and 12000 ± 700 cells/μL, respectively. While 200 mg toxin fed broilers showed a count of WBC up to 40860 ± 850 cells/μL and recorded 9000 ± 410 cells/μL of platelet count. Further, broilers treated with LpMYS6 alone revealed a lesser count in WBC compared to all other groups including control. In case of TOXB group, challenge study and TOX of pre-colonization study, a slight non-significant increase in WBC count with that of control was observed revealing no much differences within these groups. With respect to platelet count, treatment group which received LpMYS6 alone showed no differences when compared to control. Additionally, platelet count was slightly reduced in TOXB group, challenge study and FB1 treatment group (200 mg) of pre-colonization study when compared to the control.

Broilers fed with diet containing 200 mg FB1 concentration alone revealed a reduced (*$P < 0.05$) RBC count, hemoglobin concentration and per cent HCT. Broilers of pre-colonization study fed with only LpMYS6, TOXB group and challenge study showed values close to that of control. However, TOX in broilers pre-colonized with LpMYS6 reestablished the RBC count and hemoglobin concentration while the per cent HCT remained unchanged.

Serum Biochemistry

Forty-two days post-feeding, all the biochemical parameters augmented significantly ($P < 0.001$) in the serum of broilers fed with 200 mg FB1 independently compared to control (**Figure 1**). SGOT and SGPT, were high in the TOX fed with 200 mg FB1 only (**Figures 1A,B**). Treatment with TOXB also caused a significant increase in the levels of SGOT ($P < 0.001$) and SGPT ($P < 0.05$) when compared to control (**Figures 1A,B**). In contrast, the SGOT and SGPT levels were significantly reduced in the TOX (LP+TOX) of pre-colonization study administered with LpMYS6. It is notable that, in the challenge study, LpMYS6 could significantly ($P < 0.001$) alleviate the augmented serum levels of SGOT and SGPT in comparison with TOXB group and pre-colonization study (**Figures 1A,B**).

Damage to kidney was assessed by creatinine level and is depicted in the **Figure 1C**. Here, an increase in the creatinine concentration was observed in the TOXB group and 200 mg FB1-fed groups when compared to the control. In pre-colonization and challenge study, LpMYS6 significantly ($P < 0.001$) lowered the elevated levels of creatinine, however, the reduction level had no much difference within the treatment groups (**Figure 1C**). Broilers fed with FB1 toxin alone showed a significantly ($P < 0.001$) high triglyceride, cholesterol and albumin levels in the serum compared to control (**Figures 1D–F**). TOXBs and LpMYS6 each in combination with toxin lowered slightly the high levels of triglyceride and cholesterol (**Figures 1D,E**). While in case of albumin, a significant decline was noted in

TABLE 5 | Effect of *L. plantarum* MYS6 and fumonisin B1 supplemented feed on hematological indices of broilers after 42 days of feeding experiment.

Groups	WBC$10^3/\mu L$	RBC$10^6/\mu L$	Hbg/dL	HCT%	PLT$10^3/\mu L$
C	35.42 ± 3.86	2.25 ± 0.04	9.94 ± 0.18	29.16 ± 1.96	12.0 ± 0.70
LP	33.3 ± 4.85	2.09 ± 0.39	9.1 ± 1.47	28.52 ± 6.03	12.0 ± 1.94
TOX	40.86 ± 0.85	1.52 ± 0.17[a*]	7.16 ± 0.42[b*]	23.6 ± 0.07	9.0 ± 0.41
LP+TOX	38.04 ± 0.97	1.94 ± 0.09	8.40 ± 0.23	24.04 ± 1.06	10.0 ± 0.31
TOX_LP	38.58 ± 1.22	2.07 ± 0.06	9.2 ± 0.08	26.12 ± 0.66	10.0 ± 0.31
TOXB	38.9 ± 1.17	1.9 ± 0.08	8.64 ± 0.30	28.46 ± 3.15	9.2 ± 0.66

*Data are the mean ± SEM of five broiler birds per treatment group. *$P < 0.05$; [a,b]Significant when compared to control. WBC, white blood cells, RBC, red blood cells, Hb, hemoglobin, HCT, hematocrit, PLT, platelets.*

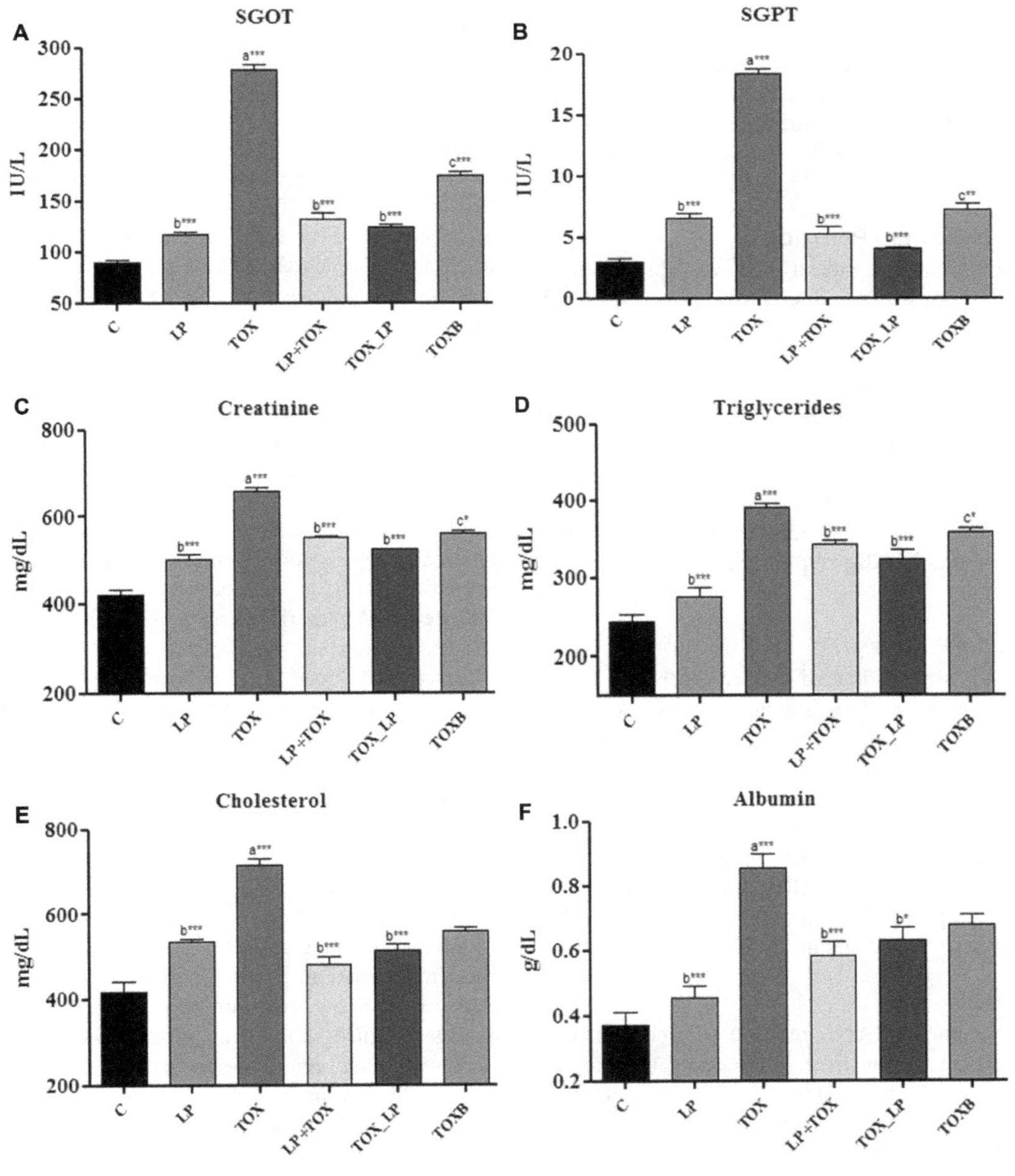

FIGURE 1 | Effect of fumonisin B1, *Lactobacillus plantarum* MYS6 and toxin binder (TOXB) on biochemical parameters of control and treatment broilers. The serum levels of **(A)** SGOT, **(B)** SGPT, **(C)** creatinine, **(D)** triglycerides, **(E)** cholesterol, and **(F)** albumin. Data are the mean ± SEM of five broiler birds per treatment group and were analyzed using one way ANOWA followed by Bonferroni *post hoc* test (*$P < 0.05$, **$P < 0.01$, ***$P < 0.001$; [a]significant when compared to control, [b]significant when compared to 200 mg FB1 toxin control, [c]significant when compared to challenge study).

broilers of pre-colonization and challenge study in comparison to TOXB group as well as broilers treated with FB1 alone (**Figure 1F**).

Markers of Oxidative Stress

Generation of ROS

Our study demonstrated a significantly high generation of ROS in liver homogenate and serum of broilers fed with FB1 alone when compared to the control group. The pre-colonization of broilers with LpMYS6 remarkably reduced the levels of ROS in liver homogenate indicating a better result when compared with the TOXB group (**Figure 2A**). Also, administering broilers with LpMYS6 and 200 mg FB1 simultaneously in challenge study showed a significant ($P < 0.01$) decline of ROS in liver homogenate than other TOX groups (**Figure 2A**). Additionally, pre-colonization of broilers with LpMYS6 in 200 mg FB1 treatment (LP+TOX) resulted in a notable ($P < 0.001$) decline of ROS level in serum. This was less than the ROS of control group and all the other treatment groups (**Figure 2B**).

Generation of Hydrogen Peroxide

A substantial elevation of free radical H_2O_2 was observed in the liver homogenate (**Figure 2C**) and serum (**Figure 2D**) of TOX group (200 mg FB1) in comparison with control. An equal and effective reduction by LpMYS6 was observed in H_2O_2 in the liver homogenate of pre-colonization and challenge study when compared to the TOXB group (**Figure 2C**). However, the levels of reduction in H_2O_2 were nonsignificant between the TOXB group and challenge study. Further, LpMYS6 was more effective in lowering the elevated levels of H_2O_2 in the serum samples of challenge study (TOX_LP) when compared with the LP+TOX group (200 mg FB1) and TOXB group (TOXB group) at $P < 0.001$ (**Figure 2D**).

Lipid Peroxidation

FB1-induced LPO was estimated as an increase in the concentration of MDA in liver homogenate and serum. In the FB1-alone-treated broilers, the concentration of MDA in liver homogenate (**Figure 2E**) and serum (**Figure 2F**) were significantly high compared to the control group. LpMYS6 in pre-colonization study and its co-administration with FB1 in challenge study reduced the levels of MDA both in liver homogenate (**Figure 2E**) and serum (**Figure 2F**) compared to the TOXB-supplemented group. But the reduction level of MDA in serum was observed to be non-significant in all the groups.

Protein Oxidation

Carbonyl content generated as a result of protein oxidation was significantly high in the liver homogenate (**Figure 2G**) ($P < 0.001$) and serum (**Figure 2H**) ($P < 0.01$) of broilers treated with FB1 alone as compared to control group. Compared to the TOXB, LpMYS6 was more effective in reverting ($P < 0.01$) the increased levels of carbonyl content in the liver homogenate to almost normal state as that of control (**Figure 2G**). Besides, LpMYS6 fed broilers of TOX_LP group (challenge study) significantly brought down the elevated levels of PCC in serum (**Figure 2H**). Interestingly, independent administration of LpMYS6 in LP group showed a slight non-significant increase in carbonyl content of serum compared to the TOXs of pre-colonization and challenge studies (**Figure 2H**).

Histopathology

The histopathological examination substantiated the FB1-induced toxicity in hepatic and renal parenchyma. The liver of control group showed a mild irregularity in the hepatocyte arrangement in hepatic cords (**Figures 3b,c**). Also, a mild infiltration of mononuclear cells in the periportal areas and sinusoidal space were noticed due to aging (**Figures 3c,d**). The liver of broilers treated with 200 mg FB1 alone showed severe disorganization in parenchyma compared to the control group revealing progressive stages of FB1 toxicity. Severe necrosis and edema (**Figure 3j**) of liver parenchyma was conspicuous. Biliary hyperplasia accompanied with inflammatory cells infiltration (**Figure 3k**) was evident of toxin insult. Additionally, liver tissue manifested extensive fibrosis surrounded by severe mononuclear cells infiltration suggestive of chronic inflammation (**Figure 3l**). Broilers fed with TOXBs showed a lower severity grade when compared to FB1 alone. Liver tissue of TOXB group displayed inflammatory cell infiltrates (**Figure 3f**), disorganized hepatic cords followed by hepatic necrosis (**Figure 3g**). Besides, moderate bile duct proliferation was observed in the liver of TOXB group (**Figure 3h**). The liver of broilers treated with LpMYS6 alone exhibited a mild hepatic disorganization with mild degeneration and focal to diffused infiltration of mononuclear cells (**Figures 3n–p**). However, LpMYS6 effectively reduced the degree of FB1 toxicity in broilers of pre-colonization (200 mg FB1 treatment) and challenge study. The liver displayed normal hepatocytes architecture though a mild to moderate hepatic disorganization (**Figure 3r**) was noticed. Severity of necrosis and edema was considerably attenuated (**Figure 3t**). A remarkable reduction in the focal inflammation and infiltration of mononuclear cells to the sinusoid was conspicuous (**Figure 3s**). The liver sections showed no fibrosis and biliary hyperplasia compared to the TOXB group and FB1 treatment alone.

Kidney sections of control group showed aging morphology involving normal renal glomeruli and Bowman's capsule space (**Figure 4a**). The increased cellularity of glomeruli and mild desquamation of tubular epithelium was observed (**Figure 4b**). Kidney sections of broilers fed with TOXB showed severe disruption of tubular epithelium and accumulation of granular casts in glomeruli (**Figure 4c**). Focal inflammation, cellular infiltration and mild edema were observed in the interstitium accompanied with distal tubular damage (**Figure 4d**). While broilers fed with 200 mg FB1 alone exhibited severe desquamation of tubular epithelium followed by destruction of renal parenchyma. Sections showed damaged architecture accompanied by acute inflammation with infiltration of inflammatory cells and massive edema (**Figure 4e**). Tubular degeneration proceeded by cytoplasmic vacuolation, fragmented cytoplasm and tubular lumen filled with eosinophilic deposits were frequently encountered as the indicators of renal tubule necrosis (**Figure 4f**). Besides necrosis, cystic glomeruli (**Figure 4g**) and series of renal tubule enlargement involving

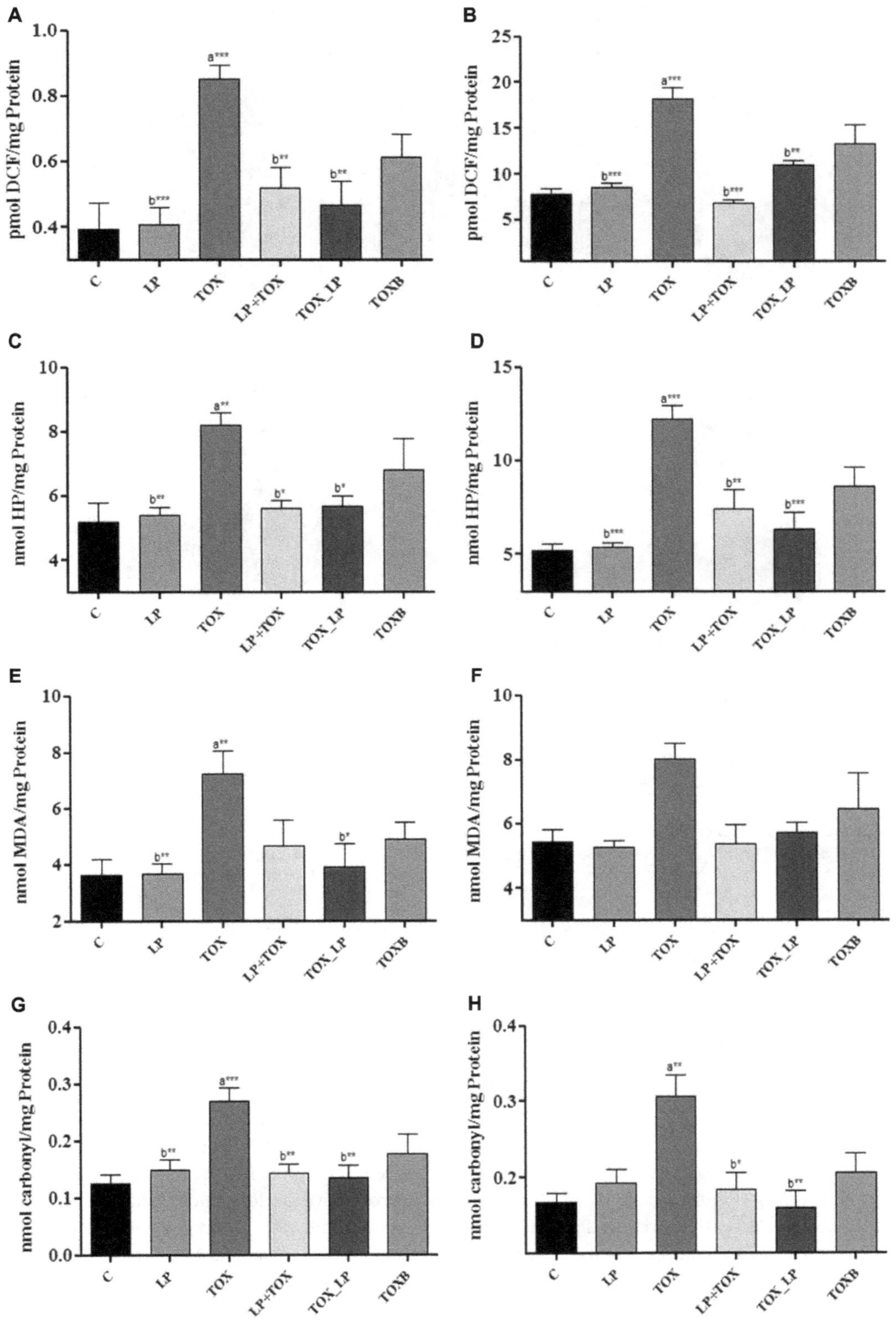

FIGURE 2 | Effect of *L. plantarum* MYS6 on fumonisin B1 induced oxidative stress in the liver homogenate and serum of control and treatment broilers. In the figure, **(A,B)** generation of ROS, **(C,D)** generation of hydrogen peroxide, **(E,F)** peroxidation of lipids, and **(G,H)** oxidation of proteins. Data are the mean ± SEM of five broiler birds per treatment group and were analyzed using one way ANOWA followed by Bonferroni *post hoc* test ($^{*}P < 0.05$, $^{**}P < 0.01$, $^{***}P < 0.001$; [a]significant when compared to control, [b]significant when compared to 200 mg FB1 toxin control).

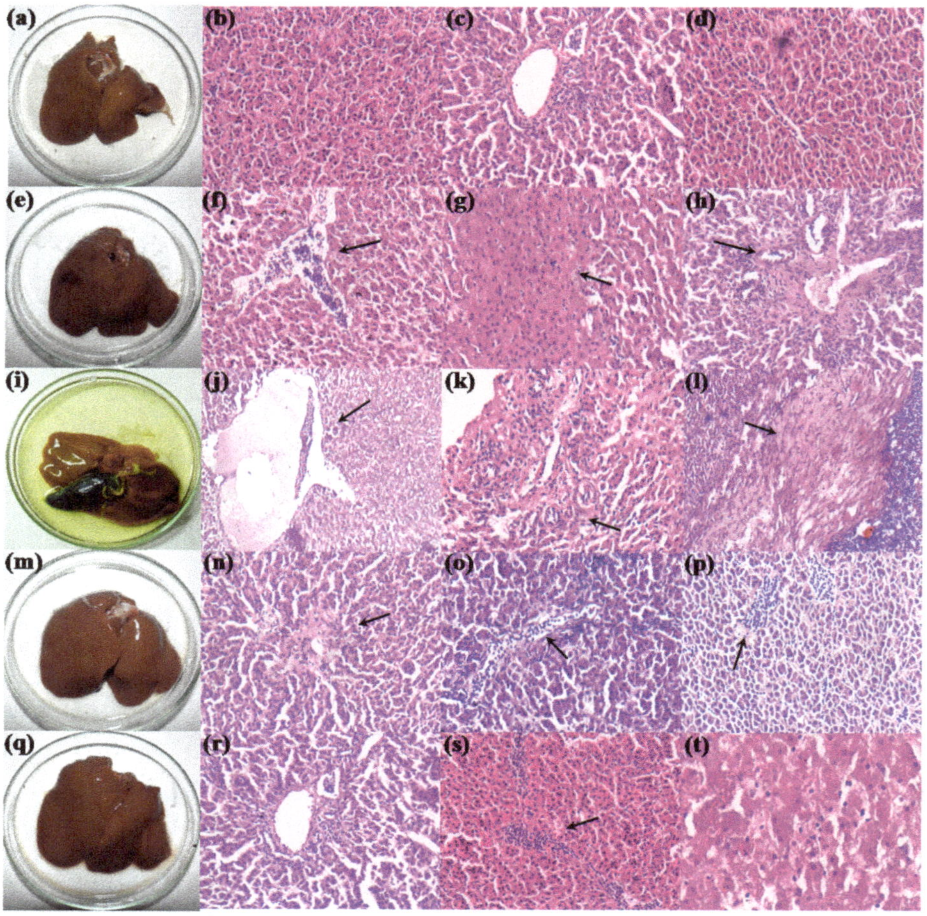

FIGURE 3 | Morphology and histopathology of hematoxylin-eosin-stained photomicrographs of liver of control and treatment broilers. **(a–d)** Control, **(e–h)** TOXB + 200 mg FB1, **(i–l)** 200 mg FB1 alone, **(m–p)** *L. plantarum* MYS6 alone, and **(q–t)** LpMYS6 + 200 mg FB1. Liver sections were observed at 400× magnification.

granular casts and vacoulation of glomeruli (**Figure 4h**) were the other morphologic severity associated with the degeneration of tissue. In contrary, kidneys of broilers treated with LpMYS6 alone depicted a normal morphology of Bowman's capsule in cortex and distal tubules yet age-related mild disruption of renal parenchyma was noticed (**Figures 4i,j**). Furthermore, treatment with LpMYS6 in pre-colonization and challenge study effectively restored the normal histology of kidney tissues. Renal tubule regeneration was clearly observed and included an array of histological changes such as karyomegaly and nuclear crowding along the affected renal tubules (**Figures 4k,l**). In addition, the severity grade of FB1 toxin was extensively reduced and no signs of edema, necrosis, cystic glomeruli, granular casts or any major abnormalities in the renal parenchyma were observed.

DISCUSSION

Fumonisin B1-induced deregulation of sphingolipid complex formation is a well-studied FB1 toxicity in animals and humans. Unlike most mycotoxins which are cyclic compounds, FB1 is a long-hydroxylated hydrocarbon chain having structural similarity to the sphingoid bases. FB1 intoxication also manifests serious consequences of oxidative stress in animals apart from the inhibition of sphinogolipid metabolism (Poersch et al., 2014). FB1 is poorly absorbed in the gastrointestinal tract unlike aflatoxins and is extensively retained as unmetabolized in the tissues such as liver and kidney. The toxin is eliminated in bile through enterohepatic recirculation and exerts its toxicity. It may also end up in the feces and as trace contaminants in urine (Shephard et al., 1994; Enongene et al., 2000). Apparently, poultry ingested with FB1 exhibit lack of appetite, low productive performance, inflamed liver, oral lesions, and immunosuppression leading to adverse health and economic status (Poersch et al., 2014). Hence protection against FB1-induced toxicity and oxidative stress in poultry becomes a prerequisite.

In our study, we observed a non-significant change in feed intake and feed conversion in the broilers treated with FB1 alone compared to control. Previous studies have reported a decrease in feed intake and feed conversion when broilers, ducks, or turkeys were ingested with feed contaminated by FB1 (Tessari et al., 2006; Benlasher et al., 2012). Further, our study showed no significant variations of body weight in broilers of treatment

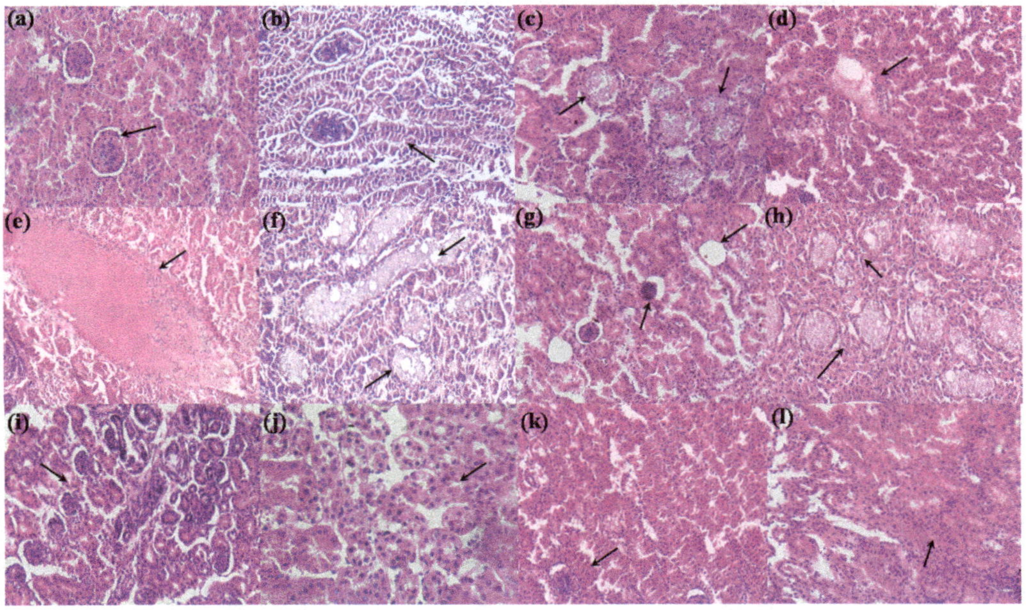

FIGURE 4 | Hematoxylin-eosin stained photomicrographs of kidney of control and treatment broilers. **(a,b)** Control, **(c,d)** TOXB + 200 mg FB1, **(e–h)** 200 mg FB1 alone, **(i,j)** *L. plantarum* MYS6 alone, and **(k,l)** LpMYS6 + 200 mg FB1. Kidney sections were observed at 400× magnification.

groups but health complications such as diarrhea and dysentery was observed in broilers fed with 200 mg FB1 per Kg feed. Earlier reports by Tran et al. (2005) and Tardieu et al. (2007) observed a reduced body weight in ducks and turkeys fed with 0–128 mg of FB1/Kg feed and 0–20 mg of FB1/Kg feed, respectively. Besides, increased relative organ weights of liver and kidney in our study marks FB1 toxicity as these organs are the sites of detoxification of many toxicants including FB1, and also the target organs for toxin effects (Voss et al., 2007). Poersch et al. (2014) also reported a significant increase in the liver weight of broilers treated with FB1 contaminated feed (100 mg/kg feed) showing its toxicity in the target organs.

With respect to hematological indices, broilers fed with 200 mg FB1-contaminated feed showed a diminished RBC count and hemoglobin ($P < 0.05$). This could be due to the toxic effects of FB1 on liver leading to haematopoietic (such as vitamins B12, folic acid, iron) suppression which eventually results in decreased synthesis of hemoglobin and erythropoietin and subsequently affect the RBC production and HCT. Our results are in accordance with the study conducted by Sobrane Filho et al. (2016), where broilers fed with diet containing a mixture of aflatoxin B1 (2 mg/kg feed) and FB1 (100 mg/kg feed) exhibited low values of erythrocyte, hemoglobin, and hematocrit compared to control while no difference was observed in the thrombocyte count. Another study by Broomhead et al. (2002) showed that the above parameters of hematology remain unaffected in broilers when treated with 25 or 50 mg/kg FB1 in diet. FB1 fed broilers in the present study showed a non-significant rise in WBC count probably due to an inflammatory response to the toxin. But Sobrane Filho et al. (2016) reported a decrease in WBC count in the broilers fed with aflatoxin B1 (2 mg/kg feed) and FB1 (100 mg/kg feed) contaminated diet. The inconsistency in the hematology results is tempting us to speculate that hematology would not be a sensitive indicator of FB1 toxicity in broilers.

Further, increased SGOT and SGPT might be the signs of damage of hepatocytes and these could be sensitive indicators of acute hepatic necrosis. In agreement with our results, Khalil et al. (2015) reported a significant increase in serum liver function markers such as alanine aminotransferase (ALT), aspartate aminotransferase (AST), and alkaline phosphatase (ALP) in Sprague–Dawley rats intoxicated with 100 and 200 mg FB1. The increased levels of cholesterol and triglyceride in our study are probable indicators of stress created in broilers due to FB1 feeding affecting lipid metabolism. Also, this could be linked to decreased feed intake and disruption of sphingolipid metabolism because of the interrelationships of these pathways. Meanwhile, a rise in the albumin in FB1-challenged broilers may be due to the damage of hepatocytes and impairment of protein synthesis. A study conducted by Cheng et al. (2006) in broilers fed with 5 and/or 15 mg FB1 showed a significant increase in serum AST, albumin, and cholesterol coupled with poor immunocompetence. Besides, increased levels of creatinine in the present study could be the result of protein catabolism or kidney affliction. A previous study by Khalil et al. (2015) reported a gradual increase in renal products such as urea, uric acid, and creatinine in rats fed with 200 mg FB1 revealing apparent kidney toxicity. Hence, our results clearly signify the damaging effects of FB1 on hepatic and renal tissues.

The FB1 toxicity in broilers was further substantiated by the assessment of oxidative stress markers in serum and liver homogenate. The accumulation of free sphingolipid bases due to FB1 toxicity induces an inhibition of complex 1 of the mitochondrial respiratory chain, CYP450, and NADPH oxidase system and therefore stimulates the generation of diverse ROS such as superoxide radical, hydrogen peroxide (Domijan and Abramov, 2011; Mary et al., 2012; Rodrigues and Gomes, 2012). The ingestion of 200 mg FB1 induced a significant increase in ROS and H_2O_2 generation, LPO marker (MDA), and carbonyl contents of protein oxidation in serum and liver homogenate in broilers. Recent studies by Theumer et al. (2010) in wistar rats and Kotan et al. (2011) in human lymphocytes indicated that generation of ROS and oxidative stress was a direct consequence of the immunotoxic effects elicited by AFB1 and FB1. Similar results on oxidative stress were observed in rats treated with AFB1 and FB1 (Hassan et al., 2014; Abdellatef and Khalil, 2016) and broiler chicks with FB1 (Poersch et al., 2014). *In vivo* studies of Wistar rats treated with 100 mg FB1, documented a significant increase in MDA level in spleen mononuclear cells, liver and kidney tissues (Theumer et al., 2010; Hassan et al., 2014). Apart from lipids, the other possible major target of oxidative damage is proteins that are further transformed into protein carbonyls. Mary et al. (2012) proposed that 48 h incubation of spleen mononuclear cells with 10 μM FB1 significantly raised the carbonyl content. Also, Domijan et al. (2007) suggested that 200 ng and 50 μg FB1 could cause oxidation of proteins in the kidney of wistar rats.

The histopathological observations of hepatic and renal tissues confirmed the abnormal serum biochemistry, oxidative stress and cellular damage induced by FB1. The intoxicated broilers marked massive destruction of hepatic and renal tissues. Tessari et al. (2006) showed severe damage of liver characterized by disorganization and megalocytosis of hepatocytes, bile duct proliferation, necrosis and inflammation and kidney sections displaying hydropic degeneration in broiler chicks exposed to 50 and 200 mg FB1. Further, Voss et al. (2007) proposed that kidney was the most sensitive organ in Sprague–Dawley and Fischer 344 rats when exposed to FB1, while in BD IX rats, liver was the main target organ.

Our study demonstrates the protective role of a probiotic strain, *L. plantarum* MYS6 (Lp MYS6) against FB1-induced toxicity and tissue damage. The LpMYS6 strain was previously characterized in our laboratory for an array of probiotic attributes, antifungal properties, FB1 detoxification by binding and extraction/purification of low molecular weight antifungal compounds (Deepthi et al., 2016). Probiotic LAB is known to act via diverse mechanisms *in vivo* which include modulation of gastrointestinal physiology by increasing the production of growth factors, competition for nutrients with enteropathogens, bioconversion of available sugars to acids, production of vitamins and organic acids, competitive exclusion for adhesive sites, beneficial immunostimulation of the gut-associated lymphoid tissue, antioxidative and anticancer/antiproliferative activities (Alberto et al., 2007; Oelschlaeger, 2010). Detoxification of mycotoxins by LAB is mainly mediated by the binding of toxin to bacterial cell and is dependent on the cell wall structural integrity of LAB.

In response to probiotic treatment, FB1-challenged broilers showed significant amelioration of toxin ill effects. Broilers of pre-colonization study exhibited a gradual increase in feed intake, body weight and FCR when compared to birds treated with toxin alone. Moreover, the broilers of challenge study showed the highest body weight among all treatment groups. Our results clearly demonstrated that LpMYS6 improved the appetite of FB1-challenged broilers thereby increasing the feed intake and body weight. A recent study by Khalil et al. (2015), reported that *L. delbrueckii* subsp. *lactis* and *Pediococcus acidilactici* significantly helped in improving the body weight and feed intake of rats after three weeks of exposure to 50, 100, and 200 mg concentrations of FB1. Also, our results are in line with the work by Gratz et al. (2006), who demonstrated that *L. rhamnosus* strain GG improved the body weight gain in rats intoxicated with AFB1. LpMYS6 was efficient in reducing the toxicity-induced weight gain in the liver, but there was no significant effect on the relative weight of kidney in all the dietary treatments. With respect to hematological parameters, LpMYS6 efficiently reestablished the RBC count and hemoglobin. The elevated levels of WBC and reduced count of PLT were restored by LpMYS6 administration. Jiang et al. (2014) showed that supplementation of yeast cell wall absorbent had a protective effect on WBC, lymphocytes, PLT, and hemoglobin in broilers fed with mycotoxin-contaminated feed. Further, oral administration of LpMYS6 significantly restored the altered levels of serum parameters such as SGOT, SGPT, creatinine, cholesterol, triglycerides and albumin, both in the pre-colonization and challenge study. The alleviated level of SGPT specifically indicates the rehabilitation of hepatocytes, and also the serum cholesterol. The reduction in elevated levels of cholesterol by LpMYS6 indicate normal lipid metabolism including sphingolipid formation and normalized feed intake. High serum creatinine is an indication of renal trauma. Our strain, LpMYS6 was efficient in reducing creatinine level which may be due to proper catabolism of dietary/tissue proteins and filtration rate in kidney. The above results indicate that LpMYS6 effectively reduced the FB1-induced hepatorenal toxicity. Khalil et al. (2015) reported that co-administration of *L. delbrueckii* subsp. *lactis* and *Pediococcus acidilactici* was efficient in normalizing ALT, AST, albumin, bilirubin levels in rats fed with 200 mg FB1-contaminated diet. Also, Jiang et al. (2014) studied that supplementation of yeast cell wall absorbent to the mycotoxin contaminated diet could significantly improve the serum levels of AST, ALT, ALP, and GGT in broiler chickens.

Furthermore, LpMYS6 effectively scavenged the elevated ROS and H_2O_2 in serum and liver homogenate. Also, the probiotic strain remarkably stabilized the altered levels of LPO and PCC in serum and tissue homogenate of liver. Administration of LpMYS6 was observed to significantly reinstate the normal morphology of liver and kidney. Deabes et al. (2012) reported a significant reduction of oxidative status in liver and kidney of aflatoxin-challenged mice treated with *L. rhamnosus* starin GG by increasing the contents of reduced glutathione (GSH) and superoxide dismutase (SOD). Further, a study by Abdellatef and Khalil (2016), demonstrated the ameliorative effects of *L. delbureckii* subsp. *lactis* DSM 20076 and *Pediococcus acidilactici* NNRL B-5627 on fumonisin B1-induced hepatoxicity and nephrotoxicity in rats.

LpMYS6 induces its protective effects probably by binding FB1 in the chicken crop or gastrointestinal tract and consequently reducing the bioavailability of FB1. This is supported by our previous observation on the *in vitro* binding ability of *L. plantarum* MYS6 to FB1 toxin wherein the per cent removal of FB1 was 32.9% and 61.7% in 2 and 4 h of incubation time, respectively (Deepthi et al., 2016). Several studies suggest that binding is the main mechanism of detoxification of mycotoxins by LAB (Gratz et al., 2007; Hathout et al., 2011; Abbes et al., 2016; Abdellatef and Khalil, 2016). However, the binding mechanism itself is not thoroughly understood. Zoghi et al. (2014) reported that probiotic LAB binds to the toxin due to the adhesive nature of S-layer proteins in their cell wall. Shetty and Jespersen (2006) suggested that carbohydrate-rich mannoproteins or glucans of LAB are involved in their binding to mycotoxins. Recently, Huang et al. (2017) suggested that *L. plantarum* C88 could effectively detoxify aflatoxin by suppressing the expression of cytochrome P450 1A2 and CYP 3A4 to decrease the production of AFBO (exo-AFB1-8,9-epoxide) and activate GST A3 through Nrf2 signaling pathways. This in turn improves GSH-conjugating activity and reduces toxin mediated oxidative stress. The majority of studies on detoxification of mycotoxins by LAB are aflatoxin-oriented with very limited data existing for LAB-mediated amelioration of FB1-induced toxicity and oxidative stress in broilers. In this context, we made an attempt to evaluate the protective effects of a potent probiotic strain, *L. plantarum* MYS6 against FB1 toxicity and oxidative stress in broilers. Our results showed that protective effects of LpMYS6 were significantly high in challenge study when compared to pre-colonization study. This indicates that the binding of FB1 occurs immediately after administration of LpMYS6 and pre-colonization of LpMYS6 might delay or decrease the binding process. Our outcome is in line with a recent finding by Huang et al. (2017) who reported that *L. plantarum* C88 effectively binds to AFB1 within 2 h post dose in mice and excreted in high levels as fecal AFB1 and lactobacilli. Nevertheless, systemic studies are still needed to understand the precise binding mechanism of FB1 to LAB.

Toxin binders are inert indigestible adsorbents widely employed in the poultry feed industry as detoxicification method. Several studies are available suggesting the application of TOXBs such as HSCAS, clay products, bentonites, zeolites, activated carbon etc (Huwig et al., 2001; Galvano et al., 2001; Avantaggiato et al., 2004; Kabak et al., 2006; Jouany, 2007; Phillips et al., 2008; Devreese et al., 2013; Agboola et al., 2015) as an effective method to minimize mycotoxin-induced toxicity. Interestingly, we found that TOXB was less effective in sequestering the toxin. Moreover, they seemed to induce oxidative stress and organ damage to some extent in our study.

In summary, the present investigation clearly demonstrates the FB1-induced toxicity, oxidative stress and vital organ damage in broilers. Oral administration of *L. plantarum* MYS6 to broilers significantly mitigated the FB1-induced toxicity and organ damage. *L. plantarum* MYS6 also significantly reinstated the imbalanced serum biochemical parameters, oxidative markers and hepatic and renal tissue damage. *L. plantarum* MYS6 was more effective in sequestering the toxin when compared to the commercially available TOXB and had protective health benefits. The protective role of *L. plantarum* MYS6 may be due to its FB1-binding capacity thereby reducing the toxin bioavailability in broilers. To the best of our knowledge, the present study is the first of its kind in employing a probiotic lactic acid bacterium to reduce the effects of FB1-induced oxidative stress and organ damage in broilers. The future prospect of the study is to understand the changes in gut microbiota, mechanism of interaction between LAB and FB1 at molecular level and developing a functional probiotic feed for broilers.

AUTHOR CONTRIBUTIONS

MYS, KSG, and BVD conceived and designed the research; BVD, RS, KPR, and ND performed the experiments and animal work; NKD supervised animal work and necropsy; BVD, RS, NKD, KSG, and MYS analyzed the data; BVD wrote the paper and MYS edited the paper.

ACKNOWLEDGMENTS

BVD acknowledges University Grants Commission for the award of RGNF research fellowship. The authors thank Central Instrumentation Facility, Institute of Excellence (IOE) for providing timely assistance. The authors thank Dr. Manjunath, Veterinary Officer, City Veterinary Hospital, Mysuru for his kind help during necropsy of broilers. We also thank Dr. Divyashree S., Dr. Nagaraja H., Dr. Shanmuga Sundaram, and Mr. Naveen Kumar for their kind help during the study.

REFERENCES

Abbes, S., Ben Salah-Abbes, J., Jebali, R., Younes, R. B., and Oueslati, R. (2016). Interaction of aflatoxin B_1 and fumonisin B_1 in mice causes immunotoxicity and oxidative stress: possible protective role using lactic acid bacteria. *J. Immunotoxicol.* 13, 46–54. doi: 10.3109/1547691X.2014.997905

Abdellatef, A. A., and Khalil, A. A. (2016). Ameliorated effects of *Lactobacillus delbrueckii* subsp. *lactis* DSM 20076 and *Pediococcus acidilactici* NNRL B-5627 on Fumonisin B1-induced Hepatotoxicity and Nephrotoxicity in rats. *Asian J. Pharm. Sci.* 11, 326–336. doi: 10.1016/j.ajps.2016.02.006

Agboola, A. F., Omidiwura, B. R. O., Odu, O., Odupitan, F. T., and Iyayi, E. A. (2015). Effect of probiotic and toxin binder on performance, intestinal microbiota and gut morphology in broiler chickens. *J. Anim. Sci. Adv.* 5, 1369–1379. doi: 10.5455/jasa.20150709085312

Alberto, M. R., Arena, M. E., and Manca de Nadra, M. C. (2007). Putrescine production from agmatine by *Lactobacillus hilgardii*: effect of phenolic compounds. *Food Control.* 18, 898–903. doi: 10.1016/j.foodcont.2006.05.006

Asrani, R. K., Katoch, R. C., Gupta, V. K., Deshmukh, S., Jindal, N., Ledoux, D. R., et al. (2006). Effects of feeding *Fusarium verticillioides* (formerly *Fusarium moniliforme*) culture material containing known levels of fumonisin B1 in Japanese quail (*Coturnix coturnix japonica*). *Poult. Sci.* 85, 1129–1135. doi: 10.1093/ps/85.7.1129

Avantaggiato, G., Havenaar, R., and Visconti, A. (2004). Evaluation of the intestinal absorption of deoxynivalenol and nivalenol by an in vitro gastrointestinal model, and the binding efficacy of activated carbon and other adsorbent materials. *Food Chem. Toxicol.* 42, 817–824. doi: 10.1016/j.fct.2004.01.004

Benlasher, E., Geng, X., Nguyen, N. T. X., Tardieu, D., Bailly, J.-D., Auvergne, A., et al. (2012). Comparative effects of fumonisins on sphingolipid metabolism and toxicity in ducks and turkeys. *Avian Dis.* 56, 120–127. doi: 10.1637/9853-071911-Reg.1

Botsoglou, N., Taitzoglou, I., Zervos, I., Botsoglou, E., Tsantarliotou, M., and Chatzopoulou, P. S. (2010). Potential of long-term dietary administration of rosemary in improving the antioxidant status of rat tissues following carbon tetrachloride intoxication. *Food Chem. Toxicol.* 48, 944–950. doi: 10.1016/j.fct.2010.01.004

Broomhead, J. N., Ledoux, D. R., Bermudez, A. J., and Rottinghaus, G. E. (2002). Chronic effects of fumonisin B1 in broilers and turkeys fed dietary treatments to market age. *Poult. Sci.* 81, 56–61. doi: 10.1093/ps/81.1.56

Cenesiz, S., Yaman, H., Ozcan, A., and Karademir, G. (2008). Effects of kefir as a probiotic on serum cholesterol, total lipid, aspartate amino transferase and alanine amino transferase activities in broiler chicks. *Med. Wet.* 64, 168–170.

Cheng, Y.-H., Ding, S.-T., and Chang, M.-H. (2006). Effect of fumonisins on macrophage immune functions and gene expression of cytokines in broilers. *Arch. Anim. Nutr.* 60, 267–276. doi: 10.1080/17450390600785079

Chiu, H. H., Tsai, C. C., Hsih, H. Y., and Tsen, H. Y. (2007). Screening from pickled vegetables the potential probiotic strains of lactic acid bacteria able to inhibit the *Salmonella* invasion in mice. *J. Appl. Microbiol.* 104, 605–612. doi: 10.1111/j.1365-2672.2007.03573.x

Deabes, M. M., Darwish, H. R., Abdel-Aziz, K. B., Farag, I. M., Nada, S. A., and Tawfek, N. S. (2012). Protective effects of *Lactobacillus rhamnosus GG* on aflatoxins-induced toxicities in male albino mice. *J. Environment. Analytic. Toxicol.* 2:132. doi: 10.4172/2161-0525.1000132

Deepthi, B. V., Poornachandra Rao, K., Chennapa, G., Naik, M. K., Chandrashekara, K. T., and Sreenivasa, M. Y. (2016). Antifungal attributes of *Lactobacillus plantarum* MYS6 against fumonisin producing *Fusarium proliferatum* associated with poultry feeds. *PLOS ONE* 11:e0155122. doi: 10.1371/journal.pone.0155122

Devreese, M., De Backer, P., and Croubels, S. (2013). Different methods to counteract mycotoxin production and its impact on animal health. *Vlaams Diergeneeskd. Tijdschr.* 82, 181–190.

Domijan, A. M., and Abramov, A. Y. (2011). Fumonisin B1 inhibits mitochondrial respiration and deregulates calcium homeostasis - Implication to mechanism of cell toxicity. *Int. J. Biochem. Cell Biol.* 43, 897–904. doi: 10.1016/j.biocel.2011.03.003

Domijan, A. M., Peraica, M., Vrdoljak, A. L., Radić, B., Žlender, V., and Fuchs, R. (2007). The involvement of oxidative stress in ochratoxin A and fumonisin B 1 toxicity in rats. *Mol. Nutr. Food Res.* 51, 1147–1151. doi: 10.1002/mnfr.200700079

Driver, A. S., Kodavanti, P. R., and Mundy, W. R. (2000). Age-related changes in reactive oxygen species production in rat brain homogenates. *Neurotoxicol. Teratol.* 22, 175–181. doi: 10.1016/S0892-0362(99)00069-0

Enongene, E. N., Sharma, R. P., Bhandari, N., Miller, J. D., Meredith, F. I., Voss, K. A., et al. (2002). Persistence and reversibility of the elevation in free sphingoid bases induced by fumonisin inhibition of ceramide synthase. *Toxicol. Sci.* 67, 173–181. doi: 10.1093/toxsci/67.2.173

Enongene, E. N., Sharma, R. P., Bhandari, N., Voss, K. A., and Riley, R. T. (2000). Disruption of sphingolipid metabolism in small intestines, liver and kidney of mice dosed subcutaneously with fumonisin B_1. *Food Chem. Toxicol.* 38, 793–799. doi: 10.1016/S0278-6915(00)00065-X

Escriva, L., Font, G., and Manyes, L. (2015). *In vivo* toxicity studies of *Fusarium* mycotoxins in the last decade: a review. *Food Chem. Toxicol.* 78, 185–206. doi: 10.1016/j.fct.2015.02.005

Fandohan, P., Gnonlonfin, B., Hell, K., Marasas, W. F. O., and Wingfield, M. J. (2005). Natural occurrence of *Fusarium* and subsequent fumonisin contamination in preharvest and stored maize in Benin, West Africa. *Int. J. Food. Microbiol.* 99, 173–183. doi: 10.1016/j/ijfoodmicro.2004.08.012

Galvano, F., Piva, A., Ritieni, A., and Galvano, G. (2001). Dietary strategies to counteract the effects of mycotoxins: a review. *J. Food Prot.* 64, 120–131. doi: 10.4315/0362-028X-64.1.120

Gerez, C. L., Torres, M. J., Font de Valdez, G., and Rollán, G. (2013). Control of spoilage fungi by lactic acid bacteria. *Biol. Control.* 64, 231–237. doi: 10.1016/j.biocontrol.2012.10.009

Gratz, S., Täubel, M., Juvonen, R. O., Viluksela, M., Turner, P. C., Mykkänen, H., et al. (2006). *Lactobacillus rhamnosus* strain GG modulates intestinal absorption, fecal excretion, and toxicity of aflatoxin B_1 in rats. *Appl. Environ. Microbiol.* 72, 7398–7400. doi: 10.1128/AEM.01348-06

Gratz, S., Wu, Q. K., El-Nezami, H., Juvonen, R. O., Mykkänen, H., and Turner, P. C. (2007). *Lactobacillus rhamnosus* strain GG reduces aflatoxin B_1 transport, metabolism, and toxicity in Caco-2 cells. *Appl. Environ. Microbiol.* 73, 3958–3964. doi: 10.1128/AEM.02944-06

Hassan, A. M., Abdel-Aziem, S. H., El-Nekeety, A. A., and Abdel-Wahhab, M. A. (2014). Panaxginseng extract modulates oxidative stress, DNA fragmentation and up-regulate gene expression in rats sub chronically treated with aflatoxin B_1 and fumonisin B_1. *Cytotechnology* 67, 861–871. doi: 10.1007/s10616-014-9726-z

Hathout, A. S., Mohamed, S. R., El-Nekeety, A. A., Hassan, N. S., Aly, S. E., and Abdel-Wahhab, M. A. (2011). Ability of *Lactobacillus casei* and *Lactobacillus reuteri* to protect against oxidative stress in rats fed aflatoxins-contaminated diet. *Toxicon* 58, 179–186. doi: 10.1016/j.toxicon.2011.05.015

Huang, L., Duan, C., Zhao, Y., Gao, L., Niu, C., Xu, J., et al. (2017). Reduction of aflatoxin B_1 toxicity by *Lactobacillus plantarum* C88: a potential probiotic strain isolated from Chinese traditional fermented food "Tofu". *PLOS ONE* 12:e0170109. doi: 10.1371/journal.pone.0170109

Huwig, A., Freimund, S., Käppeli, O., and Dutler, H. (2001). Mycotoxin detoxication of animal feed by different adsorbents. *Toxicol. Lett.* 122, 179–188. doi: 10.1016/S0378-4274(01)00360-5

International Agency for Research on Cancer [IARC] (2002). Some traditional herbal medicines, some mycotoxins, naphthalene and styrene. *IARC Monogr. Eval. Carcinog. Risks Hum.* 82, 301–366.

Jiang, S. Z., Li, Z., Wang, G. Y., Yang, Z. B., Yang, W. R., Zhang, G. G., et al. (2014). Effects of *Fusarium* mycotoxins with yeast cell wall absorbent on hematology, serum biochemistry, and oxidative stress in broiler chickens. *J. Appl. Poult. Res.* 23, 165–173. doi: 10.3382/japr.2013-00830

Jouany, J. P. (2007). Methods for preventing, decontaminating and minimizing the toxicity of mycotoxins in feeds. *Anim. Feed Sci. Technol.* 137, 342–362. doi: 10.1016/j.anifeedsci.2007.06.009

Kabak, B., Dobson, A. D. W., and Var, I. (2006). Strategies to prevent mycotoxin contamination of food and animal feed: a review. *Crit. Rev. Food Sci. Nutr.* 46, 593–619. doi: 10.1080/10408390500436185

Khalil, A. A., Abou-Gabal, A. E., Abdellatef, A. A., and Khalid, A. E. (2015). Protective role of probiotic lactic acid bacteria against dietary fumonisin B1-induced toxicity and DNA-fragmentation in sprague-dawley rats. *Prep. Biochem. Biotechnol* 45, 530–550. doi: 10.1018/10826068.2014.940969

Kotan, E., Alpsoy, L., Anar, M., Aslan, A., and Agar, G. (2011). Protective role of methanol extract of *Cetraria islandica* (L.) against oxidative stress and genotoxic effects of AFB_1 in human lymphocytes *in vitro*. *Toxicol. Ind. Health.* 27, 599–605. doi: 10.1177/0748233710394234

Levine, R. L., Garland, D., Oliver, C. N., Amici, A., Climent, I., Lenz, A. G., et al. (1990). Determination of carbonyl content in oxidatively modified proteins. *Methods Enzymol.* 186, 464–478. doi: 10.1016/0076-6879(90)86141-H

Lowry, O. H., Rosebrough, N. J., Farr, A. L., and Randall, R. J. (1951). Protein measurement using folin-phenol reagent. *J. Biol. Chem.* 193, 265–275.

Mary, V. S., Theumer, M. G., Arias, S. L., and Rubinstein, H. R. (2012). Reactive oxygen species sources and biomolecular oxidative damage induced by aflatoxin B1 and fumonisin B1 in rat spleen mononuclear cells. *Toxicology.* 302, 299–307. doi: 10.1016/j.tox.2012.08.012

Merrill, A. H., Sullards, M. C., Wang, E., Voss, K. A., and Riley, R. T. (2001). Sphingolipid metabolism: roles in signal transduction and disruption by fumonisins. *Environ. Health Perspect.* 109, 283–289. doi: 10.1289/ehp.01109s2283

Niderkorn, V., Morgavi, D. P., Pujos, E., Tissandier, A., and Boudra, H. (2007). Screening of fermentative bacteria for their ability to bind and biotransform deoxynivalenol, zearalenone and fumonisins in an in vitro simulated corn silage model. *Food Addit. Contam.* 24, 406–415. doi: 10.1080/02652030301101110

Oelschlaeger, T. A. (2010). Mechanisms of probiotic actions - A review. *Int. J. Med. Microbiol.* 300, 57–62. doi: 10.1016/j.ijmm.2009.08.005

Ohkawa, H., Ohishi, N., and Yagi, K. (1979). Assay for lipid peroxides in animal tissues by thiobarbituric acid reaction. *Anal. Biochem.* 95, 351–358. doi: 10.1016/0003-2697(79)90738-3

Phillips, T. D., Afriyie-Gyawu, E., Williams, J., Huebner, H., Ankrah, N., Ofori-Adjei, D., et al. (2008). Reducing human exposure to aflatoxin through the use of clay: a review. *Food Addit. Contam. Part A Chem. Anal. Control. Expo. Risk Assess.* 25, 134–145. doi: 10.1080/02652030701567467

Poersch, A. B., Trombetta, F., Braga, A. C. M., Boeira, S. P., Oliveira, M. S., Dilkin, P., et al. (2014). Involvement of oxidative stress in subacute toxicity induced by fumonisin B1 in broiler chicks. *Vet. Microbiol.* 1988, 6–11. doi: 10.1016/j.vetmic.2014.8.020

Riley, R. T., Enongene, E., Voss, K. A., Norred, W. P., Meredith, F. I., Sharma, R. P., et al. (2001). Sphingolipid perturbations as mechanisms for fumonisin carcinogenesis. *Environ. Health Perspect.* 109, 301–308. doi: 10.1289/ehp.01109s2301

Rodrigues, J. V., and Gomes, C. M. (2012). Mechanism of superoxide and hydrogen peroxide generation by human electron-transfer flavoprotein and pathological variants. *Free Radic. Biol. Med.* 53, 12–19. doi: 10.1016/j.freeradbiomed.2012.04.016

Sharma, D., Asrani, R. K., Ledoux, D. R., Jindal, N., Rottinghaus, G. E., and Gupta, V. K. (2008). Individual and combined effects of fumonisin B 1 and moniliformin on clinicopathological and cell-mediated immune response in Japanese quail. *Poult. Sci.* 87, 1039–1051. doi: 10.3382/ps.2007-00204

Shephard, G. S., Thiel, P. G., Sydenham, E. W., and Alberts, J. F. (1994). Biliary excretion of the mycotoxin fumonisin B1 in rats. *Food Chem. Toxicol.* 32, 489–491. doi: 10.1016/0278-6915(94)90047-7

Shetty, P. H., and Jespersen, L. (2006). *Saccharomyces cerevisiae* and lactic acid bacteria as potential mycotoxin decontaminating agents. *Trends Food Sci. Technol.* 17, 48–55. doi: 10.1016/j.tifs.2005.10.004

Sobrane Filho, S. T., Junqueira, O. M., De Laurentiz, A. C., Filardi, S., Rubio, S., and Duarte, K. F. (2016). Effects of mycotoxin adsorbents in aflatoxin B 1 - and fumonisin B 1 -contaminated broiler diet on performance and blood metabolite. *Rev. Bras. de Zootec.* 45, 250–256. doi: 10.1590/S1806-92902016000500007

Tardieu, D., Bailley, J.-D., Skiba, F., Metayer, J.-P., Grosjean, F., and Guerre, P. (2007). Chronic toxicity of fumonisins in turkeys. *Poult. Sci.* 86, 1887–1893. doi: 10.1093/ps/86.9.1887

Tessari, E. N. C., Oliveira, C. A. F., Cardoso, A. L. S. P., Ledoux, D. R., and Rottinghaus, G. E. (2006). Effects of aflatoxin B1 and fumonisin B1 on body weight, antibody titres and histology of broiler chicks. *Br. Poult. Sci.* 47, 357–364. doi: 10.1080/00071660600756071

Theumer, M. G., Cánepa, M. C., López, A. G., Mary, V. S., Dambolena, J. S., and Rubinstein, H. R. (2010). Subchronic mycotoxicoses in Wistar rats: assessment of the *in vivo* and *in vitro* genotoxicity induced by fumonisins and aflatoxin B_1, and oxidative stress biomarkers status. *Toxicology* 268, 104–110. doi: 10.1016/j.tox.2009.12.007

Todorov, S. D., Botes, M., Guigas, C., Schillinger, U., Wiid, I., Wachsman, M. B., et al. (2008). Boza, a natural source of probiotic lactic acid bacteria. *J. Appl. Microbiol.* 104, 465–477. doi: 10.1111/j.1365-2672.03558.x

Tran, S. T., Auvergne, A., Benard, G., Bailly, J.-D., Tardieu, D., Babile, R., et al. (2005). Chronic effects of fumonisin B1 on ducks. *Poult. Sci.* 84, 22–28. doi: 10.1093/ps/84.1.22

Voss, K. A., Smith, G. W., and Haschek, W. M. (2007). Fumonisins: toxicokinetics, mechanism of action and toxicity. *Anim. Feed Sci. Technol.* 137, 299–325. doi: 10.1016/j.anifeedsci.2007.06.007

Zoghi, A., Khosravi-Darani, K., and Sohrabvandi, S. (2014). Surface binding of toxins and heavy metals by probiotics. *Mini Rev. Med. Chem.* 14, 84–98. doi: 10.2174/1389557513666131211105554

20

Safety of Novel Microbes for Human Consumption: Practical Examples of Assessment in the European Union

Theodor Brodmann[1]*, Akihito Endo*[2]*, Miguel Gueimonde*[3]*, Gabriel Vinderola*[4]*, Wolfgang Kneifel*[1]*, Willem M. de Vos*[5,6]*, Seppo Salminen*[7] *and Carlos Gómez-Gallego*[7]*

[1] Department of Food Sciences and Technology, University of Natural Resources and Life Science Vienna, Vienna, Austria, [2] Department of Food and Cosmetic Science, Tokyo University of Agriculture, Hokkaido, Japan, [3] Instituto de Productos Lácteos de Asturias, Spanish Higher Research Council, Villaviciosa, Spain, [4] Instituto de Lactología Industrial (UNL-CONICET), National University of the Litoral, Santa Fe, Argentina, [5] Laboratory of Microbiology, Wageningen University and Research, Wageningen, Netherlands, [6] Immunobiology Research Program, Research Programs Unit, Faculty of Medicine, University of Helsinki, Helsinki, Finland, [7] Functional Foods Forum, Faculty of Medicine, University of Turku, Turku, Finland

***Correspondence:**
Carlos Gómez-Gallego
cargom@utu.fi

Novel microbes are either newly isolated genera and species from natural sources or bacterial strains derived from existing bacteria. Novel microbes are gaining increasing attention for the general aims to preserve and modify foods and to modulate gut microbiota. The use of novel microbes to improve health outcomes is of particular interest because growing evidence points to the importance of gut microbiota in human health. As well, some recently isolated microorganisms have promise for use as probiotics, although in-depth assessment of their safety is necessary. Recent examples of microorganisms calling for more detailed evaluation include *Bacteroides xylanisolvens, Akkermansia muciniphila*, fructophilic lactic acid bacteria (FLAB), and *Faecalibacterium prausnitzii*. This paper discusses each candidate's safety evaluation for novel food or novel food ingredient approval according to European Union (EU) regulations. The factors evaluated include their beneficial properties, antibiotic resistance profiling, history of safe use (if available), publication of the genomic sequence, toxicological studies in agreement with novel food regulations, and the qualified presumptions of safety. Sufficient evidences have made possible to support and authorize the use of heat-inactivated *B. xylanisolvens* in the European Union. In the case of *A. muciniphila*, the discussion focuses on earlier safety studies and the strain's suitability. FLAB are also subjected to standard safety assessments, which, along with their proximity to lactic acid bacteria generally considered to be safe, may lead to novel food authorization in the future. Further research with *F. prausnitzii* will increase knowledge about its safety and probiotic properties and may lead to its future use as novel food. Upcoming changes in EUU Regulation 2015/2283 on novel food will facilitate the authorization of future novel products and might increase the presence of novel microbes in the food market.

Keywords: novel microbes, safety, *Bacteroides xylanisolvens*, *Akkermansia muciniphila*, fructophilic lactic acid bacteria, *Faecalibacterium prausnitzii*

INTRODUCTION

Since ancient times, microorganisms have constituted an essential part of human nutrition and been consumed through naturally microbially fermented products containing viable bacteria, such as fermented honey, fruits, berries, and their juices and fermented products of animal origin. Without even knowing of the existence of bacteria, humans historically used them to initiate many food production processes (Selhub et al., 2014). Today, an enormous variety of fermented foods and beverages exists and provides approximately one-third of the human diet globally (Borresen et al., 2012). Certain fermented foods containing significant amounts of viable microbes, especially dairy products and fermented vegetables, are part of daily consumption by millions of people around the globe.

Studies involving new analytical technologies have generated new insights into the human and animal guts and yielded new isolates and candidates that perform special functions in this complex intestinal environment (Marchesi et al., 2016). The composition of human gut microbiota plays an important role in homeostasis and gut functionality, which are also strongly influenced by age, diet, environmental factors, disorders, diseases, and therapies. In recent decades, probiotic microorganisms have been identified as efficient modulators of intestinal microbial balance (Gómez-Gallego and Salminen, 2016). Probiotics are defined as live microorganisms that confer a health benefit to the host when administered in adequate amounts (Cammarota et al., 2014; Hill et al., 2014). These health benefits are provided through relatively common mechanisms found in the vast majority of the investigated probiotics, such as regulation of the intestinal transit, competitive exclusion of pathogens, and production of specific short chain fatty acids (SCFA). In addition, frequently observed mechanisms mostly found on a species level include vitamin synthesis, enzymatic activity, gut barrier reinforcement, and neutralization of carcinogens. The existence of a group of basic benefits shared by strains of the same species in a non-strain specific manner supports the concept of core benefits for specific species. Moreover, mechanisms described exclusively on the individual strain level provide immunological, neurological, and endocrinological effects. Such benefits in general support a healthy digestive tract and immune system (Aureli et al., 2011; Gómez-Gallego and Salminen, 2016).

Traditionally fermented foods, especially fermented dairy products, usually contain viable bacteria. The consumption of such foods is widely connected with the reduction of certain disease types (e.g., childhood obesity, type-2 diabetes, and cardiovascular diseases), improved body composition, and weight loss in adults during energy restriction (Thorning et al., 2016). The International Scientific Association for Probiotics and Prebiotics (ISAPP) panel acknowledged convincing results but also emphasized the difficulty of verifying whether the beneficial results originate from the food matrices, the (viable) microorganisms, or a combination of both. Additionally, traditional fermented foods do not qualify for the term *probiotic* because they may contain varying amounts and changing microbial species over time, and their microbiological composition is not completely known or controlled. A relevant example is traditional Kefir. The ISAPP, therefore, has proposed the term "containing live and active bacterial cultures" for traditional fermented foods (Hill et al., 2014).

Probiotics relevant to the human gut microbiota mainly belong to the genera *Lactobacillus* and *Bifidobacterium*, but several other microbial candidates, such as *Akkermansia muciniphila* and *Faecalibacterium prausnitzii*, could play roles in future probiotic products. Although, commensal gut microbes can provide beneficial health effects, the ISAPP panel suggested conducting strain-by-strain assessment until sufficient research data are available to grant probiotic status on the species level (Hill et al., 2014).

EUROPEAN UNION REGULATIONS OF MICROORGANISMS INTENTIONALLY ADDED TO FOOD

The European Union (EU) is a single-market system consisting of 28 member states and the four members of the European Free Trade Association (Iceland, Liechtenstein, Norway, and Switzerland), which are required to follow European legislation as part of the EU single market. The European Food Safety Authority (EFSA) has the mandate to assess and communicate all risks associated with the food chain in the EU. The EFSA Scientific Committees and Panels are responsible for providing scientific opinions in response to requests from the European Commission, European Parliament, and EU member states. Before the EFSA was established, risk assessment was performed by Scientific Committees assisting the Directorate General for Health and Consumers (DG SANCO). DG SANCO, re-named to DG SANTE, continues to perform a crucial regulatory role regarding microorganisms in food and feed. Standing Committees representing member states, and their interests have strong influence on the work of DG SANTE (von Wright, 2012).

Amid globalization and ongoing technical progress, the number of new food products in the EU has increased significantly, and food safety has become a growing concern. A uniform regulation for novel food was needed to ensure the protection of both European consumers and the market. The introduction of novel foods is governed by Regulation 285/97/EC (European Commission, 1997b) and Regulation 2015/2283 (European Commission, 2015), covering all foods not been used in the EU before 15 May 1997. Under Regulation 2015/2283, the EFSA, rather than competent national authorities, will perform the scientific risk assessment for novel foods; the system of individual authorization is replaced by a system of generic authorization; and the Commission will manage all applicants' files and prepares proposals for the authorization of novel foods found to be safe (European Commission, 2015). To speed decision-making, the EFSA is required to issue its opinion within 9 months of the date of receipt of a valid application.

The guidance lists general requirements for every application: (1) a description; (2) compositional data; (3) production process; (4) specifications; (5) proposed uses and use levels; and (6) anticipated intake of the novel food. Applicants also have to provide information about the absorption, distribution, metabolism, excretion, nutrition, toxicology, allergenicity, and history of use of novel foods or their source. In addition, all the novel foods that belong to the group of "foods consisting of, isolated from or produced from micro-organisms, fungi or algae" must provide the following information (EFSA Panel on Dietetic Products, 2016): (1) scientific (Latin) name (family, genus, species, strain) according to the international codes of nomenclature; (2) synonyms used interchangeably with the preferred scientific name; (3) for bacteria and yeasts (unicellular organisms), verification of the species and strain identity according to internationally accepted methods; (4) origin of the organism; and (5) if available, deposition in an officially recognized culture collection with an access number.

Qualified Presumption of Safety

EFSA introduced the concept of qualified presumption of safety (QPS) to establish a generic risk assessment approach for biological agents, with the goal to simplify and harmonize assessment of notified biological agents across the EFSA's various Scientific Panels and Units. The QPS approach also enables more focused application of the available resources to agents with higher risk potential (Leuschner et al., 2010), simplifying the assessment of low-risk microorganisms. The QPS concept is intended to establish a safety assessment for microorganisms used in feed and food production. If a specific strain notified for market authorization can unambiguously be connected to a taxonomic unit on the QPS list, the necessary safety assessment steps, if any, are indicated in the list for that taxonomic unit.

Bacteria with a previous history of safe use are usually included on the QPS list. The EFSA's Panel on Biological Hazards assesses the QPS status of a strain and declares that the assigned microorganism displays either no safety concerns or minor concerns defined and addressed with qualifications as expressed in the QPS list. Microorganisms on the QPS list, therefore, need no exhaustive safety assessment except for those specified in the QPS list.

The assessment for QPS suitability is well structured and relies on the following criteria (EFSA, 2007):

(a) Taxonomic unit: This is the most crucial part of the assessment procedure. The genus and all known species, including type species, are listed and described according to their main characteristics. The evaluated taxonomic unit must be unambiguously defined. If the assessed bacterial agent cannot be connected to any known species, it will not be recommended for the QPS list. QPS status is also denied if the taxonomic identification is insufficient.

(b) Body of knowledge: This should be related to the history of use for the assessed bacterial agent, the field of application, the existence of sufficient scientific literature about the microorganism, and the possibility to avoid potential adverse effects for humans, livestock, and the wider environment.

(c) Possible pathogenicity: The bacterial agent's lack of pathogenic and virulence properties is confirmed, and the findings must be supported by clinical data and scientific literature.

(d) Description of end use: This includes the presence and viability of the microorganism in the final product.

Most bacteria recommended for the QPS list belong to the group of Gram-positive non-sporulating bacteria. This group includes many inhabitants of the digestive tract with long histories in food and feed production. For this group, the EFSA's Scientific Committee applies a generic qualification for all taxonomic units on the list, requiring that all strains not carry any transferable antimicrobial resistance unless the final product contains no viable cells (Leuschner et al., 2010). The number of recommended Gram-negative bacteria is very low, with only one, *Gluconobacter oxydans*, on the QPS list. Many members have a long history of safe use, but safety concerns cannot be excluded. *E. coli* strain Nissle 1917, for example, has long been used as a probiotic but can cause a variety of diseases and exhibits versatile virulence mechanisms. Nevertheless, opportunistic bacteria may be placed on the QPS list with additional qualifications, but pathogenic and toxin-producing bacteria are not included.

Microorganisms whose safety properties are not fully understood are subjected to safety assessments. Such assessments need to include a distinct taxonomic classification on the species or the strain level and a comprehensive strain characterization, including whole-genome sequence analysis, to identify potential virulence and antibiotic resistance genes and their horizontal transfer capabilities. However, in the case of new and recently discovered microorganisms from previously unknown microbial groups, the availability of genome sequences might not be enough to identify potential virulence or antibiotic resistance genes. These often require comparison with available data, so functional studies on these microorganisms are needed. For accurate safety evaluation, the food business operator should include the number and the viability of microorganisms in the final product by.

The QPS approach was inspired and influenced by the American Generally Recognized As Safe (GRAS) concept, but differences exist. QPS is defined as an "assumption based on reasonable evidence" (H. C. P. Directorate-General, 2003), providing a helpful assessment tool for the EFSA but, in contrast to GRAS, offers no legal status. The EFSA is responsible for providing the burden of proof, while GRAS lays the responsibility on the food business operator. GRAS, though, requires safety assessment by independent experts to the degree that another panel of independent experts would reach the same conclusions. The QPS assessment's strong focus on the absence of acquired antibiotic resistances and virulence factors is another difference between the two concepts.

MICROORGANISMS AUTHORIZED AS NOVEL FOOD IN THE EU

Leuconostoc mesenteroides

In January 2001, the European Commission authorized market placement of a dextran preparation produced by *L. mesenteroides* as a novel food ingredient in bakery products. Puracor NV (Groot-Bijgaarden, Belgium) filed the application, and the Belgian competent authorities performed the initial assessment. The Scientific Committee for Food found that the dextran preparation by *L. mesenteroides* was safe for human consumption up to 5% in bakery products. Dextran was identified as a highly digestible bakery ingredient with similar nutritional properties as starch (European Commission, 2001).

L. mesenteroides is a Gram-positive, non-sporulating, coccoid-shaped bacterium in the order Lactobacillales. The organism is often found on the surfaces of various plant parts and is responsible for the fermentation of white cabbage into sauerkraut. *L. mesenteroides* can be also found in artisanal and industrial cheeses, possibly contributing to their safety for long-term consumption (Cibik et al., 2000; D'Angelo et al., 2017). The species can metabolize a broad range of sugars; in particular, sucrose is used to build dextran, and certain strains can produce bacteriocins with anti-listerial activity (de Paula et al., 2015).

Bacillus subtilis Natto

In April 2009, the European Commission allowed placing Vitamin K2 (menaquinone), produced by *B. subtilis* natto, in the market as a novel food ingredient under Regulation (EC) No 258/97. NattoPharma (Oslo, Norway) requested that the Irish competent authorities place *B. subtilis* natto derived Vitamin K2 in the market as a novel food ingredient to be used in foods which served particular nutritional uses and which had added vitamins and minerals (European Commission, 2009). In an initial report, the Irish competent authorities required an additional assessment, so the EFSA was requested to conduct an extended assessment. The Scientific Panel on Dietetic Products, Nutrition, and Allergies concluded that *B. subtilis* natto is a safe source of vitamin K2.

B. subtilis natto is a Gram-positive, aerobic member of the spore-forming genus *Bacillus*. This species, discovered in Japan in 1906, is responsible for production of natto, a sticky fermented soy beans. Natto, produced by *B. subtilis* natto, has long been used in the Japanese diet, so it gained Foods for Specified Health Use approval based on its health benefits from the Japanese Ministry of Health, Labor, and Welfare. *B. subtilis* has a recognized history of safe use, so the EFSA granted it QPS status (EFSA Panel on Biological Hazards, 2010).

Clostridium butyricum

In December 2014, the European Commission authorized placing in the market *C. butyricum* CBM 588 as a novel food ingredient according to Regulation (EC) No 258/97 (European Commission, 2014). The British competent authorities performed the initial assessment after Miyarisan Pharmaceutical Co. Ltd. (Tokyo, Japan) requested using *C. butyricum* on the market as a novel food ingredient used in food supplements. Some beneficial effects reported for *C. butyricum* are related to the production of SCFA and its role in lipid metabolism (Zhao et al., 2014; Shang et al., 2016). No additional assessment was necessary because further explanations provided by the applicant addressed the objections raised by member states. *C. butyricum* was authorized as novel food ingredient in food supplements at a maximum dose of 1.35×10^8 CFU per day. Intervention studies revealed the health benefits of the strain, including prevention of pouchitis in patients with ulcerative colitis and decreased incidence of side effects in patients receiving therapy for the eradication of *Helicobacter pylori* (Shimbo et al., 2005; Yasueda et al., 2016). An antibiotic resistance profile, a study for genes encoding toxins, and an animal study were conducted to ensure the safety of the strain (Isa et al., 2016). The authorized strain is a Gram-positive, spore-forming, obligate aerobic, non-pathogenic, non-genetically modified organism. The product is characterized as a white or pale gray tablet with a specific odor and sweet taste (European Commission, 2014).

Bacteroides xylanisolvens

The most recent authorization for bacteria according to Regulation (EC) No 258/97 was granted in 2015. The European Commission approved placing pasteurized milk products fermented with *B. xylanisolvens* DSM 23964 in the market as a novel food in a heat-treated, non-viable form. Details concerning *B. xylanisolvens* are discussed in the following section.

NOVEL MICROBES: DETAILS AND BACKGROUND REGARDING SAFETY

Bacteroides xylanisolvens DSM 23964

In 2015, pasteurized milk products fermented with *B. xylanisolvens* DSM 23964 were approved as a novel food under Novel Food Regulation No 258/97. Usage of this specific strain was restricted as the starter culture in the fermentation of pasteurized milk products. Only heat-treated and therefore inactivated cells of *B. xylanisolvens* were allowed in the final product (EFSA Panel on Dietetic Products, Nutrition and Allergies, 2015). In addition to the novel food evaluation, the EFSA automatically assessed *B. xylanisolvens* for admission to the QPS list. Interestingly, the EFSA revealed that the available information was not sufficient to include it in the QPS list.

The genus *Bacteroides* is a main inhabitant of the human colon, on average accounting for ~30% of intestinal microbiota, although large inter-individual variability exists (Sears, 2005). *Bacteroides* spp. is a Gram-negative, obligately anaerobic, bile resistant, non-spore forming rod originally isolated from human stool. This genus can have commensal attributes within the human body but can also promote the development of different diseases. *Bacteroides xylanisolvens* plays a major part in the fermentation and degradation of xylan and other plant fibers (Chassard et al., 2008). *Bacteroides* start colonization of the gut in the newborn child ~10 days after birth, (Gregory et al., 2015). Polysaccharides in the human diet are an important nutrition source for gut commensals, including *Bacteroides* spp. They can be metabolized into short chain fatty acids and branched chain fatty acids that are reabsorbed through the large intestine and provide an essential part of the host's daily required energy (Hooper et al., 2002).

The levels of Bacteroidetes and Firmicutes seem to be connected to obesity. Obese individuals show lower levels of Bacteroidetes and higher levels of Firmicutes in the gastro-intestinal tract. Turnbaugh and his colleagues (Turnbaugh et al., 2006) suggested that a higher Bacteroidetes/Firmicutes ratio can extract more energy from a given diet and that increased

Bacteroidetes levels in the gut led to weight loss in people with obesity.

While investigating xylan-degrading microorganisms in the human gastro-intestinal tract, Chassard et al. (2008) isolated 6 xylanolytic, Gram-negative anaerobic rods. Subsequent 16S rRNA analysis revealed that the obtained strains belonged to the genus *Bacteroides*, and after proper analysis, the 6 strains were considered to be novel species, and the researchers proposed the name *B. xylanisolvens* based on their xylan-degrading properties. The main characteristics of the designated type strain are shown in **Table 1**.

The German Federal Institute for Occupational Safety in Health (*Bundesanstalt für Arbeitsschutz und Arbeitsmedizin*, BAuA) assessed the safety of *B. xylanisolvens* as a working material (BAuA, 2011). Due to the lack of pathogenicity and diseases, the agency classified the microorganism in the lowest risk group. The recently approved strain *B. xylanisolvens DSM 23964* was first analyzed by Ulsemer and colleagues in 2011 (Ulsemer et al., 2012a,b). They isolated this strain from human feces and performed several analytical techniques to verify that it was new. Biochemical characteristics (no catalase activity, no indole production, and incapable of degrading starch), phylogenetic analysis, and DNA-DNA hybridization classified the strain as *B. xylanisolvens*. So far, the performed analyses have established no differences between the new strain and the type strain. Finally, the Random Amplification of Polymorphic DNA profile revealed significant differences, confirming the existence of the new strain *B. xylanisolvens* DSM 23964.

Scientific Opinion of the EFSA Panel on *Bacteroides xylanisolvens* DSM 23964

Following a request from the European Commission, the EFSA Panel on Dietetic Products, Nutrition and Allergies carried out additional assessment for pasteurized milk products fermented with *B. xylanisolvens* DSM 23964 as a novel food under Regulation (EC) No 258/97 (European Commission, 1997b). This strain has no history of use in the food industry, and no strain in the genus *Bacteroides* has a proven history of use in food production. The novel food status is related to low-fat and skimmed milk products fermented with *B. xylanisolvens* DSM 23964 as the starter culture. After fermentation, the product is heat treated for 1 h at 75°C, and no viable cells of *B. xylanisolvens* are found in the final product.

The relevant phenotypic and genotypic data were provided by the applicant, and the EFSA Panel considered this information regarding the characterization of *B. xylanisolvens* DSM 23964 to be sufficient. The production process was clearly described in the application, and a study to guarantee the effectiveness of the heat treatment was conducted. Consequently, the EFSA Panel deemed the applied techniques to be standardized across the dairy industry, considered that they are sufficiently described, and identified no safety concerns (EFSA Panel on Dietetic Products, Nutrition and Allergies, 2015).

The applicant also provided the anticipated intake of the product. The novel food would be marketed in liquid and semi-liquid forms in fermented, low-fat milk and skimmed milk products (fermented milk, buttermilk, yogurt, and yogurt drinks) or as a spray-dried powder (the fillings and coatings of cereals, cereal bars, fruits, and nuts). Due to a lack of European data, the applicant used consumption data from the United States. A conservative scenario was used to estimate the intake, proposing that the applicant's products would replace all existing products (e.g., yogurt and buttermilk; EFSA Panel on Dietetic Products, Nutrition and Allergies, 2015).

The applicant provided compositional data for spray-dried skimmed milk cultured with *B. xylanisolvens* DSM 23964, including an overview of relevant macronutrients. The applicant also supplied an overview of the vitamin B2, vitamin B12, free lysine, and furosine (as a marker for Maillard reaction) content to ensure that the heat treatment had no impact on these vitamins. Although, lactose content was missing from the analysis (a comparable amount to traditional products was assumed), the EFSA Panel considered consumption of the novel food to not be nutritionally disadvantageous.

The applicant also provided toxicological information about the novel food, including a study on an intraperitoneal abscess formation model in mice (Ulsemer et al., 2012b). Abscess formation is a relevant pathology because some species in the genus *Bacteroides*, such as *B. fragilis*, can induce abscesses on multiple sites in the body. *B. xylanisolvens* DSM 23964 was

TABLE 1 | General characteristics of *Bacteroides xylanisolvens*.

Phylum	Class	Order	Family	Genus	Species
Bacteroidetes	Bacteroidetes	Bacteroidales	Bacteroidaceae	*Bacteroides*	*Bacteroides xylanisolvens*
Type strain	DSM 188367 (XB1AT)				
Biosafety level	1				
Origin	Faecal sample from a healthy adult volunteer				
CHARACTERISTICS					
Morphology	Pleomorphic, Gram-negative, rod-shaped bacterium with rounded ends,				
	1.8–2.5 μm (length), 0.2–0.3 μm (width), no endospores, single or paired cells, no filaments				
Genome	Size: 6,059 kb, ORF's: 4,922, GC content: 41%				
Physiology	Chemo-organoheterotroph, mesophilic (25–42°C—optimum 38°C), pH optimum 6.8, obligate anaerobe				
	Indole negative, catalase negative, xylan positive, D-mannitol positive				
	No starch utilization				

administered in varying doses, but none of the mice developed abscesses. Human studies were also supplied to the EFSA (Ulsemer et al., 2012a,c).

Although, the applicant did not provide material regarding the allergenicity of the product, the EFSA panel judged that it would be unlikely that the allergenic potential would differ from that of other fermented dairy products. The EFSA itself had previously considered the effect of heat treatment on the allergenicity of milk (EFSA Panel on Dietetic Products EFSA Panel on Dietetic Products, Nutrition and Allergies, 2014).

QPS Evaluation of *B. xylanisolvens*

When the EFSA receives an application for a novel bacterial strain or a food product containing a novel strain, it conducts a mandatory, in-depth evaluation based on the QPS scheme. Consequently, after the EFSA Panel on Dietetic Products, Nutrition, and Allergies was asked to perform an additional assessment on *B. xylanisolvens* DSM 23964, the EFSA Panel on Biological Hazards (BIOHAZ) conducted a QPS assessment for *B. xylanisolvens* (EFSA Panel on Biological Hazards, 2014). This panel found that the published studies about *B. xylanisolvens* were not sufficient to include the organism on the QPS list, although no relevant safety concerns could be established.

The *cepA* gene in the genomic DNA of *B. xylanisolvens* DSM 23964 provides the strain with resistance to β-lactam antibiotics (Ulsemer et al., 2012b). This resistance is very common in the genus *Bacteroides* (Wexler, 2007). No mobile elements, such as conjugative transposons and plasmids, were found. The strain was also screened for 8 potential virulence genes common in other *Bacteroides* species, but none was detected, and *B. xylanisolvens* DSM 23964 showed no adhesion to Caco-2 cells in the cell culture model (Ulsemer et al., 2012b). The panel considered transfer of genes unlikely to take place due to the heat inactivation and lack of plasmids.

The panel emphasized that the body of knowledge was insufficient. *B. xylanisolvens* had no history of use in fermentation processes, and the few existing studies were limited to fermented milk products. Although, safety concerns do not seem likely, the panel found the number of published studies to be too low to definitely exclude safety issues. The pilot studies involved only small, healthy cohorts, and the administered bacterial cells were inactivated. Considering all these arguments, the panel did not recommend putting *B. xylanisolvens* on the QPS list (EFSA Panel on Biological Hazards, 2014).

Bacteroides xylanisolvens and Its Beneficial Properties

Most bacteria found in the human intestine are anaerobic. Among the many requirements for a bacterial strain to be categorized as probiotic, an essential characteristic is survival along the gastro-intestinal tract to finally provide beneficial effects for the host. *B. xylanisolvens* DSM 23964 had a survival rate of 90% after spending 3 h in simulated gastric juice and a survival rate of 96% after spending 4 h in simulated intestinal juices (Ulsemer et al., 2012b).

Immunomodulatory properties are important attributes of probiotics. The genus *Bacteroides* achieved a higher induction of mucosal IgA production than *Lactobacillus* when co-cultured with Peyer's patches lymphocytes (Yanagibashi et al., 2009).The fermentation of dietary polysaccharides with production of SCFA by *B. xylanisolvens* is connected to health-promoting effects through lower cholesterol levels, satiety stimulation, and even an anti-carcinogenic effect (Hosseini et al., 2011).

Published studies on fermented milk products containing *B. xylanisolvens* DSM 23964 are limited to inactivated bacterial cells, but by definition, probiotics need to be alive when administered to the consumer. Moreover, despite this microorganism's high survival and ability to ferment carbohydrates, these properties are irrelevant in the context of the approved product because it contains a heat-killed strain; therefore, no survival or metabolic activity is expected.

B. xylanisolvens offers several potential beneficial properties. However, its inability to bind to epithelial cells *in vitro* (Ulsemer et al., 2012b) is a major disadvantage in the assessment of probiotic properties because the capability to bind to intestinal epithelial cells in the host is a key step in probiotic activity. As well, studies with living bacteria are needed to increase the chances of acceptance as a probiotic.

Admission of *B. xylanisolvens* as a Novel Food: Impact on Other Candidates

B. xylanisolvens is only the fourth bacterium, after *L. mesenteroides*, *B. subtilis* natto, and *C. butyricum*, to be approved under Novel Food Regulation No 258/97 (European Commission, 1997b).

The positive outcome of the novel food assessment is independent from the QPS evaluation results. *B. xylanisolvens* and *C. butyricum* have not yet been included on the QPS list. It should be pointed out that during the QPS assessment, only the species itself is analyzed, and the potential food products containing the bacteria are not of interest.

Thermal inactivated bacterial form falls out of the accepted definitions of probiotics described above, because the viability of bacterial cells is an essential condition. Nevertheless, non-viable and therefore non-culturable, and immunologically active microbial cells have been reported to provide health benefits to consumers (de Almada et al., 2016) The use of killed bacteria, as long as the beneficial effect is totally or partially retained, represent and advantage when the use of live bacteria is not authorized or may be potentially harmful for some individuals such as patients with weak immune system or under inflammatory conditions (Taverniti and Guglielmetti, 2011; Tsilingiri and Rescigno, 2012). To define the use of non-viable microorganisms which, when administered in adequate amounts, confer a benefit on the consumer the term "paraprobiotic" has been proposed (Taverniti and Guglielmetti, 2011; de Almada et al., 2016), but it still is not a wide accepted and employed term by scientific community and institutions.

Several mechanistic studies have demonstrated that specific chemical compounds isolated from bacteria can induce specific immune responses (Taverniti and Guglielmetti, 2011). In these cases, the term "postbiotic" has been proposed to refer any factor resulting from the metabolic activity of a bacteria or any released bacterial molecule capable of conferring beneficial effects to the consumer in a direct or indirect way (Tsilingiri and Rescigno, 2012; de Almada et al., 2016). But, similarly with "parabiotic" concept is not an officially accepted and used term.

The acceptance of the thermal inactivated form of *B. xylanisolvens* as a novel food may pave the way for other novel microorganisms in non-viable form or novel bacterial molecules to exert positive health impacts.

Akkermansia muciniphila

The relatively newly described species *A. muciniphila* is the first discovered taxonomic member in the genus *Akkermansia*. By June 2017, there has been no evaluation according to the QPS status, which would be performed and published by EFSA. Due to the recent description of this microorganism, it has no history of use in the food industry, so it must be treated according to the Novel Food Regulation (European Commission, 1997b).

A. muciniphila was discovered in 2004 during the search for new mucus-degrading bacteria in human fecal samples. The newly isolated organism was named after Antoon Akkermans, a well-respected Dutch microbiologist who has made significant contributions to the field of microbial ecology (Belzer and De Vos, 2012). This oval-shaped, Gram-negative microorganism belongs to the phylum Verrucomicrobia. *A. muciniphila* further belongs to the class Verrucomicrobiae, the order Verrucomicrobiales, and the family Verrucomicrobiaceae. *A. muciniphila* was originally classified as a strict anaerobe, but in the same way as other anaerobic gut colonizers such as *Bacteroides fragilis* and *Bifidobacterium adolescentis*, *A. muciniphila* can tolerate small amounts of oxygen and even can use it at low oxygen concentrations (Ouwerkerk et al., 2016b). This contrasts with some of the butyrate producing bacteria that are really strict anaerobes.

Metagenomic analysis have indicated that at least 8 additional *A. muciniphila*-related species are present in the human intestine (van Passel et al., 2011). Belzer and de Vos suggested that the genus *Akkermansia* consists of 5 distinct clades (Belzer and De Vos, 2012). Four of these 5 clades are associated with *A. muciniphila*, with sequence similarity range of 80–100%.

Nearly all investigated mammals showed *Akkermansia*-related sequences in their intestinal samples. *Akkermansia*-derived sequences are not limited to mammals but also found in other vertebrates: similar sequences were detected in zebrafish and the Burmese python (Costello et al., 2010; Roeselers et al., 2011). From the latter a new species, *Akkermansia glyciniphila* was isolated and characterized from reticulated python (Ouwerkerk et al., 2016a, 2017). These ubiquitous findings suggest that *Akkermansia* played a crucial role in the early stages of vertebrata evolution and that its presence might be related to essential functions in the intestine.

Genomic analyses revealed that the single chromosome of *A. muciniphila* has 2,176 genes with a GC content of 55.8% (Donohue and Salminen, 1996). The secretome responsible for the degradation of mucin involves 61 different proteins, representing 11% of the total protein content (Belzer and De Vos, 2012).

Akkermansia is a relatively new genus, so it is expected that additional species similar to *A. muciniphila* will be found in coming years as is illustrated by the discovery of *A. glyciniphila*. It obviously has no history of use in the food sector, and its potential areas of application should be explored.

Despite the short time since the discovery of *Akkermansia*, its basic characteristics are well-known. This organism is non-motile and specialized in degrading mucin. *A. muciniphila* is anaerobe and chemo-organotroph and can use mucin as its sole nitrogen, carbon and energy source (Derrien et al., 2004). The habitat of *Akkermansia* spp. is also well-documented due to its ubiquitous occurrence in the intestines of many vertebrates (Belzer and De Vos, 2012). The general properties of *A. muciniphila* are listed in **Table 2**.

Safety Aspects

A. muciniphila is a common inhabitant of the human intestine, accounting for 1–4% of the overall colon microbiota (Derrien et al., 2008). Currently, there are no published clinical human trials in which viable cells were administered to people. Such studies have been conducted only with animal models (Everard et al., 2013). Lagier and colleagues reported two cases in humans where *A. muciniphila* accounted for up to 80% of the total

TABLE 2 | General characteristics of *Akkermansia muciniphila* -adapted from Gomez-Gallego et al. (2016).

Phylum	Class	Order	Family	Genus	Species
Verrucomicrobia	Verrucomicrobiae	Verrucomicrobiales	Verrucomicrobiaceae	*Akkermansia*	*Akkermansia muciniphila*
Type strain	MucT (ATCC BAA-835)				
Biosafety level	1				
Origin	Faecal sample from a healthy adult volunteer				
CHARACTERISTICS					
Morphology	Gram-negative, oval-shaped, non-motile				
Genome	Size: 2,664,102 bp, ORF's: 2,176, GC content: 55.8%				
Physiology	Chemo-organotrophic, anaerobic, mesophilic (20–40°C—optimum 37°C)				
	Capable of using mucin as energy, nitrogen, and carbon source; mucolytic in pure culture				
	Sulfate release in free form from mucin fermentation				

intestinal microbiota without any noticeable decline in health (Lagier et al., 2015), and there is no evidence that *A. muciniphila* is connected to any specific disease (Derrien et al., 2010).

There are general concerns because *Akkermansia* shows pathogen-like behavior. Adhesion to mucus is considered to be a crucial step during infection but is also a behavior found in several probiotics. In contrast to pathogens, *A. muciniphila*, as a mucin degrader, stays in the outer layer of the mucus and never reaches the inner layer, which is necessary for a successful infection (Gomez-Gallego et al., 2016). In addition, mucin degradation itself resembles pathogen-like behavior (Donohue and Salminen, 1996) but is regarded as a regular process in a balanced, self-renewing intestine (Gomez-Gallego et al., 2016).

Colorectal cancer patients showed a four-fold increase of *A. muciniphila* in stool samples compared to healthy subjects (Weir et al., 2013). However, patients with colorectal cancer have reduced food intake, and studies have demonstrated that fasting correlates with increased levels *of A. muciniphila* (Remely et al., 2015). In addition, colorectal cancer is related to increased cell proliferation and mucus production; therefore, it is evident that levels of the main mucus-degrading bacterium could increase in this situation (Gomez-Gallego et al., 2016).

Overall, there seem to be no specific safety concerns regarding the genus *Akkermansia* and its type strain *A. muciniphila* MucT. Potential future concerns could be eliminated through individual, case-by-case review. There are no applications so far for *A. muciniphila* and, therefore, no history of safe use, so the QPS status of this species has not yet been determined.

Akkermansia Muciniphila as Candidate for Novel Food

Currently, there are no pending applications for products containing *A. muciniphila* under Regulation (EC) 258/97 (European Commission, 1997b). *A. muciniphila* was only discovered and isolated in 2004, so comprehensive research is still needed to better understand this microorganism.

A. muciniphila was not used for human consumption to any "significant degree" in the EU before 15 May 1997. A food business operator interested in putting a product containing *A. muciniphila* in the market would have to submit an application according to the Novel Food Regulation. The European Commission published Recommendation (European Commission, 1997a) to give food companies the information needed for a successful application. In the case of *A. muciniphila*, there are still many unknown aspects that are needed for Novel Food application, as well as some limitations: (1) specification of the possible novel products which will contain *A. muciniphila*; (2) production processes to keep *A. muciniphila* alive in the final product to fulfill its potential probiotic properties; (3) anticipated human intake taking into account the lack of known intake patterns; (4) the lack of clinical trials in humans (toxicological and nutritional assessments have been conducted only with animal models); and (5) the lack of knowledge about the allergenic potential.

Based on the knowledge acquired so far, though, this microorganism could be very interesting for food companies and consumers. *A. muciniphila* is part of the gut microbiota in all humans and may display probiotic properties due to its contribution to the functional gastro-intestinal tract. In addition, current data indicate that a decline in *A. muciniphila* in the colon correlates with several diseases, such as obesity, type-2 diabetes, and inflammatory bowel disease (Png et al., 2010; Cani and Everard, 2014; Schneeberger et al., 2015). This reduction could be related with a decrease in mucus thickness. But the complex relation between *A. muciniphila* and the mucus layer remains unclear and the administration of *A. muciniphila* might stimulate the recovery of the mucus layer (Everard et al., 2013).

Recently, *A. muciniphila* has been demonstrated to provide beneficial effects even after heat treatment for 30 min at 70°C. The heat-inactivated bacteria could reduce fat mass development, insulin resistance, and dyslipidemia in obese and diabetic mice. Some membrane proteins showed stability and interaction with Toll-like receptor 2 even during the thermal process. This membrane protein also improved the gut barrier and provided ongoing beneficial effects after bacterial inactivation (Plovier et al., 2017). Like *B. xylanisolvens*, therefore, *A. muciniphila* may enter the food market in this non-viable form.

The link between obesity and decreased levels of *A. muciniphila* extends beyond rodents. A Swedish investigation showed that obese pre-school children have significantly lower levels of *A. muciniphila* than their normal-weight peers (Karlsson et al., 2012). Similarly, pre-school infants that used macrolide antibiotics showed a higher BMI than the non-antibiotic users and this was associated with a depletion of *A.muciniphila* (Korpela et al., 2016).

Despite the growing attention to *A. muciniphila*, much research is needed to gain more specific and age-restricted information. No randomized, double-blind, placebo-controlled human clinical trials have studied the effects of *A. muciniphila* intake. Most research has involved animals, and long-term studies on the human level are the next step to take. Despite the lack of information relevant to the European Commission's recommendation on novel food, the microorganism has quite promising prospects for future novel food applications, especially for its potential probiotic health benefits.

It is important to point out that *A. muciniphila* has been detected in breast tissue (Urbaniak et al., 2014) and then has been consumed by humans via breast milk (Collado et al., 2012). The question, therefore, arises whether it is necessary to prove the safety of an organism that is already part of nutrition in the early stages of life. However, the levels of viable cells in breast milk might be much lower than those added to food products. Safety concern may arise due not to the nature of *A. muciniphila* but to the levels used in food and supplements. However, assuming around 10^{13} bacteria to be present in the human intestine, an average healthy adult may carry over 10^{11} *Akkermansia* in its colon. Further discussions are needed, but for such specific cases, European legislation needs to be modified in the future. Placement of *A. muciniphila* on the QPS list under the given conditions may be complicated because a history of safe use cannot be established.

Fructophilic Lactic Acid Bacteria: New Members of the Family

Characteristics

Long before Orla-Jensen described the group of lactic acid bacteria (LAB) in 1919, humankind benefited from their positive attributes in various food production processes (von Wright, 2012). LAB are involved in various industrial fermentation processes, such as fermented milk products and sausages. Along with fermented food production, the growing sector of probiotics represents the biggest operational area for LAB.

Fructophilic lactic acid bacteria (FLAB) constitute a subgroup in the diverse LAB order. FLAB preferably use fructose as a substrate. They show poor growth on glucose, and external electron acceptors (e.g., pyruvate, oxygen, and fructose) dramatically enhance their growth. FLAB, therefore, inhabit fructose-rich niches: flowers, fruits, fermented foods, such as wine and cocoa beans, and even the gastro-intestinal tracts of insects harbor these microorganisms (Endo, 2012). The FLAB group is divided into the genera *Fructobacillus* (its type species: *F. fructosus*) and *Lactobacillus* (Endo et al., 2009).

Four *Fructobacillus* species formerly were members of the genus *Leuconostoc*, but recent analyses suggested that their unique characteristics and phylogenetic positions supported reclassification of this bacterial group (Endo and Okada, 2008). *Fructobacillus* shows a clear preference for fructose over glucose (Endo and Okada, 2008). Several findings related to metabolism, genome size, and gene losses suggest reductive evolution in *Fructobacillus* genus compared to *Leuconostoc*, providing strong support for the reclassification and renaming of *Fructobacillus* (Endo et al., 2015).

The number of species in FLAB subgroup is growing in both genera, *Fructobacillus* and *Lactobacilllus*. Fructobacillus consists of five species: *F. fructosus, F. pseudoficulneus, F. ficulneus, F. durionis,* and *F. tropaeoli* (Endo et al., 2015). *F. fructosus* and *F. pseudoficulneus* are the most frequently detected species in natural sources. These microorganisms have been isolated from figs, bananas, flowers, the honeybee gut, wine, and even taberna, a traditional beverage in Southern Mexico (Alcantara-Hernandez et al., 2010; Endo, 2012). The FLAB members in the genus *Lactobacillus* are *L. kunkeei, L. apinorum*, and *L. florum* (Neveling et al., 2012). *L. kunkeei* was originally isolated from wine and characterized as obligately FLAB (Endo et al., 2012). Interestingly, this microorganism is the major component in the gut microbiota of honeybees (Endo and Salminen, 2013). *L. apinorum* is a recently described species from honeybees, and its fructophilic characteristic were recently reported (Maeno et al., 2017). These two lactobacilli share 98.9% sequence similarity based on 16S rRNA gene sequences. The genomic characteristics of the two species, especially the gene reduction system, are similar to *Fructobacillus* spp. but not to other members of lactobacilli, suggesting that fructose-richness induced an environment-specific gene reduction in phylogenetically distant microorganisms (Maeno et al., 2016). *L. florum* was formerly the only facultatively FLAB. It is differentiated from the obligately FLAB based on the growth ratio on glucose. *L. florum* grows more slowly on glucose than fructose. Like obligately FLAB, electron acceptors enhance growth on glucose.

Practical Impact and Safety

Although, FLAB were only recently discovered, this group of microorganisms might have great potential for the food industry. LAB are generally considered to be safe and have been involved in human food production and nutrition since ancient times (von Wright, 2012). These properties might be extended to FLAB. Recent investigations detected the presence of FLAB in many different food items. For example, several *Fructobacillus* spp. have been observed during the spontaneous cocoa bean fermentation process (Lefeber et al., 2011; Papalexandratou et al., 2011), and *L. florum* has been found in grapes and wine, possibly contributing important properties from an oenological perspective (Mtshali et al., 2012).

The presence of FLAB in the gastro-intestinal tracts of bees, giant ants, tropical fruit flies, and bumblebees indicate possible probiotic characteristics (Endo, 2012), although FLAB has not been detected in vertebrates' intestines (Endo and Salminen, 2013). Bee commensal *L. kunkeei* is considered to be a candidate for honeybee probiotics and paratransgenesis. There is no clinical evidence regarding the pathogenicity of FLAB, which might be an indicator of potential safety. However, this possibility should be treated cautiously because consumers' level of exposure to this bacterial group through food is not well known. Recent studies have suggested that administration of heat-killed *L. kunkeei* YB38 has potential beneficial properties for human health, including increased bowel movements and enhanced immunoglobulin A production (Asama et al., 2015, 2016). As in the case of *B. xylanisolvens*, therefore, *L. kunkeei* might enter the food market in thermal-treated form.

Faecalibacterium prausnitzii

Fusobacterium prausnitzii is the sole member of the genus *Faecalibacterium* and a commensal bacterium of the human gut microbiota (Miquel et al., 2013). This Gram-positive, obligately anaerobe microorganism belongs to class Clostridia. It accounts for 3–5% of total fecal bacteria and, therefore, is a predominant species in human feces (Breyner et al., 2017). *F. prausnitzii* is a non-motile, non-spore-forming bacterium and extremely sensitive to oxygen (Foditsch et al., 2014). *F. prausnitzii* was initially classified as *F. prausnitzii*, but the sequence of the 16s rRNA gene established that it is only distantly related to *Fusobacterium* and more closely related to members of *Clostridium* cluster IV (Miquel et al., 2013). The general properties of *F. prausnitzii* are listed in **Table 3**.

F. prausnitzii can digest dietary fibers producing mostly butyrate, along with other SCFA (Miquel et al., 2013), and has been shown to respond to prebiotic supplementation using a mixed chain length fructan supplement and pectin (Scott et al., 2015). This microbe may play a crucial role in human health because changes in levels of *F. prausnitzii* have been associated with several gastrointestinal diseases, such as Crohn's disease, and depressive disorders (Miquel et al., 2013; Jiang et al., 2015). The microorganism also displays beneficial anti-inflammatory effects on the host, suggesting that it may be used to counterbalance the dysbiosis linked to certain diseases (Sokol et al., 2008; Jiang et al., 2015; Miquel et al., 2015). Butyrate has several beneficial effects on the host, including

TABLE 3 | General characteristics of *Faecalibacterium prausnitzii*.

Phylum	Class	Order	Family	Genus	Species
Firmicutes	Clostridia	Clostridiales	Clostridiaceae	*Faecalibacterium*	*Faecalibacterium prausnitzii*
Type strain	ATCC 27768				
Biosafety level	1				
Origin	Faecal sample from a healthy adult volunteer				
CHARACTERISTICS					
Morphology	Gram-positive, obligately anaerobe, oval-shaped, non-motile, non-spore-forming				
Genome	Size: 3.05 Mb, ORF's: 2,745, GC content: 56.4%				
Physiology	Chemo-organotrophic, anaerobic, mesophilic (optimum 37°C), pH for growth ranges between 5.7 and 6.7				
	Butyrate, D-lactate, and formate production during glucose fermentation				
	Can utilize pectin, uronic acid, and host-derived substrates for growth				

provision of an energy source for epithelial cells, induction of colonic regulatory T cells, induction of apoptosis in human colonic carcinoma cells, inhibition of inflammatory responses in intestinal biopsy specimens, and improvement of metabolic syndrome. Moreover, recent investigations have revealed possible contributions to protective mechanisms, such as self-defense against inflammatory reactions. *F. prausnitzii* has been involved in the inhibition of pro-inflammatory cytokines and the secretion of bioactive molecules which lead to blockage of the NF-κB pathway, showing protective effects in chemically induced colitis mouse models (Breyner et al., 2017). Further research with *Faecalibacterium* could increase knowledge about its probiotic effects and may lead to its future use in the food industry.

The successful use of *F. prausnitzii* as probiotic most likely will depend on the administration method. Studies related to bacterial resistance to gastric pH *in vitro* recommend oral administration of *F. prausnitzii* after feeding to avoid low gastric pH (Breyner et al., 2017). Moreover, cultivating *F. prausnitzii* is difficult even in anaerobic conditions (Miquel et al., 2013).

The inclusion of *Faecalibacterium* on the QPS list might be difficult due to its lack of a history of safe use and to the multiple antibiotic resistance genes observed in *Faecalibacterium* sp. isolates which could contribute to resistance dissemination (Breyner et al., 2017). In addition, full toxicology assays and characterization of the strain are still needed for regulatory approval (Thomas et al., 2015).

CONCLUSIONS AND OUTLOOK

Remarks on the Candidates

A brief evaluation of the benefits and drawbacks of the new microbial candidates based on existing knowledge is given in **Table 4**. Novel microbes, including many not yet assessed in humans, are increasingly proposed as potential probiotics and assessed as novel food. The introduction of these new species further challenges the traditional selection criteria because the question of their safety and efficacy arises in an untraditional manner, with no previous experience in exposure to these bacteria or their use in foods or supplements. Most probiotics belong to well-known microbial groups (lactobacilli and bifidobacteria) with long histories of safe use, which facilitates preliminary evaluation of their safety and functionality based on the available body of knowledge about these groups. However, some newly proposed probiotics were first described, cultured, and isolated during the past decade and thus present a challenge to both scientific and regulatory frontiers. Nevertheless, *A. muciniphila*, FLAB, and *F. prausnitzii* are regarded as promising candidates. The many proven and potential probiotic properties provide good opportunities for future food authorizations, but their safety in human trials still must be demonstrated.

In the context to the definition of probiotics, Plovier and colleagues made an especially interesting observation: even the pasteurized and non-replicating *Akkermansia* cells were capable of providing beneficial effects. Decreased fat-mass development, dyslipidaemia, and insulin resistance were demonstrated in obese and diabetic mice (Everard et al., 2013). This new insight might have crucial relevance and allow future authorizations because nonviable cells pose rise fewer concerns than living bacteria. Nonviable bacteria are more easily deemed safe in novel food evaluation, albeit usually in case-by-case decisions. In comparison to *B. xylanisolvens*, some information about *A. muciniphila* is still lacking. Due to the absence of practical applications, specification of the novel food and its production process and nutritional information has not yet been performed. However, there is information available about its taxonomy, culturing methods, pathogenic and toxicological nature, and nutritional assessment data in animal models (Donohue and Salminen, 1996). A major key for the approval of novel food is a sufficient number of clinical trials in humans, but *A. muciniphila* lacks enough appropriate human studies. Randomized, double-blind, placebo-controlled clinical trials, dose-response studies, and toxicological studies are still needed to, for example, establish the appropriate number of bacteria to be administered and the right matrix to provide probiotic properties. If the missing data become available, though, *A. muciniphila* has similar chances of acceptance as a novel food as the recently officially accepted *B. xylanisolvens*. Notably the EFSA positively assessed *B. xylanisolvens* although the applicant supplied only two human studies.

FLAB were also discovered and described recently, so it is challenging to predict how they might be accepted as part of future food products. Further research is needed to

TABLE 4 | Examples of potential future probiotics suggested for human use and/or assessed as novel foods in the European Union.

Bacteria species/strain	Safety assessment in European Union	Expected impact on humans	Effects (*in vitro*)	Effects (*in vivo*)	References
Clostridium butyricum/ *Clostridium butyricum* MIYAIRI 588 *Clostridium butyricum* CGMCC0313.1	Yes	Probiotic effects suggested based on Japanese studies	Butyrate production Antitumor effect Reduction on lipogenesis	SCFAs production Prevention of antibiotic-associated diarrhea (combined with *Bifidobacterium*) Protective effect on gastric ulcers Modulation of lipid profile, insulin resistance and colon homeostasis	Nakanishi et al., 2003; Shinnoh et al., 2013; Zhao et al., 2014; Wang et al., 2015; Shang et al., 2016
Bacteroides xylanisolvens/ *Bacteroides xylanisolvens* DSM 23964 *Bacteroides xylanisolvens* XB1A	Yes, but only in the pasteurized form without any viable microbes in the product	Immune protection effects suggested	Dietary fiber degradation and fermentation	Immune modulation Toxicity and safety assessment Tolerance to a regular oral intake assessment	Mirande et al., 2010; Ulsemer et al., 2012a,b,c, 2016; Li et al., 2016
Akkermansia muciniphila	Potential evaluation models suggested Novel—no EFSA evaluation available yet	Weight control, control of low-grade inflammation and prevention of type 2 diabetes	Adherence to the intestinal mucosa and effect on enterocytes	Improvement of glucose tolerance and attenuation of adipose tissue inflammation Reduction of fat-mass gain Regulation of gut inflammation, gut barrier, and gut peptide secretion Reduction of metabolic endotoxemia Attenuation of atherosclerotic lesions	Donohue and Salminen, 1996; Everard et al., 2013; Reunanen et al., 2015; Schneeberger et al., 2015; Li et al., 2016; Yassour et al., 2016
Fructophilic lactic acid bacteria: *Lactobacillus kunkeei* *Fructobacillus fructosus* *Lactobacillus florum*	Novel—no evaluation available	Selective fermentation of fructose Production of antibacterial compounds	Antibacterial activity Fructophilic properties	Reduction of microbial pathogens	Endo et al., 2009, 2010; Endo, 2012; Endo and Salminen, 2013
Faecalibacterium prausnitzii/ *Faecalibacterium prausnitzii* A2-165	Novel—no evaluation available	Beneficial anti-inflammatory effects suggested Butyric acid production	Production of anti-inflammatory compounds Inhibition of IL-17 release in human monocytes Butyrate production	Increase of plasma anti-Th17 cytokines and suppression of IL-17 levels in both plasma and colonic mucosa Normalization of altered colonic permeability Protective effect against colitis	Miquel et al., 2013; Zhang et al., 2013; Laval et al., 2015; Ulluwishewa et al., 2015; Quevrain et al., 2016

The table includes some selected examples of reported positive health effects based on in vitro and in vivo studies.

understand, for example, what differentiates this bacterium from traditional LAB and its exact relevance to the production of fermented foods. Recent studies revealed that heat-killed *L. kunkeei* possess beneficial properties, such as increased bowel movement and enhanced immunoglobulin A production (Asama et al., 2015, 2016). Their special relation to LAB, a very widely used group in the food industry, may lead to inclusion on the QPS list and novel food authorization in the future.

The growing amount of evidence supporting that the modulation of *F. prausnitzii* levels using prebiotics, probiotics, and symbiotics might have prophylactic or therapeutic applications in human health makes this bacterium interesting from the perspective of novel foods. Factors such as sensitivity to oxygen, gastric pH, and bile salts and industrial production for probiotic use need to be optimized, and toxicological assays and antibiotic resistance tests should be carefully conducted before clinical trials in humans.

The potential candidates for novel foods discussed as examples in the present work represent only a small fraction of the potential bacteria that may be included in novel foods in the future. Other potential candidates are *Eubacterium hallii* and bacteria in the genus *Roseburia*. *E. hallii* is a common inhabitant of the human gut microbiota and is known for its versatile utilization of different carbon sources. *E. hallii* can produce butyrate from lactate, acetate, and glucose and is one of the first butyrate producers in the infant gut (Pham et al., 2016). In addition, a recent study showed the impact of *E. hallii* in treating insulin resistance in a mouse model (Udayappan et al., 2016). Its early appearance in the human intestine and production of essential SCFA may enable future novel food applications in the food industry.

The genus *Roseburia* consists of five species which are Gram-positive, obligately anaerobic bacteria and motile due to the presence of subterminal flagella (Tamanai-Shacoori et al., 2017). *Roseburia* spp. are a dominant intestinal bacterial species, accounting for 2–15% of the total human gut microbiota that produce SCFA (Dostal et al., 2015). Considering the production of essential SCFA and the high levels of *Roseburia* spp. in the human microbiota, members of this genus may have great potential as future novel probiotics.

Remarks on Regulatory Aspects

Ongoing revisions of the regulations on novel food, along with the continuous updating of the QPS list, will accelerate novel food authorization and biological agent safety assessment. Both processes support the work of the EFSA and access to novel products in the food market and ensure the safety of the European consumer. The lengthy process to revise the novel food regulations has demonstrated the difficulty of changing legislation on the European level. Most decisions need to be unanimous, and it is challenging to please all member states. Although, these developments are remarkable, the EU authorization of novel food still seems more comprehensive than the GRAS concept in the United States. The precautionary principle is a fundamental pillar of environmental, food, and health policies in the EU. Prevention of any possible harm or danger to the consumer is the most important priority, especially for marketing of food containing potentially harmful bacteria. The elimination of any possible health threat, therefore, is essential before a product is allowed to enter the European market. The European consumer is the most relevant player in European legislation although companies understandably complain about such strict conditions.

Regulation (EU) 2015/2283 on novel foods (European Commission, 2015), which will come into force on January 1, 2018, is aimed at facilitating the authorization of novel food. The EFSA is responsible for the scientific risk assessment, ensuring the shift from an individual assessment by the national competent authorities to a generic assessment. The new regulation also directs the EFSA to deliver scientific opinions within 9 months after receiving all valid applications. This mandate represents enormous time savings and a significant decrease in the financial costs for food companies submitting applications. The newly introduced data protection for approved novel food authorization will also help companies successfully compete in the food market.

AUTHOR CONTRIBUTIONS

WK, SS, and CG designed the study; TB performed the bibliographical review; TB and CG drafting the manuscript; AE, GV, MG, Wd, WK, and SS contributed with the latest achievements in their field of expertise. AE, MG, GV, Wd, WK, SS, and CG interpreted the main points related with EU legislation discussed in the review for each novel bacteria. AE, MG, GV, Wd, WK, SS, and CG discussed the final version and revising them critically. All the authors give the final approval of the version to be published.

ACKNOWLEDGMENTS

CG is a recipient of the Seneca Postdoctoral Grant from the Seneca Foundation, the Regional Agency of Science and Technology of the Region of Murcia (funded by the Education and Universities Council—Autonomous Community of the Region of Murcia, Spain).

REFERENCES

Alcantara-Hernandez, R. J., Rodriguez-Alvarez, J. A., Valenzuela-Encinas, C., Gutierrez-Miceli, F. A., Castanon-Gonzalez, H., Marsch, R., et al. (2010). The bacterial community in 'taberna' a traditional beverage of Southern Mexico. *Lett. Appl. Microbiol.* 51, 558–563. doi: 10.1111/j.1472-765X.2010.02934.x

Asama, T., Arima, T. H., Gomi, T., Keishi, T., Tani, H., Kimura, Y., et al. (2015). *Lactobacillus kunkeei* YB38 from honeybee products enhances IgA production in healthy adults. *J. Appl. Microbiol.* 119, 818–826. doi: 10.1111/jam.12889

Asama, T., Kimura, Y., Kono, T., Tatefuji, T., Hashimoto, K., and Benno, Y. (2016). Effects of heat-killed *Lactobacillus kunkeei* YB38 on human intestinal environment and bowel movement: a pilot study. *Benef. Microbes* 7, 337–344. doi: 10.3920/BM2015.0132

Aureli, P., Capurso, L., Castellazzi, A. M., Clerici, M., Giovannini, M., Morelli, L., et al. (2011). Probiotics and health: an evidence-based review. *Pharmacol. Res.* 63, 366–376. doi: 10.1016/j.phrs.2011.02.006

BAuA (2011). *Begründungspapier zur Einstufung von Bacteroides xylanisolvens in Risikogruppe 1 nach* BioStoffV. Bundesanstalt für Arbeitsschutz und Arbeitsmedizin, BAuA.

Belzer, C., and De Vos, W. M. (2012). Microbes insidefrom diversity to function: the case of Akkermansia. *ISME J.* 6, 1449–1458. doi: 10.1038/ismej.2012.6

Borresen, E. C., Henderson, A. J., Kumar, A., Weir, T. L., and Ryan, E. P. (2012). Fermented foods: patented approaches and formulations for nutritional supplementation and health promotion. *Recent Pat. Food Nutr. Agric.* 4, 134–140. doi: 10.2174/2212798411204020134

Breyner, N. M., Michon, C., de Sousa, C. S., Vilas Boas, P. B., Chain, F., Azevedo, V., et al. (2017). Microbial Anti-Inflammatory Molecule (MAM) from *Faecalibacterium prausnitzii* shows a protective effect on DNBS and DSS-induced colitis model in mice through inhibition of NF-kappaB pathway. *Front. Microbiol.* 8:114. doi: 10.3389/fmicb.2017.00114

Cammarota, G., Ianiro, G., Bibbo, S., and Gasbarrini, A. (2014). Gut microbiota modulation: probiotics, antibiotics or fecal microbiota transplantation? *Intern. Emerg. Med.* 9, 365–373. doi: 10.1007/s11739-014-1069-4.

Cani, P. D., and Everard, A. (2014). *Akkermansia muciniphila*: a novel target controlling obesity, type 2 diabetes and inflammation? *Med. Sci.* 30, 125–127. doi: 10.1051/medsci/20143002003

Chassard, C., Delmas, E., Lawson, P. A., and Bernalier-Donadille, A. (2008). *Bacteroides xylanisolvens* sp. nov., a xylan-degrading bacterium isolated from human faeces. *Int. J. Syst. Evol. Microbiol.* 58(Pt 4), 1008–1013. doi: 10.1099/ijs.0.65504-0

Cibik, R., Lepage, E., and Talliez, P. (2000). Molecular diversity of leuconostoc mesenteroides and leuconostoc citreum isolated from traditional french cheeses as revealed by RAPD fingerprinting, 16S rDNA sequencing and 16S rDNA fragment amplification. *Syst. Appl. Microbiol.* 23, 267–278. doi: 10.1016/S0723-2020(00)80014-4

Collado, M. C., Laitinen, K., Salminen, S., and Isolauri, E. (2012). Maternal weight and excessive weight gain during pregnancy modify the immunomodulatory potential of breast milk. *Pediatr. Res.* 72, 77–85. doi: 10.1038/pr.2012.42

Costello, E. K., Gordon, J. I., Secor, S. M., and Knight, R. (2010). Postprandial remodeling of the gut microbiota in Burmese pythons. *ISME J.* 4, 1375–1385. doi: 10.1038/ismej.2010.71

D'Angelo, L., Cicotello, J., Zago, M., Guglielmotti, D., Quiberoni, A., and Suarez, V. (2017). Leuconostoc strains isolated from dairy products: response against food stress conditions. *Food Microbiol.* 66, 28–39. doi: 10.1016/j.fm.2017.04.001

de Almada, C. N., Almada, C. N., Martinez, R. C. R., and Sant'Ana, A. S. (2016). Paraprobiotics: evidences on their ability to modify biological responses, inactivation methods and perspectives on their application in foods. *Trends Food Sci. Technol.* 98, 56–114. doi: 10.1016/j.tifs.2016.09.011

de Paula, A. T., Jeronymo-Ceneviva, A. B., Todorov, S. D., and Penna, A. L. B. (2015). The two faces of *Leuconostoc mesenteroides* in food systems. *Food Rev. Int.* 31, 147–171. doi: 10.1080/87559129.2014.981825

Derrien, M., Collado, M. C., Ben-Amor, K., Salminen, S., and De Vos, W. M. (2008). The mucin degrader *Akkermansia muciniphila* is an abundant resident of the human intestinal tract. *Appl. Environ. Microbiol.* 74, 1646–1648. doi: 10.1128/AEM.01226-07

Derrien, M., van Passel, M. W. J., van de Bovenkamp, J. H. B., Schipper, R. G., de Vos, W. M., and Dekker, J. (2010). Mucin-bacterial interactions in the human oral cavity and digestive tract. *Gut Microbes* 1, 254–268. doi: 10.4161/gmic.1.4.12778

Derrien, M., Vaughan, E. E., Plugge, C. M., and de Vos, W. M. (2004). *Akkermansia municiphila* gen. nov., sp. nov., a human intestinal mucin-degrading bacterium. *Int. J. Syst. Evol. Microbiol.* 54, 1469–1476. doi: 10.1099/ijs.0.02873-0

Donohue, D., and Salminen, S. (1996). Safety of probiotic bacteria. *Asia Pac. J. Clin. Nutr.* 5, 25–28.

Dostal, A., Lacroix, C., Bircher, L., Pham, V. T., Follador, R., Zimmermann, M. B., et al. (2015). Iron modulates butyrate production by a child gut microbiota *in vitro*. *MBio* 6, e01453–e01415. doi: 10.1128/mBio.01453-15

EFSA (2007). *Introduction of a Qualified Presumption of Safety (QPS) Approach for Assessment of Selected Microorganisms Referred to EFSA - Opinion of the Scientific Committee.*

EFSA Panel on Biological Hazards (2014). Statement on the update of the list of QPS-recommended biological agents intentionally added to food or feed as notified to EFSA 1: Suitability of taxonomic units notified to EFSA until October 2014. *EFSA J.* 12, 1–42. doi: 10.2903/j.efsa.2014.3938

EFSA Panel on Biological Hazards (2010). Scientific Opinion on the maintenance of the list of QPS biological agents intentionally added to food and feed (2010 update). *EFSA J.* 8, 1–56. doi: 10.2903/j.efsa.2010.1944

EFSA Panel on Dietetic Products (2016). Guidance on the preparation and presentation of an application for authorisation of a novel food in the context of Regulation (EU) 2015/2283. *EFSA J.* 14, 1–24. doi: 10.2903/j.efsa.2016.4594

EFSA Panel on Dietetic Products, Nutrition and Allergies (2014). Scientific Opinion on the evaluation of allergenic foods and food ingredients for labelling purposes. *EFSA J.* 12, 1–286. doi: 10.2903/j.efsa.2014.3894

EFSA Panel on Dietetic Products, Nutrition and Allergies (2015). Scientific Opinion on the safety of 'heat-treated milk products fermented with *Bacteroides xylanisolvens* DSM 23964' as a novel food. *EFSA J.* 13, 1–18. doi: 10.2903/j.efsa.2015.3956

Endo, A. (2012). Fructophilic lactic acid bacteria inhabit fructose-rich niches in nature. *Microb. Ecol. Health Dis.* 23, 6–12 doi: 10.3402/mehd.v23i0.18563

Endo, A., Futagawa-Endo, Y., and Dicks, L. M. (2009). Isolation and characterization of fructophilic lactic acid bacteria from fructose-rich niches. *Syst. Appl. Microbiol.* 32, 593–600. doi: 10.1016/j.syapm.2009.08.002

Endo, A., Futagawa-Endo, Y., Sakamoto, M., Kitahara, M., and Dicks, L. M. T. (2010). *Lactobacillus florum* sp. nov., a fructophilic species isolated from flowers. *Int. J. Syst. Evol. Microbiol.* 60, 2478–2482. doi: 10.1099/ijs.0.019067-0

Endo, A., Irisawa, T., Futagawa-Endo, Y., Takano, K., du Toit, M., Okada, S., et al. (2012). Characterization and emended description of *Lactobacillus kunkeei* as a fructophilic lactic acid bacterium. *Int. J. Syst. Evol. Microbiol.* 62, 500–504. doi: 10.1099/ijs.0.031054-0

Endo, A., and Okada, S. (2008). Reclassification of the genus Leuconostoc and proposals of *Fructobacillus fructosus* gen. nov., comb. nov., *Fructobacillus durionis* comb. nov., *Fructobacillus ficulneus* comb. nov. and *Fructobacillus pseudoficulneus* comb. nov. *Int. J. Syst. Evol. Microbiol.* 58(Pt 9), 2195–2205. doi: 10.1099/ijs.0.65609-0

Endo, A., and Salminen, S. (2013). Honeybees and beehives are rich sources for fructophilic lactic acid bacteria. *Syst. Appl. Microbiol.* 36, 444–448. doi: 10.1016/j.syapm.2013.06.002

Endo, A., Tanizawa, Y., Tanaka, N., Maeno, S., Kumar, H., Shiwa, Y., et al. (2015). Comparative genomics of *Fructobacillus* spp. and *Leuconostoc* spp. reveals niche-specific evolution of *Fructobacillus* spp. *BMC Genomics* 16:1117. doi: 10.1186/s12864-015-2339-x

European Commission (1997a). *97/618/EC. Commission Recommendation of 29 July 1997 Concerning the Scientific Aspects and the Presentation of Information Necessary to Support Applications for the Placing on the Market of Novel Foods and Novel Food Ingredients and the Preparation of Initial Assessment Reports Under Regulation (EC) No 258/97 of the European Parliament and of the Council.*

European Commission (1997b). *R. 285/97/ERegulation, C. (EC) No. 258/97 of the European Parliament and of the Council of 27 January 1997 Concerning Novel Foods and Novel Food Ingredients.*

European Commission (2001). *E. Commission: 2001/122/EC. Commission Decision of 30 January 2001 on Authorising the Placing on the Market of a Dextran Preparation Produced by Leuconostoc mesenteroides as a Novel Food Ingredient in Bakery Products under Regulation (EC) No 258/97 of the European Parliament and of the Council (Notified Under Document Number C(2001) 174).*

European Commission (2009). *E. Commission: 2009/345/EC. Commission Decision of 22 April 2009 Authorising the Placing on the Market of Vitamin K2 (Menaquinone) from Bacillus subtilis natto as a Novel Food Ingredient under Regulation (EC) No 258/97 of the European Parliament and of the Council (Notified Under Document Number C(2009) 2935).*

European Commission (2014). *E. Commission: 2014/907/EU. Commission Implementing Decision of 11 December 2014 Authorising the Placing on the Market of Clostridium butyricum (CBM 588) as a Novel Food Ingredient under Regulation (EC) No 258/97 of the European Parliament and of the Council (Notified Under Document C(2014) 9345).*

European Commission (2015). *R. E. 2015/2283. Regulation (EU) 2015/2283 of the European Parliament and of the Council of 25 November 2015 on Novel Foods, Amending Regulation (EU) No 1169/2011 of the European Parliament and of the Council and Repealing Regulation (EC) No 258/97 of the European Parliament and of the Council and Commission Regulation (EC) No,1852/2001.*

Everard, A., Belzer, C., Geurts, L., Ouwerkerk, J. P., Druart, C., Bindels, L. B., et al. (2013). Cross-talk between *Akkermansia muciniphila* and intestinal epithelium controls diet-induced obesity. *Proc. Natl. Acad. Sci. U.S.A.* 110, 9066–9071. doi: 10.1073/pnas.1219451110

Foditsch, C., Santos, T. M., Teixeira, A. G., Pereira, R. V., Dias, J. M., Gaeta, N., et al. (2014). Isolation and characterization of *Faecalibacterium prausnitzii* from calves and piglets. *PLoS ONE* 9:e116465. doi: 10.1371/journal.pone.0116465

Gomez-Gallego, C., Pohl, S., Salminen, S., De Vos, W. M., and Kneifel, W. (2016). *Akkermansia muciniphila*: a novel functional microbe with probiotic properties. *Benef. Microbes* 7, 571–584. doi: 10.3920/BM2016.0009

Gómez-Gallego, C., and Salminen, S. (2016). Novel probiotics and prebiotics: how can they help in human gut microbiota dysbiosis? *Appl. Food Biotechnol.* 3, 72–81. doi: 10.22037/afb.v3i2.11276

Gregory, K. E., LaPlante, R. D., Shan, G., Kumar, D. V., and Gregas, M. (2015). Mode of birth influences preterm infant intestinal colonization with bacteroides over the early neonatal period. *Adv. Neonatal Care* 15, 386–393. doi: 10.1097/ANC.0000000000000237

H. C. P. Directorate-General (2003). *Working Document on a Generic Approach to the Safety Assessment of Micro-Organisms Used in Feed/Food and Feed/Food Production.* Available online at: https://ec.europa.eu/food/sites/food/files/safety/docs/sci-com_scf_out178_en.pdf

Hill, C., Guarner, F., Reid, G., Gibson, G. R., Merenstein, D. J., Pot, B., et al. (2014). The International Scientific Association for Probiotics and Prebiotics consensus statement on the scope and appropriate use of the term probiotic. *Nat. Rev. Gastroenterol. Hepatol.* 11, 506–514. doi: 10.1038/nrgastro.2014.66

Hooper, L. V., Midtvedt, T., and Gordon, J. I. (2002). How host-microbial interactions shape the nutrient environment of the mammalian intestine. *Annu. Rev. Nutr.* 22, 283–307. doi: 10.1146/annurev.nutr.22.011602.092259

Hosseini, E., Grootaert, C., Verstraete, W., and Van de Wiele, T. (2011). Propionate as a health-promoting microbial metabolite in the human gut. *Nutr. Rev.* 69, 245–258. doi: 10.1111/j.1753-4887.2011.00388.x

Isa, K., Oka, K., Beauchamp, N., Sato, M., Wada, K., Ohtani, K., et al. (2016). Safety assessment of the Clostridium butyricum MIYAIRI 588(R) probiotic strain including evaluation of antimicrobial sensitivity and presence of Clostridium toxin genes *in vitro* and teratogenicity *in vivo*. *Hum. Exp. Toxicol.* 35, 818–832. doi: 10.1177/0960327115607372

Jiang, H., Ling, Z., Zhang, Y., Mao, H., Ma, Z., Yin, Y., et al. (2015). Altered fecal microbiota composition in patients with major depressive disorder. *Brain Behav. Immun.* 48, 186–194. doi: 10.1016/j.bbi.2015.03.016

Karlsson, C. L., Önnerfält, J., Xu, J., Molin, G., Ahrné, S., and Thorngren-Jerneck, K. (2012). The microbiota of the gut in preschool children with normal and excessive body weight. *Obesity* 20, 2257–2261. doi: 10.1038/oby.2012.110

Korpela, K., Salonen, A., Virta, L. J., Kekkonen, R. A., Forslund, K., Bork, P., et al. (2016). Intestinal microbiome is related to lifetime antibiotic use in Finnish pre-school children. *Nat. Commun.* 7:10410. doi: 10.1038/ncomms10410

Lagier, J. C., Hugon, P., Khelaifia, S., Fournier, P. E., La Scola, B., and Raoult, D. (2015). The rebirth of culture in microbiology through the example of culturomics to study human gut microbiota. *Clin. Microbiol. Rev.* 28, 237–264. doi: 10.1128/CMR.00014-14

Laval, L., Martin, R., Natividad, J. N., Chain, F., Miquel, S., Desclee de Maredsous, C., et al. (2015). *Lactobacillus rhamnosus* CNCM I-3690 and the commensal bacterium *Faecalibacterium prausnitzii* A2-165 exhibit similar protective effects to induced barrier hyper-permeability in mice. *Gut Microbes* 6, 1–9. doi: 10.4161/19490976.2014.990784

Lefeber, T., Gobert, W., Vrancken, G., Camu, N., and De Vuyst, L. (2011). Dynamics and species diversity of communities of lactic acid bacteria and acetic acid bacteria during spontaneous cocoa bean fermentation in vessels. *Food Microbiol.* 28, 457–464. doi: 10.1016/j.fm.2010.10.010

Leuschner, R. G. K., Robinson, T. P., Hugas, M., Cocconcelli, P. S., Richard-Forget, F., Klein, G., et al. (2010). Qualified presumption of safety (QPS): a generic risk assessment approach for biological agents notified to the European Food Safety Authority (EFSA). *Trends Food Sci. Technol.* 21, 425–435. doi: 10.1016/j.tifs.2010.07.003

Li, M., Li, G., Shang, Q., Chen, X., Liu, W., Pi, X. E., et al. (2016). *In vitro* fermentation of alginate and its derivatives by human gut microbiota. *Anaerobe* 39, 19–25. doi: 10.1016/j.anaerobe.2016.02.003

Maeno, S., Dicks, L., Nakagawa, J., and Endo, A. (2017). *Lactobacillus apinorum* belongs to the fructophilic lactic acid bacteria. *Biosci. Microb. Food Health.* doi: 10.12938/bmfh.17-008

Maeno, S., Tanizawa, Y., Kanesaki, Y., Kubota, E., Kumar, H., Dicks, L., et al. (2016). Genomic characterization of a fructophilic bee symbiont *Lactobacillus kunkeei* reveals its niche-specific adaptation. *Syst. Appl. Microbiol.* 39, 516–526. doi: 10.1016/j.syapm.2016.09.006

Marchesi, J. R., Adams, D. H., Fava, F., Hermes, G. D., Hirschfield, G. M., Hold, G., et al. (2016). The gut microbiota and host health: a new clinical frontier. *Gut* 65, 330–339. doi: 10.1136/gutjnl-2015-309990

Miquel, S., Beaumont, M., Martín, R., Langella, P., Braesco, V., and Thomas, M. (2015). A proposed framework for an appropriate evaluation scheme for microorganisms as novel foods with a health claim in Europe. *Microb. Cell Fact.* 9, 14–48. doi: 10.1186/s12934-015-0229-1

Miquel, S., Martin, R., Rossi, O., Bermudez-Humaran, L. G., Chatel, J. M., Sokol, H., et al. (2013). *Faecalibacterium prausnitzii* and human intestinal health. *Curr. Opin. Microbiol.* 16, 255–261. doi: 10.1016/j.mib.2013.06.003

Mirande, C., Kadlecikova, E., Matulova, M., Capek, P., Bernalier-Donadille, A., Forano, E., et al. (2010). Dietary fibre degradation and fermentation by two xylanolytic bacteria *Bacteroides xylanisolvens* XB1AT and Roseburia intestinalis XB6B4 from the human intestine. *J. Appl. Microbiol.* 109, 451–460. doi: 10.1111/j.1365-2672.2010.04671.x

Mtshali, P. S., Divol, B., and du Toit, M. (2012). Identification and characterization of Lactobacillus florum strains isolated from South African grape and wine samples. *Int. J. Food Microbiol.* 153, 106–113. doi: 10.1016/j.ijfoodmicro.2011.10.023

Nakanishi, S., Kataoka, K., Kuwahara, T., and Ohnishi, Y. (2003). Effects of high amylose maize starch and Clostridium butyricum on microbiota and formation metabolism in colonic of azoxymethane-induced aberrant crypt foci in the rat colon. *Microbiol. Immunol.* 47, 951–958. doi: 10.1111/j.1348-0421.2003.tb03469.x

Neveling, D. P., Endo, A., and Dicks, L. M. (2012). Fructophilic *Lactobacillus kunkeei* and *Lactobacillus brevis* isolated from fresh flowers, bees and bee-hives. *Curr. Microbiol.* 65, 507–515. doi: 10.1007/s00284-012-0186-4

Ouwerkerk, J. P., Aalvink, S., Belzer, C., and de Vos, W. M. (2016a). *Akkermansia glycaniphila* sp. nov., an anaerobic mucin-degrading bacterium isolated from reticulated python faeces. *Int. J. Syst. Evol. Microbiol.* 66, 4614–4620. doi: 10.1099/ijsem.0.001399

Ouwerkerk, J. P., Koehorst, J. J., Schaap, P. J., Ritari, J., Paulin, L., Belzer, C., et al. (2017). Complete genome sequence of *Akkermansia glycaniphila* strain Pyt^T, a mducin-degrading specialist of the reticulated python gut. *Genome Announc.* 5:e01098-16. doi: 10.1128/genomeA.01098-16

Ouwerkerk, J. P., van der Ark, K. C., Davids, M., Claassens, N. J., Robert Finestra, T., de Vos, W., et al. (2016b). Adaptation of *Akkermansia muciniphila* to the oxic-anoxic interface of the mucus layer. *Appl. Environ. Microbiol.* 82, 6983–6993. doi: 10.1128/AEM.01641-16

Papalexandratou, Z., Vrancken, G., De Bruyne, K., Vandamme, P., and De Vuyst, L. (2011). Spontaneous organic cocoa bean box fermentations in Brazil are characterized by a restricted species diversity of lactic acid bacteria and acetic acid bacteria. *Food Microbiol.* 28, 1326–1338. doi: 10.1016/j.fm.2011.06.003

Pham, V. T., Lacroix, C., Braegger, C. P., and Chassard, C. (2016). Early colonization of functional groups of microbes in the infant gut. *Environ. Microbiol.* 18, 2246–2258. doi: 10.1111/1462-2920.13316

Plovier, H., Everard, A., Druart, C., Depommier, C., Van Hul, M., Geurts, L., et al. (2017). A purified membrane protein from *Akkermansia muciniphila* or the pasteurized bacterium improves metabolism in obese and diabetic mice. *Nat. Med.* 23, 107–113. doi: 10.1038/nm.4236

Png, C. W., Lindén, S. K., Gilshenan, K. S., Zoetendal, E. G., McSweeney, C. S., Sly, L., et al. (2010). Mucolytic bacteria with increased prevalence in IBD mucosa augment *in vitro* utilization of mucin by other bacteria. *Am. J. Gastroenterol.* 105, 2420–2428. doi: 10.1038/ajg.2010.281

Quevrain, E., Maubert, M. A., Sokol, H., Devreese, B., and Seksik, P. (2016). The presence of the anti-inflammatory protein MAM, from *Faecalibacterium prausnitzii*, in the intestinal ecosystem. *Gut.* 65:882. doi: 10.1136/gutjnl-2015-311094

Remely, M., Hippe, B., Geretschlaeger, I., Stegmayer, S., Hoefinger, I., and Haslberger, A. (2015). Increased gut microbiota diversity and abundance of *Faecalibacterium prausnitzii* and Akkermansia after fasting: a pilot study. *Wien. Klin. Wochenschr.* 127, 394–398. doi: 10.1007/s00508-015-0755-1

Reunanen, J., Kainulainen, V., Huuskonen, L., Ottman, N., Belzer, C., Huhtinen, H., et al. (2015). *Akkermansia muciniphila* adheres to enterocytes and strengthens the integrity of the epithelial cell layer. *Appl. Environ. Microbiol.* 81, 3655–3662. doi: 10.1128/AEM.04050-14

Roeselers, G., Mittge, E. K., Stephens, W. Z., Parichy, D. M., Cavanaugh, C. M., Guillemin, K., et al. (2011). Evidence for a core gut microbiota in the zebrafish. *ISME J.* 5, 1595–1608. doi: 10.1038/ismej.2011.38

Schneeberger, M., Everard, A., Gomez-Valades, A. G., Matamoros, S., Ramirez, S., Delzenne, N. M., et al. (2015). *Akkermansia muciniphila* inversely correlates with the onset of inflammation, altered adipose tissue metabolism and metabolic disorders during obesity in mice. *Sci. Rep.* 5:16643. doi: 10.1038/srep16643

Scott, K. P., Antoine, J. M., Midtvedt, T., and van Hemert, S. (2015). Manipulating the gut microbiota to maintain health and treat disease. *Microb. Ecol. Health Dis.* 26:25877. doi: 10.3402/mehd.v26.25877

Sears, C. L. (2005). A dynamic partnership: celebrating our gut flora. *Anaerobe* 11, 247–251. doi: 10.1016/j.anaerobe.2005.05.001

Selhub, E. M., Logan, A. C., and Bested, A. C. (2014). Fermented foods, microbiota, and mental health: ancient practice meets nutritional psychiatry. *J. Physiol. Anthropol.* 33:2 doi: 10.1186/1880-6805-33-2

Shang, H., Sun, J., and Chen, Y. Q. (2016). Clostridium butyricum CGMCC0313.1 modulates lipid profile, insulin resistance and colon homeostasis in obese mice. *PLoS ONE* 11:e0154373. doi: 10.1371/journal.pone.0154373

Shimbo, I., Yamaguchi, T., Odaka, T., Nakajima, K., Koide, A., Koyama, H., et al. (2005). Effect of *Clostridium butyricum* on fecal flora in *Helicobacter pylori* eradication therapy. *World J. Gastroenterol.* 11, 7520–7524. doi: 10.3748/wjg.v11.i47.7520

Shinnoh, M., Horinaka, M., Yasuda, T., Yoshikawa, S., Morita, M., Yamada, T., et al. (2013). *Clostridium butyricum* MIYAIRI 588 shows antitumor effects by enhancing the release of TRAIL from neutrophils through MMP-8. *Int. J. Oncol.* 42, 903–911. doi: 10.3892/ijo.2013.1790

Sokol, H., Pigneur, B., Watterlot, L., Lakhdari, O., Bermudez-Humaran, L. G., Gratadoux, J. J., et al. (2008). *Faecalibacterium prausnitzii* is an anti-inflammatory commensal bacterium identified by gut microbiota analysis of Crohn disease patients. *Proc. Natl. Acad. Sci. U.S.A.* 105, 16731–16736. doi: 10.1073/pnas.0804812105

Tamanai-Shacoori, Z., Smida, I., Bousarghin, L., Loreal, O., Meuric, V., Fong, S. B., et al. (2017). *Roseburia* spp.: a marker of health? *Future Microbiol.* 12, 157–170. doi: 10.2217/fmb-2016-0130

Taverniti, V., and Guglielmetti, S. (2011). The immunomodulatory properties of probiotic microorganisms beyond their viability (ghost probiotics: proposal of paraprobiotic concept). *Genes Nutr.* 6, 261–274. doi: 10.1007/s12263-011-0218-x

Thomas, L. V., Suzuki, K., and Zhao, J. (2015). Probiotics: a proactive approach to health. A symposium report. *Br. J. Nutr.* 114(Suppl. 1), S1–S15. doi: 10.1017/S0007114515004043

Thorning, T. K., Raben, A., Tholstrup, T., Soedamah-Muthu, S. S., Givens, I., and Astrup, A. (2016). Milk and dairy products: good or bad for human health? An assessment of the totality of scientific evidence. *Food Nutr. Res.* 60:32527. doi: 10.3402/fnr.v60.32527

Tsilingiri, K., and Rescigno, M. (2012). Postbiotics: what else? *Benef. Microbes* 4, 101–107. doi: 10.3920/BM2012.0046

Turnbaugh, P. J., Ley, R. E., Mahowald, M. A., Magrini, V., Mardis, E. R., and Gordon, J. I. (2006). An obesity-associated gut microbiome with increased capacity for energy harvest. *Nature* 444, 1027–1031. doi: 10.1038/nature05414

Udayappan, S., Manneras-Holm, L., Chaplin-Scott, A., Belzer, C., Herrema, H., Dallinga-Thie, G. M., et al. (2016). Oral treatment with. *Npj Biofilms Microb.* 2, 1–10. doi: 10.1038/npjbiofilms.2016.9

Ulluwishewa, D., Anderson, R. C., Young, W., McNabb, W. C., van Baarlen, P., Moughan, P. J., et al. (2015). Live *Faecalibacterium prausnitzii* in an apical anaerobic model of the intestinal epithelial barrier. *Cell. Microbiol.* 17, 226–240. doi: 10.1111/cmi.12360

Ulsemer, P., Toutounian, K., Kressel, G., Goletz, C., Schmidt, J., Karsten, U., et al. (2016). Impact of oral consumption of heat-treated *Bacteroides xylanisolvens* DSM 23964 on the level of natural TFα-specific antibodies in human adults. *Benef. Microbes* 6:16. doi: 10.3920/BM2015.0143

Ulsemer, P., Toutounian, K., Kressel, G., Schmidt, J., Karsten, U., Hahn, A., et al. (2012a). Safety and tolerance of *Bacteroides xylanisolvens* DSM 23964 in healthy adults. *Benef. Microbes* 3, 99–111. doi: 10.3920/BM2011.0051

Ulsemer, P., Toutounian, K., Schmidt, J., Karsten, U., and Goletz, S. (2012b). Preliminary safety evaluation of a new *Bacteroides xylanisolvens* isolate. *Appl. Environ. Microbiol.* 78, 528–535. doi: 10.1128/AEM.06641-11

Ulsemer, P., Toutounian, K., Schmidt, J., Leuschner, J., Karsten, U., and Goletz, S. (2012c). Safety assessment of the commensal strain *Bacteroides xylanisolvens* DSM 23964. *Regul. Toxicol. Pharmacol.* 62, 336–346. doi: 10.1016/j.yrtph.2011.10.014

Urbaniak, C., Cummins, J., Brackstone, M., MacKlaim, J. M., Gloor, G. B., Baban, C. K., et al. (2014). Microbiota of human breast tissue. *Appl. Environ. Microbiol.* 80, 3007–3014. doi: 10.1128/AEM.00242-14

van Passel, M. W. J., Kant, R., Zoetendal, E. G., Plugge, C. M., Derrien, M., Malfatti, S., et al. (2011). The genome of *Akkermansia muciniphila*, a dedicated intestinal mucin degrader, and its use in exploring intestinal metagenomes. *PLoS ONE* 6:e16876. doi: 10.1371/journal.pone.0016876

von Wright, A. (2012). Microbes for human and animal consumption. *Benef. Microorg. Agric. Food Environ.* 27–40 doi: 10.1079/9781845938109.0027

Wang, F.-Y., Liu, J.-M., Luo, H.-H., Liu, A.-H., and Jiang, Y. (2015). Potential protective effects of *Clostridium butyricum* on experimental gastric ulcers in mice. *World J. Gastroenterol.* 21, 8340–8351. doi: 10.3748/wjg.v21.i27.8340

Weir, T. L., Manter, D. K., Sheflin, A. M., Barnett, B. A., Heuberger, A. L., and Ryan, E. P. (2013). Stool microbiome and metabolome differences between colorectal cancer patients and healthy adults. *PLoS ONE* 8:e70803. doi: 10.1371/journal.pone.0070803

Wexler, H. M. (2007). Bacteroides: the good, the bad, and the nitty-gritty. *Clin. Microbiol. Rev.* 20, 593–621. doi: 10.1128/CMR.00008-07

Yanagibashi, T., Hosono, A., Oyama, A., Tsuda, M., Hachimura, S., Takahashi, Y., et al. (2009). Bacteroides induce higher IgA production than Lactobacillus by increasing activation-induced cytidine deaminase expression in B cells in murine Peyer's patches. *Biosci. Biotechnol. Biochem.* 73, 372–377. doi: 10.1271/bbb.80612

Yassour, M., Lim, M. Y., Yun, H. S., Tickle, T. L., Sung, J., Song, Y. M., et al. (2016). Sub-clinical detection of gut microbial biomarkers of obesity and type 2 diabetes. *Genome Med.* 8:17. doi: 10.1186/s13073-016-0271-6

Yasueda, A., Mizushima, T., Nezu, R., Sumi, R., Tanaka, M., Nishimura, J., et al. (2016). The effect of *Clostridium butyricum* MIYAIRI on the prevention of pouchitis and alteration of the microbiota profile in patients with ulcerative colitis. *Surg Today* 46, 939–949. doi: 10.1007/s00595-015-1261-9

Zhang, X., Shen, D., Fang, Z., Jie, Z., Qiu, X., Zhang, C., et al. (2013). Human gut microbiota changes reveal the progression of glucose intolerance. *PLoS ONE* 8:e71108. doi: 10.1371/journal.pone.0071108

Zhao, X., Guo, Y., Liu, H., Gao, J., and Nie, W. (2014). *Clostridium butyricum* reduce lipogenesis through bacterial wall components and butyrate. *Appl. Microbiol. Biotechnol.* 98, 7549–7557. doi: 10.1007/s00253-014-5829-x

Permissions

All chapters in this book were first published by Frontiers; hereby published with permission under the Creative Commons Attribution License or equivalent. Every chapter published in this book has been scrutinized by our experts. Their significance has been extensively debated. The topics covered herein carry significant findings which will fuel the growth of the discipline. They may even be implemented as practical applications or may be referred to as a beginning point for another development.

The contributors of this book come from diverse backgrounds, making this book a truly international effort. This book will bring forth new frontiers with its revolutionizing research information and detailed analysis of the nascent developments around the world.

We would like to thank all the contributing authors for lending their expertise to make the book truly unique. They have played a crucial role in the development of this book. Without their invaluable contributions this book wouldn't have been possible. They have made vital efforts to compile up to date information on the varied aspects of this subject to make this book a valuable addition to the collection of many professionals and students.

This book was conceptualized with the vision of imparting up-to-date information and advanced data in this field. To ensure the same, a matchless editorial board was set up. Every individual on the board went through rigorous rounds of assessment to prove their worth. After which they invested a large part of their time researching and compiling the most relevant data for our readers.

The editorial board has been involved in producing this book since its inception. They have spent rigorous hours researching and exploring the diverse topics which have resulted in the successful publishing of this book. They have passed on their knowledge of decades through this book. To expedite this challenging task, the publisher supported the team at every step. A small team of assistant editors was also appointed to further simplify the editing procedure and attain best results for the readers.

Apart from the editorial board, the designing team has also invested a significant amount of their time in understanding the subject and creating the most relevant covers. They scrutinized every image to scout for the most suitable representation of the subject and create an appropriate cover for the book.

The publishing team has been an ardent support to the editorial, designing and production team. Their endless efforts to recruit the best for this project, has resulted in the accomplishment of this book. They are a veteran in the field of academics and their pool of knowledge is as vast as their experience in printing. Their expertise and guidance has proved useful at every step. Their uncompromising quality standards have made this book an exceptional effort. Their encouragement from time to time has been an inspiration for everyone.

The publisher and the editorial board hope that this book will prove to be a valuable piece of knowledge for researchers, students, practitioners and scholars across the globe.

List of Contributors

Miroslav Dinić, Jovanka Lukić, Jelena Djokić, Ivana Strahinić, Nataša Golić and Jelena Begović
Laboratory for Molecular Microbiology, Institute of Molecular Genetics and Genetic Engineering, University of Belgrade, Belgrade, Serbia

Marina Milenković
Department of Microbiology and Immunology, Faculty of Pharmacy, University of Belgrade, Belgrade, Serbia

Arantxa López-López, Anny Camelo-Castillo, María D. Ferrer, Áurea Simon-Soro and Alex Mira
Department of Health and Genomics, Center for Advanced Research in Public Health, FISABIO Foundation, Valencia, Spain

Paulraj Kanmani and Haruki Kitazawa
Food and Feed Immunology Group, Laboratory of Animal Products Chemistry, Graduate School of Agricultural Science, Tohoku University, Sendai, Japan
Livestock Immunology Unit, International Education and Research Center for Food and Agricultural Immunology, Graduate School of Agricultural Science, Tohoku University, Sendai, Japan

Patricia Clua and Susana Alvarez
Immunobiotics Research Group, Tucuman, Argentina
Laboratory of Immunobiotechnology, Reference Centre for Lactobacilli (CERELA-CONICET), Tucuman, Argentina

Julio Villena
Food and Feed Immunology Group, Laboratory of Animal Products Chemistry, Graduate School of Agricultural Science, Tohoku University, Sendai, Japan
Immunobiotics Research Group, Tucuman, Argentina
Laboratory of Immunobiotechnology, Reference Centre for Lactobacilli (CERELA-CONICET), Tucuman, Argentina

Maria G. Vizoso-Pinto
Faculty of Medicine, INSIBIO (UNT-CONICET), National University of Tucuman, Tucuman, Argentina

Cecilia Rodriguez
Laboratory of Genetics, Reference Centre for Lactobacilli (CERELA-CONICET), Tucuman, Argentina

Vyacheslav Melnikov
Gabrichevsky Institute of Epidemiology and Microbiology, Moscow, Russia
Central Research Institute of Epidemiology, Moscow, Russia

Hideki Takahashi
Laboratory of Plant Pathology, Graduate School of Agricultural Science, Tohoku University, Sendai, Japan
Plant Immunology Unit, International Education and Research Center for Food and Agricultural Immunology, Graduate School of Agricultural Science, Tohoku University, Sendai, Japan

Ye Wang
Institute of Genetic Engineering, Jinan University, Guangzhou, China
Guangdong Provincial Key Laboratory of Gastroenterology, Department of Gastroenterology, Institute of Gastroenterology, Nanfang Hospital, Southern Medical University, Guangzhou, China

Yang Bai and Fachao Zhi
Guangdong Provincial Key Laboratory of Gastroenterology, Department of Gastroenterology, Institute of Gastroenterology, Nanfang Hospital, Southern Medical University, Guangzhou, China

Yafang Tan, Yanping Han, Xiaoyi Wang, Zongmin Du, Ruifu Yang and Yujing Bi
State Key Laboratory of Pathogen and Biosecurity, Beijing Institute of Microbiology and Epidemiology, Beijing, China

Huimin Deng and Zhengchao Li
Guangdong Provincial Key Laboratory of Gastroenterology, Department of Gastroenterology, Institute of Gastroenterology, Nanfang Hospital, Southern Medical University, Guangzhou, China
State Key Laboratory of Pathogen and Biosecurity, Beijing Institute of Microbiology and Epidemiology, Beijing, China

Yangyang Liu
Guangzhou ZhiYi biotechnology Co. Ltd., Guangzhou, China

Rizwana Parveen Rani and Abraham David Ravindran
Department of Biology, The Gandhigram Rural Institute - Deemed University, Gandhigram, India

Marimuthu Anandharaj
Biodiversity Research Center, Academia Sinica, Taipei, Taiwan

Racha El Hage, Emma Hernandez-Sanabria and Tom Van de Wiele
Center for Microbial Ecology and Technology, Faculty of Bioscience Engineering, Ghent University, Ghent, Belgium

Masaki Ishii
Genome Pharmaceuticals Institute Co. Ltd., Tokyo, Japan

Satoshi Nishida
Genome Pharmaceuticals Institute Co. Ltd., Tokyo, Japan
Laboratory of Microbiology, Graduate School of Pharmaceutical Sciences, The University of Tokyo, Tokyo, Japan
Department of Microbiology and Immunology, Teikyo University School of Medicine, Tokyo, Japan

Kazuhisa Sekimizu
Genome Pharmaceuticals Institute Co. Ltd., Tokyo, Japan
Laboratory of Microbiology, Graduate School of Pharmaceutical Sciences, The University of Tokyo, Tokyo, Japan
Teikyo University Institute of Medical Mycology, Tokyo, Japan

Yayoi Nishiyama and Shigeru Abe
Teikyo University Institute of Medical Mycology, Tokyo, Japan

Irfan A. Rather and Yong-Ha Park
Department of Applied Microbiology and Biotechnology, School of Biotechnology, Yeungnam University, Gyeongsan, South Korea

Vivek K. Bajpai and Young-Kyu Han
Department of Energy and Materials Engineering, Dongguk University, Seoul, South Korea

Yun Suk Huh
Department of Biological Engineering, Inha University, Incheon, South Korea

Eijaz A. Bhat
Department of Biochemistry, Yeungnam University Gyeongsan, South Korea

Jeongheui Lim and Woon K. Paek
National Science Museum, Ministry of Science, ICT and Future Planning, Daejeon, South Korea

Philippe Langella and Luis G. Bermúdez-Humarán
INRA, Commensal and Probiotics-Host Interactions Laboratory, Micalis Institute, AgroParisTech, Paris, France

Miguel A. Rodriguez-Carvajal
Department of Organic Chemistry, Universidad de Sevilla, Sevilla, Spain

Thibault Allain
INRA, Commensal and Probiotics-Host Interactions Laboratory, Micalis Institute, AgroParisTech, Paris, France
UMR 7245, Muséum National d'Histoire Naturelle, Centre National de la Recherche Scientifique, Sorbonne Universités, Paris, France

Soraya Chaouch, Marie-Agnès Travers, Philippe Grellier and Isabelle Florent
UMR 7245, Muséum National d'Histoire Naturelle, Centre National de la Recherche Scientifique, Sorbonne Universités, Paris, France

Myriam Thomas, Isabelle Valle and Bruno Polack
INRA, Ecole Nationale Vétérinaire d'Alfort, BIPAR, ENVA, ANSES, UMR, Université Paris-Est, Champs-sur-Marne, France
INRA, Laboratoire de Santé Animale, BIPAR, ENVA, ANSES, UMR, Maisons-Alfort, France

Yasuo Ono
Department of Microbiology and Immunology, Teikyo University School of Medicine, Tokyo, Japan

Nuria Castro-Bravo, Claudio Hidalgo-Cantabrana, Patricia Ruas-Madiedo and Abelardo Margolles
Department of Microbiology and Biochemistry of Dairy Products, Instituto de Productos Lácteos de Asturias - Consejo Superior de Investigaciones Científicas, Villaviciosa, Spain

David Rios-Covian, Nuria Salazar, Miguel Gueimonde and Clara G. de los Reyes-Gavilan
Department of Microbiology and Biochemistry of Dairy Products, Instituto de Productos Lácteos de Asturias, Consejo Superior de Investigaciones Científicas (IPLA-CSIC), Villaviciosa, Asturias, Spain

Federico Baruzzi, Silvia de Candia, Laura Quintieri and Leonardo Caputo
Institute of Sciences of Food Production, National Research Council of Italy (ISPA-CNR), Bari, Italy

Francesca De Leo
Institute of Biomembranes, Bioenergetic and Molecular Biotechnologies, National Research Council of Italy (IBIOM-CNR), Bari, Italy

Jason B. Navarro, Lauren Mashburn-Warren, Lauren O. Bakaletz and Steven D. Goodman
Center for Microbial Pathogenesis, The Research Institute at Nationwide Children's Hospital, Columbus, OH, USA

Joshua B. Simpson
Department of Chemistry, College of Arts and Sciences, University of North Carolina, Chapel Hill, NC, United States

Michael T. Bailey
Center for Microbial Pathogenesis, The Research Institute at Nationwide Children's Hospital, Columbus, OH, USA
Wexner Medical Center, Institute for Behavioral Medicine Research, The Ohio State University, Columbus, OH, USA

Jason W. Arnold, Jakub Kwintkiewicz and M. Andrea Azcarate-Peril
Division of Gastroenterology and Hepatology, Department of Medicine, Microbiome Core Facility, Center for Gastrointestinal Biology and Disease, School of Medicine, University of North Carolina, Chapel Hill, NC, United States

Patrice D. Cani
Walloon Excellence in Life Sciences and Biotechnology (WELBIO), Metabolism and Nutrition Research Group, Louvain Drug Research Institute, Université catholique de Louvain, Brussels, Belgium

Willem M. de Vos
Laboratory of Microbiology, Wageningen University, Wageningen, Netherlands
Immunobiology Research Program, Research Programs Unit, Department of Bacteriology and Immunology, University of Helsinki, Helsinki, Finland

Katarina VeljovicVeljović, Nikola Popović, Marija Miljković , Maja Tolinački, Amarela Terzić -Vidojević and Milan Kojić
Institute of Molecular Genetics and Genetic Engineering, University of Belgrade, Belgrade, Serbia

Philippe Langella and Luis G. Bermúdez-Humarán
Commensal and Probiotics-Host Interactions Laboratory, Micalis Institute, Institut National de la Recherche Agronomique, AgroParisTech, Jouy-en-Josas, France

Thibault Allain, Rebeca Martín, Chantal Bridonneau, Véronique Robert, Sylvie Hudault, Florian Chain, Olivier Berteau, Jean M. Chatel, Luis G. Bermúdez-Humarán, Muriel Thomas and Philippe Langella
Commensal and Probiotics-Host Interactions Laboratory, Micalis Institute, Institut National de la Recherche Agronomique, AgroParisTech, Jouy-en-Josas, France
UMR7245, Muséum National d'Histoire Naturelle, Centre National de la Recherche Scientifique, Sorbonne-Universités, Paris, France

Soraya Chaouch, Isabelle ValléeSoraya Chaouch, Philippe Grellier and Isabelle Florent
UMR7245, Muséum National d'Histoire Naturelle, Centre National de la Recherche Scientifique, Sorbonne-Universités, Paris, France
Myriam Thomas, Myriam Thomas and Isabelle Vallée
JRU BIPAR, ANSES, Ecole Nationale Vétérinaire d'Alfort, INRA, Université Paris-Est, Animal Health Laboratory, Maisons-Alfort, France

André G. Buret
Department of Biological Sciences, University of Calgary, Calgary, AB, Canada

Bruno Polack
JRU BIPAR, Ecole Nationale Vétérinaire d'Alfort, ANSES, INRA, Université Paris-Est, Maisons-Alfort, France

Jeffrey Roach
Research Computing, University of North Carolina, Chapel Hill, NC, United States

Sylvie Miquel
Commensals and Probiotics-Host Interactions Laboratory, Micalis Institute, Institut National de la Recherche Agronomique, AgroParisTech, Université Paris-Saclay, Jouy-en-Josas, France
Université Clermont Auvergne, Centre National de la Recherche Scientifique UMR 6023 Laboratoire Microorganismes: Génome et Environnement, Clermont-Ferrand, France

Leandro Benevides
Commensals and Probiotics-Host Interactions Laboratory, Micalis Institute, Institut National de la Recherche Agronomique, AgroParisTech, Université Paris-Saclay, Jouy-en-Josas, France
Department of General Biology, Federal University of Minas Gerais, Belo Horizonte, Brazil

Vasco Azevedo
Department of General Biology, Federal University of Minas Gerais, Belo Horizonte, Brazil

Willem M. de Vos
Laboratory of Microbiology, Wageningen University and Research, Wageningen, Netherlands
Immunobiology Research Program, Research Programs Unit, Faculty of Medicine, University of Helsinki, Helsinki, Finland

Harry Sokol
Commensals and Probiotics-Host Interactions Laboratory, Micalis Institute, Institut National de la Recherche Agronomique, AgroParisTech, Université Paris-Saclay, Jouy-en-Josas, France
AVENIR Team Gut Microbiota and Immunity Equipe de Recherche Labélisée (ERL), Institut National de la Santé et de la Recherche Médicale U1157/UMR7203, Faculté de Médecine Saint-Antoine, Université Pierre et Marie Curie, Paris, France
Service de Gastroentérologie, Hôpital Saint-Antoine, Assistance Publique—Hôpitaux de Paris, Paris, France

B. V. Deepthi, Rakesh Somashekaraiah, K. Poornachandra Rao, N. Deepa and M. Y. Sreenivasa
Department of Studies in Microbiology, University of Mysore, Mysuru, India

N. K. Dharanesha
Animal Disease Diagnostic Laboratory and Information Centre, Institute of Animal Health and Veterinary Biologicals, Karnataka Veterinary, Animal and Fisheries Sciences University (KVAFSU), Mysuru, India

Miguel Gueimonde
Instituto de Productos Lácteos de Asturias, Spanish Higher Research Council, Villaviciosa, Spain

Gabriel Vinderola
Instituto de Lactología Industrial (UNL-CONICET), National University of the Litoral, Santa Fe, Argentina

Seppo Salminen and Carlos Gómez-Gallego
Functional Foods Forum, Faculty of Medicine, University of Turku, Turku, Finland

K. S. Girish
Department of Studies and Research in Biochemistry, Tumkur Universty, Tumkur, India

Theodor Brodmann and Wolfgang Kneifel
Department of Food Sciences and Technology, University of Natural Resources and Life Science Vienna, Vienna, Austria

Akihito Endo
Department of Food and Cosmetic Science, Tokyo University of Agriculture, Hokkaido, Japan

Index

www.ingramcontent.com/pod-product-compliance
Lightning Source LLC
LaVergne TN
LVHW082132200926
848484LV00008B/2045